120.00

369 0289223

Library
~~ital

~~ ~~n below.

Controversies in knee surgery

Controversies in orthopaedic surgery

Volumes in the series:

Controversies in hip surgery
Bourne

Controversies in total knee replacement
Laskin

Controversies in knee surgery
Williams and Johnson

Controversies in knee surgery

Edited by
Riley J. Williams

Assistant Professor and Attending Orthopedic Surgeon
Hospital for Special Surgery
Cornell University Medical College, New York NY, USA

and

David P. Johnson

Consultant Orthopaedic Surgeon
St Mary's Hospital, Bristol, UK

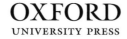
OXFORD
UNIVERSITY PRESS

This book has been printed digitally and produced in a standard specification
in order to ensure its continuing availability

OXFORD
UNIVERSITY PRESS

Great Clarendon Street, Oxford OX2 6DP

Oxford University Press is a department of the University of Oxford.
It furthers the University's objective of excellence in research, scholarship,
and education by publishing worldwide in

Oxford New York

Auckland Cape Town Dar es Salaam Hong Kong Karachi
Kuala Lumpur Madrid Melbourne Mexico City Nairobi
New Delhi Shanghai Taipei Toronto
With offices in
Argentina Austria Brazil Chile Czech Republic France Greece
Guatemala Hungary Italy Japan South Korea Poland Portugal
Singapore Switzerland Thailand Turkey Ukraine Vietnam

Oxford is a registered trade mark of Oxford University Press
in the UK and in certain other countries

Published in the United States
by Oxford University Press Inc., New York

ISBN 978-0-19-852066-5

Printed and bound by CPI Antony Rowe, Eastbourne

Contents

List of contributors *xi*

Part 1. Primary Anterior Cruciate Ligament
(ACL) Reconstruction

1

What is the natural history of ACL injury in the athletic individual? *3*
Paolo Aglietti and Francesco Giron

2

Does ACL reconstruction prevent articular degeneration? The ACL risk equation *15*
Paul H. Marks, Kurt P. Droll, and Michelle Cameron

3

Primary ACL reconstruction: what are the best methods of fixation for grafts used in ACL reconstruction surgery? *37*
Charles H. Brown

4

Bone-tendon-bone autograft ACL reconstruction is the most effective surgical option for restoring anterior knee stability following ACL injury *57*
Scott D. Mair and Darren L. Johnson

5

Implications of tunnel widening in the ACL reconstructed knee *67*
Mark G. Clatworthy

6

Primary ACL reconstruction: does gender affect outcome following ACL reconstruction surgery? *83*
Brian M. Crites and Leigh Ann Curl

7

Lactic and glycolic acid-based bioresorbable polymeric materials in ACL reconstruction *97*
Michel Vert

8

Bio-absorbable interference screws in ACL reconstruction *109*
David P. Johnson and Jason L. Koh

9

The physiology of bone-tendon healing must be considered for successful ACL reconstruction rehabilitation *129*
Deryk G. Jones and J.-K. Francis Suh

10

The evolution of rehabilitation for ACL reconstruction *151*
K. Donald Shelbourne and Michael D. Dersam

11

ACL reconstruction in the skeletally immature: indications, methodology and concerns *167*
George A. Paletta

12

Indications for ACL reconstruction in the over-forty age group *185*
John Bartlett

Part 2. Revision ACL Reconstruction

13

Graft options for revision ACL surgery – which is the most effective? *193*
Eric W. Carson, Alonzo Sexton, and Deryk G. Jones

14

One stage versus two stage revision ACL reconstruction: indications and techniques *211*
Giancarlo Puddu and Guglielmo Cerullo

Part 3. Medial Collateral Ligament

15

Medial collateral ligament repair at the time of primary ACL reconstruction: when and why *229*
Joseph H. Guettler and Laurence D. Higgins

Part 4. Lateral Collateral Ligament/Posterolateral Corner

16

Acute repair of the posterolateral structures of the knee results in superior clinical outcomes compared to the current methods of reconstruction *255*
Answorth A. Allen and Victor Lopez Jr

17

Reconstruction methods for the lateral side of the knee: what we do *273*
Christopher J. Wahl and Russell F. Warren

Part 5. Arthritic ACL Deficient Knees

18

Arthritis in the ACL deficient knee: what is the best approach? *303*
Riley J. Williams and David P. Johnson

19

Arthritic ACL-deficient knees – is there increased patient morbidity following combined high tibial osteotomy/ACL reconstruction? *329*
Christoph B. Marti and Roland P. Jakob

Part 6. Posterior Cruciate Ligament (PCL)

20

Natural history of PCL injuries *343*
K. Donald Shelbourne and Cary Guse

21

PCL reconstruction: is it necessary following PCL rupture? *359*
Todd M. Herrenbruck and John A. Bergfeld

22

PCL reconstruction: the double-bundle method is most effective for restoring posterior tibiofemoral laxity *375*

Andrew A. Amis

Part 7. Meniscus and Cartilage Injury

23

Meniscus and cartilage injury: does meniscal allograft transplantation prevent articular cartilage degeneration? *387*

Scott A. Rodeo

24

Indications, preservation, and implant techniques for meniscal allograft transplantation *407*

Ewoud van Arkel

25

Microfracture arthroplasty is an effective means to treat full thickness cartilage lesions of the knee *425*

J. Richard Steadman, William G. Rodkey, and Karen K. Briggs

26

Autologous chondrocyte transplantation can effectively treat most articular cartilage lesions of the knee? *439*

Mats Brittberg and Lars Peterson

27

Fresh osteochondral allograft transplantation for the treatment of hyaline cartilage defects: is this a viable surgical alternative? *455*

Beth E. Shubin Stein and Riley J. Williams

Part 8. Complex Knee Injury

28

Is it best to surgically address all injured ligaments in the acute injury period? *477*

Rene Verdonk and Fredrik Almqvist

29

Chronic multi-ligament knee injuries are best treated using osteotomies about the knee *489*

Tarik Ait Si Selmi, Philippe Neyret, G. Schuck de Freitas, T. Lootens, and L. Jacquot

30

Indications and outcomes of acute, simultaneous ACL and PCL reconstruction *511*

Hussein A. Elkousy, Jon K. Sekiya, and Christopher D. Harner

31

Knee motion loss: why does it happen and what does one do about it? *529*

Thomas P. Branch and Jon E. Browne

Index *547*

Contributors

Paolo Aglietti MD
First Orthopaedic Clinic
University of Florence
Florence
Italy

Tarik Ait Si Selmi
Hôpital de la Croix Rousse
Centre Livet
Lyon
France

Answorth A. Allen MD
Assistant Professor of Orthopedic Surgery
Weil Medical College of Cornell University
Assistant Attending Physician
The Hospital for Special Surgery
New York, NY
USA

Fredrik Almqvist MD PHD
Ghent University Hospital
Ghent
Belgium

Andrew A. Amis DSC
Professor of Orthopaedic Biomechanics
Departments of Mechanical Engineering and
   Musculoskeletal Surgery
Imperial College of Science, Technology and
   Medicine
London, UK

Ewoud van Arkel PHD
Department of Orthopaedic Surgery
MCH Westeinde Hospital
The Hague
The Netherlands

John Bartlett MBBS FRACS
1/210 Burgundy Street
Heidelberg 3084
Melbourne, Victoria
Australia

John A. Bergfeld MD
Head, Section of Sports Medicine
Department of Orthopaedics
The Cleveland Clinic Foundation
Cleveland, OH
USA

Thomas P. Branch MD
2665 N Decatur Road
Suite 640
Decatur, GA
USA

Karen K. Briggs
Steadman Hawkins Clinic and
   Steadman Hawkins Sports Medicine
   Foundation
Vail, CO
USA

Mats Brittberg
Cartilage Research Unit
Göteborg University
Department of Orthopaedics
Kungsbacka Hospital
Kungsbacka
Sweden

Charles H. Brown Jr. MD
Department of Orthopaedic Surgery
Brigham and Women's Hospital
Harvard Medical School
Boston, MA
USA

Jon E. Browne
6675 Holmes
Suite 400
Kansas City, MO
USA

Michelle Cameron MD
Surgical Staff
Rocky Mountain Orthopaedic Specialists
Canada

Eric W. Carson MD
Resurgens Orthopaedics
Atlanta, GA
USA

Guglielmo Cerullo MD
Orthopaedic Surgeon
Clinica Valle Giulia
Rome
Italy

Mark G. Clatworthy FRACS
Middlemore Hospital
Auckland
New Zealand

Brian M. Crites MD
Assistant Professor
Department of Orthopaedics
University of Maryland
Baltimore, MD
USA

Leigh Ann Curl MD
Assistant Professor
Johns Hopkins Department of Orthopaedic
  Surgery
Johns Hopkins Bayview Medical Center
Baltimore, MD
USA

Michael D. Dersam MD
Methodist Sports Medicine Center
Indianapolis, IN
USA

Kurt P. Droll MSC MD
Resident, Division Orthopaedic Surgery
University of Toronto
Toronto
Canada

Hussein A. Elkousy MD
Fondren Orthopedic Group
Sugarland, TX
USA

Francesco Giron MD
First Orthopaedic Clinic
University of Florence
Florence
Italy

Joseph H. Guettler MD
24255 13 Mile Road
Suite 100
Bingham Farms, MI
USA

Cary Guse MD
Department of Orthopaedic Surgery
Indiana University School of Medicine
Indianapolis, IN
USA

Christopher D. Harner MD
Blue Cross of Western Pennsylvania
  Professor and Director
Center for Sports Medicine
University of Pittsburgh Medical Center
3200 South Water Street
Pittsburgh, PA
USA

Todd M. Herrenbruck MD
Orthopaedic Sports Medicine Fellow
Section of Sports Medicine
Department of Orthopaedics
The Cleveland Clinic Foundation
Cleveland, OH
USA

Laurence D. Higgins MD
Duke Sports Medicine
Duke University Medical Center
Durham, NC
USA

L. Jacquot
Hôpital de la Croix Rousse
Centre Livet
Lyon
France

Roland P. Jakob
Service de Chirurgie Orthopaedique
Hôpital Cantonal
Fribourg
Switzerland

Darren L. Johnson MD
Professor and Chairman
Section of Sports Medicine
University of Kentucky
Lexington, KY
USA

David P. Johnson MD MB ChB FRCS(ORTH)
Consultant Orthopaedic Surgeon
St. Mary's Hospital
Clifton
Bristol, UK

Deryk G. Jones MD
Department of Orthopaedic Surgery
Tulane University
New Orleans, LA
USA

Jason L. Koh MD
Attending Physician
Orthopaedic Surgery
Northwestern Memorial Hospital
Chicago, IL
USA

T. Lootens
Hôpital de la Croix Rousse
Centre Livet
Lyon
France

Victor Lopez Jr. BS
Research Assistant
Sports Medicine and Shoulder Service
The Hospital for Special Surgery
New York, NY
USA

Scott D. Mair MD
Assistant Professor
Section of Sports Medicine
University of Kentucky
Lexington, KY
USA

Paul H. Marks BSC MD FRCSC
Surgical Staff
Orthopaedic and Arthritic Institute
Sunnybrook and Women's College
Hospital Science Centre
and Assistant Professor
Department of Surgery
University of Toronto
Toronto
Canada

Christoph B. Marti
Orthopädie/Traumatologie
Spital des Sensebizirks
Maggenberg
Tafers
Switzerland

Philippe Neyret
Hôpital de la Croix Rousse
Centre Livet
Lyon
France

George A. Paletta Jr. MD
Washington University School of
   Medicine
Orthopaedic Surgery Department
St. Louis, MO
USA

Lars Peterson
Gothenburg Medical Center
Gothenburg
Sweden

Giancarlo Puddu
Orthopaedic Surgeon
Clinica Valle Giulia
Rome
Italy

Scott A. Rodeo MD
Sports Medicine and Shoulder Service
The Hospital for Special Surgery
New York, NY
USA

William G. Rodkey
Steadman Hawkins Clinic and
  Steadman Hawkins Sports Medicine
  Foundation
Vail, CO
USA

G. Schuck de Freitas
Hôpital de la Croix Rousse
Centre Livet
Lyon
France

Jon K. Sekiya MD
Center for Sports Medicine
University of Pittsburgh Medical Center
Pittsburgh, PA
USA

Alonzo Sexton MD
Emory University School of Medicine
Atlanta, GA
USA

K. Donald Shelbourne MD
Methodist Sports Medicine Center
Indianapolis, IN
USA

Beth E. Shubin Stein MD
Sports Medicine and Shoulder Service
Hospital for Special Surgery
New York, NY
USA

J. Richard Steadman
Steadman Hawkins Clinic and
  Steadman Hawkins Sports Medicine
  Foundation
Vail, CO
USA

J.-K. Francis Suh PHD
Departments of Orthopaedic Surgery and
  Biomedical Engineering
Tulane University
New Orleans, LA
USA

Rene Verdonk MD PHD
Ghent University Hospital
Belgium

Michel Vert MSC DSC
Faculty of Pharmacy
University of Montpellier
Montpellier
France

Christopher J. Wahl MD
Center for Orthopedics
Hamden, CT
USA

Russell F. Warren MD
Attending Surgeon
Sports Medicine and Shoulder Service
Hospital for Special Surgery
New York, NY
USA

Riley J. Williams MD
Attending Surgeon
Sports Medicine and Shoulder Service
Hospital for Special Surgery
New York, NY
USA

Part 1. Primary Anterior Cruciate Ligament (ACL) Reconstruction

1

What is the natural history of ACL injury in the athletic individual?

Paolo Aglietti and Francesco Giron

Several studies have attempted to define the disability, associated pathologies, and degenerative changes of the knee after an isolated untreated lesion of the anterior cruciate ligament (ACL). However, this is a controversial issue because most of these studies do not reflect the true natural history of the ACL-deficient knee, due to the fact that only symptomatic knees have been observed. A comprehensive natural history study should include a sufficiently large number of patients who are evaluated for the first time at the time of injury without selection or bias. A thorough documentation and assessment of the injury is required. The ACL lesion and the associated meniscal, chondral, and ligament pathology should be documented both clinically and arthroscopically. The patients should be followed prospectively for long enough to assess the change in symptoms over a relevant period of time and the functional impairment which results. The analysis would include documentation of the progression of the instability and laxity, the need for further surgery, the development of meniscal tears, and degenerative changes of the joint. If reliable prognostic factors were identified by such natural history studies, then they may be used for the acute injured patient to determine the optimal method of management for any particular injury. Unfortunately many studies are of short or incomplete follow-up, without objective documentation or flawed by inconsistent and varying treatment between cases. Nevertheless, even in studies where the documentation is incomplete, often important information can be provided on the functional impairment, the incidence of associated meniscal or cartilage pathology, and the effectiveness of rehabilitation regimens.

Functional impairment

The disability that follows an ACL lesion has been variously assessed and interpreted. In 1962, Smillie (1962) stated that 'if ruptures of the ACL are the most common ligament injuries . . . they

3

are not the most important'. Later, Hughston and Barrett (1983), reviewing 93 knees that underwent surgery for an anteromedial rotatory instability, came to the conclusion that the ACL-deficient knee is subject to meniscal tears and joint deterioration as a result of not recognizing the full extent of the initial injury. They emphasized the importance of the medial meniscus, the meniscotibial ligaments, and the posterior oblique ligament.

More recently the attention has been focused on ACL insufficiency as the main cause of symptoms. McDaniel and Dameron (1980) in a retrospective study on 50 ACL-deficient patients with an average follow-up of 10 years found that 46 per cent of the patients following ACL rupture had no restriction in function because of the knee. Nevertheless, 4 per cent of patients had had to give up all sports activity because of the knee injury. Thirty-eight per cent of patients had to decrease or modify their sports participation, and 12 per cent were no longer interested in sports. Furthermore, 69 per cent of the knees experienced giving way episodes, and 36 per cent complained of pain. The worst results were associated with pronounced thigh atrophy and bilateral meniscectomy. In this study, however, the return to sports activities as the principal criteria for failure has been overemphasized and the type of sport undertaken was not adequately documented. Many of the patients continued to participate in vigorous activities despite symptoms of giving way and swelling.

Noyes et al. (1983a) reviewed 103 symptomatic isolated chronic ACLs in young athletes at an average of five and half years after the initial injury. Thirty-five per cent of them had a reinjury within six months, 51 per cent within one year, and 80 per cent stated that their symptoms increased after reinjury. Most of the patients (67 per cent) had severe disability due to twisting and pivoting activities, but moderate to severe disability was also noted in a further 31 per cent during walking and in 44 per cent during daily living activities. Pain, swelling, and giving way were present in roughly one-third of the cases during walking and increased to almost two-thirds of the patients during strenuous activities. A history of undergoing meniscectomy increased the incidence of pain and swelling symptoms two- to fourfold. Swelling was more frequent in patients who had a longer interval since the original injury. The same authors investigated the possibility of improving the symptoms with a course of rehabilitation, activity modification and knee bracing (Noyes et al., 1983b) in 84 patients. The patients were on average 28 years old, had sustained the original injury eight years previously, and were evaluated after a 3-year follow-up. The results showed that roughly one-third of the patients improved with non-operative management and could participate in daily living and recreational activities with minimal or no symptoms. This group had increased their activity level above pretreatment levels. However these knees could not be considered normal, since the symptoms were experienced during strenuous sports activities. A third of patients remained about the same, with similar symptoms and an activity level that was just below that required for recreational sports. One-third of the patients became worse over the course of the study, and failed the rehabilitation complaining of significant symptoms that prevented any sports and were present in daily living activities. It was not possible to predict from the beginning which knee would benefit from the treatment. The key to success seemed to be the willingness of the patient to modify their activity levels in order to avoid giving way and reinjuries. The authors concluded that patients 'who continued athletics despite reinjuries, literally destroyed their knee joints'.

Giove et al. (1983), investigated the effects of a rehabilitation course for chronic ACL injury in 24 men. The rehabilitation was based on strengthening of the hamstring muscles. The program progressed from isometric exercises through isotonic and isokinetic exercises until the hamstrings were as strong as the quadriceps of the involved limb and stronger than the uninvolved side. After completing a sports participation survey it was found that 12 per cent of the patients had no restrictions, 46 per cent were able to undertake full activity with minor symptoms, 33 per cent had reduced the activity level and complained of moderate to severe symptoms, 8 per cent could not perform any sporting activity. The ability to participate differed significantly among the various sports. While most of the patients were able to participate in non-contact non-pivoting sports without significant symptoms, the same was not true for pivoting non-contact or even worse, in pivoting contact sports. None of the patients could play football and volleyball without restrictions. High participation levels were seen only in subjects with hamstrings/quadriceps ratios over 100 per cent. This study supports the hypothesis that hamstring strengthening is helpful in restoring function following ACL injury, provided that twisting, pivoting and jumping activities are avoided.

The importance of hamstring strength was also investigated by Walla et al. (1985) in 38 athletes with chronic ACL instability at an average interval of five and half years from injury. During this time 81 per cent of the patients had experienced significant reinjury, and 61 per cent had undergone a meniscesctomy. At the time of follow-up only 32 per cent of patients could participate in strenuous activities without symptoms. Fewer problems were encountered in cutting manoeuvres in patients who could completely control the pivot-shift by active contraction of their hamstrings, and especially so in patients who could do so in spite of being distracted (reflex control). No correlation was found between hamstring strength and participation level. It was concluded that the capability of the hamstring control over the pivot-shift strongly correlates with patient's function. Based on these findings, muscular coordination is an important predictor of success of conservative treatment, more than the degree of laxity or pivot-shift.

Similarly Fowler and Regan (1987) treated with arthroscopy and a three-week rehabilitation course a group of 51 chronic ACL-deficient knees for continuing symptoms, such as instability (78 per cent) and locking (22 per cent). Meniscal surgery, including partial meniscectomy and meniscal suture, was performed in 43 per cent of the patients. With an average follow-up of 18 months from surgery, only 17 per cent returned to full participation in pivoting sports, 22 per cent participated in pivoting sports with some restrictions, 26 returned to some form of sport not involving pivoting manoeuvres, and 35 per cent did not participate in sports. Patients with good muscular condition returned to a higher sports participation level. In conclusion, while 65 per cent of the patients returned to some form of sport activity, only 10 obtained the preinjury level of competition. The knees with meniscal tear showed a more favourable outcome compared to those with pure symptoms of instability.

Pattee *et al.* (1989) prospectively evaluated 49 untreated ACL lesions at an average follow-up of five and half years. An ACL reconstruction was performed on 18 per cent of the knees during the follow-up period. In the remaining 40 patients, 20 per cent returned to their preinjury sports activity level without restrictions, and 25 per cent functioned at the same level but with symptoms, some patients requiring bracing. Seventeen patients (43 per cent) had diminished their athletic level, while five (12 per cent) had given up all sports. Pain was present in 60 per cent of the patients and swelling occurred in 40 per cent after vigorous activities. On physical examination, 27 patients (87 per cent) had pivot-shifts. The side to side difference in anterior tibial translation (KT-1000 arthrometer) was only 3 mm on average. Despite the fact that several knees with minor laxity were included in this group of patients due to the selection process, only 20 per cent returned to full preinjury athletic activity with minimal or no symptoms.

In 1990, Barrack *et al.* (1990) presented a study on 72 complete ACL lesions in soldiers treated non-operatively. The study was retrospective, but all the patients were seen in acute phase and the diagnosis was confirmed by arthroscopy. The three-year follow-up overall results were fair or poor in 69 per cent of the knees. In this group of young active patients, 88 per cent of the knees were symptomatic, 64 per cent complained of giving way, 61 per cent of swelling, and 81 per cent of pain; 60 per cent had to discontinue or change sport. Few patients could perform jumping, turning, or cutting activities, and 48 per cent had difficulties with stair climbing. Most of the patients (83 per cent) with a bilateral meniscectomy at the initial arthroscopy had fair or poor results. A reconstruction was necessary in 35 per cent of the knees, and knees with meniscal tears were more likely to need a reconstruction. This study supports the contention that poor results may be expected in active individuals with a documented ACL lesion and a positive pivot-shift. The military status decreased the possibility of modifing their lifestyle and thus lessen the symptoms.

Bonamo *et al.* (1990) investigated the natural history of the ACL-deficient knee in 79 recreational athletes who underwent arthroscopic non-ligamentous surgery. The interval from injury to surgery was variable, and 20 per cent were in the acute phase. Meniscal surgery was performed in 67 per cent of the knees and articular cartilage debridement in 27 per cent. A postoperative rehabilitation programme was instituted with the goal of obtaining less than 10 per cent deficiency in strength, power, and endurance compared to the contralateral leg. With an average follow-up of 52 months, symptoms were infrequent for the activities of daily living, but 73 per cent complained of instability and 47 per cent of frank giving way during sports. Pain and swelling were present during sports activities in 27 per cent and 30 per cent, respectively. Only 5 per cent resumed the preinjury level of sport participation, 55 per cent had to modify it slightly, while 40 per cent modified it significantly. A detailed survey of the participation in different sports revealed that participation was related to the amount of lateral movement and pivoting required with a low rate of return to pivoting sports like basketball. Reinjury occurred in 37 per cent of the patients, and the incidence of reinjury was inversely related to the age of the patient. After a follow-up period of over four years, quadriceps and hamstring strength deficit, pivot-shift grades $2+$ or $3+$, occurrence of a significant reinjury and repeat arthroscopy were associated with a higher incidence of poor results. In this study, 20 per cent had had or were planning to have an ACL reconstruction by the end of the study. This paper suggests that no advantage can be expected by repeating arthroscopy without ligament reconstruction, for continued problems in an ACL-deficient knee.

Recently Scavenius *et al.* (1999) performed a retrospective study on 70 surgically verified ACL ruptures treated conservatively. During the follow-up period 25 patients underwent a secondary ACL reconstruction, setting the failure rate of the initial non-operative treatment at 37 per cent. After an average interval of seven years 33 patients went through a detailed clinical examination. In all of the reviewed patients there was a decline in median Lysholm score from a score of 100 prior to the injury, to 86 at follow-up, and a decrease in median Tegner values from seven to five at follow-up. Only three patients returned to preinjury sports activity level. According to the ESSKA classification, the number of 'cutting-sports performers' declined dramatically from 24 to two. All but one patient ascribed their decline in activity to their knee status. The objectively measured antero-posterior translocations were significantly higher on the injured knee compared to the healthy knee ($P < 0.05$). Intermittent rest pain was suffered by 63 per cent of the patients. During the time from inclusion until follow-up, 13 patients (39 per cent) sustained an additional ipsilateral knee lesion, most commonly a tear of the medial meniscus. This data confirmed that in ACL-deficient patients the overall outcome of the conservative treatment is not satisfactory and is mainly characterized by a low frequency of return to unrestricted preinjury level of function, and by an high level of symptomatic instability resulting in a high proportion of secondary ACL reconstructions.

Radiographic degenerative changes

Radiographic degenerative changes following an ACL injury have been reported in 20–88 per cent of cases (Arnold *et al.*, 1979; Kannus and Jarvinen, 1987; Lynch *et al.*, 1983, McDaniel and Dameron, 1980; Noyes *et al.*, 1983a; Pattee *et al.*, 1989; Satku *et al.*, 1986; Sherman *et al.*, 1988; Walla *et al.*, 1985; Gillquist and Messner, 1999).

McDaniel and Dameron (1980) in an average 10-year follow-up study of untreated ACL injuries found a normal knee to be present in only 25 per cent of the cases. Minimal changes were recorded in a further 54 per cent of the knees. Medial joint line narrowing was present in 15 per cent, while frank arthritis was present in 6 per cent of knees. A definite relationship was found between osteoarthritis and a varus deformity, medial meniscectomy, and a medial joint space narrowing.

Noyes *et al.* (1983a) evaluated the radiographic changes in 91 chronic symptomatic ACL-deficient knees. At an average follow-up of five and a half years 25 per cent had minimum arthritis, 19 per cent moderate, and 2 per cent severe. A strong correlation was found between severity of the changes and the amount of time elapsed since the injury. No definite relationship between the presence of degenerative changes and a history of meniscectomy was shown. Since knees without meniscectomy developed radiographic changes similar to those that had meniscectomy, the authors suggested that extensive meniscal tears and loss of function may have occurred without surgical removal of the meniscus itself.

Walla *et al.* (1985), in their study on 38 athletes with chronic ACL instability at an average follow-up of five years, reported moderate to severe changes in 23 per cent of the athletes injured less than five years prior to the study and in 66 per cent of those injured over five years earlier. Severe degenerative changes and lateral rim sign were more frequent in knees with a previous meniscectomy.

Satku *et al.* (1986) reported on 49 chronic ACL injuries followed for an average of six years. After meniscectomy, moderate to severe degenerative changes were present in 16 per cent of the knees followed less than five years and in 52 per cent of those followed more than five years. In five knees without previous meniscectomy, but with meniscal symptoms, moderate to severe degenerative changes were present in each case. An arthroscopy performed in two cases confirmed the presence of extensive meniscal tears with loss of meniscal function. None of the nine patients with intact menisci and no evidence of meniscal injury had more than very mild changes on their radiographs. Overall moderate and severe changes were present in 31 per cent and 8 per cent of the knees, respectively.

The authors concluded that loss of meniscal function due to either meniscectomy or extensive meniscal tears plays an important role in the progressive degeneration of the cruciate-deficient knee joint.

Kannus and Jarvinen (1987) in an average follow-up of eight years found that a definite post-traumatic arthritis was evident in 70 per cent of the 49 evaluated knees, and two knees required a proximal tibial osteotomy to correct the varus deformity. Narrowing of the medial and lateral joint lines was present in 39 per cent and 33 per cent of the knees, respectively. Osteophytes in the medial femoral condyle and the medial tibial plateau were present in 55 per cent and 49 per cent respectively.

In a detailed study by Sherman *et al.* (1988) on degenerative changes in the ACL-deficient knee a new rating system was developed to separately record peripheral and degenerative changes. A group of 127 chronic symptomatic ACL-deficient knees was studied with an average follow-up of 79 months; 37 per cent of the knees were followed more than five years. The patients were divided into six groups according to the presence of demonstrated meniscal tears, previous meniscectomy, and collateral ligament insufficiency. Pheripheral changes (osteophytes) were more frequent than degenerative changes (including joint narrowing, subchondral sclerosis, cysts, angular deformity, and loose bodies). More than one pheripheral change occurred in 92 per cent of the knees, while only 36 per cent had more than one degenerative change. The radiographic score had significantly decreased in knees with longer intervals since the original injury and in cases which had undergone a previous meniscectomy. Knees with known retained meniscal tears showed less degeneration than knees with a prior meniscectomy. When the different groups were analysed separately with regard to the effects of time from the original injury, it was found that within 10 years all the groups had similar low radiographic scores, whilst radiographic degeneration was evident in 65 per cent of the knees with a time interval longer than 10 years. This per centage increased to 83 per cent in those patients with an interval longer than 20 years. The authors concluded that peripheral and degenerative changes should be separately recorded and that only the latter are unequivocal signs of osteoarthritis. In the ACL-deficient knee periarticular peripheral osteophytic changes manifest themselves earlier than would otherwise be the case; whereas osteoarthritic degeneration requires a longer time interval to take place. The progression of the ACL-deficient knee toward osteoarthritis was confirmed, and meniscectomy and collateral ligament insufficiency hasten this course. With follow-up longer than 10 years, however, no difference was evident between those knees which had undergone a menisectomy compared to those which had not.

Recently Shirakura *et al.* (1995) prospectively evaluated 46 ACL-deficient recreational athletes at an average follow-up of five years. Radiographic examinations at follow-up exhibited differences between the injured and uninjured knees in 32 per cent of the knees. Using Fairbank's criteria, eight knees (17 per cent) had Grade I osteoarthritic changes. Four knees had diffuse osteopenia of the tibia, femur, and patella, in comparison to the uninjured side. The authors concluded that in cases of ACL injury, an early diagnosis and some modification of activity, accompanied by comprehension of the characteristics of the anterior cruciate ligament-deficient knee, prevent reinjury, late meniscectomy, and ultimately degenerative osteoarthritis.

In conclusion, the radiological literature shows that there is evidence following chonic ACL injury that peripheral changes and osteophytes are an early change, followed by other more significant degenerative changes such as joint space narrowing. The process may take years and the progression is related to the activity level of the patients, but certainly it is accelerated by undertaking a meniscectomy or the presence of extensive meniscal tears resulting in loss of meniscal function. Standard anteroposterior weight-bearing film is not the most sensitive detector of early cartilage degeneration, since the affected area is frequently located more posteriorly on the femoral condyles. The postero-anterior flexion weight-bearing view has been shown to be more sensitive and specific.

Meniscal and chondral lesions

Is generally believed that the presence of a meniscal lesion as well as articular cartilage degeneration in the ACL-deficient knee indicates a more severe and progressed form of instability. Several authors have found a correlation between degenerative changes and a previous meniscectomy both in the conservatively treated ACL-deficient knees (McDaniel and Dameron, 1980; Noyes et al., 1983a; Pattee et al., 1989; Satku et al., 1986; Sherman et al., 1988; Walla et al., 1985; Gillquist and Messner, 1999) and in the ACL-reconstructed joint (Lynch et al., 1983; Aglietti et al., 1997; Jomha et al., 1999; Shelbourne and Gray, 2000). Articular cartilage or chondral lesion has been frequently reported in the presence of chronic ACL laxity, and the degree, size and site is important when planning an ACL reconstruction. Some of the meniscal and chondral lesion are the results of the initial trauma, while others develop during the repetitive episodes of giving way.

Indelicato and Bittar (1985) compared the incidence of meniscal and chondral lesions in 44 acute and 56 chronic ACL lax knees. The incidence of lesions of the medial meniscus, lateral meniscus, and of both menisci was 60, 32, and 23 per cent, respectively, in acute and 80, 36, and 24 per cent, respectively, in chronic injuries. Chondral fractures were seen in 23 of the acute knees and chondromalacia of the femoral condyles in 54 per cent of the chronic laxities. This study supports the degenerative effect of repetitive injuries of the knee. The incidence of meniscal tears increased from 77 per cent in the acute knees to 91 per cent in the chronic injuries.

Pattee *et al.* (1989), reporting their experience on the conservative treatment in 68 acute ACL tears, found at arthroscopy a tear of the medial meniscus in 51 per cent of the cases, of the lateral meniscus in 43 per cent, and of both menisci in 27 per cent.

Similarly Cerabona *et al.* (1988) reported the incidence and type of meniscal tears in a group of 102 acute ACL injuries, as observed at arthrotomy. The patients were divided in two groups: 67 knees had an 'isolated' ACL tear while the remaining 35 had a concomitant tear of the collateral ligaments. The incidence of tears of the medial meniscus, lateral meniscus, or both menisci was 21, 18, and 3 per cent, respectively, in the isolated ACL tear group and 31, 20, and 3 per cent, respectively, in the other group. The predominant medial meniscus tear was a peripheral and longitudinal type of lesion (71 per cent), while radial or complex tear lesions predominated in the lateral meniscus. Meniscal suture was performed in 75 per cent of the medial meniscus tears but in only 27 per cent of the lateral.

The meniscal and cartilage pathology was also investigated by Fowler and Regan (1987) in their study on chronic ACL-deficient knees. Most of the knees (78 per cent) underwent arthroscopy because of persisting symptoms of giving way, while in the remaining knees locking was the chief complaint. Tears of the medial meniscus and lateral meniscus were reported with the same frequency (37 per cent), although partial excision was more frequently performed medially (63 per cent) than laterally (26 per cent). Degenerative changes were noted with similar frequency in the medial and lateral compartment (12 per cent), but were more frequent in the patello-femoral joint (21 per cent).

In a group of 500 chronic ACL-insufficient knees Conteduca *et al.* (1991) found an incidence of cartilage degeneration in the medial, lateral and patellofemoral compartments of 29, 7, and 5 per cent, respectively. A significantly higher incidence of cartilage degeneration was reported in knees with previous surgery, in competitive compared to occasional athletes, in knees with an interval of more than two years since the original injury and in those with greater laxity.

In 1993, Aglietti and Buzzi (1993) reported on the incidence of associate meniscal and chondral pathology in a series of 100 chronic ACL-deficient knees undergoing ACL reconstruction. The interval between injury to surgery was 40 months on average and the knees were thoroughly inspected by arthroscopy. A previous medial meniscectomy was performed in 13 knees, a lateral in seven, and a bilateral in four. A tear of the medial meniscus was found at arthroscopy in 56 knees, whereas a lateral meniscus tear was noted in 36 cases. Longitudinal tears were the most common lesions in both medial (89 per cent) and lateral meniscus (50 per cent). Including previous surgery and surgery at the time of reconstruction there were only 20 knees with intact menisci, while a tear of the medial, lateral, or both menisci were present in 38, 12, and 30 per cent of the knees, respectively.

The Outerbridge classification (Outerbridge, 1961) was employed to record separately cartilage lesions of the medial, lateral, and patellofemoral compartment. The incidence of cartilage pathology of grades I, II, and III in the medial compartment was 13, 12, and 5 per cent, respectively; in the lateral compartment, 10, 7, and 0 per cent, respectively; and in the patellofemoral joint, 8, 4, and 1 per cent, respectively.

There was a significantly higher incidence of knees with intact menisci when the interval between injury to surgery was less than five years. No correlation was found between the incidence of meniscal tears and the grade of instability. There was a significant correlation between cartilage degeneration in the tibiofemoral compartment and length of interval between injury and surgery. More cartilage changes were evident in the medial compartment of knees with a torn medial meniscus. These results should be considered representative of the pathology encountered in the most symptomatic laxities which required reconstruction. A lower incidence of meniscal lesions was found in a comparable group of 85 acute isolated ACL injuries with comparable criteria: 11 per cent for medial meniscus, 16.5 per cent for lateral, and 9 per cent for both menisci. No chondromalacic changes were present in acute knees, but there was a 2 per cent incidence of osteochondral fractures of the lateral femoral condyle. This data supports the concept of increasing meniscal and cartilage damage due to repetitive episodes of giving way and continued instability.

Conclusion

In a review of the literature of several studies with follow-up times between 5 to 20 years, Gillquist and Messner (1999) reported that radiographic arthrosis significantly increased after all knee injuries compared with the uninjuried joint of the same patient. Partial or total ruptures of the ACL without major concomitant injuries seem to increase the risk tenfold (15 to 20 per cent incidence of arthrosis) compared with age-matched, uninjured population. Fifty to seventy per cent of the patients with complete ACL rupture and associated injuries have radiographic changes after 15 to 20 years. Thus, an ACL injury combined with a significant meniscus tear or other knee ligament injuries results in arthrosis in most patients. Ten to 20 years after ACL injury, arthrosis often presents as slight joint space reduction or is not associated with major clinical symptoms. The progression of the arthrosis is slow, and in some cases the condition seems to remain stable. Time is an important determinant for the degree of arthrosis, and other significant symptoms requiring treatment may be delayed and only encountered over 30 years from the initial trauma.

References

Aglietti P, Buzzi R (1993). Chronic anterior cruciate ligament injuries. In Insall J, Windsor RE, Scott WN, Kelly AM, Aglietti P (eds) *Surgery of the Knee*, pp. 425–504. Second ed, Churchill Livingstone, New York.

Aglietti P, Buzzi R, Giron F, Simeone AJ, Zaccherotti G (1997). Arthroscopic-assisted anterior cruciate ligament reconstruction with the central third patellar tendon. A 5–8-year follow-up. *Knee Surgery Sports Traumatology and Arthroscopy*, 5, 138–144.

Arnold JA, Coker TP, Heaton LM, Park JP, Harris WD (1979). Natural history of anterior cruciate tears. *American Journal of Sports Medicine*, 7, 305–313.

Barrack RL, Bruckner JD, Kneisl J, Inman WS, Alexander AH (1989). The outcome of nonoperatively treated complete tears of the anterior cruciate ligament in active young adults. *Clinical Orthopaedics and Related Researches*, 259, 192–199.

Bonamo JJ, Fay C, Firestone T (1990). The conservative treatment of the anterior cruciate deficient knee. *American Journal of Sports Medicine*, 18, 618–623.

Cerabona F, Sherman MF, Bonamo JR, Sklar J (1988). Patterns of meniscal injury with acute anterior cruciate ligaments tears. *American Journal of Sports Medicine*, 16, 603–609.

Conteduca F, Ferretti A, Mariani PP, Puddu G, Perugia L (1991). Chondromalacia and chronic anterior instabilities. *American Journal of Sports Medicine*, 19, 119–123.

Fowler PJ, Regan WD (1987). The patients with symptomatic chronic anterior cruciate ligament insufficiency: results of minimal arthroscopic surgery and rehabilitation. *American Journal of Sports Medicine*, 15, 321–325.

Gillquist J, Messner K (1999). Anterior cruciate ligament reconstruction and the long-term incidence of gonarthrosis. *Sports Medicine*, 27, 143–156.

Giove TP, Miller SJ, Kent BE, Sanford TL, Garrick JG (1983). Non-operative treatment of the torn anterior cruciate ligament. *Journal of Bone and Joint Surgery*, 65-A, 184–191.

Hughston JC, Barrett GR (1983). Acute anteromedial rotatory instability: long-term results of surgical repair. *Journal of Bone and Joint Surgery*, 65-A, 145–153.

Indelicato PA, Bittar ES (1985). A perspective of lesion associated with ACL insufficiency of the knee: A review of 100 cases. *Clinical Orthopaedics and Related Researches*, 198, 77–80.

Jomha NM, Borton DC, Clingekeffer AJ, Pinczewski LA (1999). Long-term osteoarthritic changes in anterior cruciate ligament reconstructed knees. *Clinical Orthopaedics and Related Researches*, 358, 188–193.

Kannus P, Jarvinen M (1987). Conservatively treated tears of the anterior cruciate ligament: Long-term follow-up result. *Journal of Bone and Joint Surgery*, 69-A, 1007–1012.

Lynch MA, Henning CE, Glick KR Jr (1983). Knee joint surface changes: Long-term follow-up meniscus tear treatment in stable anterior cruciate ligament reconstructions. *Clinical Orthopaedics and Related Researches*, 172, 148–153.

McDaniel WJ, Dameron TB (1980). Untreated ruptures of the anterior cruciate ligament: a follow-up study. *Journal of Bone and Joint Surgery*, 62-A, 696–705.

Noyes FR, Mooar PA, Matthews DS, Butler DL (1983a). The symptomatic anterior cruciate-deficient knee. I. The long term functional disability in athletically active individuals. *Journal of Bone and Joint Surgery*, 65-A, 154–162.

Noyes FR, Matthews DS, Mooar PA, Grood ES (1983b). The symptomatic anterior cruciate-deficient knee. II. The results of rehabilitation, activity modification and counselling on functional disability. *Journal of Bone and Joint Surgery*, 65-A, 163–174.

Outerbridge RE (1961). The etiology of chondromalacia patellae. *Journal of Bone and Joint Surgery*, 43-B, 752–757.

Pattee GA, Fox JM, Del Pizzo W, Friedman MJ (1989). Four to ten year follow-up of unreconstructed anterior cruciate ligament tears. *American Journal of Sports Medicine*, 17, 430–435.

Satku K, Kumar VP, Ngoi SS (1986). Anterior cruciate ligament injuries: To counsel or to operate? *Journal of Bone and Joint Surgery*, 68-B, 458–461.

Scavenius M, Bak K, Hansen S, Norring K, Jensen KH, Jorgensen U (1999). Isolated total ruptures of the anterior cruciate ligament: A clinical study with long-term follow-up of 7 years. *Scandinavian Journal of Medicine and Science in Sports*, 9, 114–119.

Shelbourne KD, Gray T (2000). Results of anterior cruciate ligament reconstruction based on meniscus and articular cartilage status at the time of surgery. Five- to fifteen-year evaluation. *American Journal of Sports Medicine*, 28, 446–452.

Sherman MF, Warren RF, Marshall JL, Savatsky GJ (1988). A clinical and radiographical analysis of 127 anterior cruciate insufficient knees. *Clinical Orthopaedics and Related Researches*, 227, 229–237.

Shirakura K, Terauchi M, Kizuki S, Moro S, Kimura M (1995). The natural history of untreated anterior cruciate tears in recreational athletes. *Clinical Orthopaedics and Related Researches*, 317, 227–236.

Smillie IS (1962). *Injuries of the knee joint*. Livingstone, Edinburgh.

Walla DJ, Albright JP, Mc Auley E, Martin RK, Eldridge V, El-Khoury G (1985). Hamstring control and the unstable anterior cruciate ligament-deficient knee. *American Journal of Sports Medicine*, 13, 34–39.

2

Does ACL reconstruction prevent articular degeneration? The ACL risk equation

Paul H. Marks, Kurt P. Droll, and Michelle Cameron

Introduction

Osteoarthritis is found more commonly in the knee than in any other weight-bearing joint in the human body. Individuals with anterior cruciate ligament (ACL) insufficiency have been found to have a slightly higher risk for developing osteoarthritis in the knee compared to the general population. Several risk factors have been implicated in the development of osteoarthritis in the ACL-deficient knee including concomitant meniscal pathology, osteochondral pathology, impaired proprioception, and biochemical mediators. The following article reviews the evidence pertaining to the above risk factors. In addition, in an effort to aid in the future prognosis of post-traumatic OA, we propose that an 'ACL risk equation' be developed that would express the overall osteoarthritis risk quantitatively and would include all of the pertinent risk factors.

Osteoarthritis (OA) is one of the most common diseases in the world, and it has been estimated that 10 per cent of the general population of North America suffers from this disorder (Cunningham and Kelsey 1984). OA, also known as degenerative joint disease, is found more commonly in the knee than in any other weight-bearing joint in the human body (Slemenda 1992). The principal pathologic features of this disease include progressive focal degradation of the articular cartilage lesion and at the joint margins (i.e. osteophytes) (Brandt 1985). These structural changes in the knee can manifest clinically as joint pain, stiffness, crepitation, loss of motion, and enlargement. Consequently, OA in the knee joint may significantly impair lower extremity function, thus making it extremely disabling and detrimental to overall quality of life. For example, individuals with knee OA have been reported to be twice as likely as those free of OA to have limitations in physical functioning such as traveling up or down stairs or engaging in 'heavy chores' (Davis *et al.* 1991). From an economic perspective, it has been postulated that the annual cost of OA in the USA is 82 billion dollars (Centers for Disease Control 2003). Since the knee is the most common site, it is without a doubt responsible for a large proportion of this financial burden. As a result, OA of the knee joint is a major public health problem worldwide.

Despite OA of the knee being relatively prevalent in the population, the etiology and prognostic factors for this disease are poorly understood. Several studies however have implicated anterior cruciate ligament (ACL) insufficiency as a precursor for degenerative change in the knee (Sherman *et al.* 1988; Giove *et al.* 1983; Pattee *et al.* 1989; and Hawkins *et al.* 1986). These studies reported that individuals with chronic ACL deficiency are at a significantly higher risk for developing OA as compared to the general population. Anterior cruciate ligament insufficiency is a relatively common condition. Neilson and Yde (1991) reported an ACL injury rate of 0.3 per 1000 inhabitants in Denmark during a one-year period among a community of 256,000 inhabitants (i.e. 76 ACL injuries). Another population based study from San Diego Kaiser Health Plan evaluated knee injuries over a three-year period from among 280,000 inhabitants. The rate of ACL injury was reported to be 0.34 per 1000 individuals (Miyaska *et al.* 1991). As expected, rupture of the ACL is a more common event in athletes. A large proportion of ACL ruptures occur while participating in sporting activities, principally those that involve deceleration, twisting, cutting, and jumping movements. In a study of ski injuries, Feagin and associates (Feagin *et al.* 1987) reported 72 ACL injuries per 100,000 skier days and estimated over 100,000 ACL injuries in the United States per year from skiing alone. In addition, a football injury study reported 42 ACL injuries per 1000 players which extrapolated into a 16 per cent chance of ACL injury in a four year collegiate career and a 100-fold increase risk for ACL injury compared with the general population (Hewson and Mendini 1986). As reported in the Kaiser study sport activities such as football, baseball, soccer, basketball, and skiing accounted for approximately 78 per cent of the ACL injuries sustained while participating in sports (Miyaska *et al.* 1991). Consequently, many individuals rupture their ACL each year, which results in an increased likelihood of becoming disabled with OA in the future.

The natural history of the ACL-deficient knee has yet to be completely elucidated. Therefore, much debate exists regarding the relationship between osteoarthritis and the anterior cruciate ligament-deficient knee. In addition to pain and swelling (Noyes *et al.* 1983) previous studies have documented that ACL rupture often leads to joint instability (Hawkins *et al.* 1986; Feagin and Curl 1976). Consequently, this data has provided the impetus for many researchers to postulate that repetitive anterior tibial subluxation episodes under weight-bearing conditions can cause intraarticular damage to structures such as the articular cartilage, menisci, joint capsule and ligamentous restraints. This results in additive trauma and progressive deterioration of the joint and in turn, OA (Johnson *et al.* 1992). Many researchers such as Lynch and Henning (1998) are convinced of this causal relationship and state that 'degenerative arthritis in the ACL-deficient knee is inevitable'. However, controversy surrounds this topic because several studies do not directly support this theory. Ferretti *et al.* (1991) and more recently, Daniel and associates (1994) reported that individuals who underwent ligament reconstruction acutely have an overall higher likelihood of developing arthrosis in the affected knee. This suggests that the etiology of the osteoarthritic changes seen after ACL rupture is multifactorial, and not solely due to biomechanical disturbances. Therefore the purpose of this paper is to outline several risk factors which have been implicated to play a role in the development of OA in the ACL-deficient knee such as concomitant meniscal pathology, osteochondral pathology, impaired proprioception, and biochemical mediators in the knee joint.

Meniscal pathology

Structure and function of normal meniscus

The menisci are crescent shaped wedges of fibrocartilage located between the condyles of the femur and tibia (Figure 2.1). These structures are composed primarily of Type I collagen (accounts for 90 per cent of total collagen within meniscus), and other components which are found in much smaller quantities such as non-collagenous protein, proteoglycans, and interstitial fluid (McDevitt and Webber 1989). The vascular supply of the menisci originates predominantly from the inferior and superior lateral and medial

Fig. 2.1

Anterior view of right knee showing gross anatomy of the cruciate ligaments and menisci. ACL – anterior cruciate ligament, PCL – posterior cruciate ligament, mfl – meniscal femoral ligament of Humphry.

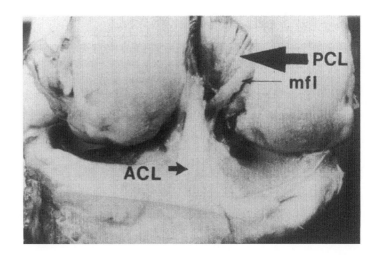

geniculate arteries. The degree of peripheral vascular penetration however, has been found to be only 10–30 per cent of the outer width of the adult meniscus (Arnoczky and Warren 1982). Therefore the majority of the meniscus is avascular, which profoundly influences its ability to heal from injury. Several studies have shown that the menisci have a characteristic pattern of collagen fibre orientation. The majority of collagen fibres are aligned in a circumferential fashion, yet there are some that are oriented radially, particularly at the meniscal surfaces (Bullough *et al.* 1970; Ahmed and Burke 1983). Thus, the biomechanical functions of the meniscus stem from the physical properties of this matrix.

The menisci were for many years believed to be simply vestigial structures. However, a large body of evidence from the last few decades has suggested that the meniscus serves a variety of significant functions. Biomechanical studies have established that the meniscus has an important role as a load-bearing structure, for it has been reported that 50 per cent to 85 per cent of the compressive load of the knee joint is transmitted through the meniscus (Ahmed and Burke 1983). In addition, the viscoelastic properties of menisci allow them to function as shock absorbers in dampening the load generated during weight-bearing activity (Johnson and Pope 1978). As a result, intact menisci transmit load and absorb energy, thus protecting the articular surfaces from compressive stress. In the kinematics of a normal knee, there is both sliding and rolling motion of the femur on the tibia. This is accomplished by articulating a rounded femoral condyle with a relatively flattened tibial plateau. As a result, only a small region of the femur is in direct contact with the tibia. Therefore the menisci decrease joint incongruity by filling in the space between the tibia and the femur (Simon *et al.* 1973). By increasing joint congruity, the menisci are able to assist in joint stability by deepening the articular surfaces of the tibial plateau (Smillie 1971). This is particularly relevant in the ACL-deficient knee, for Levy and associates (1982) showed that the posterior horn of the medial meniscus acts as a posterior wedge and thus serves as a secondary restraint to anterior tibial translation. Furthermore, during joint motion the menisci contribute to joint lubrication by spreading synovial fluid over the articular surfaces, and during weight-bearing serve to compress nutrients in the articular cartilage (Renstrom and Johnson 1990).

Prevalence and pattern of meniscal injury in ACL-deficient knees

Anterior cruciate ligament-insufficiency is associated with a high rate of concomitant meniscal lesions. In acute ACL-deficiency, the incidence of meniscal tears has been reported to range from 41 per cent to 77 per cent (DeHaven 1980; Noyes *et al.* 1980; Woods and Chapman 1984; Indelicato and Bittar 1985; Hirshman *et al.* 1990;

Shelbourne and Nitz 1991; Paletta *et al.* 1992). In contrast, the reported rated of meniscal injury in the intact ACL knee is 15 per cent to 25 per cent (Noyes *et al.* 1980; DeHaven 1980). In the chronic ACL-deficient knee, the incidence of meniscal damage is reported to be even higher, with rates ranging from 73 per cent–98 per cent (Indelicato and Bittar 1985; Warren and Marshall 1978; McDaniel and Dameron 1980; Noyes *et al.* 1983; Fowler and Regan 1987). Woods and Chapman (1984) compared a group of patients with chronic injuries to a group with acute injuries and reported that the incidence of meniscal tears almost doubled (88 per cent vs. 45 per cent respectively). Therefore, some meniscal injuries occur at the time of initial injury, while others may result from recurrent giving way episodes long after the ACL was disrupted.

The reported incidence of medial versus lateral meniscus injured has been described. While the type of injury is obviously influenced by the mechanism of injury, lateral meniscal tears are more common in acute ACL ruptures (Fowler and Regan 1987; Cooper *et al.* 1990) and medial tears predominate with chronic insufficiency (Woods and Chapman 1984; Indelicato and Bittar), indicating continued injury to the medial meniscus over time due to knee instability. In the chronic setting, MacIntosh has called the ACL the 'watchdog' of the medial meniscus (personal communication). In both the acute and chronic ACL-deficiency situation, the peripheral posterior horns of the meniscus are at greatest risk of tearing and account for more than half of the meniscal injuries identified (Thompson and Fu 1993). However, differences in the type of meniscal tear are evident depending upon whether it is located in the medial or lateral meniscus. A peripheral longitudinal tear is the most common medial meniscal lesion, while the lateral meniscus is more at risk for radial tear (Cerabona *et al.* 1998). The type of meniscal tear and its association with osteoarthritis will be discussed subsequently.

Meniscal pathology and osteoarthritis of the ACL-deficient knee

The role of meniscal lesions in the pathogenesis of OA in the knee continues to be the focus of considerable discussion. Loss or damage of this structure has been associated with an accelerated development of OA (McDaniel and Dameron 1980; Fairbank 1948; Satku *et al.* 1986). Fairbank, in his classic paper from 1948 (Fairbank 1948) described post-meniscectomy (i.e. removal of meniscus) roentgenographic changes that included joint space narrowing, osteophyte development, and flattening of the femoral articular surface. He reported these changes were present in 50–66 per cent of the knees studied after meniscectomy and in only 5 per cent of the contralateral knees. Consequently, Fairbank was one of the first to postulate that loss of the load-bearing role of the meniscus leads to degenerative changes. An example of roentgenographic degenerative change of the knee is presented in Figure 2.2.

The importance of an intact meniscus is the prevention of OA in an ACL-deficient knee has been well documented. Sherman and associates (1988) reported a significantly higher incidence of degenerative change in ACL-insufficient knees with prior meniscectomy compared to those without meniscectomy. This is in agreement with the findings of several authors (Lynch and Henning 1998; Noyes *et al.* 1983; Sommerlath 1989). Furthermore, individuals who had both menisci removed were reported to have a higher frequency of OA than individuals with unilateral meniscectomy or meniscal repair (Sommerlath 1989). In addition, Sommerlath and Gillquist (1987) found in a seven-year follow-up of subjects with intact ligaments that degenerative arthritis occurs more frequently in patients with total meniscectomy than in those with only partial meniscectomy.

Meniscectomy has been shown to profoundly affect the manner in which load-bearing occurs in the knee joint. As a result of partial or total meniscectomy the contact area between the tibia and femur is decreased approximately 30 per cent to 50 per cent (Kurosawa *et al.* 1980). Consequently, the reduced contact area increases the stresses of compression and shear across the articular cartilage likely resulting in degenerative change (DeHaven 1990).

The progression of articular degeneration in the knee can also be influenced simply by having a meniscal injury, without a history of meniscal surgery. Satku and associates (1986) reported that all ACL-deficient subjects with clinical evidence of meniscal injury but no meniscectomy had degenerative change in the knee. However, not all meniscal tears are associated with damage of the articular cartilage. Unstable tears, such as bucket-handle, longitudinal with broken handles, and complex tears have been shown to correlate

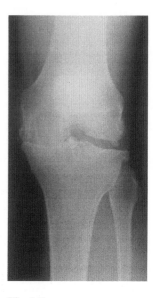

Fig. 2.2

Plain radiographs of the knee demonstrating severe degenerative disease in the medial compartment.

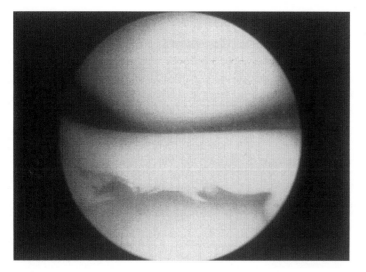

Fig. 2.3

Arthroscopic view of the knee revealing a displaced 'bucket-handle' medial meniscal tear.

with an increased incidence of OA (Lynch and Henning 1998; Lewandrowski *et al.* 1997). Figure 2.3 illustrates a classic bucket-handle tear of the meniscus. Nevertheless, it has been demonstrated that damaged menisci still distribute some load and these knees are less likely to have OA complications than those knees treated with partial or total meniscectomy (Casscells 1978; Lynch *et al.* 1983). Consequently, the risk of degeneration appears to be influenced by the degree of meniscal pathology and as a result, the primary goal of management is to preserve the meniscus if at all possible.

Osteochondral pathology

Prevalence and patterns of osteochondral pathology in ACL-deficient knees

The increasing utilization of magnetic resonance imaging (MRI) and arthroscopy in the management of musculoskeletal trauma have allowed investigators to reliably identify lesions of articular cartilage and bone within the knee joint (Vellet *et al.* 1991; Engebretsen *et al.* 1993; Lahm *et al.* 1998). These lesions were previously not visualized on routine roentgenograms. An acute rupture of the ACL has been shown to be associated with damage to both these structures in the knee (Bray and Dandy 1989; Indelicato 1983).

The reported incidence of chondral injury in the acutely ruptured ACL knee ranges from 18–46 per cent (Daniel 1994; Lynch *et al.* 1983; Bray and Dandy 1990; Indelicato 1983; Hardacker *et al.* 1990; and Spindler *et al.* 1983). These studies commonly defined articular cartilage injuries as any chondromalacia, fractures, impaction, creases, or fissures upon observation; an example of which can be seen in Figure 2.4. Furthermore, the medial compartment has been reported to be more at risk of sustaining damage than the lateral

Fig. 2.4

Arthroscopic view of the knee demonstrating severe degenerative disease down to eburnated bone on the tibial surface.

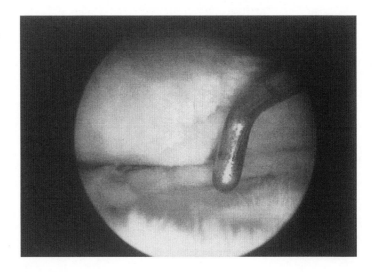

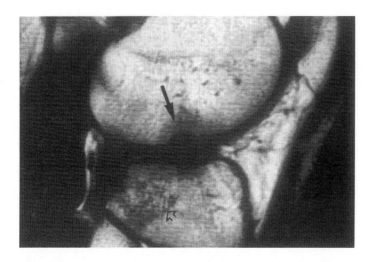

Fig. 2.5
T1-weighted magnetic resonance image showing sites of osseous injury of the anterior aspect of the lateral femoral condyle (closed arrow) and the posterior aspect of the lateral tibial plateau (open arrow).

compartment (Daniel *et al.* 1994; Hirshman *et al.* 1990). However, the two studies which analysed the location of the chondral injury did so three months after the injury. Therefore it is possible that these studies did not accurately document articular damage at time of injury but rather subsequent damage due to altered pathomechanics (i.e. giving out episodes) of the ACL-deficient knee.

In 1989, Mink and Deutsch (1989) coined the term 'bone bruise' to describe post-traumatic subcortical regions of altered signal intensity in the femur and/or tibia on T1- and T2-weighted MRI images. The lesions on T1-weighted images are characterized by decreased signal intensity while on T2-weighted images there is a corresponding increase in signal intensity (Figure 2.5). These 'bone bruises' were subsequently classified by Vellet and colleagues (1991) according to their architectural appearance, their spatial relationship with cortical bone, and their short-term osteochondral sequelae. There is general agreement that the pathogenesis of these identifiable lesions on MRI results from microtrabecular fracture. This bone injury and its sequelae, i.e. haemorrhage, edema, and inflammation, are responsible for the abnormal signals seen on imaging (Mink and Deutsch 1989). The reported incidence of bone bruises with acute ACL rupture is even higher than that observed for articular cartilage injury. Several studies have revealed that approximately 80 per cent of patients with a complete tear of their ACL have concomitant bone bruises (Vellet *et al.* 1991; Spindler *et al.* 1983; Speer *et al.* 1992; Rosen *et al.* 1991). Bone bruises are evident in many sites within the knee joint, however approximately 80 per cent occur in the lateral compartment (Spindler *et al.* 1983; Graf *et al.* 1993). The sulcus terminalis of the lateral femoral condyle and the posterior tibial plateau are the most common areas involved. The high frequency of bone bruises in the lateral compartment of an acute ACL-deficient knee suggests that the mechanism of injury includes anterior subluxation, increased internal rotation of the tibia,

Fig. 2.6

Image of the knee in a patient who had an acute rupture of the anterior cruciate ligament. This lateral view demonstrates the impact of the lateral femoral condyle on the posterior aspect of the lateral tibial plateau.

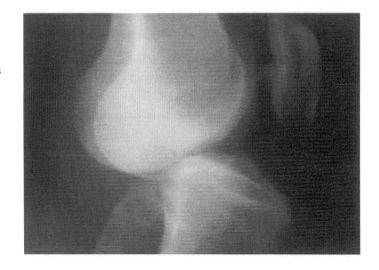

and a valgus stress. This would position the lateral femoral condyle over the posterior edge of the lateral tibial plateau as (Figure 2.6). With subsequent valgus stress, impaction of these structures occurs resulting in localized osseous contusions (Speer *et al.* 1992). In addition, bone scintigraphy has confirmed the location and presence of bone bruises in acute ligamentous knee injuries (Marks *et al.* 1992).

Osteochondral pathology and osteoarthritis of the ACL-deficient knee

Direct chondral injuries such as those identified by arthroscopy have been shown to initiate the process of OA (Arnoczky *et al.* 1991). This has been postulated to occur due to the limited ability of articular cartilage to repair itself. The impaired ability to heal stems from the lack of blood supply and also from the ability of articular cartilage chondrocytes to form adequate new tissue (Martin 1994). The severity of chondral injury appears to play a role in the progression of OA, as demonstrated by animal model studies. Injuries graded as 'superficial' may cause death of cells surrounding the injury, however they do not necessarily lead to OA unless there is accompanying joint incongruity (Arnoczky *et al.* 1991). Deep penetrating injuries on the other hand heal inadequately, for the defect fills in with cartilaginous tissue that is not articular cartilage but rather a mixture of hyaline and fibrocartilage. Consequently, this new tissue does not remain intact over time and thus contributes to the future development of cartilage degeneration (Mankin 1982). With regards to the ACL-deficient knee, repeated episodes of anterior subluxation can exacerbate existing articular cartilage damage (Mankin 1982). Thus, the chondral lesion accompanying the acute rupture of the ACL may provide a focus for deterioration of the articular cartilage.

The natural history of bone bruises and their pathodegenerative implications within the knee joint remains largely unknown. Bone bruises represent a blunt injury to the overlying articular cartilage, subchondral bone, and inner marrow. Because of their relatively high occurrence in acute ACL injuries they have generated a renewed interest in the etiology of post-traumatic knee OA. A number of animal model studies have investigated this possible relationship. Mankin (1982) reported that a single, supraphysiological blow to the surface of canine knee articular cartilage which exceeds a critical threshold serves as a precursor for OA. Whether the trauma experienced at the time of ACL trauma is significant enough to exceed this threshold remains unknown. Donohue and associates (1983) have noted that blunt trauma to adult canine articular cartilage produced changes in its histological, biochemical, and ultrastructural characteristics without articular surface disruption. In addition, they showed that it may be weeks or months before surface abnormalities become apparent. Consequently, the articular cartilage could be damaged yet appear normal on arthroscopic evaluation immediately following injury and degenerative change may not become visibly apparent until much time later. This is consistent with clinical results reported by Graf and associates (1993) and Mink and Deutsch (1989) who stated that there was no correlation between the location of bone bruises on MRI and articular cartilage damage in acute ACL-deficient knees.

There is a lack of data concerning this topic from human studies in the literature, however Vellet and associates (1991) prospectively studied bone bruises and acute ACL tears. They reported that bone bruises localized in the medullary area (i.e. reticular) resolved completely within three months, however lesions characterized by their contiguity with the adjacent cortical bone (i.e. geographic) had evidence of osteochondral sequelae at follow-up 6–12 months later. These changes included subcortical sclerosis, cartilage thinning, cartilage loss, and cortical impaction.

Coen and associates (1996) have recently reported a phenomenon they have termed 'dimpling' that describes a softening of articular cartilage overlying an occult osseous injury. The cartilage transiently indents after gentle placement of a probe. The long-term sequela of dimpling is unknown. However, it may prove to be an early prognostic indicator of OA. Researchers have postulated that the mechanism for post-traumatic OA from a bone bruise is that the subchondral bone heals via callous formation which results in a stiffer construct than the previous normal bone. The decreased compliance of the new subchondral bone would require the articular cartilage to absorb more of the compressive forces and thus possibly lead to degenerative change (Rosen *et al.* 1991). The minimal evidence published to date nevertheless indicates that blunt trauma to the articular cartilage, even when not visible on initial inspection, may have profound effects on future cartilage integrity.

Impaired proprioception

Proprioception in the normal knee

Recently, it has become apparent that most intraarticular and periarticular knee joint structures, in addition to their mechanical function, also play an important role in knee proprioception (Kennedy *et al.* 1982; Zimney 1988). Proprioception is considered a specialized variation of the sensory modality of touch and encompasses the sensations of joint movement (i.e. kinesthesia) and position (i.e. joint position sense) (Lephart *et al.* 1992). Proprioception in the knee has been shown to be provided by mechanoreceptors localized in the muscle, tendon, skin, capsule and ligaments (Kennedy *et al.* 1982; Zimney 1988). Recent neuroanatomical studies have demonstrated specialized mechanoreceptors such as Ruffini endings, Golgi tendon organs, and Pacinian corpuscles in the human ACL. These mechanoreceptors respond to mechanical deformation (e.g. tension) of the tissue and serve to translate the stimulus into specific neuronal signal(s) (Shutte 1987). They have been found to be more active at the extreme ranges of motion and also responsible for initiating reflex contraction about the knee joint; both properties of which may serve a protective or stabilizing role (Kennedy *et al.* 1982; Solomonow *et al.* 1987). Consequently, the ACL provides important neurologic feedback to the central nervous system which directly mediates joint position sense and protective muscular stabilization reflexes about the joint (Lephart *et al.* 1995; Solomonow *et al.* 1987). Therefore, a lack of afferent input from these mechanoreceptors may contribute to the progressive functional decline of the knee joint.

Impaired proprioception and osteoarthritis in the ACL-deficient knee

A significant deterioration in the proprioception of the knee joints occurs with an ACL rupture compared to the non-injured contralateral knee joint or an age-matched control group has been well documented by several investigators (Barrack *et al.* 1989; MacDonald *et al.* 1996; Corrigan *et al.* 1992; Beard *et al.* 1993; and Barrett *et al.* 1991). As mentioned previously, complete ACL insufficiency, and thus loss of this ligament's mechanical function, creates an unstable knee. Loss of ACL proprioceptive function, as originally proposed by Kennedy and associates (1982), is thought to contribute to this increasing instability over time through loss of the dynamic stabilizing reflexes. If this were the case, then proprioceptive loss would be expected to be present acutely as well as chronically. If loss of the ACL simply results in loss of passive restraint, which leads over time to mechanical stretching of capsular structures, and thus to a possible change in response of capsular receptors, loss of proprioceptive ability would be expected chronically but not acutely. Barrack and associates (1989) and MacDonald and associates (1996) showed no difference in proprioception deficits between knees with acute and chronic injuries, thus suggesting that proprioceptive loss can also be a cause of increased joint laxity and not just the result of it.

Appropriately coordinated and timed muscle coactivation normally attenuates load across the articular cartilage. Muscle activity is a critical determinant of the mechanical stiffness of the joint, which relates to its ability to resist disturbances and to maintain articular congruence (Johansson *et al.* 1991). Afferent signals from mechanoreceptors in the ACL have been shown to initiate joint-protective muscular reflexes. Joint instability occurs when there is a lack of muscular reflex stabilization of the knee is associated with a diminished sensory feedback mechanism, which causes a latent motor response of the hamstring muscles. Beard and associates (1993) reported in 1993 that reflex hamstring contraction latency is significantly slower in ACL-deficient knees than in the contralateral non-injured knee. Furthermore, they claimed the greater the latency, the greater the instability. This data suggested that the loss of proprioceptive input from the ruptured ACL, evident as the longer response time required for the ACL-hamstring reflex are to become active, contributes significantly to the functional instability of the knee. This corroborates with Kennedy's original theory.

The relationship between impaired proprioception and osteoarthritis has been minimally evaluated. Barrett and associates (1991) reported that joint position sense was impaired in a cohort of patients with osteoarthritic knees, however this was not a longitudinal study and therefore it is difficult to conclude that the loss of position sense causes OA or is a consequence of it or both. Many osteoarthritic patients have an abnormal wide-based gait but it may not necessarily be related to the pain experienced. Instead it may be due to the loss of proprioception. The abnormal gait has been proposed by some authors to result from an effort to maximize proprioceptive input (Barrett *et al.* 1991; Stauffer *et al.* 1997). A similar effect is observed in the ACL-deficient knee. The gait of a patient with an ACL-deficient knee is designed to prevent excessive anterior displacement of the tibia, and is reported to result from abnormal proprioception (Barrett *et al.* 1991; Berchuk *et al.* 1990). After an ACL rupture, proprioception must arise from other intact structures within the knee joint. However, the ACL-deficient knee has been shown to move in a non-physical axis (resulting in alterations in gait and movement) (Berchuk *et al.* 1990). Thus the remaining proprioceptive output is non-physiological disorganized. Consequently, patients feel the knee to be unstable because cortical interpretation and analysis of knee position is disturbed. Therefore, the lack of proprioceptive feedback resulting from a rupture of the ACL leads to poor spatial and temporal coordination of muscle activity and limb position. This is characterized clinically by joint instability and an abnormal gait. As a result, this causes an increased, repetitive, poorly distributed load across the joint surface, which leads to progressive degenerative change in the knee (Barrett 1991; Sharma and Pai 1997). Longitudinal studies are required in order to fully elucidate the relationship between impaired proprioception and OA in ACL-deficient knees.

Biochemical mediators

Biochemistry of articular cartilage

Articular cartilage is a highly differentiated tissue consisting of four major components: chondrocytes, Type II collagen, proteoglycan, and water. The three latter components form the extracellular matrix (ECM) of the cartilage, the conformation of which provides the property of resilience. As a result, the articular cartilage located in the knee joint is able to resist load-bearing forces (Maroudas *et al.* 1986). Chondrocytes, although few in number, play a key role in matrix homeostasis. Matrix integrity is maintained through the regulation of degradative and synthetic events. This regulation is mediated by biological agents known as cytokines. Cytokines are polypeptides released by living cells, which act as local intercellular messengers to regulate host cell function (Nathan and Sporn 1991). Specifically, catabolic cytokines act on chondrocytes and synovial cells to induce production of matrix degrading enzymes, such as metalloproteases. This is normally balanced by anabolic cytokines, which act on chondrocytes to induce production of cartilage matrix (Westacott and Sharif 1996). This process is schematically outlined in Figure 2.7. Alterations in the concentrations of any of the components responsible for this homeostasis may shift the equilibrium in favour of either overproduction of matrix proteins or to net degradation.

Biochemical mediator of OA in an ACL-deficient knee

The reported frequency of post-traumatic OA following ACL injury has been rather variable. This has led researchers to postulate that endogenous factors, in addition to mechanical factors, contribute to the development of knee OA. Osteoarthritis is characterized by slow changes in matrix metabolism. Initially there is an increase in water content of cartilage implying a failure in the elastic restraint of the collagen network. Shortly afterward, an increased turnover of proteoglycans occurs followed by an eventual net loss of proteoglycans from the ECM as catabolic events dominate over anabolic events (Heinegard and Oldberg 1989; Mankin and Brandt 1992). Therefore, an imbalance between the anabolic and catabolic events occurs in OA, resulting in the loss of cartilage matrix. The role of cytokines in this process has received particular attention due to their function, as described above in regulating articular cartilage matrix homeostasis. The intraarticular cytokines most commonly implicated in the pathogenesis of

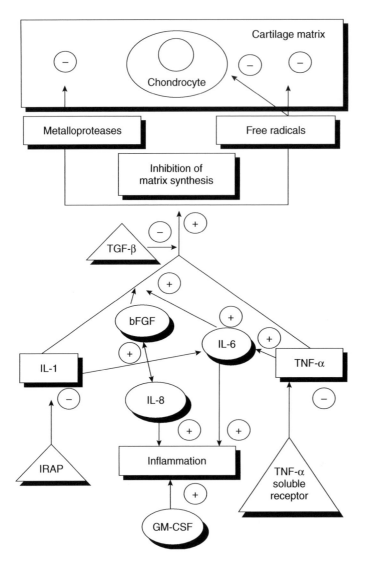

Fig. 2.7
The effects of synovial fluid cytokines on articular chondrocytes and cartilaginous matrix. Cytokines exert their effects on cartilage components indirectly through the production of free radicals which damage both the chondrocyte and the matrix; suppression of cartilage matrix synthesis by the chondrocyte; and promotion of production of metalloproteases which catabolize the cartilage matrix. IL – interleukin; TNF – tumour necrosis factor; GM-CSF – granulocyte/macrophage-colony stimulating factor; IRAP – interleukin-1-receptor antagonist protein; bFGF – basic fibroblast growth factor; TGF – transforming growth factor.

OA have been interleukin (IL)-1, 6, and 8, interleukin-1-receptor antagonist protein (IL-1Ra), tumour necrosis factor alpha (TNF-α), and granulocyte/macrophage-colony stimulating factor (GM-CSF).

Interleukin-1 exists in two isoforms – alpha (α) and beta (β), and they both have the biological ability to suppress the synthesis of Type II collagen which is a major constituent of articular cartilage matrix (Arner and Pratta 1989). Furthermore, IL-1 promotes the resorption of the cartilage matrix by inducing the production of specific matrix degrading enzymes known as metalloproteases (Pelletier *et al.* 1991). IL-1 also stimulates chondrocytes and synoviocytes to produce IL-6, which is believed to act as a cofactor for the inhibition of proteoglycan synthesis by IL-1 (Neitfeld *et al.* 1990). The cytokine

IL-1Ra has been shown to antagonize the activity of both isoforms of IL-1 (Seckinger *et al.* 1987). This is accomplished because IL-1Ra is a specific antagonist that competitively inhibits binding of IL-1 to its receptors. IL-1Ra is further characterized as having no intrinsic agonist activity (Carter *et al.* 1990). Consequently, IL-1Ra can neutralize the catabolic effects of IL-1a and IL-1b.

The actions of TNF-α are very similar to those observed with IL-1. Tumour necrosis factor-alpha is a macrophage derived cytokine that also promotes the degradation of cartilage, and suppresses the synthesis of cartilage proteoglycans (Saklatuala 1989). Like IL-1, TNF-α stimulates the secretion of IL-6 from chondrocytes. Furthermore, increased synthesis of IL-1 and metalloprotease has been shown to promote intraarticular inflammation, which results in the production of more IL-1 and TNF-α (Pelletier *et al.* 1991). Therefore, these latter cytokines induce cartilage degradation indirectly via their inflammatory properties.

Only recently have researchers investigated the role of intraarticular cytokines in the pathogenesis of post-traumatic OA. Several researchers have reported that IL-1a levels do not change in acute or chronic ACL-deficient knees compared to uninjured knees (Cameron *et al.* 1994; Marks and Cameron 1998). However, levels of IL-1b have been shown to increase after an acute ACL injury and they remain elevated, approximately fourfold when compared to uninjured knees, in the chronic setting (Marks and Cameron 1998). The level of chondroprotective IL-1Ra is also increased acutely however there is only a slight increase, if at all, observed in chronic knees (Cameron *et al.* 1994; Marks and Cameron 1998). This suggests the loss of an important chondroprotective cytokine in subjects with chronic ACL-deficiency. The chronic absence of IL-1Ra may allow IL-1 to act unabated and thus inflict more damage to the articular cartilage. Increased expression of IL-1 receptors on OA chondrocytes suggests that only small amounts of IL-1a or b, such as those levels seen normally, are needed to trigger catabolic enzyme production in OA joints (Roos *et al.* 1995). The levels of TNF-α have been reported to increase acutely and while their levels fall over several weeks they still remain elevated compared to uninjured knee values (Cameron *et al.* 1994; Marks and Cameron 1998). This suggests that TNF-α may play a role in chronic cartilage loss after ACL rupture. High levels of IL-6 and 8 have been noted in the acute phase of ACL injury but they have been shown to fall back to the normal range by three months after injury. Conversely, the concentration of GM-CSF has been shown to remain near the normal range acutely, however it elevates in the chronic setting (Cameron 1994). This suggests that IL-6 and 8 play a role in acute inflammation while GM-CSF assists in propagating chronic chondral destruction. Recent work by Marks and Cameron (1998) demonstrated increased expression of IL-1b and TNF-α with increasing grades of chondrosis in a chronic ACL-deficient knee. Furthermore, they showed decreasing IL-1Ra levels with increasing grades of chondrosis. This suggests that certain cytokine profiles are associated with greater risk for developing post-traumatic OA in the ACL-deficient knee.

Summary and future work

The etiology of degenerative change in the knee following rupture of the ACL remains uncertain. The development of osteoarthritis in the ACL-deficient knee is a complex process with many factors likely contributing to its initiation and/or perpetuation. The role of biomechanical, neuroanatomical, and biochemical factors in the development of knee OA was the focus of this paper. Along with instability of the knee, the degree of meniscal pathology has been well established as having a profound influence on modifying OA risk. Of all the meniscal pathologies, meniscectomy, partial or total, appears to present the greatest OA risk, more so than damaged or repaired menisci. The magnitude of risk is illustrated by the fact that if a meniscectomy is performed, the development of OA is independent of the stabilization achieved with ACL reconstruction (Ferretti *et al.* 1991). Consequently, preservation of the meniscus should be a primary goal of management. Occult osseous lesions or bone bruises represent traumatic injuries to bone. They occur in more than 80 per cent of individuals with complete ruptures of the ACL, and have been shown to have degenerative osteochondral sequelae. Therefore, MRI-detected bone bruises are an important variable to consider. In addition, an ACL-insufficient knee has been shown to have deficits in proprioceptive function. This results in alterations in gait with resulting modifications in weight-bearing loads in the knee joint, which may lead to degenerative changes. The role of cytokines in promoting cartilage degradation has recently received attention. Individuals with relatively high concentrations of chondrodestructive cytokines, such as IL-1b and TNF-α, and correspondingly low levels of chondroprotective cytokines such as IL-1Ra are at increased risk for developing post-traumatic OA in the ACL-deficient knee.

It is important to understand is that all the risk factors mentioned above do not act in isolation, but rather interact with each other to produce the degenerative changes. Moreover, other endogenous factors such as increasing age (less than 60) (Roos *et al.* 1995) , obesity (Lynch and Henning 1998), abnormal alignment of the knee joint (Coventry 1973), genetic predisposition (Ala-Kokko *et al.* 1990), and high levels of activity (Lynch and Hennning 1998), although not profiled in this paper, have also been implicated as risk factors for knee OA. Therefore, many factors may contribute to OA and orthopaedic surgeons need to be aware of all the possible risks in order to determine the proper prognosis for OA after ACL rupture. Consequently, in an effort to aid in the future prognosis of post-traumatic OA, we propose

Fig. 2.8

Proposed ACL risk equation. OA risk as a function of documented risk factors.

$$OA\ (risk) = f(C_1X_1 + C_2X_2 + C_3X_3 + C_4X_4 + C_5X_5 + C_6X_6 + \cdots)$$

$C = $ Risk coefficient
$X_1 = $ ACL instability
$X_2 = $ Meniscal pathology
$X_3 = $ Bone bruise (MRI)
$X_4 = $ Cytokine abnormalities
$X_5 = $ Impaired proprioception
$X_6 = $ Other

that an 'ACL risk equation' be developed which would express overall osteoarthritis risk quantitatively. This proposed equation would be a function of all the pertinent risk factors (Figure 2.8). To properly generate the ACL risk equation, a multiple-variable analysis investigating the degree of interaction among these risk factors (which ultimately produce post-traumatic OA) is necessary. The ability to determine an individual's level of OA risk would aid the surgeon in tailoring pre- and postoperative management. In addition, novel therapeutic strategies may be subsequently developed, such as gene therapy, in order to counteract or neutralize the relevant factors and thus protect the ACL-insufficient knee from degenerative changes.

References

Ahmed AM and DL Burke (1983). In-vitro measurements of static pressure distribution in synovial joints: I. Tibial surface of the knee. *J Biomech Eng.* 105: 216–225.

Ala-Kokko L, Baldwin CT, Moskowitz RW, *et al.* (1990). Single base mutation in the type II procollagen gene (COL2A1) as a cause of primary osteoarthritis associated with a mild chondraodysplasia. *Proc Natl Acad Sci USA.* 87: 6565–6568.

Arner EC and MA Pratta (1989). Independent effects of interleukin-1 on proteoglycan breakdown, proteoglycan synthesis, and prostaglandin E2 release from cartilage in organ culture. *Arthritis Rheum.* 32: 288–297.

Arnoczky SP and RF Warren (1982). Microvaculature of the human meniscus. *Am J Sports Med.* 10: 90–95.

Arnoczky SP, Skyhar MJ, Wickiewicz TL (1991). In JB McGinty (ed.) *Basic Science of the Knee. Operative Arthroscopy.* Raven Press: New York, pp. 155–192.

Barrack R, Skinner HB, Buckley SL (1989). Proprioception in the anterior cruciate deficient knee. *Am J Sports Med.* 17: 1–6.

Barrett DS, Cobb AG, Bentley G (1991). Joint proprioception in normal, osteoarthritic and replaced knees. *J Bone Joint Surg.* 73B: 53–56.

Barrett DS (1991). Proprioception and function after anterior cruciate reconstruction. *J Bone Joint Surg.* 73B: 883–837.

Beard DJ, Kyberg PG, Ferguson CM, *et al.* (1993). Proprioception after rupture of the anterior cruciate ligament. An objective indication in the need of surgery? *J Bone Joint Surg.* 75B: 311–315.

Berchuk M, Andriacchi TP, Bach BR, *et al.* (1990). Gait adaptations by patients who have a deficient anterior cruciate ligament. *J Bone Joint Surg.* 72A: 871–877.

Brandt KD (1985). In WN Kelley, ED Harris and RS Sledge (eds) *Osteoarthritis: Clinical patterns and pathology. Textbook of Rheumatology.* 2nd Edition. WB Saunders: Philadelphia, pp. 1432–1448.

31

Bray RC and DJ Dandy (1989). Meniscal lesions and chronic anterior cruciate ligament deficiency. Meniscal tears occurring before and after reconstruction. *J Bone Joint Surg.* 71B: 128–130.

Bullough PG, Munuera L, Murphy J, *et al.* (1970). The strength of menisci of the knee as it relates to their fine structure. *J Bone Joint Surg.* 52(3): 564–567.

Cameron ML, Buchgraber A, Paessler HH, *et al.* (1994). The natural history of the anterior cruciate ligament-deficient knee. *Am J Sports Med.* 25: 750–754.

Cameron ML, Fu FH, Paessler HH, *et al.* (1994). Synovial fluid cytokine concentrations as possible prognostic indicators in the ACL-deficient knee. *Knee Surg, Sports Traumatol, Arthroscopy.* 2: 38–44.

Carter DB, Beibert MR, Dunn CJ (1990). Purification, cloning, expression and biological characterization of an interleukin-1 receptor antagonist protein. *Nature.* 344: 633–638.

Casscells SW (1978). *Arthroscopic and Cadaver Knee Investigations.* Symposium on arthroscopy and arthrography of the knee. American Academy of Orthopaedic Surgeons. Mosby: St. Louis, pp. 122–141.

Centers for Disease Control and Prevention: Targeting Arthritis; The Nation's Leading Cause of Disability. (2003) Department of Health and Human Services. U.S. Government Atlanta, Georgia.

Cerabona F, Sherman M, Bonamo J, *et al.* (1998). Patterns of meniscal injury with acute anterior cruciate ligament tears. *Am J Sports Med.* 16: 603–609.

Coen MJ, Caborn DNM, Johnson DL (1996). The dimpling phenomenon: articular cartilage injury overlying an occult osteochondral lesion at the time of anterior cruciate ligament reconstruction. *Arthroscopy.* 12: 502–505.

Cooper DE, Arnoczky SP, Warren RF (1990). Arthroscopic meniscal repair. *Clin Sports Med.* 9: 589–607.

Corrigan JP, Cashmen WF, Brady MP (1992). Proprioception in the cruciate deficient knee. *J Bone Joint Surg.* 74B: 247–250.

Coventry MB (1973). Osteotomy about the knee for degenerative and rheumatoid arthritis: indications, operative technique and results. *J Bone Joint Surg.* 55A: 23–48.

Cunningham LS and Kelsey JL (1984). Epidemiology of musculoskeletal impairments and associated disability. *Am J Public Health.* 74: 574–579.

Daniel DM, Stone ML, Dobson BE, *et al.* (1994). Fate of the ACL-injured patient. A prospective outcome study. *Am J Sports Med.* 22: 632–644.

Davis MA, Ettinger WH, Neuhaus JM, *et al.* (1991). Knee osteoarthritis and physical functioning: evidence from NHANES I epidemiologic follow-up study. *J Rheumatol.* 18: 591–598.

DeHaven KE (1980). The diagnosis of acute knee injuries with hemarthrosis. *Am J Sports Med.* 8: 9–14.

DeHaven KE (1990). *The role of the meniscus.* In JW Ewing (ed.) *Articular Cartilage and Knee Joint Function. Basic Science and Arthroscopy.* Raven Press: New York, pp. 103–115.

Donohue JM, Buss D, Oegema TR Jr, *et al.* (1983). The effects of indirect trauma on adult canine articular cartilage. *J Bone Joint Surg.* 65A: 948–957.

Engebretsen L, Arendt E, Fritts HM (1993). Osteochondral lesions and cruciate ligament injuries. MRI in 18 knees. *Acta Orthop Scand.* 64: 434–436.

Fairbank TJ (1948). Knee joint changes after meniscectomy. *J Bone Joint Surg.* 30B: 664–670.

Feagin JA Jr and WW Curl (1976). Isolated tear of the anterior cruciate ligament: 5-year follow-up study. *Am J Sports Med.* 4: 95–100.

Feagin JA Jr, Lambert KL, Cunningham RR, *et al.* (1987). Consideration of the anterior cruciate ligament injury in skiing. *Clin Orthop.* 216: 13–18.

Ferretti A, Conteduca F, De Carli A, *et al.* (1991). Osteoarthritis of the knee after ACL reconstruction. *Int Orthop.* 15: 367–371.

Fowler PJ and Regan WP (1987). The patient with symptomatic chronic anterior cruciate ligament insufficiency: Results of minimal arthroscopic surgery and rehabilitation. *Am J Sports Med.* 15: 321–325.

Giove TP, Miller SJ III, Kent BE, *et al.* (1983). Nonoperative treatment of the torn anterior cruciate ligament. *J Bone Joint Surg.* 65A: 184–192.

Graf BK, Cook DA, DeSmet AA, *et al.* (1993). 'Bone bruises' on magnetic resonance imaging evaluation of anterior cruciate ligament injuries. *Am J Sports Med.* 21: 220–223.

Hardacker WT, Garrett WE Jr, Bassett FH III (1990). Evaluation of acute traumatic hemarthrosis of the knee joint. *South Med J.* 83: 640–644.

Hawkins RJ, Misamore GW, Merrit TR (1986). Follow up of the acute non-operated isolated anterior cruciate ligament tears. *Am J Sports Med.* 14: 205–210.

Heinegard D and Oldberg A (1989). Structure and biology of cartilage and bone matrix noncollagenous macromolecules. FASEB 3: 2042–2054.

Hewson GF and Mendini RA (1986). Prophylactic knee bracing in college football. *Am J Sports Med.* 14: 262–266.

Hirschman HP, Daniel D, Miyasaka K (1990) The fate of unoperated knee ligament injuries. In D Daniel (ed.) *Knee Ligaments Structure Function. Injury and Repair.* Raven Press: New York, pp. 481–503.

Indelicato PA and ES Bittar. A perspective of lesions associated with anterior ligament insufficiency of the knee. *Clin Orthop.* 1985:77–80.

Indelicato PA (1983). Nonoperative treatment of complete tears of the medial collateral ligament of the knee. *J Bone Joint Surg.* 65A: 323–329.

Johansson H, Sjølander P, Sojka P (1991). A sensory role for the cruciate ligaments. *Clin Orthop.* 268: 161–178.

Johnson RJ and Pope MH (1978). *Functional Anatomy of the Meniscus.* Symposium on reconstruction of the knee. American Academy of Orthopaedic Surgeons. Mosby: St. Louis, p.3.

Johnson RJ, Beynnon BD, Nichols CE, *et al.* (1992). The treatment of injuries of the anterior cruciate ligament. *J Bone Joint Surg.* 74A: 140–148.

Kennedy JC, Alexander IJ, Hayes KC (1982). Nerve supply of the human knee and its functional importance. *Am J Sports Med.* 10: 329–335.

Kurosawa H, Fukubayashi T, Nakajima H (1980). Load-bearing mode of the knee: Physical behavior of the knee joint with and without menisci. *Clin Orthop.* 149: 283–290.

Lahm A, Erggelet C, Steinwachs M, *et al.* (1998). Articular and osseous lesions in recent ligament tears: arthroscopic changes compared with magnetic resonance imaging findings. *Arthroscopy.* 14: 597–604.

Lephart SM, Fu FH, Borsa PA, *et al.* (1995). Proprioception of the knee and shoulder joint in normal, athletic, capsuloligamentous pathological, and post-reconstruction individuals. *Orthop Trans.* 18: 1157.

Lephart SM, Kicher MS, Fu FH, *et al.* (1992). Proprioception following anterior cruciate ligament reconstruction. *J Sport Rehabil.* 1: 188–196.

Levy IM, Torzilli DA, Warren RF (1982). The effect of medial meniscectomy on anterior-posterior motion of the knee. *J Bone Joint Surg.* 64A: 883–888.

Lewandrowski K-U, Muller J, Schollmeier G (1997). Concomitant meniscal and articular cartilage lesions in the femorotibial joint. *Am J Sports
Med.* 25: 486–494.

Lynch MA and CE Henning (1998). Osteoarthritis in the ACL-deficient
knee. In J Feagin (ed.) *The Crucial Ligament.* Churchill Livingstone:
New Jersey, pp. 385–391.

Lynch MA, Henning CE, Glick KR Jr (1983). Knee joint surface changes.
Clin Orthop. 172: 148–153.

MacDonald PB, Hedden D, Pacin O, *et al.* (1996). Proprioception in anterior cruciate ligament-deficient and reconstructed knees. *Am J Sports
Med.* 24: 774–778.

Mankin HJ and Brandt KD (1992). Biochemistry and metabolism of cartilage in osteoarthritis. In R Moskowitz (ed.) *Osteoarthritis. Diagnosis
and Medical Surgical Management.* 2nd Edition. Saunders: Philadelphia,
pp. 109–154.

Mankin HJ (1982). Current concepts review: the response of articular cartilage to mechanical injury. *J Bone Joint Surg.* 64A: 460–466.

Marks PH and ML Cameron (1998). Inflammatory cytokine profiles correlate with the degree of chondrosis in the chronic anterior cruciate
ligament deficient knee. (Personal communication).

Marks PH, Goldenberg JA, Vezina WC, *et al.* (1992). Subchondral bone
infractions in acute ligamentous knee injuries demonstrated on bone
scintigraphy and magnetic resonance imaging. *J Nuclear Medicine.* 33:
516–520.

Maroudas A, Mizrahi J, Katz EP, *et al.* (1986). Physiochemical properties
and functional behaviour of normal and osteoarthritic human cartilage. In K Kvettner (ed.) *Articular Cartilage Biochemistry.* 3rd Edition.
Raven Press: New York.

Martin DF (1994). Pathomechanics of knee osteoarthritis. *Med Sci Sports
Exerc.* 26: 1429–1434.

McDaniel WJ and Dameron TB (1980). Untreated ruptures of the anterior
cruciate ligament. A follow-up study. *J Bone Joint Surg.* 62A: 696–705.

McDevitt CA and Webber RJ (1989). The ultrastructure and biochemistry
of meniscal cartilage. *Clin Orthop.* 252: 8–18.

Mink JH and Deutsch AL (1989). Occult cartilage and bone injuries of the
knee: detection, classification, and assessment with MR imaging.
Radiology. 170: 823–829.

Miyaska KC, Daniel DM, Stone ML, *et al.* (1991). The incidence of
knee ligament injuries in the general population. *Am J Knee Surg.*
4: 3–8.

Nathan C and Sporn M (1991). Cytokines in context. *J Cell Biol.* 113:
981–986.

Neilson AB and Yde J (1991). Epidemiology of acute knee injuries:
a prospective hospital investigation. *J. Trauma.* 31: 1644–1648.

Neitfeld JJ, Wilbrink B, Helle M, *et al.* (1990). Interleukin-1 induced
interleukin-6 is required for the inhibition of proteoglycan synthesis
by interleukin-1 in human cartilage. *Arthritis Rheum.* 33: 1695–1701.

Noyes FR, Basset RW, Grood ES, *et al.* (1980). Arthroscopy in acute traumatic hemarthrosis of the knee: incidence of anterior cruciate tears
and other injuries. *J Bone Joint Surg.* 62A: 687–695.

Noyes FR, Mooar PA, Matthews DS, *et al.* (1983). The symptomatic anterior cruciate deficient knee: I. The long term functional disability in
athletically active individuals. *J Bone Joint Surg.* 65A: 154–162.

Paletta GA Jr, Levine DS, O'Brien SJ, *et al.* (1992). Patterns of meniscal
injury associated with acute anterior cruciate ligament injuries in
skiers. *Am J Sports Med.* 20: 542–547.

Pattee GA, Fox JM, Del Pizzo W, et al. (1989). Four to ten year follow-up of unreconstructed anterior cruciate ligament tears. *Am J Sports Med.* 17: 430–435. 65A: 154–162.

Pelletier JP, Roughley PJ, DiBattista JH, et al. (1991). Are cytokines involved in osteoarthritis pathophysiology? *Semin Arthritis Rheum.* 20 (suppl. 2): 12–25.

Renstrom P and Johnson RJ (1990). Anatomy and biomechanics of the menisci. *Clin Sports Med.* 9: 523–538.

Roos H, Adalberth T, Dahlberg L, et al. (1995). Osteoarthritis of the knee after injury to the anterior cruciate ligament or meniscus: the influence of time and age. *Osteoarthritis Cartilage.* 3: 261–267.

Rosen MA, Jackson DW, Berger PE (1991). Occult osseous lesions documented by magnetic resonance imaging associated with anterior cruciate ligament ruptures. *Arthroscopy.* 7: 45–51.

Saklatuala J (1989). Tumour necrosis factor-alpha stimulates resorption and inhibits synthesis of proteoglycan in cartilage. *Nature.* 322: 547–549.

Satku K, Kumar VP, Ngoi SS (1986). Anterior cruciate ligament injuries. To counsel or to operate. *J Bone Joint Surg.* 68B: 458–461.

Schutte MJ, Dabezies EJ, Zimney ML, et al. (1987). Neural anatomy of the human anterior cruciate ligament. *J Bone Joint Surg.* 69A: 243–247.

Seckinger P, Williamson K, Balavione JF (1987). A urine inhibitor of interleukin-1 activity affects both interleukin-1a and 1b but not tumour necrosis factor-a. *J Immunol.* 139: 1541–1545.

Sharma L and YC Pai (1997). Impaired proprioception and osteoarthritis. *Curr Opin Rheumatol.* 9: 253–258.

Shelbourne KD and Nitz PA (1991). The O'Donoghue triad revisited-combined knee injuries involving anterior cruciate and medial collateral ligament tears. *Am J Sports Med.* 19: 474–477.

Sherman MF, Warren RF, Marshall JL, et al. (1988). A clinical and raidographical analysis of 127 anterior cruciate insufficient knees. *Clin Orthop.* 227: 229–237.

Simon WH, Freidenberg S, Richardson S (1973). Joint congruence: a correlation of joint congruence and thickness of articular cartilage in dogs. *J Bone Joint Surg.* 55A: 1614.

Slemenda CW (1992). The epidemiology of osteoarthritis of the knee. *Curr Opin Rheumatol.* 4: 546–551.

Smillie JS (1971). *Injuries of the Knee Joint,* 4th edn. Churchhill Livingstone: Edinburgh, p. 68.

Solomonow M, Baratta R, Zhou BH, et al. (1987). The synergistic action of the anterior cruciate ligament and thigh muscles in maintaining joint stability. *Am J Sports Med.* 15: 207–213.

Sommerlath K and Gillquist J (1987). Knee function after meniscus repair and total meniscectomy. A 7-year follow-up study. *Arthroscopy.* 3: 166–169.

Sommerlath K (1989). The importance of the meniscus in unstable knees: a comparative study. *Am J Sports Med.* 17: 773–777.

Speer KP, Spritzer CE, Bassett FH III, et al. (1992). Osseous injury associated with acute tears of the anterior cruciate ligament. *Am J Sports Med.* 20: 382–389.

Spindler KP, Schlis JP, Bergfeld JA, et al. (1983). Prospective study of osseous, articular, and meniscal lesions in recent anterior cruciate ligament tears by magnetic resonance imaging and arthroscopy. *Am J Sports Med.* 23: 77–81.

Stauffer RN, Chao EYS, Gyøry AN. (1997). Biomechanical gait analysis of the diseased knee joint. *Clin Orthop.* 126: 246–255.

Thompson WO and Fu FH (1993). The meniscus in the cruciate-deficient knee. *Clin Sports Med.* 12: 771–796.

Vellet AD, Marks PH, Fowler PJ, *et al.* (1991). Occult post-traumatic osteochondral lesions of the knee: prevalence, classification, and short term sequelae evaluated with MR imaging. *Radiology.* 178: 271–276.

Warren RF and Marshall J (1978). Injuries of the anterior cruciate and medial collateral ligaments of the knee. *Clin Orthop.* 136: 191–197.

Westacott CI and Sharif M (1996). Cytokines in osteoarthritis: mediators or markers of joint destruction? *Semin Arthritis Rheum.* 25: 254–272.

Woods GM and Chapman DR (1984). Repairable posterior menisco-capsular disruption in anterior cruciate ligament injuries. *Am J Sports Med.* 12: 381–385.

Zimney ML (1988). Mechanoreceptors in articular tissues. *Am J Anat.* 182: 16–32.

Primary ACL reconstruction: what are the best methods of fixation for grafts used in ACL reconstruction surgery?

Charles H. Brown

Introduction

Rigid initial graft fixation is critical to the success of ACL reconstruction. Attaining rigid initial graft fixation minimizes elongation and prevents failure at the graft fixation sites during cyclical loading of the knee prior to biological incorporation of the ACL graft (Butler 1987; Holden *et al.* 1988). Current 'accelerated' ACL postoperative rehabilitation programmes emphasize early joint motion, early closed-chain muscle strengthening, and early weight bearing (Shelbourne and Nitz 1990). Such postoperative rehabilitation regimens place high demands on the unincorporated ACL graft. Holden *et al.* (1988) have shown that graft fixation rather than the strength of the ACL graft tissue is the weak link during the early postoperative period. However, at the present time it is unknown how much force is applied to the ACL graft and graft fixation sites with activities performed in the early postoperative period. Noyes *et al.* (1984) have hypothesized that normal activities of daily living apply up to 454 N (100 lb) of force to the ACL graft and graft fixation sites. Morrison (1968, 1969, 1970) using force plate and gait analysis has estimated that the loads in the ACL during activities of daily living range from 27 N (ascending ramp) to 445 N (descending stairs).

Currently, bone-patellar tendon-bone and multiple stranded hamstring tendon autografts are the tissues most commonly used to replace a torn ACL (Fu *et al.* 2000). At the present time, graft fixation techniques for these tissues involves fixing soft tissue or bone blocks inside a bone tunnel or at the femoral or tibial cortical surfaces at a distance from the joint line (Brand *et al.* 2000b). Although the initial strength and stiffness of both bone-patellar tendon-bone (Noyes *et al.* 1984; Cooper *et al.* 1993; Muellner *et al.* 1998), and four-strand hamstring tendon grafts (Hamner *et al.* 1999) have been reported to be higher than that of the normal young human ACL (Woo *et al.* 1991), there are significant differences in fixation site healing among these graft tissues.

It is generally accepted that bone-to-bone healing occurs faster than soft tissue to bone healing. In a sheep model, Walton (1999) demonstrated osseous integration of the bone blocks of a bone-patellar tendon-bone graft into the bony tunnel walls at six weeks. However, at four weeks a fibrous union between the soft tissue of the graft and bone tunnel wall led to no difference in failure load if the interference screw was present or removed before testing.

Detailed knowledge about the biology and healing time frame of soft tissue to bone is still evolving. Rodeo *et al.* (1993) in a dog model using a long extensor tendon graft that was inserted into an extra-articular bone tunnel demonstrated that it took approximately 8 to 12 weeks for the peripheral fibers of the tendon graft to heal to the bone tunnel wall. In this animal model, tendon-to-bone healing occurred via the progressive development and maturation of a fibrous interface between the soft tissue graft and bone tunnel wall which was bridged by Sharpey-like fibers. The strength of this interface was found to increase with time, and the 12 week specimens were found to fail at the grip or at the mid-substance of the tendon graft.

Weiler *et al.* (2002) have recently examined the healing stages of an Achilles tendon ACL reconstruction in a sheep model using direct tendon-to-bone interference fixation at the ACL anatomic attachment sites with bioabsorbable poly-(D,L-lactide) interference screws. Histologic findings at six weeks demonstrated a tendon-bone junction with only a partial fibrous interzone (FIZ) between the graft and bone tunnel wall. Sharpey-like fibers were located mainly in areas where a FIZ developed between the graft tissue and bone. In areas where the FIZ developed there was immature woven bone and large amounts of noncalcified osteoid. The nine weeks specimens demonstrated that almost all gaps along the graft-bone interface were filled with woven bone. At 12 weeks, a mature, con-tinuous graft-bone interface with Sharpey's-like fibers was present. At 1 year the graft-bone interface had the appearance of a normal direct ligament insertion with a transition zone consisting of miner-alized cartilage and fibrocartilage. Based on their results, Weiler *et al.* (2002) concluded that anatomic interference fit fixation of a soft-tissue graft promotes direct tendon-to-bone formation. However, they were uncertain whether this result occurred because of decreased graft-tunnel motion or blockage of synovial fluid access.

Due to slower fixation site healing, graft fixation techniques for soft tissue ACL grafts should be able to withstand cyclic loads for a longer period of time without significant elongation occurring at the graft fixation sites if an 'accelerated' postoperative rehabilitation protocol is to be used. Howell and Hull (1998) have recommended that fixation methods that either fail, are of low stiffness, or exces-sively slip at loads <500 N should be avoided when using an aggressive rehabilitation program in knees reconstructed with hamstring tendon grafts until clinical studies have established the safety of these fixation methods.

Patellar tendon graft

Due to its high initial tensile strength and stiffness (Noyes *et al.* 1984; Cooper *et al.* 1993; Muellner *et al.* 1998), early fixation site healing (Walton 1999), predictable ability to restore stability, and reports by many authors of good and excellent short, medium, and long term results (Aglietti *et al.* 1992, 1997; Buss *et al.* 1993; Bach *et al.* 1994, 1998; Shelbourne and Nitz 1990; Shelbourne and Gray 1997), the bone-patellar tendon-bone autograft is considered by many surgeons to be the 'gold standard' for replacement of a torn ACL, and is currently the most commonly used autograft tissue. However, donor-site morbidity remains a problem for the patellar tendon autograft (Kartus *et al.* 1997, 1999, 2001).

The most popular fixation method for bone-patellar tendon-bone grafts utilizes fully threaded metal or bioabsorbable interference screws. The use of interference screws is based largely on work performed by Kurosaka and colleagues in this area (Kurosaka *et al.* 1987). These authors demonstrated superior fixation strength and stiffness of bone-patellar tendon-bone grafts fixed with a custom-designed large diameter 9.0 mm fully threaded screw in human cadaveric knees. Subsequent studies have shown that the initial fixation properties of bone-tendon-bone grafts are influenced by the following factors:

1   gap size (graft tunnel size match)
2   bone quality (host and graft bone plug)
3   screw size
4   screw length
5   screw divergence.

In the laboratory evaluation of interference screw fixation of bone-patellar tendon-bone grafts, the gap size between the bone block and bone tunnel and bone quality appear to be the most critical factors. Kurosaka *et al.* (1987) reported that making the size of the patellar and tibial bone blocks close to the size of the bone tunnels was extremely important 'in obtaining a solid fixation'. Using a porcine experimental model, Reznik *et al.* (1990) demonstrated that bone quality and gap size significantly influenced the ultimate failure load of bone blocks fixed in 10 mm bone tunnels with 7 mm screws. When the gap between the bone block and bone tunnel wall was 4 mm or more, increasing the screw diameter to 9 mm increased the failure load by 97 per cent. However, when the gap was >4 mm and a 9 mm screw used, the results were inferior to using a 7 mm screw with a gap <4 mm.

Fithian *et al.* (1992) investigated the effect of gap size on graft fixation strength and recommended use of 7 mm screws when the gap size was less than 2 mm, and 9 mm screws for gap sizes between 2–4 mm. Suture/post fixation was recommended when the gap size exceeded 6 mm. Similar conclusions and recommendations have been made by Butler *et al.* (1994), who recommended that a 7 or 9 mm screw be used for a gap sizes of 1–2 mm, and a 9 mm screw for a gap size of 3–4 mm. These authors recommended that for gap sizes >5 mm that it might be beneficial to 'back up' a 9 mm screw with post fixation.

Using human cadaveric knees of various ages, Cassim *et al.* (1993) demonstrated that the fixation strength of bone-tendon-bone patellar tendon grafts fixed in the proximal tibia and distal femur was influenced primarily by gap size and screw diameter. When the gap size was <1 mm and a 9 × 30 mm screw used, the mean ultimate failure load was 1060 N. The failure load for the tibia was on average 15 per cent lower than that of the femur. Placement of the screw on the cancellous or cortical side of the bone block and endoscopic placement versus rear-entry placement did not influence fixation strength. Specimens with a mean age of 79 years demonstrated a decrease in failure load to <42 per cent of the load achieved using specimens with a mean age of 35 years. The lower failure loads reported in the tibia and older specimens are a reflection of lower bone mineral density.

Weak or osteoporotic bone provides inadequate purchase for interference screw fixation of bone-tendon-bone grafts (Butler 1987). Brown *et al.* (1996b) evaluated the fixation strength of bone-patellar tendon-bone grafts using bovine specimens, young human specimens (33–52 years), and elderly human specimens (68–81 years). In this study, the mean failure load for the elderly specimens was approximately 50 per cent of those values noted in bovine and young human specimens. Brand *et al.* (2000a) have demonstrated that the bone mineral density of the proximal tibia in humans is significantly less than that of the distal femur. This finding is one of the explanations for the lower fixation strength of tibial versus femoral fixation using interference screws (Brand *et al.* 2000b).

Compared to the influence of gap size and bone mineral density, the fixation properties of interference screw fixation of bone-tendon-bone grafts appears to be less dependent on screw size and length. Using elderly human cadaveric specimens, Brown *et al.* (1993a) found no significant difference in the fixation strength of bone-patellar tendon-bone grafts fixed in the distal femur using endoscopically inserted 7 mm screws and 9 mm screws inserted using a rear-entry technique. Hulstyn *et al.* (1993) using a bovine femur-bone-patellar tendon bone-tibia model found no significant difference in fixation strength between 7 and 9 mm screws. These authors also found no significant difference in fixation strength between 7 × 20 mm and 7 × 30 mm screws, and 9 × 20 mm and 9 × 30 mm screws. Screw diameter and length had no significant effect on graft stiffness. The most common site of fixation failure was on the tibial side. However,

Kohn and Rose (1994) using human cadaveric knees (mean age, 30 years), reported that both femoral and tibial fixation using 9 mm screws was stronger compared to 7 mm screws. They recommended against the use of 7 mm screws for tibial fixation. Gerich *et al.* (1997) demonstrated superior tibial fixation strength comparing 9 $\times$ 30 mm screws with 9 $\times$ 20 mm, and 7 $\times$ 30 mm screws.

Divergence of the interference screw from the bone block and the axis of the bone tunnel can occur with both rear-entry and endo-scopic techniques. The incidence of screw divergence appears to be more common with endoscopic ACL reconstruction (Lemos *et al.* 1993); this phenomenon occurs more frequently during femoral bone plug fixation (Dworsky *et al.* 1996). Based on clinical studies, screw divergence $<30°$ does not seem to have a significant effect on the clinical outcome (Dworsky *et al.* 1996). Using a porcine experi-mental model, Jomha *et al.* (1993) reported no significant difference in femoral fixation strength with endoscopically inserted screws with screw divergence up to 10°. However, there was a significant drop in femoral fixation strength with screw divergence = 20°. Pierz *et al.* (1995) using porcine tibias demonstrated that interference screws inserted to simulate a rear-entry femoral fixation technique or tibial bone block fixation resulted in a significant decrease in fixation strength from 0° to 15° and 15° to 30° of divergence. Interference screws inserted to simulate an endoscopic technique resulted in a significant decrease in fixation strength only at 30° of divergence. These authors concluded that optimal interference screw fixation occurs when the screw is placed parallel to the bone block and bone tunnel. However, minor degrees of divergence from parallel will affect the fixation strength of femoral screws inserted through a rear-entry technique and tibial fixation screws compared to femoral screws inserted using an endoscopic technique.

Although metal interference screws are commonly used, they do possess certain disadvantages. Metal interference screws can distort MRI images, potentially injure the graft during insertion, or com-plicate revision ACL surgery. Bioabsorbable interference screws have been proposed as a method to eliminate these potential com-plications (Barber *et al.* 1995). Several biomechanical studies have compared the initial fixation strength of bioabsorbable interference screws and conventional metal interference screws in animal and human cadaveric models (Abate *et al.* 1998; Caborn *et al.* 1997; Walton 1999; Weiler *et al.* 1998). In general these biomechanical studies have shown that most bioabsorbable screws provide similar fixation strength and stiffness to a conventional metal interference screw. However, Pena *et al.* (1996) using middle age (mean age 42 years) human cadaveric knees reported lower fixation strengths for first and second-generation bioabsorbable screws compared to metal screws. There have been no significant differences in the clin-ical results of bioabsorbable versus metal screws (Barber *et al.* 1995; Marti *et al.* 1997). Concerns with bioabsorbable interference screws have focused largely on the issues of screw breakage (Barber *et al.* 1995; Johnson 1998), and biocompatibility (Weiler *et al.* 2000). Screw breakage has largely been addressed by designing screws and screw drivers that allow the insertion torque to be distributed along the entire length of the screw, and decreasing the insertion torque by notching the tunnel or using a tap.

Foreign body reactions have been reported with the use of highly crystalline polyglycolide polymers (Böstman 1992; Bucholz *et al.* 1994; Casteleyn *et al.* 1992; Weiler *et al.* 1996, 2000). Other materials such as polylactide and its copolymers and stereocopolymers have been reported to have better biocompatibility (Bucholz *et al.* 1994; Casteleyn *et al.* 1992; Weiler *et al.* 1996, 2000). However, Martinek and Friederich (1999) have reported a case of tibial and pretibial cyst formation 8 months following an ACL reconstruction using a bone-patellar tendon-bone autograft in which the tibial bone block was fixed with a 6 × 23 mm bioabsorbable interference screw made of poly-D,L-lactide. To my knowledge, such reactions have not been reported with titanium interference screws. Further long-term clinical studies are needed to prove the safety and biocompatibility of bioabsorbable interference screws.

At the present time, most ACL reconstructions are performed using an endoscopic technique which eliminates the need for a lateral thigh incision thus improving cosmesis; it also decreases postoperative pain and quadriceps muscle weakness. However, when the endoscopic technique is used to perform an ACL reconstruction with a bone-tendon-bone graft, potential circumstances can arise in which the distal bone block protrudes out of the tibial tunnel. This occurrence precludes the use of interference screw fixation on the tibial side. In these situations, alternative tibia fixation techniques such as staples or suture/post fixation must be utilized. This graft-tunnel mismatch most commonly occurs when the patellar tendon graft is 'too long' for the drilled tibial length. This situation is most commonly encountered when the total length of the bone-patellar tendon-bone graft is >105 mm, or when a bone-patellar tendon-bone allograft which has been harvested from a tall person is used. Staple fixation of the protruding bone block into a bone trough has been shown to provide satisfactory initial fixation (Gerich *et al.* 1997). However, the staples are often prominent resulting in local irritation and the need for hardware removal. Graft-tunnel mismatch can be eliminated in some cases by drilling a steeper or longer tibial tunnel. However, a too steep tibial tunnel may not allow transtibial drilling of an anatomic femoral tunnel to be performed.

Another potential problem associated with the endoscopic technique which also precludes interference screw fixation is a 'blow-out' of the posterior wall of the femoral tunnel. Converting to a two-incision rear-entry technique is the most common method of dealing with this occurrence. An alternative endoscopic femoral fixation method which can eliminate graft-tunnel mismatch is the

EndoButton (Brown and Steiner 1994; Lyons and Graf 1998). The EndoButton technique allows the surgeon to safely recess the femoral bone block up into the femoral tunnel, thus shortening the amount of graft to be contained in the tibial tunnel. Since secure fixation with the EndoButton technique relies on the implant anchoring on the femoral cortex, EndoButton fixation can be utilized in situations where a blow-out of the posterior femoral cortex occurs and interference screw fixation is precluded. Brown *et al.* (1996a) have demonstrated that the fixation strength of the femur-patellar tendon graft-tibia complex using a EndoButton femoral fixation technique in elderly cadaveric knees compares favorably with interference screw fixation. Limitations of the EndoButton technique are related to the stiffness of the connecting sutures, and knot slippage.

Guidelines and recommendations for fixation of patellar tendon grafts

Two-incision technique

Femoral fixation: 8 or 9 mm diameter metal screws, length 20–25 mm. Bioabsorbable screws can be used; however, the higher insertion torque generated by the insertion of the screw against the hard cortex of distal femur may result in a higher incidence of screw breakage compared to bioabsorbable screws inserted using an endoscopic technique. If the gap between the bone block and bone tunnel is greater than 4 mm, suture post fixation or plastic buttons should be utilized.

Tibial fixation: avoid use of 7 mm screws. Use 8 or 9 mm screws, length 20–25 mm. For gap sizes >4 mm consider suture/post or button fixation. In soft bone or situations where low insertion torque is encountered consider backing up the interference screw fixation by tying sutures around a fixation post.

Endoscopic technique

Femoral fixation: 7 or 8 mm diameter metal or bioabsorbable screws, length 20–25 mm. For bioabsorbable screws review and use manufacturer's suggestions regarding tapping or notching the bone tunnel to minimize the risk of screw breakage. EndoButton is used in the case of long grafts to avoid graft-tunnel mismatch, and blow-out of the posterior wall.

Tibial fixation: 8 or 9 mm metal or bioabsorbable screws, length 20–25 mm. Use bone trough and staples or suture/post fixation for graft-tunnel mismatch.

Hamstring tendon grafts

Due to the reported lower donor site morbidity, the use of multiple stranded hamstring tendon grafts for ACL reconstruction has increased rapidly in the last few years (Brown *et al.* 1993b). Concerns about the use of hamstring tendon grafts for ACL reconstruction have focused largely on the issues of: (1) initial graft strength; (2) initial graft fixation strength; (3) the biology of soft-tissue-to-bone healing; and (4) radiographic tunnel enlargement. In order to more closely approximate the tensile properties of the young human ACL (Woo *et al.* 1991), multiple stranded hamstring tendon grafts are currently recommended (Brown *et al.* 1993b). Hamner *et al.* (1999) have demonstrated that the initial failure load and stiffness of equally tensioned doubled semitendinosus and gracilis hamstring tendon grafts is additive, and is greater than that of 10 mm central-third patellar tendon grafts (Noyes *et al.* 1984; Cooper *et al.* 1993; Muellner *et al.* 1998), and the young human ACL (Woo *et al.* 1991). It is important to note in this laboratory biomechanical study, that when there was no attempt to maintain equal tension in all four graft limbs, the tensile properties of the doubled gracilis and semitendinosus graft construct was not significantly different from that of a doubled semitendinosus graft (Figure 3.1). Equally tensioning in this study was achieved by looping the axilla of the folded grafts around a post which allowed the tendons to slide, and applying equal weight to the sutures on the free ends of the graft.

The optimal fixation method for hamstring tendon grafts remains controversial. Steiner *et al.* (1994) assessed the tensile properties of hamstring and patellar tendon fixation techniques in elderly human cadaveric knees. This study demonstrated that the initial failure load of some hamstring fixation techniques was higher than those reported for patellar tendon grafts fixed with interference screws. However, the stiffness of the hamstring fixation techniques was lower and the displacement to failure significantly longer compared to

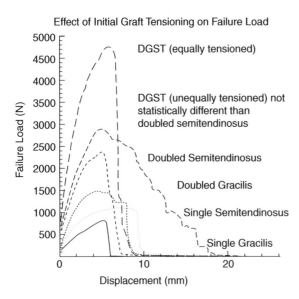

Fig. 3.1
Load-elongation curves for paired human hamstring tendon grafts. The load-elongation curves demonstrate that doubling a single strand gracilis or semitendinosus tendon graft doubles the failure load and stiffness. The failure load of equally tensioned combined double gracilis and semitendinosus tendons (DGST) is equal to the failure load of a doubled semitendinosus tendon graft plus the failure load of a doubled gracilis tendon graft. However, when no attempt is made to equally tension all four strands of a DGST graft, the failure load and stiffness are not significantly different from that of a doubled semitendinosus tendon graft. All strands of a four-strand hamstring tendon graft must be under equal tension for the composite to have its optimal strength and stiffness.

Fig. 3.2
Commonly used hamstring tendon graft femoral fixation techniques

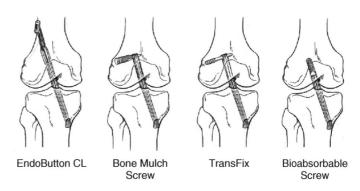

EndoButton CL   Bone Mulch Screw   TransFix   Bioabsorbable Screw

patellar tendon grafts fixed with interference screws. The hamstring fixation techniques in this study utilized AO ligament washers and suture/post fixation and required a two-incision technique.

In 2004, the most commonly used femoral fixation methods for hamstring tendon grafts include:

1 EndoButton CL
2 Cross-pins
3 Bioabsorbable interference screws (Figure 3.2).

These current graft fixation techniques allow hamstring tendon ACL reconstructions to be performed utilizing an endoscopic technique. Of these fixation techniques, only the EndoButton CL and cross-pin techniques where the cross-pin is inserted through the loop of all graft limbs will allow the tendons to slide, and potentially allow equal tension to be applied to all strands of the graft. Interference screw fixation or techniques which involve suturing the limbs of the graft together prior to tensioning and femoral fixation do not allow the graft limbs to slide, and therefore are unlikely to allow for the possibility of equally tensioning all grafts limbs. Based on the biomechanical study of Hamner *et al.* (1999), such fixation techniques will not maximize the initial tensile properties of four-strand hamstring tendon grafts, and will result in a graft construct whose initial tensile properties are not significantly different from that of a doubled semitendinosus graft.

Höher *et al.* (1998, 1999) have suggested that hamstring fixation techniques that fix the graft closer to the anatomic attachment sites of the normal ACL (aperture fixation) are preferable, and will result in less longitudinal motion of the ACL graft in the bone tunnel under cyclic loading conditions (bungee-effect) compared to fixation techniques which fix the graft away from the normal anatomic attachment sites (suspensory fixation). It has been proposed that aperture fixation increases the stiffness of the graft fixation-bone complex by shortening the length of the ACL graft between the graft fixation sites. This concept is based on the biomechanical study of Ishibashi *et al.* (1997) which showed improvement in anterior tibial translation and internal tibial rotation of the femur-bone-patellar tendon-tibia complex when the site of tibial fixation was located in a more proximal versus distal location.

However, To *et al.* (1999) have suggested that the results of the Ishibashi *et al.* (1997) study may have resulted from using tibial fixation methods which may have had different stiffness. They postulated that the difference in knee kinematics and *in situ* graft forces was caused by using staple fixation for the distal fixation method, which has less stiffness than interference screws which were used for the proximal fixation method. Using a springs-in-series analysis, they demonstrated that the stiffness of the graft fixation-bone complex is influenced more by the stiffness of the graft fixation method than the length of the ACL graft. They recommended that the best way to increase the stiffness of the graft fixation-bone complex is to increase the stiffness of the ACL graft fixation methods rather than shortening the length of the ACL graft. Based on this analysis, aperture fixation methods would not seem to offer any mechanical advantage over suspensory fixation methods that have similar stiffness.

Longitudinal motion of the hamstring tendon graft along the axis of the bone tunnel under cyclic loading conditions has been proposed as one of the main mechanisms responsible for radiographic tunnel enlargement (Höher *et al.* 1998). Radiographic tunnel enlargement has been reported to be more common following the use of hamstring tendon autografts compared to patellar tendon autografts (L'Insalata *et al.* 1997; Clatworthy *et al.* 1999; Webster *et al.* 2001). It has been hypothesized that graft-tunnel motion along the axis of the bone tunnel may impair biological incorporation of the hamstring tendon graft into the bone tunnels causing subsequent bone tunnel enlargement (Höher *et al.* 1998). The higher incidence of bone tunnel enlargement following hamstring tendon ACL reconstructions is thought to reflect the longer time required for soft tissue-to-bone healing, and the lower stiffness of hamstring fixation techniques.

Short term clinical studies by Clatworthy *et al.* (1999), Jansson *et al.* (1999), Nebelung *et al.* (1998), and Webster *et al.* (2001) have shown no correlation of tunnel enlargement with KT-1000 values or clinical outcome. However, the long term clinical significance of radiographic tunnel enlargement remains unknown. Tunnel enlargement may complicate revision ACL surgery because of the need to bone graft the enlarged bone tunnels as the first stage of a two stage procedure.

Brown *et al.* (1999) have compared the initial tensile properties, slippage, and graft-tunnel motion under cyclic loading from 50–250 N with the load applied parallel to the axis of the femoral bone tunnel of some commonly performed femoral ACL hamstring tendon graft fixation techniques. This experimental model used middle-aged human cadaveric knees (mean age = 46 years), and doubled gracilis and semitendinosus tendon grafts sized to the nearest 0.5 mm. In this study the EndoButton CL (1345 ± 179 N), and cross-pin fixation with the Bone Mulch Screw (977 ± 238 N) and

TransFix (934 w ± 296 N) were the strongest hamstring femoral fixation techniques. Although the mean failure load (562 ± 69 N) of hamstring tendon grafts fixed with 8 × 23 mm bioabsorbable screws exceeded the estimated loads experienced by the ACL during the early postoperative period, 4 of 11 (36 per cent) of the hamstring tendon grafts fixed with bioabsorbable screws failed before reaching 1000 cycles. There were no failures under cycling loading when the hamstring tendon grafts were fixed using an EndoButton CL or cross-pins. Hamstring tendon grafts fixed with bioabsorbable screws resulted in twice the amount of slippage compared to grafts fixed with the EndoButton CL and cross-pin techniques. Weiler *et al.* (2001) have recently shown that the fixation strength, stiffness, and slippage under cyclic loading of hamstring tendon grafts fixed with bioabsorbable interference screws can be improved by the addition of the EndoPearl device.

The stiffest hamstring fixation techniques resulted when the hamstring tendon grafts were fixed with bioabsorbable screws and cross-pins. We found no significant difference in the stiffness of 10 mm patellar tendon grafts fixed with 7 × 25 mm metal interference screws and hamstring tendon grafts fixed with bioabsorbable screws and the two cross-pin techniques. Unpublished work from our laboratory has demonstrated that the stiffness of the femur-EndoButton CL-hamstring tendon complex is dependent on the length of the connecting loop. The stiffness for the 20 mm continuous loop was 179 N/mm and dropped to 118 N/mm when a 35 mm loop was used. The length of the femoral tunnel and therefore the continuous loop length are dependent on the external position of the tibial tunnel and the flexion angle of the knee when drilling the femoral guide pin (Brown and Sklar 1999). With proper surgical technique it is usually possible to obtain continuous loop lengths of 15–20 mm.

There was no significant difference in graft-tunnel motion between the various hamstring fixation techniques, or between the various hamstring fixation techniques and patellar tendon grafts fixed with metal interference screws. Suspensory fixation of hamstring tendon grafts using cross-pins and aperture fixation with bioabsorbable interference screws which had similar stiffness in our study resulted in identical amounts of graft tunnel motion. Our data supports the hypothesis of To *et al.* (1999), that the mechanical behavior of the graft fixation-bone complex is influenced more by the stiffness of the graft fixation method rather than the length of the ACL graft. Although it has been suggested that aperture fixation of hamstring tendon grafts with bioabsorbable screws may decrease tunnel enlargement, Höher *et al.* (1998) and Clatworthy (2001) has demonstrated that tunnel enlargement cannot be decreased by:

1 avoiding the use of suspensory fixation techniques
2 using a stiffer fixation construct
3 or fixing the graft closer to the joint line.

These findings suggest that biomechanical factors are not the primary etiology of tunnel enlargement, and that biological causes probably play a significant role.

Tibial fixation is the weaker fixation site for both patellar tendon and hamstring tendon grafts (Hulstyn *et al.* 1993; Steiner *et al.* 1994). Tibial fixation is weaker primarily because of the lower bone mineral density of the proximal tibia compared to the distal femur (Brand *et al.* 2000a), and also due to the fact that the line of applied force to the ligament grafts and graft fixation sites is parallel to the axis of the tibial tunnel. Brand *et al.* (2000a) have shown that the fixation strength of four-strand hamstring tendon grafts fixed with bioabsorbable interference screws is directly related to local bone mineral density. Commonly used tibial fixation methods for hamstring tendon grafts include:

1 Staples
2 Ligament washers
3 Suture/post
4 Bioabsorbable interference screws
5 IntraFix Tibial Anchor
6 WasherLoc
7 Rapid-Fix (Figure 3.3).

Due to their ease of insertion and low profile eliminating the need for hardware removal, bioabsorbable interference screws have become an increasingly popular method of tibial fixation for hamstring tendon grafts. However, of the currently available hamstring tendon tibial fixation techniques, interference screw fixation is most dependent on bone quality, and precise sizing of the tendon graft diameter to the bone tunnel size (Brand *et al.* 2000a, b; Steenlage *et al.* 1999).

Unpublished data from our lab for hamstring tendon grafts fixed with 9 × 23 mm bioabsorbable screws in human cadaveric knees

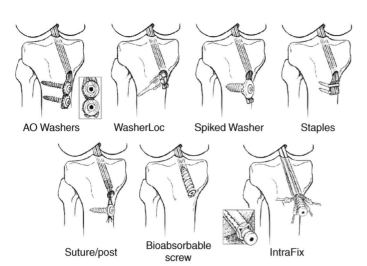

AO Washers   WasherLoc   Spiked Washer   Staples

Suture/post   Bioabsorbable screw   IntraFix

Fig. 3.3
Commonly used hamstring tendon graft tibial fixation techniques. Adapted from Operative Techniques in Sports Medicine, 7, 4, 199. WS Saunders.

(mean age = 48 years) cyclically loaded from 50–250 N demonstrated a mean failure load of 527 N, stiffness of 290 N/mm. However, 31 per cent of the hamstring tendon grafts fixed with bioabsorbable screws failed before completing 1000 cycles. The strongest tibial fixation methods resulted when the hamstring tendon grafts were fixed using two AO ligaments washers in a figure-of-eight fashion, the WasherLoc, and the IntraFix tibial anchor. The stiffest tibial fixation methods resulted when the hamstring tendon grafts were fixed with two AO spiked ligament washers, 9 mm bioabsorbable screws, and the WasherLoc.

Magen *et al.* (1999) compared the tensile properties of six tibial fixation methods in porcine tibias and human tibias from donors with a mean age of 35 years. The strongest and stiffest tibial fixation methods in human bone resulted when the gracilis and semitendinosus tendons were long enough to be secured under two AO spiked ligament washers or fixed with the WasherLoc. Tibial fixation using interference screws in human bone performed significantly worse compared to animal bone. The authors suggested that a higher yield load and less slippage could be achieved by using fixation methods that anchored in cortical bone more distally in the tibial tunnel or on the tibial cortex rather than the less cancellous bone inside the tibial tunnel with an interference screw.

Recommendations for hamstring tendon graft fixation

Femoral fixation

At the present time, cross-pin fixation techniques are the stiffest fixation method, and the EndoButton CL the strongest. The stiffness of the femur-EndoButton CL-hamstring tendon graft complex is dependent on the length of the EndoButton CL. Stiffness of the EndoButton CL technique can be maximized by keeping the length of the continuous loop as short as possible or by adding supplemental interference screw fixation. The stiffness of the hybrid EndoButton CL + interference screw fixation method is dictated by the stiffness of interference screw fixation (255 N/mm) and is independent of the length of the EndoButton CL loop. Hamstring tendons fixed with cross-pins and the EndoButton CL result in the least amount of slippage. Although bioabsorbable screw fixation (aperture fixation) has become a popular fixation technique, Brown *et al.* (1999) have demonstrated a high failure rate under cyclic loading and almost twice the amount of slippage compared to cross-pin techniques or the EndoButton CL. The cyclic properties of interference screw fixation of hamstring tendon grafts can be improved by using the EndoPearl (Weiler *et al.* 2001). At the present time, the EndoButton CL or cross-pin techniques (Bone Mulch Screw and TransFix) appear to be the most reliable and predictable femoral fixation techniques for hamstring tendon ACL grafts. These two femoral fixation techniques are also currently the only ones which allow for the possibility of equal tensioning of all grafts limbs.

Tibial fixation

Unpublished data from our lab using a cyclic testing protocol demonstrated that tibial fixation with bioabsorbable screw is stiff, but weaker than fixation with spiked ligament washers, suture/post, the WasherLoc, or the IntraFix. In our testing, bioabsorbable screws had a high failure rate under cyclic loading. Based on the high failure rate under cyclic loading that we experienced, strong consideration should be given to backing up bioabsorbable screw fixation when the insertion torque is low or when used in soft bone. Suture/post fixation is reliable (no cyclic failures) but has lower stiffness. AO spiked ligament washers are strong, stiff, but prominent, and require a longer graft to insure that all limbs of the graft are fixed under both washers. The IntraFix is low profile, strong, stiff, and reliable (no cyclic failures in our testing), but requires good bone quality. The WasherLoc is strong and stiff, but requires coring out of the anterior tibial cortex. At the present time, tibial fixation with two AO ligament washers, the WasherLoc, and the IntraFix tibial anchor appear to be the strongest, stiffest, most reliable tibial fixation methods.

General conclusions

Although differences in specimen type and age, and biomechanical testing protocols make it difficult to compare the results of one fixation study with another, it is possible to arrive at some general conclusions regarding ACL graft fixation:

1 All present methods of ACL graft fixation are significantly weaker and less stiff than ACL replacement grafts.
2 The tibial fixation site is the weakest link.
3 The primary parameters which govern the fixation strength of interference screws are: bone quality, the gap between the bone tunnel and bone block, screw diameter and length, and screw divergence.
4 Interference screw fixation using metal or bioabsorbable interference screws appears to be the optimal method at the present time for fixation of bone-patellar tendon-bone grafts.
5 There is little consensus on the optimal fixation method for hamstring tendon grafts.
6 At the present time, the EndoButton CL and cross-pin techniques appear to be the strongest, stiffest, and most reliable femoral fixation techniques for hamstring tendon grafts.
7 Femoral fixation of hamstring tendon grafts using bioabsorbable interference screws is popular, but slippage remains a problem.

8   Tibial fixation for hamstring tendon grafts remains a challenge.
9   There is no clinical data to support the notion that the tunnel widening phenomena observed following after hamstring ACL reconstruction can be decreased by using interference screws at the tunnel aperture.

References

Abate JA, Fadale PD, Hulstyn MJ, *et al.* (1998). Initial fixation strength of polylactic acid interference screws in anterior cruciate ligament reconstruction. *Arthroscopy*, 14, 278–284.

Aglietti P, Buzzi R, D'Andria S, Zaccherotti G (1992). Arthroscopic anterior cruciate ligament reconstruction with patellar tendon graft. *Arthroscopy*, 8, 510–516.

Aglietti P, Buzzi R, Giron F, Simeone AJ, Zaccherotti G (1997). Arthroscopic-assisted anterior cruciate ligament reconstruction with the central third patellar tendon. A 5–8 year follow-up. *Knee Surg Sports Traumatol Arthros*, 5, 138–149.

Bach BB, Tradonsky S, Bojchuk J, Levy ME, Bush-Joseph CA, Khan NH (1998). Arthroscopically assisted anterior cruciate ligament reconstruction using patella tendon autograft. Five- to nine-year follow-up evaluation. *Am J Sports Med*, 26, 20–29.

Bach BB, Jones GT, Sweet FA, Hager CA (1994). Arthroscopy-assisted anterior cruciate ligament reconstruction using patellar tendon substitution. Two- to four-year follow-up results. *Am J Sports Med*, 22, 758–767.

Barber FA, Elrod BF, McGuire DA, Paulos LE (1995). Preliminary results of an absorbable interference screw. *Arthroscopy*, 11, 537–548.

Böstman OM (1992). Intense granulomatous inflammatory lesions associated with absorbable internal fixation devices made of polyglycolide in ankle fractures. *Clin Ortho*, 278, 193–199.

Brand JC, Pienkowski D, Steenlage E, Hamilton D, Johnson DL, Caborn DNM (2000a). Interference screw fixation of a quadrupled hamstring tendon graft is directly related to bone mineral density and insertion torque. *Arthroscopy*, 28, 705–710.

Brand JC, Weiler A, Caborn DNM, Brown CH, Johnson DL (2000b). Graft fixation in cruciate ligament reconstruction. *Am J Sports Med*, 28, 761–774.

Brown CH, Hecker AT, Hipp JA, Myers ER, Hayes WC (1993a). The biomechanics of interference screw fixation of patellar tendon anterior cruciate ligament grafts. *Am J Sports Med*, 21, 880–886.

Brown CH, Steiner ME, Carson EW (1993b). The use of hamstring tendons for anterior cruciate ligament reconstruction: technique and results. *Clin Sports Med*, 12, 723–756.

Brown CH, Steiner ME (1994). Anterior cruciate ligament injuries. In J Siliski (ed.) *Traumatic Disorders of the Knee*, pp. 247–253. Springer-Verlag: New York.

Brown CH, Sklar JH, Hecker AT, Hayes WC (1996a). Biomechanics of endoscopic anterior cruciate ligament graft fixation. Presented at the second World Congress on Sports Trauma/American Orthopaedic Society for Sports Medicine 22nd Annual Meeting, Buena Vista, FL.

Brown CH, Sklar JH (1999). Endoscopic anterior cruciate ligament reconstruction using doubled gracilis and semitendinosus tendons and endobutton femoral fixation. *Oper Tech Sports Med*, 7, 201–213.

Brown CH, Wilson DR, Hecker AT, Ferragamo M (1999). Comparison of hamstring and patellar tendon femoral fixation: cyclic load. *Book of*

Abstracts and Outlines, 25th Annual Meeting American Orthopaedic Society for Sports Medicine, Traverse City, MI, pp. 413–414.

Brown GA, Peña F, Grøntvedt T, Labadie D, Engebretsen L (1996b). Fixation strength of interference screw fixation in bovine, young human, and elderly human cadaver knee: influence of insertion torque, tunnel-bone block gap, and interference. *Knee Surg Sports Tramatol Arthrosc*, 3, 238–249.

Bucholz RW, Henry S, Henley MB (1994). Fixation with bioabsorbable screws for the treatment of fractures of the ankle. *J Bone Joint Surg*, 76A, 319–324.

Buss DD, Warren RF, Wickiecwicz TL, Galinat BJ, Panariello R (1993). Arthroscopically assisted reconstruction of the anterior cruciate ligament with the use of autogenous patellar-ligament grafts. *J Bone Joint Surg*, 75A, 1346–1355.

Butler DL (1987). Evaluation of fixation methods in cruciate ligament reconstruction. *Instr Course Lect*, 23, 173–183.

Butler JC, Branch TP, Hutton WC (1994). Optimal graft fixation – the effect of gap size and screw size on bone plug fixation in ACL reconstruction. *Arthroscopy*, 10, 524–529.

Caborn DNM, Urban WP, Johnson DL *et al.* (1997). Biomechanical comparison between bioscrew and titanium alloy interference screws for bone-patellar tendon-bone graft fixation in anterior cruciate ligament reconstruction. *Arthroscopy*, 13, 229–232.

Casteleyn PP, Handelberg F, Haentjens P (1992). Biodegradable rods versus kirschner wire fixation of wrist fractures. A randomized study. *J Bone Joint Surg*, 74B, 858–861.

Cassim A, Lobenhoffer P, Gerich T, Tscherne H (1993). The fixation strength of the interference screw in anterior cruciate ligament replacement as a function of technique and experimental setup. *Trans Ortho Res Soc*, 18, 31.

Clatworthy MG, Annear P, Bulow JU, Bartlett RJ (1999). Tunnel widening in anterior cruciate ligament reconstruction: a prospective evaluation of hamstring and patellar grafts. *Knee Surg Sports Traumatol Arthrosc*, 7, 138–145.

Clatworthy MG (2001). Tunnel widening in hamstring ACL reconstruction: a prospective clinical and radiographic evaluation of four different fixation techniques. *American Orthopaedic Society for Sports Medicine Specialty Day*, San Francisco CA, pp. 127.

Cooper DE, Deng XH, Burstein AL, Warren RF (1993). The strength of central third patellar tendon graft. A biomechanical study. *Am J Sports Med*, 21, 818–824.

Dworsky BS, Jewell BF, Bach BR (1996). Interference screw divergence in endoscopic anterior cruciate ligament reconstruction. *Arthroscopy*, 12, 45–49.

Fu FH, Bennett CH, Ma CB, *et al.* (2000). Current trends in anterior cruciate ligament reconstruction. Part II. Operative procedures and clinical correlations. *Am J Sports Med*, 28, 124–130.

Fithian DC, Daniel DM, Casanave A (1992). Fixation in knee ligament repair and reconstruction. *Oper Tech Ortho*, 2, 63–70.

Gerich TG, Cassim A, Lattermann C, Lobenhoffer HP (1997). Pullout strength of tibial graft fixation in anterior cruciate ligament replacement with patellar tendon graft: interference screw versus staple fixation in human knees. *Knee Surg Traumatol Arthrosc*, 5, 84–88.

Hamner DL, Brown CH, Steiner ME, Hecker AT, Hayes WC (1999). Hamstring tendon grafts for reconstruction of the anterior cruciate ligament: biomechanical evaluation of the use of multiple strands and tensioning techniques. *J Bone Joint Surg*, 81A, 549–552.

Höher J, Möller HD, Fu FH (1998). Bone tunnel enlargement after anterior cruciate ligament reconstruction: fact or fiction? *Knee Surg Sports Traumatol Arthrosc*, 6, 231–240.

Höher J, Livesay GA, Ma CB, Withrow JD, Fu FH, Woo SL-Y (1999). Hamstring graft motion in the femoral bone tunnel when using titanium button/polyester tape fixation. *Knee Surg Sports Traumatol Arthrosc*, 7, 215–219.

Howell SM, Hull ML (1998). Aggressive rehabilitation using hamstring tendons. Graft construct, tibial tunnel placement, fixation properties, and clinical outcome. *Am J Knee Surg*, 11, 120–127.

Hulstyn M, Fadale PD, Abate J, Walsh WR (1993). Biomechanical evaluation of interference screw fixation in a bovine patellar bone-tendon-bone autograft complex for anterior cruciate ligament reconstruction. *Arthroscopy*, 9, 417–424.

Holden JP, Grood ES, Butler *et al.* (1988). Biomechanics of fascia lata ligament replacement: early postoperative changes in the goat. *J Ortho Res*, 6, 639–647.

Ishibashi Y, Rudy TW, Livesay GA, Stone JD, Fu FH, Woo SL-Y (1997). The effect of anterior cruciate ligament graft fixation site at the tibia on knee stability: evaluation using a robotic testing system. *Arthroscopy*, 13, 177–182.

Jansson KA, Harilainen A, Sandelin J, Karjalainen PT, Aronen HJ, Tallroth K (1999). Bone tunnel enlargement after anterior cruciate ligament reconstruction with the hamstring autograft and endo-button fixation technique. *Knee Surg Sports Traumatol Arthrosc*, 7, 290–295.

Johnson DP (1998). Operative complications from the use of biodegradable Kurosaka screw. *J Bone Joint Surg*, 80B(Supp 1), 103.

Jomha NM, Raso J, Leung P (1993). Effect of varying angles on the pull-out strength of interference screw fixation. *Arthroscopy*, 9, 580–583.

Kartus J, Stener S, Lindahl S, *et al.* (1997). Factors affecting donor-site morbidity after anterior cruciate ligament reconstruction using bone-patellar tendon-bone autografts. *Knee Surg Sports Traumatol Arthrosc*, 5, 222–228.

Kartus J, Magnusson L, Stener S, Brandson S, *et al.* (1999). Complications following arthroscopic anterior cruciate ligament reconstruction. A 2–5 year follow-up of 604 patients with special emphasis on anterior knee pain. *Knee Surg Sports Traumatol Arthrosc*, 7, 2–8.

Kartus J, Movin T, Karlsson J (2001). Donor-site morbidity and anterior knee problems after anterior cruciate ligament reconstruction using autografts. *Arthroscopy*, 17, 971–980.

Kohn D, Rose C (1994). Primary stability of interference screw fixation: influence of screw diameter and insertion torque. *Am J Sports Med*, 22, 334–338.

Kurosaka M, Yoshiya S, Andrish JT (1987). A biomechanical comparison of different surgical techniques of graft fixation in anterior cruciate ligament reconstruction. *Am J Sports Med*, 15, 225–229.

Lemos MJ, Albert J, Simon T, Jackson DW (1993). Radiographic analysis of femoral interference screw placement during ACL reconstruction: endoscopic versus open technique. *Arthroscopy*, 9, 154–158.

L'Insalata JC, Klatt B, Fu FH, Harner CD (1997). Tunnel expansion following anterior cruciate ligament reconstruction: a comparison of hamstring and patellar tendon autografts. *Knee Surg Sports Traumatol Arthrosc*, 5, 234–238.

Lyons PM, Graf BK (1998). Pearls and pitfalls of EndoButton fixation. *Tech Ortho*, 13, 299–305.

Magen HE, Howell SM, Hull ML (1999). Structural properties of six tibial fixation methods for anterior cruciate ligament soft tissue grafts. *Am J Sports Med*, 27, 35–43.

Marti C, Imhoff AB, Bahrs C, *et al.* (1997). Metallic versus bioabsorbable interference screw for fixation of bone-patellar tendon-bone autograft in arthroscopic anterior cruciate ligament reconstruction. A preliminary report. *Knee Surg Sports Traumatol Arthrosc*, 5, 225–226.

Martinek V, Friederich NF (1999). Case report. Tibial and pretibial cyst formation after anterior cruciate ligament reconstruction with bioabsorbable interference screw fixation. *Arthroscopy*, 15, 317–320.

Morrison JB (1968). Bioengineering analysis of force actions transmitted by the knee joint. *Biomed Eng(April)*, 164.

Morrisson JB (1969). Function of the knee joint in various activities. *Biomed Eng*, 4, 573–580.

Morrisson JB (1970). The mechanics of the knee joint in relation to normal walking. *J Biomech*, 3, 51–61.

Muellner T, Reihsner T, Mrkonjic W, *et al.* (1998). Twisting of patellar tendon grafts does not reduce their mechanical properties. *J Biomech*, 31, 311–315.

Nebelung W, Becker R, Merkel M, Ropke M (1998). Bone tunnel enlargement after anterior cruciate ligament reconstruction with semitendinosus tendon using EndoButton fixation on the femoral side. *Arthroscopy*, 14, 810–815.

Noyes FR, Butler DL, Grood ES, Zernicke RF, Hefzy MS (1984). Biomechanical analysis of human ligament grafts used in knee-ligament repairs and reconstructions. *J Bone Joint Surg*, 66A, 344–352.

Peña F, Grøntvedt T, Brown GA, Aune AK, Engebretsen L (1996). Comparison of failure strength between metallic and absorbable interference screws. Influence of insertion torque, tunnel-bone block gap, bone mineral density, and interference. *Am J Sports Med*, 24, 329–334.

Pierz K, Baltz M, Fulkerson J (1995). The effect of Kurosaka screw divergence on the holding strength of bone-tendon-bone graft. *Am J Sports Med*, 23, 332–335.

Reznik AM, Davis JL, Daniel DM (1990). Optimizing interference fixation for cruciate ligament reconstruction. *Trans Ortho Res Soc*, 15, 519.

Rodeo SA, Arnoczky SP, Torzilli PA, Hidaka C, Warren RF (1993). A biomechanical and histological study in the dog. *J Bone Joint Surg*, 75A, 1795–1803.

Shelbourne KD, Nitz P (1990). Accelerated rehabilitation after anterior cruciate ligament reconstruction. *Am J Sports Med*, 18, 292–299.

Shelbourne KD, Gray T (1997). Anterior cruciate ligament reconstruction with autogenous patellar tendon graft followed by accelerated rehabilitation. A two- to nine-year follow-up. *Am J Sports Med*, 25, 786–795.

Steenlage E, Brand JC, Caborn D, *et al.* (1999). Interference screw fixation of a quadrupled hamstring graft is improved with precise match of tunnel to graft diameter. *Arthroscopy*, 15, 59.

Steiner ME, Hecker AT, Brown CH, Hayes WC (1994). Anterior cruciate ligament graft fixation: comparison of hamstring and patellar tendon grafts. *Am J Sports Med*, 22, 240–242.

To JT, Howell SM, Hull ML (1999). Contributions of femoral fixation methods to the stiffness of anterior cruciate ligament replacement at implantation. *Arthroscopy*, 15, 379–387.

Walton M (1999). Absorbable and metal interference screws; comparison of graft security during healing. *Arthroscopy*, 15, 818–826.

Webster KE, Feller JA, Hameister KA (2001). Bone tunnel enlargement following anterior cruciate ligament reconstruction: a randomized comparison of hamstring and patellar tendon grafts with 2 years follow-up. *Knee Surg Sports Traumatol Arthrosc*, 9, 86–91.

Weiler A, Helling H-J, Kirch U, *et al.* (1996). Foreign-body reaction and the course of osteolysis after polyglycolide implants for fracture fixation. Experimental study in sheep. *J Bone Joint Surg*, 78B, 369–376.

Weiler A, Windhagen HJ, Raschke MJ, Laumeyer A, Hoffmann RFG (1998). Biodegradable interference screw fixation exhibits pull-out force and stiffness similar to titanium screw. *Am J Sports Med*, 26, 119–128.

Weiler A, Hoffmann RFG, Stähelin AC, Helling HJ, Südkamp NP (2000). Biodegradable implants in sports medicine: the biological base. *Arthroscopy*, 16, 305–321.

Weiler A, Richter CM, Schmidmaier G, Kandziora F, Südkamp NP (2001). The endopearl device increases fixation strength and eliminates construct slippage of hamstring tendon grafts with interference screw fixation. *Arthroscopy*, 17, 353–359.

Weiler A, Hoffmann RFG, Bail JH, Rehm O, Südkamp NP (2002). Tendon healing in a bone tunnel. Part II: histological analysis after biodegradable interference fit fixation in a model of anterior cruciate ligament reconstruction in a sheep. *Arthroscopy*, 18, 124–135.

Woo SL-Y, Hollis JM, Adams DJ, Lyon RM, Takai S (1991). Tensile properties of the human femur-anterior cruciate-ligament tibia complex. The effect of specimen age and orientation. *Am J Sports Med*, 19, 217–225.

4

Bone-tendon-bone autograft ACL reconstruction is the most effective surgical option for restoring anterior knee stability following ACL injury

Scott D. Mair and Darren L. Johnson

The amount of attention given to reconstruction of the anterior cruciate ligament (ACL) in the recent orthopaedic literature has been remarkable. It is estimated that more than 2000 scientific articles, numerous reviews and chapters regarding the ACL have been published (Frank and Jackson 1997). In the early 1980s, ACL reconstruction was generally considered only in young, high-level athletes with demonstrated knee instability that precluded their participation in athletic endeavors. As the benefits of ACL reconstruction in improving functional stability of the knee have been reported, the procedure has become increasingly common. Currently, it is estimated that over 100,000 (ACL) reconstruction procedures are performed annually in the United States alone (Brown and Carson 1999).

Given the tremendous number of performed ACL reconstructions, and the preponderance of recently published literature on this topic, one might expect that it would now be very clear to knee surgeons just how the symptomatic ACL-deficient knee is best treated. Instead, there are few subjects in orthopaedics that produce as much controversy. It seems that as the annual number of ACL reconstructions performed has increased, so too has the number of methods proposed to repair this ligament. Controversy remains regarding patient selection, surgical techniques, graft fixation, and graft selection. Despite all the knowledge gained over the last twenty years, the subject of graft selection elicits the most heated debate in sports medicine circles.

Why does the graft selection controversy persist? In essence, it seems that while numerous graft sources produce good results, no one graft choice is without drawbacks, morbidity or risk. Currently accepted graft options include autogenous cental-third patellar tendon, hamstring tendons (semitendinosus and gracilis), quadriceps tendon, and allografts. Each of these grafts has distinct advantages and disadvantages. In evaluating each graft choice there are many factors, but the primary considerations involve the ability of the graft to restore knee stability, along with the avoidance of donor site morbidity. Given that each patient undergoing ACL reconstruction has different goals and concerns, it is reasonable that the choice of graft should be individualized to the patient. It is the goal of this chapter to outline the reasons that patellar tendon autograft remains the best choice in the majority of patients undergoing ACL reconstruction.

Knee stability – patellar tendon versus hamstrings

The primary goal of ACL reconstruction is to restore stability to the knee. In doing so, it is hoped that patients are able to return to their desired activity level. In numerous articles, as well as the hearts and minds of many knee surgeons, the bone-patellar tendon-bone (BTB) construct is considered the 'gold standard' for ACL reconstruction. One would expect that in order to justify a change to another graft option, the scientific literature would demonstrate that significant improvements in knee stability and functional outcome are associated with the used of other graft materials. However, this has not been the case. It is our contention that grafts sources, other than the BTB autografts, come and go on a cyclical basis. We feel that the BTB graft has withstood the test of time and represents the most logical choice for ACL reconstruction in the majority of symptomatic ACL-deficient patients.

Recently, the most frequent debate involves the comparison of outcomes observed following ACL reconstruction using autograft patellar tendon and hamstring tendon grafts. These two graft sources are the most commonly utilized grafts in the United States. In fact, some recent surveys suggest that hamstrings have become the most commonly performed graft. Recent polls at the annual meetings of the American Orthopaedic Society for Sports Medicine and the Arthoscopy Association of North America have found that up to 60 per cent of surgeons consider hamstrings their first choice of graft for ACL reconstructions (Carson 1999). However, if hamstrings have supplanted patellar tendon from 'gold standard' to silver, it is not because they have been shown to improve knee stability or knee outcome.

Numerous studies comparing results of patellar tendon and hamstring ACL reconstructions have been published. In assessing knee stability, both objective (KT-1000 arthrometry) and subjective measures (knee outcome scores) of treated patients are typically reported. A review of the results of these studies finds that, on the topic of post-reconstruction knee stability, most studies fall into one of two groups – those studies that found no difference between hamstring and patellar tendon reconstructed knees, and those studies that found a trend or statistically proven better stability in the patellar tendon group. We are unable to find a single study that shows any evidence of improved knee stability using hamstrings over patellar tendon grafts for ACL reconstruction.

Several studies have noted an increase in laxity, as documented by instrumented arthrometer testing, in patients undergoing ACL reconstruction with hamstring grafts compared to patellar tendon grafts. A prospective randomized study with mean three year follow-up found manual maximum KT-1000 side-to-side difference of 2.1 + 2.0 mm in patients undergoing reconstruction with patellar tendon (Anderson et al. 2001). In those patients where hamstrings were utilized, KT-1000 values were 3.1 + 2.3 mm, a statistically greater amount of laxity. Several other studies have found an increase in instrumented measures of laxity in hamstring reconstructions as compared to patellar tendon (Feagin et al. 1997; Feller and Webster 2002; Otero and Hutcheson 1993). Increased laxity by clinical exam in hamstring tendon grafts compared to patellar tendon grafts has been described (Otero and Hutcheson 1993). A prospective study found that knee laxity was increased in female ACL-deficient patients who underwent hamstring tendon ACL reconstruction compared to a matched group of patellar reconstructed knees; no difference between hamstring and patellar tendon reconstructions was noted in male patients (Corry et al. 1999). Several other studies have found no significant difference in laxity in comparing these two types of reconstruction.

While stabilization of the knee is the primary reason to perform ACL reconstruction, differences in objective knee laxity would not necessarily be of concern if functional results remained similar between differing ACL graft sources. Several studies have noted the increased likelihood of a return to preinjury activity levels after ACL reconstruction with patellar tendon autograft compared to hamstring tendons. In a prospective study of a group of patients undergoing reconstruction for chronic ACL injury, a return to sports participation was more frequently observed in those patients who underwent patellar tendon reconstruction compared to those who underwent hamstring tendon reconstruction (80 vs. 43 per cent, $P < 0.01$) (Aglietti et al. 1994). In a study analyzing female patients, those who underwent hamstring tendon ACL reconstruction were less likely to return to preinjury activity levels as defined by Tegner scores (Hamstring group: 5.17, Patellar tendon group: 6.59) at a mean two year follow-up interval (Barrett et al. 2002). Another report found that there was a significantly greater return to level I (strenuous) IKDC (International Knee Documentation Committee) sporting activity in patients undergoing patellar tendon reconstruction compared to hamstrings, despite the finding of higher donor-site morbidity in the BTB group (Corry et al. 1999).

Many studies have found no significant differences in overall knee function or return to sports when patellar tendon and hamstring reconstructions are compared. However, in treating high level athletes, a premium is placed upon ability to return to sport and it

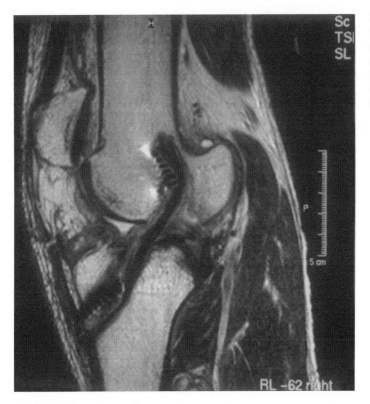

Fig. 4.1

Patellar tendon autograft ACL reconstruction four months after surgery. This MRI performed in the plane of the ACL shows that the graft is incorporating well.

remains clear where the allegiance of the typical sports medicine surgeons lies with regard to graft choice. During the 1998–99 season, a survey of 31 head team physicians in the National Football League was performed. When asked about graft preference for ACL reconstruction, patellar tendon autograft was the overwhelming choice (Bradley *et al.* 2002). This graft was favored by 30 of 31 (97 per cent) physicians in the acute setting, and 29 of 31 (94 per cent) in a chronic situation. Only one physician used hamstring autograft in both settings, and one other chose patellar tendon allograft for the chronically ACL-deficient knee. All other physicians stated that patellar tendon autograft was performed in all cases. When a predictable return to high-demand activities is desired, patellar tendon remains the graft of choice (Figure 4.1).

Graft fixation

One of the primary reasons why bone-patellar tendon-bone ACL reconstructions 'feel' more like the native ACL competent knee is likely related to the ability of the surgeons to achieve bony fixation within a bone tunnel. It has been demonstrated that during the first two months following surgical reconstruction of the ACL, the most common cause of graft failure is loss of graft fixation. As such, the initial graft fixation must be strong enough to withstand *in vivo* forces during the early postoperative period (Frank and Jackson 1997). In addition, fixation should be as close to the joint line as possible, as this enhances the stiffness of the graft construct, and limits the length of graft which may elongate during the early rehabilitation period. At comparable loads, a longer graft undergoes more overall strain (Frank and Jackson 1997). In a porcine ACL reconstruction model, graft fixation that was distant to the joint line resulted in significantly more anterior knee laxity compared to graft fixation that was placed near the joint line (Ishibashi *et al.* 1997). A biomechanical comparison of cadaveric patellar tendon and hamstring tendons found that more anatomic reconstruction techniques provided significantly higher structural properties, and smaller losses of fixation compared with extracortical fixation for both types of grafts (Scheffler *et al.* 2002).

The bone-patellar tendon-bone ACL graft allows for strong (greater than 450 N) bone to bone fixation with interference screws, placed near the articular surface (Figure 4.2). While numerous new techniques have been developed for fixation of soft tissue grafts, no single technique fulfills both of those criteria, particularly on the tibial side. On the femoral side, techniques that employ the use of cross-pin fixation provide strong fixation of hamstring grafts near the joint line. However, on the tibia, soft tissue fixation is more of a problem. Interference screws that are designed to be used with soft tissue grafts do facilitate achieving graft fixation near the articular surface, but soft tissue grafts that are fixed in this manner may still slip

Fig. 4.2
Bone-tendon-bone ACL reconstruction allows for rigid fixation with interference screws.

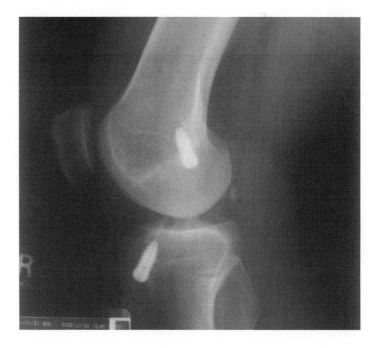

despite the use of an appropriately sized interference screw (Scheffler *et al.* 2002). Other tibial fixation techniques, such as staples or screw and washer constructs, remain distant from the articular surface, and increase the likelihood of the application of excessive strain loads to the graft during the postoperative period.

Tunnel expansion

Gradual expansion of tunnels over time can occur with all types of grafts (Fu *et al.* 1999). The clinical significance of this finding is unknown, and no studies have shown a direct correlation between tunnel expansion and knee laxity. Concerns exist as to whether this bone resorption negatively affects clinical outcome over the long-term. Futhermore, if bone tunnel expansion occurs and a patient has a recurrence of symptomatic knee instability, these expanded tunnels may further complicate achieving a successful revision ACL reconstruction. Staged revision reconstruction may be necessary to correct bony loss, thus further exposing affected patients to repeated surgical risks.

Several studies have found an increased degree of tunnel expansion following ACL reconstruction using hamstring autografts compared to patellar tendon autografts (Clatworthy *et al.* 1999; L'Insalata *et al.* 1997; Webster *et al.* 2001). Significant differences in tunnel expansion have been observed between these two types of grafts on both the femoral and tibial side. It has been hypothesized that tunnel expansion may be increased when fixation of the graft is distant to the joint line, as this configuration allows for more motion of the graft in the sagittal plane during knee motion (L'Insalata *et al.* 1997). With repeated cycling of the knee, it is possible that the described graft motion may lead to the bone tunnel expansion with many soft tissue grafts. However, one study has compared tunnel enlargement in hamstring and patellar tendon grafts; in this study, patients were followed for a minimum of two years and an Endobutton (distant) fixation was utilized in both groups (Webster *et al.* 2001). A significantly greater increase in femoral tunnel width was found in the hamstring group compared to the patellar tendon group. Thus, increased tunnel expansion in knees undergoing hamstring ACL reconstruction may not be entirely related to fixation issues. Tunnel expansion appears to be less of a problem in the knee reconstructed with bone-patellar tendon-bone autograft (Figure 4.3).

Allografts

The use of allograft tissue, grafts harvested from human donors, in ACL reconstruction has increased in recent years. The primary advantage of allograft tissue is the elimination of the potential for morbidity at the donor harvest site. One of the major concerns of

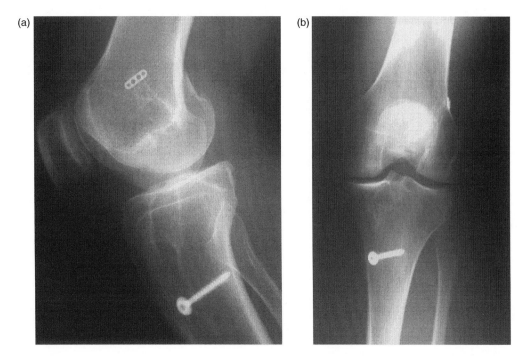

Fig. 4.3

AP and lateral radiographs of a knee 14 months after ACL reconstruction with hamstrings. Fixation is distal to the joint, and significant tunnel lysis is present on both the femoral and tibial side.

allograft use is the potential for viral or bacterial transmission. Careful donor screening and sterile procurement of allograft tissue are the best methods of preventing contamination. While extremely rare, transmission of HIV, hepatitis, and bacterial infection have occurred with allograft use, and patients must be counseled about this risk.

Concerns also exist with regard to the retention of tensile properties in allografts. This is an area of controversy, as there are studies showing similar outcomes after allograft ACL reconstruction as compared to autogenous grafts (Noyes and Barber-Westin 1996; Shino *et al.* 1986). However, one published report found only a 53 per cent rate of functional stability after allograft reconstruction in patients undergoing surgery for a chronically unstable knee (Noyes *et al.* 1994). In a study done in goats, knees reconstructed with allografts were found to have increased laxity, lower ultimate tensile load, and delayed biological incorporation as compared to autograft (Jackson *et al.* 1993). In general, allografts are reserved for multiple ligament reconstruction, revision surgery, or for lower demand patients (Fu *et al.* 1999).

Donor site morbidity

The primary concern relating to the choice of patellar tendon autograft for ACL reconstruction is the potential for morbidity associated with harvest of the graft. Major postoperative complications to the extensor mechanism of the knee, patella fracture or patellar tendon rupture, have been reported. However, while these complications are frequently mentioned, they are extremely rare. In a review of the literature, comprised of 19 studies, with a total of 1466 patella tendon autograft ACL reconstructions, two such complications were noted (Nedeff and Bach 2001).

A more commonly seen problem associated with harvest of the central third of the patellar tendon is anterior knee pain. The incidence of this problem has been reported, and varies between 3 and 50 per cent (Fu *et al.* 2000; Nedeff and Bach 2001). The definition of what constitutes anterior knee pain varies greatly in these series. It should also be noted that anterior knee pain has been documented in 22 per cent of ACL-deficient patients who do not undergo surgery, and can also occur in patients undergoing hamstring reconstruction (Buss *et al.* 1995). Thus, not all anterior knee pain can be ascribed to graft harvest. Certainly, anterior knee pain after patellar tendon ACL reconstruction cannot be completely discounted, but in the majority of cases it is relatively mild.

The incidence of anterior knee pain after graft harvest is considerably less than it was in the late 1980s (Nedeff and Bach 2001). It is postulated that more aggressive postoperative rehabilitation programs result in a very low incidence of these symptoms (Shelbourne and Trumper 1997). The popularity of accelerated rehabilitation programs, emphasizing early weight-bearing, quadriceps activation, knee extension, and patellar mobility have contributed to an improvement in postoperative outcomes. It has also been found that grafting the donor defect in the patella can reduce the incidence of postoperative patellar pain (Martin *et al.* 1996).

The incidence of donor site problems related to hamstring ACL reconstruction is quite low, but this graft is not completely without potential for morbidity. Pain in the area of the harvest is very rare. Most studies have found that hamstring strength returns to normal by six months after harvest of the semitendinosus and gracilis, though one study noted a persistent deficit in hamstring peak torque (Marder *et al.* 1991). It has been reported that internal rotation strength at the knee is permanently diminished after hamstring ACL reconstruction (Viola *et al.* 2000).

Summary

Several different options are available in choosing a graft for ACL reconstruction, and all generally produce satisfactory results. Ideally, the sports medicine surgeon is comfortable with the different graft options and can individualize the choice to the needs of each particular patient. In certain patients, such as those with pre-existing patellofemoral pain, or relatively low demands on the knee, patellar tendon may not be the best option for an ACL graft. Conversely, in high-level athletes where a premium is placed on restoring stability, in female patients with generalized ligamentous laxity, or in the chronic or revision setting, patellar tendon is the graft of choice. The bone-patellar tendon-bone autograft has stood the test of time and deserves to be described as the 'gold standard' to which other graft options should be compared. In an extensive review of the literature, Nedeff and Bach found 19 studies which reported on the results of arthroscopically-assisted patella tendon autograft ACL reconstruction with minimum two year follow-up (Nedeff and Bach 2001). Of the eight series that reported subjective patient satisfaction, the worst result was a 91 per cent satisfaction rate. Clearly, the patellar tendon autograft has been proven to consistently restore knee stability, and provides a high rate of patient satisfaction. Patellar tendon is the best graft choice in the majority of patients undergoing ACL reconstruction.

References

Aglietti P, Buzzi R, Zaccherotti G, DeBiase P (1994). Patellar tendon versus doubled semitendinosus and gracilis tendons for anterior cruciate ligament reconstruction. *American Journal of Sports Medicine*, 22(2), 211–7.

Anderson AF, Snyder RB, Lipscomb AB Jr (2001). Anterior cruciate ligament reconstruction. A prospective randomized study of three surgical methods. *American Journal of Sports Medicine*, 29(3), 272–9.

Barrett GR, Noojin FK, Hartzog CW, Nash CR (2002). Reconstruction of the anterior cruciate ligament in females: a comparison of hamstring versus patellar tendon autograft. *Arthroscopy*, 18(1), 46–54.

Bradley JP, Klimkiewicz JJ, Rytel MJ, Powell JW (2002). Anterior cruciate ligament injuries in the National Football League: epidemiology and current treatment trends among team physicians. *Arthroscopy*, 18(5), 502–9.

Brown CH Jr and Carson EW (1999). Revision anterior cruciate ligament surgery. *Clinics in Sports Medicine*, 18, 109–35.

Buss DD, Min R, Skyhar M, Galinat B, Warren RF, Wickiewicz TL (1995). Nonoperative treatment of acute anterior cruciate ligament injuries in a selected group of patients. *American Journal of Sports Medicine*, 23, 160–5.

Carson EW (1999). Fact, myth, or common sense: anterior cruciate ligament reconstruction graft selection. *Orthopedics*, 22(6), 567–8.

Clatworthy MG, Annear P, Bulow JU, Bartlett RJ (1999). Tunnel widening in anterior cruciate ligament reconstruction: a prospective evaluation of hamstring and patella tendon grafts. *Knee Surgery Sports Traumatology Arthroscopy*, 7(3), 138–45.

Corry IS, Webb JM, Clingeleffer AJ, Pinczewski LA (1999). Arthroscopic reconstruction of the anterior cruciate ligament. A comparison of patellar tendon autograft and four-strand hamstring tendon autograft. *American Journal of Sports Medicine*, 27(3), 444–54.

Feagin JA Jr, Wills RP, Lambert KL, Mott HW, Cunningham RR (1997). Anterior cruciate ligament reconstruction. Bone-patella tendon-bone versus semitendinosus anatomic reconstruction. *Clinical Orthopaedics*, 341, 69–72.

Feller JA and Webster KE (2003). A randomized comparison of patellar tendon and hamstring tendon anterior cruciate ligament reconstruction. *American Journal of Sports Medicine*, 31(4), 564–73.

Frank CB and Jackson DW (1997). The science of reconstruction of the anterior cruciate ligament. *Journal of Bone and Joint Surgery*, 79-A, 1556–76.

Fu FH, Bennett CH, Lattermann C, Ma CB (1999). Current trends in anterior cruciate ligament reconstruction. Part 1: biology and biomechanics of reconstruction. *American Journal of Sports Medicine*, 27, 821–30.

Fu FH, Bennett CH, Ma CB, Menetrey J, Lattermann C (2000). Current trends in anterior cruciate ligament reconstruction. Part 2: operative procedures and clinical correlations. *American Journal of Sports Medicine*, 28, 124–30.

Ishibashi Y, Rudy TW, Livesay GA, *et al.* (1997). The effect of anterior cruciate ligament graft fixation site at the tibia on knee stability: evaluation using a robotic testing system. *Arthroscopy*, 13, 177–82.

Jackson DW, Grood ES, Goldstein JD, *et al.* (1993). A comparison of patellar tendon autograft and allograft used for anterior cruciate ligament reconstruction in the goat model. *American Journal of Sports Medicine*, 21, 176–85.

L'Insalata JC, Klatt B, Fu FH, Harner CD (1997). Tunnel expansion following anterior cruciate ligament reconstruction: a comparison of hamstring and patellar tendon autografts. *Knee Surgery Sports Traumatology Arthroscopy*, 5(4), 234–8.

Marder RA, Raskind JR, Carroll M (1991). Prospective evaluation of arthroscopically assisted anterior cruciate ligament reconstruction. Patellar tendon versus semitendinosus and gracilis tendons. *American Journal of Sports Medicine*, 19, 478–84.

Martin RP, Galloway MT, Daigneault JP, Goehner K (1996). Patellofemoral pain following anterior cruciate ligament reconstruction: bone grafting the patellar defect. American Academy of Orthopaedic Surgeons annual meeting.

Nedeff DD and Bach BR (2001). Arthroscopic anterior cruciate ligament reconstruction using patellar tendon autografts. *American Journal of Knee Surgery*, 14(4), 243–58.

Noyes FR and Barber-Westin SD (1996). Reconstruction of the anterior cruciate ligament with human allograft. Comparison of early and later results. *Journal of Bone and Joint Surgery*, 78-A, 524–37.

Noyes FR, Barber-Westin SD, Roberts CS (1994). Use of allografts after failed treatment of rupture of the anterior cruciate ligament. *Journal of Bone and Joint Surgery*, 76-A, 1019–31.

Otero AL and Hutcheson L (1993). A comparison of the doubled semitendinosus/gracilis and central third of the patellar tendon autografts in arthroscopic anterior cruciate ligament reconstruction. *Arthroscopy*, 9(2), 143–8.

Scheffler SU, Sudkamp NP, Gockenjan A, Hoffmann RF, Weiler A (2002). Biomechanical comparison of hamstring and patellar tendon graft anterior cruciate ligament reconstruction techniques: the impact of fixation level and fixation method under cyclic loading. *Arthroscopy*, 18(3), 304–15.

Shelbourne KD and Trumper RV (1997). Preventing anterior knee pain after anterior cruciate ligament reconstruction. *American Journal of Sports Medicine*, 25, 41–7.

Shino K, Kimura T, Hirose H, Inoue M, Ono K (1986). Reconstruction of the anterior cruciate ligament by allogeneic tendon graft. An operation for chronic ligamentous insufficiency. *Journal of Bone and Joint Surgery*, 68-B, 739–46.

Viola RW, Sterett WI, Newfield D, Steadman JR, Torry MR (2000). Internal and external tibial rotation strength after anterior cruciate ligament reconstruction using ipsilateral semitendinosus and gracilis tendon autografts. *American Journal of Sports Medicine*, 28(4), 552–5.

Webster KE, Feller JA, Hameister KA (2001). Bone tunnel enlargement following anterior cruciate ligament reconstruction: a randomized comparison of hamstring and patellar tendon grafts with 2-year follow-up. *Knee Surgery Sports Traumatology Arthroscopy*, 9(2), 86–91.

5

Implications of tunnel widening in the ACL reconstructed knee

Mark G. Clatworthy

Introduction

Tunnel widening was first described in the early 1990s with bone-patella-bone (BPB) grafts (Fahey and Indelicato 1994; Peyrache *et al.* 1996; Linn *et al.* 1993; Roberts *et al.* 1991; Jackson *et al.* 1990). Widening was most marked with ethylene oxide sterilized allografts (Jackson *et al.* 1990; Roberts *et al.* 1991). In the late 1990s Insalata and Harner (Insalata *et al.* 1997) and Clatworthy *et al.* (1999) demonstrated significantly greater tunnel widening with hamstring grafts. These findings caused great concern for knee surgeons as these findings were reported at a time of increasing popularity for hamstring grafts. The Clatworthy study (Clatworthy *et al.* 1999) showed no correlation with a poor result but only 38 patients were evaluated. In a small study of 28 patients Nebelung (Nebelung *et al.* 1998) also showed no correlation. Tunnel widening was attributed to the new suspensory fixation devices developed in the mid-1990s for hamstring fixation.

In this chapter we will evaluate the incidence and clinical outcome of tunnel widening with different grafts and fixation devices, assess the theories proposed for tunnel widening, and discuss the ramification of this phenomenon.

Tunnel widening studies

The initial tunnel widening studies evaluated tunnels on plain radiographs. A cortical line demarcating the tunnel wall is seen on the postoperative radiograph between four and six months. The tunnel wall is most clearly seen with hamstring grafts (Figure 5.1). The tunnel may be more difficult to see with BPB grafts. The tunnel diameter is compared with the diameter of the drill used intra-operatively to determine a change in diameter or area of the tunnel.

Many studies have described tunnel widening in ACL reconstruction with BPB grafts (Fahey and Indelicato 1994; Peyrache *et al.* 1996;

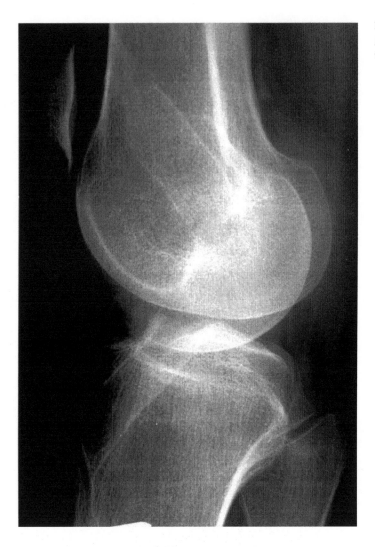

Fig. 5.1
Marked expansion of the
tunnels with a hamstring graft.

Linn *et al.* 1993; Roberts *et al.* 1991; Jackson *et al.* 1990; Nakayama *et al.* 1998; Zijl *et al.* 2000). Most studies have concentrated on the proximal aspect of the tibial tunnel where the rectangular patella tendon lies within the cylindrical tunnel (Figure 5.2). Tunnel widening has been most commonly reported with allografts (Fahey and Indelicato 1994; Jackson *et al.* 1990; Linn *et al.* 1993; Roberts *et al.* 1991). Fahey and Indelicato (1994) showed a significant difference in bone tunnel enlargement in allografts (1.2 mm) compared with autografts (0.26 mm). In contrast Hoher *et al.* (1998) and Zijl *et al.* (2000) demonstrated no significant difference between allograft and autograft tissue sources for ACL surgery. Cystic changes have been noted in the tunnels of patients with ethylene oxide treated patella tendon allografts (Roberts *et al.* 1991; Jackson *et al.* 1990). Linn *et al.* (1993) demonstrated striking tunnel widening in some

Fig. 5.2

Marked widening of the tibial tunnel with a BPB.

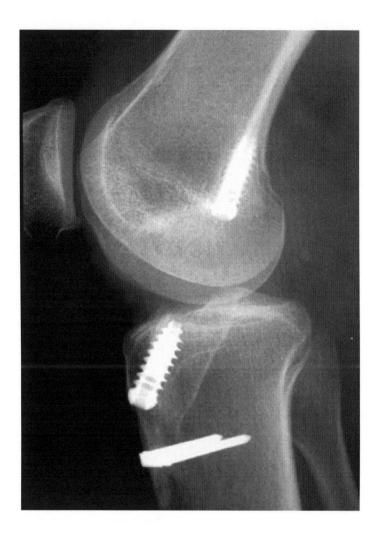

patients treated with Achilles tendon allografts. Less marked tunnel widening has been demonstrated in patients with autogenous patella tendon grafts (Nakayama *et al.* 1998; Peyrache *et al.* 1996).

As the tunnel walls are often difficult to delineate on plain radiographs CT and bone scintigraphy studies have enabled researchers to better evaluate tunnel widening in patients with a BPB ACL reconstruction. Fink *et al.* (2001) prospectively evaluated changes in the tibial bone tunnel of 34 patients using CT over a two year period. CT scans were performed at 1 and 6 weeks and at 3, 6, 12, and 24 months postoperatively. The tibial bone tunnel was measured in the sagittal and coronal planes at five different levels. The diameters of the tibial tunnel increased an average overall by 30.6 per cent in the sagittal plane and 16.4 per cent in the coronal plane within two years. The enlargement was significantly higher in the mid portion of the tunnel, which resulted in a uniform

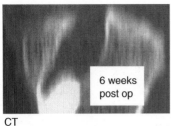

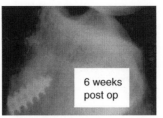

CT   Plain Radiograph

Fig. 5.3
CT demonstration of tunnel with BPB grafts.

cavity-type appearance. The percentage of change in tunnel size was significantly higher within the first six weeks following surgery compared with all other time intervals. The authors comment on the inaccuracy of plain films for measuring tunnels and demonstrate cases where plain films underestimate the degree of tunnel widening (Figure 5.3). Muren *et al.* (2001) reported similar findings. Tibial condyle bone mineral density, bone ingrowth and changes in diameter in the tibia bone tunnel were studied with quantified computed tomography postoperatively and after 1, 3, 6, and 12 months in ten patients. They found no sign of bone ingrowth in the form of increased bone mineral density in the bone tunnels in any of the patients. The tunnel diameter increased in all patients during the first postoperative months. After one year, five patients had a smaller diameter than at the first postoperative examination, two had the same diameter as immediately after surgery and two patients had a larger diameter. A sclerotic zone developed in all patients along the perimeter of the tunnel during the 3–6 months of follow-up. They conclude they found no growth of bone into the tunnel and tendinous part of the graft during the first postoperative year.

Hogervorst *et al.* (2000) examined tibial bone tunnels with bone scans at two years in 68 patients. Scan uptake at the tibial tunnel was increased in 29 per cent of patients. Marked increase of scintigraphic uptake was associated with tibial tunnel enlargement of more than 35 per cent and a graft length in the tibial tunnel over 14 mm. Scan uptake was correlated to tunnel enlargement and tunnel enlargement was correlated to graft length inside the tibial tunnel. Scintigraphy indicated the enlarged tibial tunnels are filled with remodeling bone. Tibial fixation location influenced ligament healing inside the tunnel: they concluded that the return of osseous homeostasis at the tibial tunnel can take more than two years when fixation is more than 14 mm below the joint.

Tunnel widening with hamstring grafts was first described by L'Insalata and Harner (L'Insalata *et al.* 1997). They compared 30 patients with a BPB graft fixed with metal interference screws with 30 patients with a hamstring graft utilizing an Endobutton for femoral fixation and sutures around a post for tibial fixation. One surgeon performed the surgery and patients underwent a uniform rehabilitation protocol. They reported significantly greater tunnel widening in the AP and lateral x-ray for hamstring grafts compared to BPB reconstruction. In a similar study Clatworthy *et al.* (1999) reported comparable results. The mean increase in femoral tunnel area in the hamstring group was 100.4 per cent compared with a *decrease* of 25 per cent in the BPB group. In the tibial tunnel, the mean increase in the hamstring group was 73.9 per cent compared with a decrease of 2.1 per cent in the patella tendon group. A recent comparative study by Webster *et al.* (2001) reports similar results. Interestingly in both studies patients received suspensory fixation for the patella tendon and hamstring grafts. In Clatworthy's study a Mitek Anchor was used and in Webster's an Endobutton.

Two further studies have reported on tunnel widening with hamstring grafts. Simonian *et al.* (2000) compared tunnel widening in patients receiving a hamstring graft with one incision trans-tibial technique with an Endobutton with a two incision technique fixed with screws and washers. Greater widening was seen in the one incision technique. Segawa *et al.* (2001) correlated tunnel widening in hamstring patients with the position of the tibial tunnel and angle of the femoral tunnel. They demonstrated greater tunnel widening if the tibial tunnel is anterior, and if there is a greater angle to the femoral tunnel. The authors conclude that the main factors associated with tunnel enlargement are the locations and angles of the tunnels. The windshield-wiper motion of the graft may be enhanced by changing tension in the graft due to tunnel malposition. An acute femoral tunnel angle may increase the mechanical stress on the anterior margin of the femoral tunnel.

Etiology

The proposed etiology for tunnel widening can be divided into two broad categories: biomechanical and biological. The most commonly held theories contend that mechanical factors lead to excess motion in the graft, which in turn results in bony tunnel expansion. This phenomena has been termed the 'bungee cord theory' (Hoher *et al.* 1998, 1999, 2000; To *et al.* 1999). Tunnel widening is attributed to excessive graft tunnel motion secondary to suspensory fixation devices such as from an Endobutton or suture anchor. A second theory proposed for the biomechanical etiology of tunnel widening is the 'windscreen wiper theory' (Hoher *et al.* 2000). In this mechanism, tunnel widening is attributed to the graft oscillating from a distant point of fixation resulting in cone-shaped tunnels, where the wide end of the cone abuts the intraarticular space.

These theories are based on the cadaver work of Hoher *et al.* Their initial study (Hoher *et al.* 1999) determined the relative motion of a quadruple hamstring graft within the femoral bone tunnel under tensile loading. Six graft constructs were prepared from the semitendinosus and gracilis tendons of human cadavers and were fixed with a titanium button and polyester tape within a bone tunnel in a cadaveric femur. Three different lengths of polyester tape

(15, 25, and 35 mm loops) were evaluated. Graft-tunnel motion was found to range from 0.7 ± 0.2 to 3.3 ± 0.2 mm, and significant increases in graft-tunnel motion were observed with increasing tensile loads. Shorter tape length (15 mm) resulted in significantly less motion when compared to longer tape length (35 mm). They concluded that graft-tunnel motion is significant and should be considered when using this fixation technique. A shorter distance between the tendon tissue and the titanium button is recommended to minimize the amount of graft-tunnel motion.

In a subsequent study (Hoher *et al.* 1998) they compared quadrupled semitendinosus tendon fixed with titanium button/polyester tape and suture/screw post (Graft A) and a double semitendinosus and double gracilis tendon fixed with a cross-pin and two screws over washers (Graft B). Elongation of the graft construct in response to 100 cycles of loading (20–150 N) was 1.8 and 0.6 per cent of the original length for Grafts A and B, respectively. However, after a series of five cyclic loading tests, the residual permanent elongation for each construct was 3.8 ± 1.2 and 0.3 ± 0.2 mm, a significant difference between the two graft constructs. Further analysis found more than 90 per cent of the permanent elongation occurred in the proximal and distal regions of Graft A, which consisted of polyester tape tied to a titanium button (proximal) and sutures tied around a screw post (distal). The tensile load-to-failure tests also revealed significant differences ($P < 0.05$) between the two graft constructs. Linear stiffness was 32 ± 1 and 119 ± 19 N/mm and ultimate load was 415 ± 36 and 658 ± 128 N for Grafts A and B, respectively. For Graft A, the polyester tape consistently failed; for Graft B, slippage or tearing from the washers was the mode of failure. They concluded that a quadruple-hamstring graft fixed over a cross-pin proximally and with metal washers distally has less permanent elongation in response to cyclic loading and has structural properties superior to those of a graft construct that includes suture and tape material.

In a similar study To *et al.* (1999) evaluated the stiffness of three femoral fixation devices – a button, anchor and post. They reported the stiffness of the femur-button-graft complex averaged 23 ± 2 N/mm, the femur-anchor-graft complex averaged 25 ± 3 N/mm, and the femur-post with bone graft-graft complex averaged 225 ± 23 N/mm ($P = 0.0001$). The knot in the suture loop was the least stiff component and determined the stiffness when the raft was fixed with both the button and anchor.

All papers expressed concern about the excessive graft tunnel motion and recommended stiffer fixation constructs. In response to these concerns Smith and Nephew developed the Endobutton Continuous Loop which was a significantly stiffer construct and surgeons started using interference screws and securing the graft directly to the tibia rather than use sutures around a post.

Charlie Brown (Brand *et al.* 2000) recently evaluated the more modern fixation constructs. He compared graft tunnel motion utilizing BPB grafts fixed with metal interference screws and sutures tied around a button with hamstring grafts fixed with Endobutton CL, Endobutton with Mersilene tape, Bioscrew, Transfix and Bone Mulch Screw. The BPB with sutures tied around a button had significantly greater tunnel motion than all other groups with no significant difference between other groups.

The second school of thought is that tunnel widening is due to biological factors. Postoperative MRI scans have demonstrated synovial fluid tracking between the graft and bone tunnel wall. Cytokines capable of directly or indirectly affecting bone resorption have been identified in normal synovial fluid (Komiya *et al.* 1992; Schmalzried *et al.* 1997). Evaluation of the synovial fluid following an ACL disruption shows significant increases in the osteolytic cytokines IL-6, IL-8 and TNFα. Sub-acutely, the levels of the protective cytokine IRAP drops (Cameron *et al.* 1997), (Cameron *et al.* 1994). There is also the probable release of cytokines at the time of graft necrosis that ultimately results in revascularization. It has been proposed that cytokines released at the time of ACL injury and graft necrosis may lead to osteolysis through the action of proteolytic enzymes.

In a recently completed study (Clatworthy *et al.* 2001), we were able to put these biomechanical theories to the test by evaluating four different hamstring fixation methods:

1   Bioabsorbable aperture fixation – Bioscrew (Arthrex Inc., Naples, Fl)
2   Metal aperture fixation – RCI screw (Smith and Nephew)
3   Stiff construct – Bone Mulch Screw femoral fixation (Arthrotek) and staples tibial fixation (Richards)
4   Elastic fixation – Endobutton and Mersilene tape femoral fixation (Smith and Nephew) and staples tibial fixation (Richards)

The study group comprised 79 patients undergoing Bioscrew fixation under Jens Buelow in Phorzheim Germany, 57 patients with RCI screw fixation by Leo Pinczewski in Sydney, Australia, 42 patients receiving the Bone Mulch Screw and staples from Steven Howell in California, USA and 64 patients from the Fowler Kennedy Clinic in London, Canada with an Endobutton and staples. All patients received an isolated arthroscopic doubled semitendinosus and gracilis ACL reconstruction and a similar accelerated rehabilitation program. All patients were evaluated for tunnel widening at a minimum of one year postoperatively with magnification adjusted AP and lateral radiographs using Scion Image software. The hypotheses for biomechanical theories of tunnel widening to hold true were:

1   Tunnel widening will be decreased by
    (i)   eliminating the bungy cord phenomenon
    (ii) utilizing a stiffer fixation construct – Bone Mulch Screw and Staples
    (iii) applying aperture graft fixation – Bioscrew and RCI screw

2   Tunnel widening will be predominantly in the primary plane of
    movement
    (i) the sagittal plane

Tunnel widening with the different fixation techniques were as
follows:

Bioscrew   139 per cent
RCI Screw   94 per cent
Bone Mulch Screw and Staples   77 per cent
Endobutton and Staples   59 per cent

There was a significant difference between the four fixation methods (ANOVA $P = 0.001$). Evaluation of the plane of tunnel movement showed that for the Bioscrew, RCI Screw and Endobutton
staple groups, there was no significant difference in widening
between the sagittal and coronal plane. In the Bone Mulch
Screw/Staple group there was more widening in the coronal plane
than the sagittal plane. Widening was circumferential rather than
sagittal, and tunnel shape was principally linear. Thus, all hypotheses proposed were refuted. This study suggests that tunnel widening
can not solely be explained by the use of an elastic fixation construct. There is huge variation in tunnel widening between patients,
even among patients treated with similar grafts, fixation method,
surgeon and rehabilitation protocol (Figure 5.4). We propose that
biological variation in graft/tendon bone tunnel healing is responsible for this observation.

In a similar study, Feller et al. (2002) also demonstrated greater
tunnel widening in hamstring ACL reconstruction when Bioscrews
were compared with an Endobutton and sutures to a post construct.
In a recent study, Buelow et al. (2002) provide further understanding
of the role graft fixation techniques play in the etiology of tunnel
widening. To determine whether tunnel enlargement can be
decreased by fixing the graft close to the joint line with a stiffer fixation construct, the authors compared 'anatomical' (one absorbable
interference screw-femur, and bicortical fixation using two absorbable

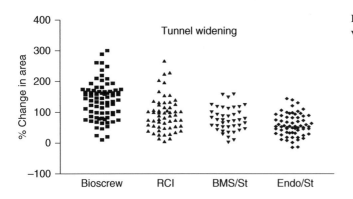

Fig. 5.4
Variation in tunnel widening.

interference screws-tibia) with extra cortical fixation techniques (Endobutton femoral fixation, and suture fixation (2 # 6 Ethibonds) over a post and washer at the tibia). Sixty patients were evaluated over a two year period. Radiographs of the operated knee were obtained immediately, 6 months, and 24 months following ACL reconstruction. In the 'anatomical' group the immediately postoperative bone tunnel area was 75 per cent larger than the initial tunnel area, after six months it was increased another 31 per cent, and between 6 and 24 months it remained basically unchanged. In the 'extra cortical' group there was no significant enlargement immediately postoperatively, but after six months the tunnel width was 65 per cent larger than the initial area of drill and graft size, and between 6 and 24 months it decreased to 47 per cent.

In an ongoing MRI study Pinczewski (2002) is also showing that the insertion of a metal RCI screw alone results in a 75 per cent enlargement of the tunnel. Clatworthy *et al.* (2001) did not adjust for the initial enlargement that occurs with the insertion of an interference screw in their calculations. Adjustment of their data shows there is similar initial tunnel enlargement for all four fixation techniques used in that study: Bioscrew 64 per cent, RCI Screw 57 per cent, Bone Mulch Screw + Staples 77 per cent, Endobutton + Staples 59 per cent (ANOVA $P = 0.22$). In summary insertion of an interference screw not only compresses the graft but causes significant bony tunnel expansion. Over a six month period, tunnel widening occurs with all fixation techniques. Clatworthy *et al.* (2001) demonstrated no difference between four fixation techniques; Buelow *et al.* (2002) showed less widening with anatomical fixation.

Timing of tunnel widening

The timing of tunnel widening is best evaluated by CT and MRI studies as tunnel walls are not clearly seen on radiographs until four months following ACL surgery. Fink *et al.* (2001) evaluated the progression of tunnel widening in patients with a BPB graft using sequential CT scans. These authors showed that most of the observed tunnel expansion occurs within the first six weeks following surgery. Buelow (2002) performed sequential MRI scans in 10 patients at 2 days, 6 weeks, 12 weeks and 6 months to assess tunnel size. He observed that most of the tunnel widening occurred early, but that tunnel expansion continued to progress through six months. Studies that have used radiographs to assess tunnel size have reported similar findings. Peyarche *et al.* (1996) analyzed 44 patients treated for ACL deficiency using an autogenous bone patella bone graft at 3, 6, 12, 24 and 36 months using x-rays. This study showed that tunnel enlargement was evident at three months following ACL surgery. The tunnel diameter did not significantly change from three months to two years, and then decreased in size between 2–3 years. In a randomized prospective study comparing hamstring and patella tendon grafts Webster *et al.* (2001) showed no progression of tunnel widening between four months and two years with both patella tendon and hamstring grafts. These studies demonstrate that some tunnel widening occurs at the time of graft-host healing.

Graft/bone tunnel healing

There is one published report (human cases) that describes the healing of tendon grafts within a bone tunnel. Pinczewski *et al.* (1997) evaluated two patients who had early mid-substance graft failure of a four strand hamstring tendon graft that was secured with round headed interference screws. These failures occurred at 12 and 15 weeks. These patients were revised with a patella tendon graft enabling a trephine biopsy of the tibial tunnel. Histology demonstrated collagen fiber continuity resembling Sharpey's fibers at the tendon bone junction. The histology finding from this report support the findings of Liu and Rodeo in animals. Liu *et al.* (1997) outlined the early morphologic phenomenon of tendon to bone healing in the rabbit. They demonstrated over a six week period reorganization of scar tissue into an interface that resembled Sharpey's fibers. Rodeo *et al.* (1993) evaluated the histology and pull out strength of tendon-to-bone in a dog model. They also demonstrated Sharpey's fibers. Biomechanically they showed mid-substance tendon rupture rather than bone tendon interface failure beyond twelve weeks.

The described animal studies utilized an extra-articular model, and are thus not directly applicable to the clinical scenario following intraarticular reconstruction of the ACL. As the bone-tendon healing described by Rodeo and Liu did not include an intraarticular component, these healing grafts were not exposed to synovial fluid or the cytokines that are typically released into a joint following an ACL disruption (Cameron *et al.* 1997, 1994). Another animal model was developed by Grana *et al.* that included an intraarticular graft reconstruction in rabbits (Blickenstaff *et al.* 1997; Grana *et al.* 1994). These authors evaluated a semitendinosus ACL reconstruction in rabbit by performing histology and biomechanical testing up to one year. Their first paper (Grana *et al.* 1994) evaluated healing up to 12 weeks. Histologically they showed a similar but slower process than Liu *et al.* (1997). Biomechanically they demonstrated dramatic decreases in the strength over the first nine weeks with an improvement at 12 weeks. Their second paper (Blickenstaff *et al.* 1997) followed the ACL-reconstructed rabbits for a year. Maturation of the tendon tunnel interface was complete at six months, however, at one year, large differences still persisted in the strength and stiffness of the graft compared with the normal semi-tendinosus tendon and native ACL. All these models describe the development of a fibrous interzone that undergoes a maturation process leading to the development of an indirect type of ligament

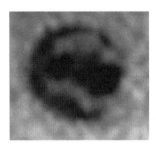

Fig. 5.5

Axial MRI of tendon/tunnel construct. Dark tendon surrounded by intermediate signal (fibrous interzone) surrounded by cortical rim of bone.

insertion. These animal studies are consistent with MRI evaluation of patients. Axial slices show the tendons centrally surrounded by intermediate signal tissue which is likely to be the fibrous interzone (Figure 5.5).

Weiler *et al.* (2002) describes the development of a direct tendon insertion where there is compression of the ACL graft from an interference screw using a sheep model. Clatworthy and Walton (2002) have just completed a study evaluating tunnel widening in a sheep model. The objective of the study was to determine the true tunnel diameter by measuring the histological section; then to compare these measurements with plain radiographs and MRI scans to determine whether we accurately measure tunnel diameter. Ten sheep underwent a split extensor digitorum tendon ACL reconstruction secured with endobuttons at the femoral and tibial tunnel exits. The sheep were then sacrificed at six months. Plain radiographs were only able to evaluate the tibial tunnel with accuracy. Tunnel widening was 95 per cent on radiographs. Axial MRI scan tunnel widening was 70 per cent for the femoral tunnel and 120 per cent for the tibial tunnel. These findings were consistent with human studies. Histologically, we found that there was a cortical rim of bone of varying thickness surrounding the graft (Figure 5.6). Tunnel measurements were made within this cortical rim. We found a 19 per cent decrease in femoral tunnel area and a 4 per cent decrease in tibial tunnel area. Axial MRI scan measurements were then repeated to measure within the cortical rim. Tunnel widening was −3 per cent for the femoral tunnel and 27 per cent for the tibial tunnel. From this study, we concluded that tunnel widening has been overstated as we have included this observed cortical rim of bone in our measurements.

Fig. 5.6

Histology of specimen of sheep ACL. Rim of cortical bone surrounding tendon.

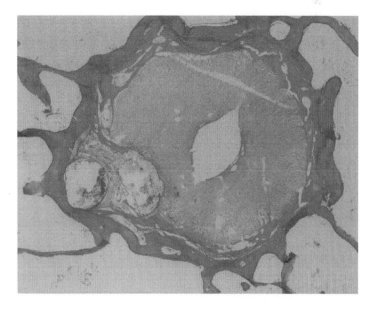

Clinical significance of tunnel widening

To date no study has been able to correlate poor clinical outcome with tunnel widening. Six studies have evaluated BPB grafts (Fahey and Indelicato 1994; Fink *et al.* 2001; Fu and Schulte 1996; Nakayama *et al.* 1998; Peyrache *et al.* 1996; Zijl *et al.* 2000). Five studies had less then 68 patients while Fahey's study evaluated 143 patients. Nebelung's study (Nebelung *et al.* 1998) was the first study to correlate tunnel widening in hamstring grafts with laxity and clinical outcome. Only twenty eight patients were evaluated, and there was no correlation between increased laxity and a poor result. Five further studies (Clatworthy *et al.* 1999; Buelow *et al.* 2002; Segawa *et al.* 2001; Simonian *et al.* 2000; Webster *et al.* 2001) also show no correlation between laxity and clinical outcome. However, it is important to note that the patient numbers are small, ranging from 33 to 87 patients.

In another study, Clatworthy *et al.* (2001) evaluated 242 patients and correlated KT–1000 arthrometer findings, Cincinnati Knee Score and IKDC score with tunnel widening. Again, there was no correlation between increased knee laxity and poor outcome/function following ACL reconstruction. The Pearson correlation coefficients and *P*-values demonstrate no correlation All outcome measures show a negative correlation.

KT 1000 Arthrometer	$r = -0.01628$, $P = 0.8151$
IKDC Score	$r = -0.08875$, $P = 0.2013$
Cincinnati Knee Score	$r = -0.1223$, $P = 0.1143$

I believe that we can now be confident that there is no correlation with tunnel widening and a poor outcome. However the presence of tunnel widening is not a benign condition, especially in cases where revision ACL reconstruction is necessary. Significant tunnel widening may necessitate the use of a two stage approach: initial stage of graft removal and bone grafting followed by revision ACL reconstruction.

Summary

In the published literature, tunnel widening following ACL reconstruction has not been shown to negatively influence clinical outcome. Thus, it would appear that the only true significance of this 'problem' is in those cases where revision ACL reconstruction is considered. Studies from our institution have detected the presence of a cortical rim of bone that surrounds the matured ACL graft. As described methods of tunnel widening evaluation have usually included this cortical rim in the calculation of tunnel widening, we contend that the degree of widening described in many published studies is excessive.

Tunnel widening was initially blamed on the use of suspensory-cortical fixation devices such as the Endobutton or post and washer constructs. However, numerous reports have demonstrated that tunnel widening occurs with all fixation devices and graft types. Using anatomical fixation devices may decrease the progression of tunnel widening, however the use of those devices needed for this type of construct significantly expands the tunnel at the time of surgery. ACL surgeons must decide whether it is worth trading off an initially larger tunnel for the possible advantage of the direct tendon insertions that often result following the use of these anatomic fixation devices. There is a huge variation in tunnel widening between patients despite them undergoing a similar procedure with the same graft, fixation device, surgeon and rehabilitation protocol. This suggests biological variation in the graft tunnel healing process that is probably unique to each individual who undergoes ACL reconstruction surgery.

References

Blickenstaff, K. R., Grana, W. A., and Egle, D. 1997, 'Analysis of a semitendinosus autograft in a rabbit model', *Am. J. Sports Med.*, vol. 25, no. 4, pp.554–559.

Brand, J., Jr., Weiler, A., Caborn, D. N., Brown, C. H., Jr., and Johnson, D. L. 2000, 'Graft fixation in cruciate ligament reconstruction', *Am. J. Sports Med.*, vol. 28, no. 5, pp.761–774.

Buelow, J. U. 2002, An MRI investigation of tunnel widening. Personal communication.

Buelow, J-U., Siebold, R., and Ellermann, A. 2002, A prospective evaluation of tunnel enlargement in anterior cruciate ligament reconstruction with hamstrings: extracortical versus anatomical fixation. *Knee. Surg. Sports Traumatol. Arthrosc*, vol. 10, no. 5, pp. 289–293.

Cameron, M., Buchgraber, A., Passler, H., Vogt, M., Thonar, E., Fu, F., and Evans, C. H. 1997, 'The natural history of the anterior cruciate ligament-deficient knee. Changes in synovial fluid cytokine and keratan sulfate concentrations', *Am. J. Sports Med.*, vol. 25, no. 6, pp.751–754.

Cameron, M. L., Fu, F. H., Paessler, H. H., Schneider, M., and Evans, C. H. 1994, 'Synovial fluid cytokine concentrations as possible prognostic indicators in the ACL-deficient knee', *Knee. Surg. Sports Traumatol. Arthrosc.*, vol. 2, no. 1, pp.38–44.

Clatworthy, M. G., Buelow, J. U., Pinczewski, L. A., Seibold, R., Howell, S. M., Amendola, A., Al Sayyad, M., and Fowler, P. 2001, Tunnel Widening in Hamstring ACL Reconstruction: A prospective clinical and radiographic evaluation of four different fixation techniques. AOSSM Speciality Day, Abstract.

Clatworthy, M. G. and Walton, M. 2002, A radiological and histological evaluation of tunnel widening in a sheep model, Unpublished Work.

Clatworthy, M. G., Annear, P., Buelow, J. U., and Bartlett, R. J. 1999, 'Tunnel widening in anterior cruciate ligament reconstruction: a prospective evaluation of hamstring and patella tendon grafts', *Knee. Surg. Sports Traumatol. Arthrosc.*, vol. 7, no. 3, pp.138–145.

Fahey, M. and Indelicato, P. A. 1994, 'Bone tunnel enlargement after anterior cruciate ligament replacement', *Am. J. Sports Med.*, vol. 22, no. 3, pp.410–414.

Feller, J. A., Webster, K. E., and Hameister, K. A. 2002, Bioabsorbable versus metallic tibial fixation in ACL reconstruction: a clinical and radiographic study. ACL Study Group.

Fink, C., Zapp, M., Benedetto, K. P., Hackl, W., Hoser, C., and Rieger, M. 2001, 'Tibial tunnel enlargement following anterior cruciate ligament reconstruction with patellar tendon autograft', *Arthroscopy*, vol. 17, no. 2, pp.138–143.

Fu, F. H. and Schulte, K. R. 1996, 'Anterior cruciate ligament surgery 1996. State of the art?', *Clin. Orthop.*, 325, pp.19–24.

Grana, W. A., Egle, D. M., Mahnken, R., and Goodhart, C. W. 1994, 'An analysis of autograft fixation after anterior cruciate ligament reconstruction in a rabbit model', *Am. J. Sports Med.*, vol. 22, no. 3, pp.344–351.

Hogervorst, T., van der Hart, C. P., Pels Rijcken, T. H., and Taconis, W. K. 2000, 'Abnormal bone scans of the tibial tunnel 2 years after patella ligament anterior cruciate ligament reconstruction: correlation with tunnel enlargement and tibial graft length', *Knee. Surg. Sports Traumatol. Arthrosc.*, vol. 8, no. 6, pp.322–328.

Hoher, J., Livesay, G. A., Ma, C. B., Withrow, J. D., Fu, F. H., and Woo, S. L. 1999, 'Hamstring graft motion in the femoral bone tunnel when using titanium button/polyester tape fixation', *Knee. Surg. Sports Traumatol. Arthrosc.*, vol. 7, no. 4, pp.215–219.

Hoher, J., Moller, H. D., and Fu, F. H. 1998, 'Bone tunnel enlargement after anterior cruciate ligament reconstruction: fact or fiction?', *Knee. Surg. Sports Traumatol. Arthrosc.*, vol. 6, no. 4, pp.231–240.

Hoher, J., Scheffler, S. U., Withrow, J. D., Livesay, G. A., Debski, R. E., Fu, F. H., and Woo, S. L. 2000, 'Mechanical behavior of two hamstring graft constructs for reconstruction of the anterior cruciate ligament', *J. Orthop. Res.*, vol. 18, no. 3, pp.456–461.

Jackson, D. W., Windler, G. E., and Simon, T. M. 1990, 'Intraarticular reaction associated with the use of freeze-dried, ethylene oxide-sterilized bone-patella tendon-bone allografts in the reconstruction of the anterior cruciate ligament', *Am. J. Sports Med.*, vol. 18, no. 1, pp.1–10.

Komiya, S., Inoue, A., Sasaguri, Y., Minamitani, K., and Morimatsu, M. 1992, 'Rapidly destructive arthropathy of the hip. Studies on bone resorptive factors in joint fluid with a theory of pathogenesis', *Clin. Orthop.*, 284, pp.273–282.

Linn, R. M., Fischer, D. A., Smith, J. P., Burstein, D. B., and Quick, D. C. 1993, 'Achilles tendon allograft reconstruction of the anterior cruciate ligament-deficient knee', *Am. J. Sports Med.*, vol. 21, no. 6, pp.825–831.

L'Insalata, J. C., Klatt, B., Fu, F. H., and Harner, C. D. 1997, 'Tunnel expansion following anterior cruciate ligament reconstruction: a comparison of hamstring and patellar tendon autografts', *Knee. Surg. Sports Traumatol. Arthrosc.*, vol. 5, no. 4, pp.234–238.

Liu, S. H., Panossian, V., al-Shaikh, R., Tomin, E., Shepherd, E., Finerman, G. A., and Lane, J. M. 1997, 'Morphology and matrix composition during early tendon to bone healing', *Clin. Orthop.*, 339, pp. 253–260.

Muren, O., Brosjo, E., Dahlstedt, L., Dahlborn, M., and Dalen, N. 2001, 'No bone ingrowth into the tibia tunnel in anterior cruciate ligament-reconstructed patients: a 1-year prospective quantified CT study of 10 patients reconstructed with an autologous bone-patellar tendon-bone graft', *Acta Orthop. Scand.*, vol. 72, no. 5, pp.481–486.

Nakayama, Y., Shirai, Y., Narita, T., and Mori, A. 1998, 'Enlargement of bone tunnels after anterior cruciate ligament reconstruction', *Nippon Ika Daigaku Zasshi*, vol. 65, no. 5, pp.377–381.

Nebelung, W., Becker, R., Merkel, M., and Ropke, M. 1998, 'Bone tunnel enlargement after anterior cruciate ligament reconstruction with semi-tendinosus tendon using Endobutton fixation on the femoral side', *Arthroscopy*, vol. 14, no. 8, pp.810–815.

Peyrache, M. D., Djian, P., Christel, P., and Witvoet, J. 1996, 'Tibial tunnel enlargement after anterior cruciate ligament reconstruction by autogenous bone-patellar tendon-bone graft', *Knee. Surg. Sports Traumatol. Arthrosc.*, vol. 4, no. 1, pp.2–8.

Pinczewski, L. A. 2002, An MRI evaluation of tunnel widening. Personal communication.

Pinczewski, L. A., Clingeleffer, A. J., Otto, D. D., Bonar, S. F., and Corry, I. S. 1997, 'Integration of hamstring tendon graft with bone in reconstruction of the anterior cruciate ligament', *Arthroscopy*, vol. 13, no. 5, pp.641–643.

Roberts, T. S., Drez, D. J., McCarthy, W., and Paine, R. 1991, 'Anterior cruciate ligament reconstruction using freeze-dried, ethylene oxide-sterilized, bone-patellar tendon-bone allografts. Two year results in thirty-six patients [published erratum appears in Am J Sports Med 1991 May-Jun; 19(3):272]', *Am. J. Sports Med.*, vol. 19, no. 1, pp.35–41.

Rodeo, S. A., Arnoczky, S. P., Torzilli, P. A., Hidaka, C., and Warren, R. F. 1993, 'Tendon-healing in a bone tunnel. A biomechanical and histological study in the dog', *J. Bone Joint Surg. Am.*, vol. 75, no. 12, pp.1795–1803.

Schmalzried, T. P., Akizuki, K. H., Fedenko, A. N., and Mirra, J. 1997, 'The role of access of joint fluid to bone in periarticular osteolysis. A report of four cases', *J. Bone Joint Surg. Am.*, vol. 79, no. 3, pp.447–452.

Segawa, H., Omori, G., Tomita, S., and Koga, Y. 2001, 'Bone tunnel enlargement after anterior cruciate ligament reconstruction using hamstring tendons', *Knee. Surg. Sports Traumatol. Arthrosc.*, vol. 9, no. 4, pp.206–210.

Simonian, P. T., Erickson, M. S., Larson, R. V., and O'kane, J. W. 2000, 'Tunnel expansion after hamstring anterior cruciate ligament reconstruction with 1-incision EndoButton femoral fixation', *Arthroscopy*, vol. 16, no. 7, pp.707–714.

To, J. T., Howell, S. M., and Hull, M. L. 1999, 'Contributions of femoral fixation methods to the stiffness of anterior cruciate ligament replacements at implantation', *Arthroscopy*, vol. 15, no. 4, pp.379–387.

Webster, K. E., Feller, J. A., and Hameister, K. A. 2001, 'Bone tunnel enlargement following anterior cruciate ligament reconstruction: a randomised comparison of hamstring and patellar tendon grafts with 2-year follow-up', *Knee. Surg. Sports Traumatol. Arthrosc.*, vol. 9, no. 2, pp.86–91.

Weiler, A., Hoffmann, R. F., Bail, H. J., Rehm, O., and Sudkamp, N. P. 2002, 'Tendon healing in a bone tunnel. Part II: Histologic analysis after biodegradable interference fit fixation in a model of anterior cruciate ligament reconstruction in sheep', *Arthroscopy*, vol. 18, no. 2, pp.124–135.

Zijl, J. A., Kleipool, A. E., and Willems, W. J. 2000, 'Comparison of tibial tunnel enlargement after anterior cruciate ligament reconstruction using patellar tendon autograft or allograft', *Am. J. Sports Med.*, vol. 28, no. 4, pp.547–551.

6

Primary ACL reconstruction: does gender affect outcome following ACL reconstruction surgery?

Brian M. Crites and Leigh Ann Curl

Introduction

Injury to the ACL and subsequent reconstruction is very common in the clinical practice of orthopaedic surgery. Approximately 75,000 ACL injuries occur each year in the United States, with 50,000 reconstructions performed annually.[1, 2] The majority of ACL injuries occur by a non-contact mechanism during sporting activities;[3, 4] it has been established that females have a much higher incidence of ACL injury than males, particularly in the sports of basketball and soccer.[2, 5–8] Calculated rates of injury range from 2.4–9.5 times higher.[9, 10] The increased risk in females has been seen in high school,[11, 12] recreational,[13, 14] collegiate,[9] and elite[15] athletic populations. Thus, skill level does not seem to be a factor.

The reason for this gender difference in risk of ACL injury is the current focus of much research. The likely explanation for this observed gender disparity is multifactorial with both 'intrinsic' and 'extrinsic' factors playing a role.[9] Extrinsic factors include the shoe – surface interface, lower extremity muscular strength, and neuromuscular control. Intrinsic factors include limb alignment, joint laxity, femoral notch dimension, ligament size, and hormonal influences. While the focus of current research is targeted towards the identification of causative factors so that subsequent preventative strategies may be devised, it is less clear what role these variables may have on the ultimate outcome in females following reconstructive surgery: assuming that not all intrinsic or extrinsic factors can be altered by surgery or training, what role do they play in the outcome of ACL reconstructive surgery? Furthermore, do females have a higher failure rate, compared to males, following surgical reconstruction of the ACL? The authors will attempt to address these questions in this treatise.

Intrinsic factors

Femoral notch dimension and ligament size

The relationship between the intercondylar notch width and native ACL size and the role that this relationship plays in ACL injury has been summarized in a recent extensive review by Arendt.[16] Arendt reviewed 15 papers on the relationship of notch size or notch width index and ligament size to ACL injury. Gender was explored as a variable in 9 of the 15 studies. Overall, significant limitations and inconsistencies were noted among the studies due to variation in population size, population source (cadaveric specimen, acute vs. chronic injury, bilateral vs. unilateral injury), and measurement techniques (plain radiographs, CT, direct caliper measurement). The limitations were such that the study conclusions were varied and the resulting evidence was not sufficient to establish a firm association between gender, notch width, ACL size, and ACL injury. However, Arendt did state that the available literature supported some general conclusions:

1 Females have smaller notches than males
2 Notch width in patients with unilateral ACL injury is generally less than noninjured control subjects
3 Notch width in patients with a history of bilateral ACL injury is generally less than patients with unilateral ACL injury.

The potential role that a small notch might play in elevating the risk of injury remains purely conjectural. One theory is that a small notch may result in a 'mechanical impingement' on the ACL during lower extremity internal rotation and hyperextension. A second theory is that a small notch houses a smaller, and thus 'weaker', ligament that may be at greater risk of injury during activity. While both theories are purely speculative, if such a relationship does exist it would have a direct implication for surgical reconstruction. Surgical notchplasty widens the small notch and therefore could theoretically be used to decrease the risk of postoperative reinjury following ACL reconstruction. The application of larger ACL grafts could also potentially decrease this same risk.

The extent of surgical notchplasty performed at the time of ACL reconstruction is highly variable. Some surgeons advocate making a typical anterior to posterior femoral notch resection that facilitates a view of the 'over-the-top position'; others advocate a minimal notch resection that merely allows for palpation of the posterior femur using a hooked or curved instrument. Multiple studies have addressed the relationship of tibial graft positioning relative to the superior aspect of the notch to avoid graft impingement in extension.[17–19] However, there are few studies that have explored the variables of notchplasty size and notch-width index and their effect upon ACL reconstruction outcome. Markolf et al.[20] evaluated the effect of notchplasty on graft force, pretensioning, and excursion in a cadaveric model. Their study found that a larger notchplasty resulted in a requirement for higher graft pretension to restore functional anteroposterior knee stability, thus raising the theoretical concern for long-term graft compromise or failure. Mann et al.[21] evaluated ten ACL reconstruction patients using CT scanning at one-year postoperatively to assess the effect of notchplasty on post-reconstruction notch width. All patients did well clinically, and CT scans demonstrated only a small amount of bony regrowth in all but two patients at one year. The authors concluded that, when bone is resected intraoperatively to prevent graft impingement, notch width can be expected to reform to a 'small degree'. The authors also felt that this regrowth did not result in subsequent graft failure. To these authors' knowledge, there is no evidence to support the notion that a wide notchplasty will reduce the risk of ultimate graft failure, in either male or female patients.

Graft options for cruciate reconstruction include allograft and autograft tissues, with autologous central third patellar tendon and quadrupled hamstrings being the most common source.[22, 23] The central third patellar tendon is the most common tissue used to reconstruct the ACL, with most surgeons utilizing a 10–11 mm graft.[24, 25] Shelbourne et al.[26] reported on 714 consecutive patients and found that there was no difference in the re-rupture rate between men and women following reconstruction with 10 millimeter patellar autografts. The authors theorized that the use of the same size graft could be responsible for the similar failure rates noted in both males and females.

There are numerous reports of excellent long-term results using patellar tendon.[27–30] However, hamstring tendon reconstructions are gaining recent popularity because of the development of improved soft-tissue fixation, the observation that these patients experience less postoperative pain, and some surgeon's desire to avoid the extensor mechanism as a graft source.[31, 32] While results similar to patellar tendon have been reported for reconstructions using hamstring grafts,[33–35] some surgeons are hesitant to use hamstring tendon reconstructions in females. There is considerable concern about the potential small size of the semitendinosus and gracilis tendons in the female patient; intuitively, surgeons believe that a small initial graft will result in an increased risk of subsequent graft failure. Others cite graft remodeling including hypertrophy in response to load as a standard postoperative phenomenon that renders the size of the initial graft less important. There are no published studies that have compared the precise size of the hamstring tendon construct with ultimate outcome following surgery in either men or women. Additionally, accepting that many females are 'quadriceps dominant' (as discussed below under neuromuscular factors), surgical harvest of the hamstrings may further compromise the protective agonistic action of the hamstring tendons. Loss of this protective effect could result in an increased risk of ACL reinjury following surgery. Persistent hamstring strength deficits have been

85

demonstrated following reconstruction with quadrupled semitendinosus and gracilis.[36, 37]

The choice of graft tissue remains a critical decision that requires a thorough understanding of the complex factors involved in making an appropriate selection for the individual patient.[38] When comparing outcomes in males versus females, there is no consensus as to the 'best' graft based on gender as a variable alone.

Hormonal influence

Hormone receptor proteins for estrogen and progesterone have been identified in ACL tissues, suggesting that female sex hormones may play a role in ligament composition and function.[39–41] Laboratory studies have demonstrated that the collagen-producing fibroblasts of the ACL are influenced by variations in hormone levels: increasing estrogen levels decrease collagen synthesis[42, 43] while progesterone acts as an antagonist to the effects of estrogen.[44] High levels of estrogen have been associated with reduced strength of the ACL.[45] Furthermore, some authors have identified a relationship between the phase of the menstrual cycle and the occurrence of ACL injury in females. Wojtys et al. noted that the majority of ACL injuries in females occurred during the ovulatory phase of the menstrual cycle (days 10 to 14) which is the phase at which estrogen levels surge.[46] Other studies have failed to confirm this relationship.[15]

Overall, controversy persists as to whether the systemic hormone fluctuations of estrogen and progesterone that occur during the menstrual cycle influence the mechanical properties of the in vivo ACL and subsequently adversely affect the risk of injury in female athletes. To the authors' knowledge, while much research continues in this area, no studies have addressed the potential influence of these hormones during the postoperative period in which graft incorporation and 'ligamentization' occurs.

Muscular strength and neuromuscular control

The non-contact mechanisms of ACL injury have been extensively studied. Boden et al.[3] studied 90 athletes with ACL tears and found that 72 per cent of the injuries were non-contact; this study found that deceleration was a critical component in 53 per cent of the injured knees. These authors noted that deceleration occurred at an average knee flexion of 23 degrees. This figure is alarmingly close to the 25 degree flexion point in the study by Shoemaker et al.[47] at which the anterior tibial force was maximized and at which point the ACL experienced the highest loads. During knee flexion and deceleration, like that which occurs during landing from a jump or pivoting, the quadriceps muscle functions in an eccentric fashion. The quadriceps is the major antagonist of the ACL, and quadriceps activation results in increasing forces across the ACL.[48] Huston and Wotjys[49] demonstrated that, on average, female athletes have a neuromuscular pattern of initial quadriceps recruitment, as opposed to males who demonstrate initial hamstring recruitment during activity. Furthermore, the time to peak hamstring activity is longer in females. Thus, this 'quadriceps first' pattern of muscle activation, if it occurs during deceleration from a jump or pivot, may place increased stress on the ACL and consequently increase the risk of injury.

The presence of gender differences in neuromuscular function has been demonstrated by a number of authors.[49-51] This remains an active area of research as clinicians seek to discover preventative strategies for ACL injury.[52, 53] While various authors[54-57] have shown promising early results with training programs designed to lessen the incidence of ACL injury in females, it is less clear if the standard regimen of physical therapy typically utilized following acute cruciate reconstruction results in the elimination of the 'quadriceps first' pattern of muscle recruitment: if a 'quadriceps first' pattern of muscle activation persisted following cruciate reconstruction, a higher risk of injury could possibly persist into the postoperative period. While there is abundant literature on rehabilitation protocols following reconstruction,[58, 59] to the authors' knowledge, no studies have yet specifically addressed the potential persistence of a quadriceps dominant recruitment pattern following surgery.

Review of the literature

The literature is not uniform in how the success of ACL reconstruction is determined. Clinical outcome can be measured in many ways.[60] Subjective and objective functional outcome surveys, postoperative pain, ligament laxity testing, physical exam parameters, strength, radiological criteria, return to sport, and re-rupture rates have all been used to measure the success of ACL reconstruction.[61] The importance of each factor is relative, and all are likely valid contributors to the final overall outcome following ACL reconstruction. With this in mind, we will review the available studies of ACL reconstruction as they relate to the differences between males and females utilizing various outcome measures.

Results – no gender difference

As mentioned previously, Shelbourne et al.[26] reported on 714 consecutive patients and found that there was no difference in the re-rupture rate between males and females following reconstruction with 10 millimeter patellar autografts. They theorized that the use of the same size graft could be responsible for the similar failure rates.

When strength is evaluated postoperatively, Natri et al.[62] found a 9–20 per cent extension strength deficit in 119 patients at an average of four years following ACL reconstruction. However, there was no correlation with this strength deficit and gender. Hofmeister et al.[63] also found mild residual weakness in the quadriceps and hamstring muscles in their series of 22 adolescent females; this did not seem to affect the overall outcome. All of their patients were subjectively satisfied with the surgery. Seven patients returned to competitive sports. The mean Lysholm score was 94 and the International Knee Documentation Committee (IKDC) scores were normal in 40 per cent and nearly normal in 60 per cent of the patients. Laxity testing postoperatively with KT-1000 revealed that 90 per cent had a side-to-side difference of 3 mm or less. They concluded that the mild muscular weakness did not alter a successful functional outcome.

Wiger et al.[64] evaluated the results of arthroscopic ACL reconstruction in male and female competitive athletes. There were 133 females and 296 males who were all reconstructed with bone-patellar tendon-bone autografts with interference screw fixation. Average follow-up was 38 months. They found no statistical difference between males and females with regard to IKDC scores, Lysholm scores, subjective anterior knee pain, subjective satisfaction, KT-1000 testing, or return to preinjury activity. They concluded that the results were comparable in males and females.

In a similar study comparing results and complications of ACL surgery in females versus males, Barber-Westin et al.[65] reported on 47 females and 47 males who were well matched in regards to age, sports activity, articular cartilage lesions, and chronicity of injury. All 94 patients had reconstruction with bone-patellar tendon-bone autografts. There was no statistically significant difference between the two groups in complications or overall outcome. The overall failure rate was 6 per cent for the females and 4 per cent for the males. One interesting finding was that the incidence of patellofemoral crepitus in females was only one half of that noted in the male patients.

In a two year follow-up study Barrett et al.[66] examined the outcomes of female patients who underwent ACL reconstruction and compared the use of hamstring tendons to bone-patellar tendon-bone autograft. With failure defined as KT-1000 results of greater than 5 mm side-to-side difference, 2+ Lachman, 1+ or greater pivot shift, or revision surgery, these authors found no statistical difference in patient outcome between the two grafts. The failure rate was 23 per cent for the hamstring group and 8 per cent for the patellar tendon group. These are comparable to other series for ACL results.

Siegel and Barber-Westin[67] published their results of arthroscopic ACL reconstruction utilizing quadruple looped hamstring tendons in 82 patients with an average follow-up of 43 months. Thirty-four of the patients were females. There was no statistical difference in outcome with regard to sex of the patients. Eighty-three percent of the patients returned to sports and 92 per cent of the patients subjectively rated their knee as normal or very good. Ferrari et al.[68] performed a retrospective review of ACL reconstruction in 200 patients, of which 63 were women. The authors compared the outcome of the male patients to the female patients. All patients received bone-patellar tendon-bone autograft and had the surgery performed by the same surgeon. There was no statistical difference with regard to gender noted in the follow-up Lachman or pivot shift test. There was also no gender difference in the number of patients with a side-to-side difference of 5 mm or greater on KT-1000 testing. Knee scores consisting of Tegner, Lysholm, Cincinnati, and modified HSS systems failed to demonstrate a significant difference between males and females. There was also no difference between the incidence of donor site morbidity or patellofemoral crepitus. Subjective patient satisfaction was 96 per cent for the females and 98 per cent for the males. The authors concluded that there was no basis for using gender as factor in the decision to perform ACL reconstructive surgery.

When assessing the presence of anterior knee pain, Tsuda et al.[69] found no statistical difference between 39 females compared to 36 males. The incidence of anterior knee pain was 22 per cent in the males and 13 per cent in the females. The authors advocated using two transverse incisions for the graft harvest and bone grafting the bony defects of the donor sites.

Results – gender difference

Noojin et al.[70] compared the results of females and males who had the ACL reconstructed with quadrupled hamstring tendon. The average follow-up was 40 months. There were 39 females and 26 males. They found that there was no statistical difference in the presence of patellofemoral crepitus or effusion on follow-up examination. There was no difference in the Lysholm knee scores, but Tegner scoring revealed that more males returned to their preinjury activity level than females. Likewise, there was no difference in KT-1000 testing results, but Lachman and pivot shift examinations did reveal significant differences. There were 31 per cent of the females with a 1+ Lachman compared to 7 per cent of the males, and 7 per cent of the females had a positive pivot shift compared to none of the men. Both of these physical exam differences were statistically significant. In the female group there was also a significant higher incidence of loss of terminal extension compared to the contralateral leg. The overall failure rate was also statistically different between the two groups. Females had a failure rate of 23 per cent compared to 4 per cent in males. The authors speculated that this higher failure rate could be partially due to the females having smaller hamstring tendons as subjectively noted by the surgeon at the time of surgery; unfortunately, graft size was not objectively measured. In addition, a visual analog test was given with regard to pain in the knee and females had both a higher frequency and intensity of pain compared to the males.

In another study females were found to have a greater incidence of significant postoperative pain compared to males.[71] Taenzer et al. found that females reported statistically higher pain scores on post-operative day one with activity and at rest compared to men. They also found that significantly fewer females were able to perform independent straight-leg raises on postoperative day one and two when compared to males. However, there was no difference in the amount of narcotic medication used throughout the study. Importantly, while postoperative pain levels were higher in females, the study did not evaluate the ultimate functional outcomes in males vs. females.

In a study by Corry et al.[72] that compared patellar tendon auto-graft with quadrupled hamstring autograft, anterior tibial transla-tion, as measured by KT-1000, did demonstrate significantly higher laxity in the females who underwent ACL reconstruction. Compared to their male counterparts, female patients from both the hamstring and patellar tendon groups demonstrated increased knee laxity at the follow-up interval. However, the presence of increased objective lax-ity did not correlate with final activity level, IKDC scores, or Lysholm scores. The poor correlation between KT-1000 results and functional outcome has also been noted by Snyder-Mackler et al.[73] and Tyler et al.[74]

The development of patellofemoral osteoarthritis has been implic-ated in poor functional outcomes in patients following ACL recon-struction by a study by Jarvela et al.[75] In their study on results of ACL reconstruction with multi-strand semitendinosus tendons ver-sus bone-patellar tendon-bone, Muneta et al.[76] found that mostly females in either group had a positive patellofemoral grind test. The authors postulated that this physical finding may be one factor that negatively influences the outcome of female patients following ACL reconstruction.

Conclusion

For females, both the risk and incidence of ACL injury is higher than that observed for males of similar activity levels. Moreover, those females who participate in the cutting edge sports, such as basketball and soccer, are particularly vulnerable. Soccer and basket-ball may account for up to two thirds of the ACL injuries in females between the ages of 25 and 35 years.[2] The recognition of this ele-vated injury risk has prompted research dedicated to further elucidating these risk factors so that preventative measures may be taken to decrease ACL injury rates in females. At the time of writ-ing, there is no consensus regarding to the exact cause(s) of this ele-vated risk. However most clinicians would agree that it is likely a multifactorial problem, combining both extrinsic and intrinsic factors. The difference in neuromuscular lower extremity control between males and females has shown early promise as a potential avenue for ACL injury prevention in females.

Despite the growing number of female participants in collegiate and professional sports, the recognition of a higher risk of ACL injury in females, and the ultimate need for reconstructive surgery in light of these injuries, surprisingly few studies have focused on the results of ACL reconstruction specifically in female patients. While a few studies have shown significant differences for various outcome parameters, the majority of studies available support the conclusion that gender does not affect outcome in surgical reconstruction of the ACL. Unfortunately, the majority of research papers evaluating the clinical outcome of various ACL reconstruction techniques continue to include a preponderance of male subjects. Additionally, the level of activity and the specific sport that the subjects have returned to have varied. As was the case with elucidating the increased incidence of ACL injury in females compared to males, the disparity in the outcome of following ACL surgery, if it exists, may become apparent if sport-specific return and reinjury rates are investigated. As more and more women become active in competitive athletics the numbers of reconstructions will inevitably increase. This will allow more follow-up studies and hopefully a clearer understanding of this growing problem.

References

1. Daniel, D.M., *et al.*, Instrumented measurement of anterior knee laxity in patients with acute anterior cruciate ligament disruption. *Am J Sports Med*, 1985. 136: 401–407.
2. Garrick, J. and R. Requa, Anterior cruciate ligament injuries in men and women: How common are they?, in L. Griffin (ed.) *Prevention of Noncontact ACL Injuries*, 2001, America Academy of Orthopaedic Surgeons: Rosemont, Illinois. 1–9.
3. Boden, B.P., *et al.*, Mechanisms of anterior cruciate ligament injury. *Orthopedics*, 2000. 23(6): 573–578.
4. Noyes, F.R., *et al.*, The symptomatic anterior cruciate deficient knee: Part I: Long-term functional disability in athletically active individuals. *J Bone Joint Surg*, 1983. 65A2: 154–162.
5. Dehaven, K.E. and D. Lintner, Athletic injuries: comparison by age, sport, and gender. *Am J Sports Med*, 1986. 14(3): 218–224.
6. Ferretti, A., *et al.*, Knee ligament injuries in volleyball players. *Am J Sports Med*, 1992. 20(2): 203–207.
7. Gray, J., *et al.*, A survey of injuries to the anterior cruciate ligament of the knee in female basketball players. *Int J Sports Med*, 1985. 6(6): 314–316.
8. Engstrom, B. and C. Johansson, Soccer injuries among elite female players. *Am J Sports Med*, 1991. 19(4): 372–375.
9. Arendt, E. and R. Dick, Knee injury patterns among men and women in collegiate basketball and soccer. NCAA data and review of literature. *Am J Sports Med*, 1995. 23(6): 694–701.

10. Gwinn, D.E., *et al.*, The relative incidence of anterior cruciate ligament injury in men and women at the United States Naval Academy. *Am J Sports Med*, 2000. 28(1): 98–102.

11. Powell, J.W. and K.D. Barber-Foss, Sex-related injury patterns among selected high school sports. *Am J Sports Med*, 2000. 28(3): 385–391.

12. Messina, D.F., W.C. Farney, and J.C. DeLee, The incidence of injury in Texas high school basketball: A prospective study among male and female athletes. *Am J Sports Med*, 1999. 27(3): 294–299.

13. Lindenfeld, T.N., *et al.*, Incidence of injury in indoor soccer. *Am J Sports Med*, 1994. 22(3): 364–371.

14. Bjordal, J.M., *et al.*, Epidemiology of anterior cruciate ligament injuries in soccer. *Am J Sports Med*, 1997. 25(3): 341–345.

15. Myklebust, G., *et al.*, A prospective cohort study of anterior cruciate ligament injuries in elite Norwegian team handball. *Scand J Med Sci Sports*, 1998. 8(3): 149–153.

16. Arendt, E., Relationship between notch-width index and risk of non-contact ACL injury, in L.Y. Griffin (ed.), *Prevention of Noncontact ACL Injuries*. 2001, American Academy of Orthopaedic Surgeons: Rosemont, Illinois. 1–9.

17. Howell, S.M., *et al.*, The relationship between the angle of the tibial tunnel in the coronal plane and loss of flexion and anterior laxity after anterior cruciate ligament reconstruction. *Am J Sports Med*, 2001. 29(5): 567–574.

18. Yaru, N., D. Daniel, and D. Penner, The effect of tibial attachment site on graft impingement in an anterior cruciate ligament reconstruction. *Am J Sports Med*, 1992. 20(2): 217–220.

19. Miller, M.D. and A.D. Olszewski, Posterior tibial tunnel placement to avoid anterior cruciate ligament graft impingement by the intercondylar roof. An *in vitro* and *in vivo* study. *Am J Sports Med*, 1997. 25(6): 818–822.

20. Markolf, K.L., *et al.*, Biomechanical effects of femoral notchplasty in anterior cruciate ligament reconstruction. *Am J Sports Med*, 2002. 30(1): 83–89.

21. Mann, T.A., *et al.*, The natural history of the intercondylar notch after notchplasty. *Am J Sports Med*, 1999. 27(2): 181–188.

22. Fu, F.H., *et al.*, Current trends in anterior cruciate ligament reconstruction: Part 1. Biology and biomechanics of reconstruction. *Am J Sports Med*, 1999. 27(6): 821–830.

23. Fu, F.H., *et al.*, Current trends in anterior cruciate ligament reconstruction: Part II. Operative procedures and clinical correlations. *Am J Sports Med*, 2000. 28(1): 124–130.

24. McKernan, D. and L. Paulos, Graft selection, in F.H. Fu, C.D. Harner, and K.G. Vince (eds), *Knee Surgery*, 1994, Williams & Wilkins: Baltimore, MD. 667–678.

25. Shelbourne, K.D., *et al.*, Correlation of remaining patellar tendon width with quadriceps strength after autogenous bone-patellar tendon-bone anterior cruciate ligament reconstruction. *Am J Sports Med*, 1994. 22(6): 774–777.

26. Shelbourne, K.D., T.J. Davis, and T.E. Klootwyk, The relationship between intercondylar notch width of the femur and the incidence of anterior cruciate ligament tears. A prospective study. *Am J Sports Med*, 1998. 26(3): 402–408.

27. Howe, J.E., *et al.* Anterior cruciate ligament reconstruction using quadriceps patellar tendon graft. Part 1. Long term followup. *Am J Sports Med*, 1991. 19(5): 447–457.

28. O'Brien, S.J., *et al.*, Reconstruction of the chronically insufficient anterior cruciate ligament with the central third of the patellar ligament. *J Bone Joint Surg*, 1991. 73A(2): 278–286.

29. Jarvela, T., *et al.*, Bone-patellar tendon-bone reconstruction of the anterior cruciate ligament. A long-term comparison of early and late repair. *Int Orthop*, 1999. 23(4): 227–231.
30. Fu, F.H. and K.R. Schulte, Anterior cruciate ligament surgery 1996. State of the art? *Clin Orthop*, 1996. 325: 19–24.
31. Anderson, A.F., R.B. Snyder, and A.B. Lipscomb Jr., Anterior cruciate ligament reconstruction. A prospective randomized study of three surgical methods. *Am J Sports Med*, 2001. 29(3): 272–279.
32. Brown, C.H. Jr., M.E. Steiner, and E.W. Carson, The use of hamstring tendons for anterior cruciate ligament reconstruction. Technique and results. *Clin Sports Med*, 1993. 12(4): 723–756.
33. Erikksson, K., *et al.*, A comparison of quadruple semitendinosus and patellar tendon grafts in reconstruction of the anterior cruciate ligament. *J Bone Joint Surg*, 2001. 83B(3): 348–354.
34. Allen, A.D., *et al.*, Assessment of the endoscopic semitendinosus/gracilis autograft procedure with interference screw fixation for reconstruction of the anterior cruciate ligament. *Orthopedics*, 2001. 24(4): 347–353.
35. Beard, D.J., *et al.*, Hamstrings vs patella tendon for anterior cruciate ligament reconstruction: A randomized controlled trial. *Knee*, 2001. 8(1): 45–50.
36. Coombs, R. and T. Cochrane, Knee flexor strength following anterior cruciate ligament reconstruction with the semitendinosus and gracilis tendons. *Int J Sports Med*, 2001. 22(8): 618–622.
37. Keays, S.L., *et al.*, Muscle strength and function before and after anterior cruciate ligament reconstruction using semitendinosus and gracilis. *Knee*, 2001. 8(3): 229–234.
38. Bartlett, R.J., M.G. Clatworthy, and T.N. Nguyen, Graft selection in reconstruction of the anterior cruciate ligament. *J Bone Joint Surg*, 2001. 83B(5): 625–634.
39. Liu, S.H., *et al.* Primary immunolocalization of estrogen and progesterone target cells in the human cruciate ligament. *J Orthop Res*, 1996. 14(4): 526–533.
40. Sciore, P., C.B. Frank, and D.A. Hart, Identification of sex hormone receptors in human and rabbit ligaments of the knee by reverse transcription-polymerase chain reaction: Evidence that receptors are present in tissue from both male and female subjects. *J Orthop Res*, 1998. 16(5): 604–610.
41. Slauterbeck, J.R. and D.M. Hardy, Sex hormones and knee ligament injuries in female athletes. *Am J Med Sci*, 2001. 322(4): 196–199.
42. Yu, W.D., *et al.*, Combined effects of estrogen and progesterone on the anterior cruciate ligament. *Clin Orthop*, 2001. 383: 268–281.
43. Liu, S.H., *et al.*, Estrogen affects the cellular metabolism of the anterior cruciate ligament. *Am J Sports Med*, 1997. 25(5): 704–709.
44. Samuel, C.S., *et al.*, The effect of relaxin on collagen metabolism in the nonpregnant rat pubic symphysis: The influence of estrogen and progesterone in regulating relaxin activity. *Endocrinology*, 1996. 137(9): 3884–3890.
45. Slauterbeck, J., *et al.*, Estrogen level alters the failure load of the rabbit anterior cruciate ligament. *J Orthop Res*, 1999. 17(3): 405–408.
46. Wojtys, E.M., *et al.*, Association between the menstrual cycle and anterior cruciate ligament injuries in female athletes. *Am J Sports Med*, 1998. 26(5): 614–619.
47. Shoemaker, S.C., *et al.*, Quadriceps/anterior cruciate graft interaction: An in vivo study of joint kinematics and anterior cruciate ligament graft tension. *Clin Orthop*, 1993. 294: 379–390.
48. Arms, S.W., *et al.*, The biomechanics of anterior cruciate ligament rehabilitation and reconstruction. *Am J Sports Med*, 1984. 12(1): 8–18.

49. Huston, L.J. and E.M. Wojtys, Neuromuscular performance characteristics in elite female athletes. *Am J Sports Med*, 1996. 24(4): 427–436.

50. Bell, D.G. and I. Jacobs, Electro-mechanical response times and rate of force development in males ans females. *Med Sci Sports Exerc*, 1986. 18(1): 31–36.

51. Winter, E.M. and F.B. Brooks, Electromechanical response times and muscle elasticity in men and women. *Eur J Appl Physiol Occup Physiol*, 1991. 63(2): 124–128.

52. Hewett, T.E., *et al.*, The effect of neuromuscular training the incidence of knee injury in female athletes: A prospective study. *Am J Sports Med*, 1999. 27(6): 699–706.

53. Teitz, C., Video analysis of ACL injuries, in L.Y. Griffin (ed.) *Prevention of Noncontact ACL Injuries*, 2001, American Academy of Orthopaedic Surgeons: Rosemont, Illinois. 87–92.

54. Griffins, N., *et al.*, Injury prevention of the anterior cruciate ligament in AOSSM Annual Meeting. 1989. Traverse City, Michigan.

55. Hewett, T., J. Raccoon, and T.N. Lindenfeld, A prospective study of the effect of neuromuscular training on the incidence of knee injury in female athletes in AOSSM Annual Meeting. 1998. Vancouver, British Columbia.

56. Caraffa, A., *et al.*, Prevention of anterior cruciate ligament injuries in soccer: A prospective controlled study of proprioceptive training. *Knee Surg Sports Traumatol Arthrosc*, 1996. 4(1): 19–21.

57. Cerulli, G., *et al.*, Proprioceptive training and prevention of anterior cruciate ligament injuries in soccer. *J Orthop Sports Phys Ther*, 2001. 31(11): 655–660.

58. Shelbourne, K.D. and G.A. Rowdon, Anterior cruciate ligament injury. The competitive athlete. *Sports Med*, 1994. 17(2): 132–140.

59. Risberg, M.A., *et al.*, Design and implementation of a neuromuscular training program following anterior cruciate ligament reconstruction. *J Orthop Sports Phys Ther*, 2001. 31(11): 620–631.

60. Johnson, D.S. and R.B. Smith, Outcome measurement in the ACL deficient knee – what's the score? *Knee*, 2001. 8(1): 51–57.

61. Nedeff, D.D. and B.R. Bach Jr., Arthroscopic anterior cruciate ligament reconstruction using patellar tendon autografts: A comprehensive review of contemporary literature. *Am J Knee Surg*, 2001. 14(4): 243–258.

62. Natri, A., *et al.*, Isokinetic muscle performance after anterior cruciate ligament surgery. Long-term results and outcome predicting factors after primary surgery and late-phase reconstruction. *Int J Sports Med*, 1996. 17(3): 223–228.

63. Hofmeister, E.P., *et al.*, Results of anterior cruciate ligament reconstruction in the adolescent female. *J Pediatr Orthop*, 2001. 21(3): 302–306.

64. Wiger, P., *et al.*, A comparison of results after arthroscopic anterior cruciate ligament reconstruction in female and male competitive athletes. A two- to five-year follow-up of 429 patients. *Scand J Med Sci Sports*, 1999. 9(5): 290–295.

65. Barber-Westin, S.D., F.R. Noyes, and M. Andrews, A rigorous comparison between the sexes of results and complications after anterior cruciate ligament reconstruction. *Am J Sports Med*, 1997. 25(4): 514–526.

66. Barrett, G.R., *et al.*, Reconstruction of the anterior cruciate ligament in females: A comparison of hamstring versus patellar tendon autograft. *Arthroscopy*, 2002. 18(1): 46–54.

67. Siegel, M.G. and S.D. Barber-Westin, Arthroscopic-assisted outpatient anterior cruciate ligament reconstruction using the semitendinosus and gracilis tendons. *Arthroscopy*, 1998. 14(3): 268–277.

68. Ferrari, J.D., *et al.*, Anterior cruciate ligament reconstruction in men and women: An outcome analysis comparing gender. *Arthroscopy*, 2001. 17(6): 588–596.

69. Tsuda, E., *et al.*, Techniques for reducing anterior knee symptoms after anterior cruciate ligament reconstruction using a bone-patellar tendon-bone autograft. *Am J Sports Med*, 2001. 29(4): 450–456.

70. Noojin, F.K., *et al.*, Clinical comparison of intraarticular anterior cruciate ligament reconstruction using autogenous semitendinosus and gracilis tendons in men versus women. *Am J Sports Med*, 2000. 28(6): 783–789.

71. Taenzer, A.H., C. Clark, and C.S. Curry, Gender affects report of pain and function after arthroscopic anterior cruciate ligament reconstruction. *Anesthesiology*, 2000. 93(3): 670–675.

72. Corry, I.S., *et al.*, Arthroscopic reconstruction of the anterior cruciate ligament: A comparison of patellar tendon autograft and four-strand hamstring tendon autograft. *Am J Sports Med*, 1999. 27(3): 444–454.

73. Snyder-Mackler, L., *et al.*, The relationship between passive joint laxity and functional outcome after anterior cruciate ligament injury. *Am J Sports Med*, 1997. 25(2): 191–195.

74. Tyler, T.F., *et al.*, Association of KT-1000 measurements with clinical tests of knee stability 1 year following anterior cruciate ligament reconstruction. *J Orthop Sports Phys Ther*, 1999. 29(9): 540–545.

75. Jarvela, T., *et al.*, The incidence of patellofemoral osteoarthritis and associated findings 7 years after anterior cruciate ligament reconstruction with a bone-patellar tendon-bone autograft. *Am J Sports Med*, 2001. 29(1): 18–24.

76. Muneta, T., *et al.*, Effects of aggressive early rehabilitation on the outcome of anterior cruciate ligament reconstruction with multi-strand semitendinosus tendon. *Int Orthop*, 1998. 22(6): 352–356.

7

Lactic and glycolic acid-based bioresorbable polymeric materials in ACL reconstruction

Michel Vert

Introduction

There are a few polymers that have been recognized in the literature as degradable in a mammalian organism. These polymers derived from glycolic acid (GA) and from L- and D- lactic acid (L-LA and D-LA) enantiomers, and were introduced in the field of biomaterials in the 1960s. They are still the most attractive compounds regarding applications as matrices implanted for temporary therapeutic devices in human surgical and pharmacological therapies. Though polymer chemists started paying attention to glycolic and lactic acid-based polymers (PLAGA) almost 30 years earlier, it is only in the 1950s that high molecular weight PLAGA polymers with exploitable mechanical properties appeared, thanks to advances in polymer synthesis and, especially, in ring opening polymerization (Lowe 1954; Kleine and Kleine 1959). The first member of the PLAGA family (Table 7.1) that was commercialized was the homopolymer of GA also named polyglycolic acid or PGA (Frazza and Schmitt 1971).

The PGA compound is a good fiber-forming polymer that degrades rapidly in aqueous media, including animal body fluids. It generates moderate inflammatory response in the case of tiny devices like threads. These properties are the main reasons for the rapid development of GA-based sutures, currently known as Dexon® or Ercedex® (pure PGA) and Vicryl® or Galactine 910® (GA copolymer with a small amount of LA), in the 1970s (Kronenthal 1974; Salthouse and Matlaga 1976). At the same time, the main structural, degradation and biocompatibility characteristics of PLAGA homo and copolymers were identified (Kulkarni et al. 1966; Cutright et al. 1974; Reed and Guilding 1981). However, the first generations of GA-rich polymers could hardly fulfill the requirements of devices used in bone surgery such as screws, plates, nails, etc., mostly because of too rapid loss of mechanical properties

Table 7.1 The PLAGA family, compositions, and acronyms

Poly(glycolic acid)—PGA	$-\!\left[O-CH_2-CO\right]_n\!-$
Poly(L-lactic acid)—PLA$_{100}$	$-\!\left[O-\underset{\underset{CH_3}{\mid}}{\overset{\overset{H}{\mid}}{C}}-CO\right]_n\!-$
Poly(lactic acid)— stereocopolymers PLA$_x$	$-\!\left[O-\underset{\underset{CH_3}{\mid}}{\overset{\overset{H}{\mid}}{C}}-CO\right]_m\!\left[O-\underset{\underset{H}{\mid}}{\overset{\overset{CH_3}{\mid}}{C}}-CO\right]_p\!-$
Poly(L-lactic acid-co-glycolic acid)—PLA$_x$GA$_{100\,-\,x}$	$-\!\left[O-\underset{\underset{CH_3}{\mid}}{\overset{\overset{H}{\mid}}{C}}-CO\right]_m\!\left[O-CH_2-CO\right]_p\!-$
Poly(L-lactic-co-D-lactic-co-glycolic acids) terpolymers— PLA$_x$GA$_y$	$-\!\left[O-\underset{\underset{CH_3}{\mid}}{\overset{\overset{H}{\mid}}{C}}-CO\right]_m\!\left[O-\underset{\underset{H}{\mid}}{\overset{\overset{CH_3}{\mid}}{C}}-CO\right]_p\!\left[O-CH_2-CO\right]_q\!-$

and degradation. Fortunately, people realized also that LA-rich polymers were more resistant to aqueous media than GA-rich ones, and thus had a better potential for applications in bone surgery (Kulkarni *et al.* 1971). Examples of promising bone tissue healing were reported, especially in the case of slightly stressed sites (Sedel *et al.* 1978; Vert *et al.* 1984). However structural and degradation characteristics of LA-rich polymers and copolymers turned out to be rather complex because of the presence of an asymmetric carbon atom in the LA molecule and because of the fact that high molecular weight polymers of this type had to be synthesized by ring opening of a cyclic dimer of chiral LA, thus introducing the repeating units that form polymer chains by pair (Lillie and Schultz 1975; Chabot *et al.* 1983).

It is in 1981 that a decisive breakthrough changed the perspectives, that is, when we showed for the first time that properly synthesized, purified, and processed LA-rich polymers could retain 90 per cent of their initial mechanical properties beyond 1 year, that is, for a period of time compatible with the reconstruction of bone provided that mechanical stresses were not too high (Vert *et al.* 1981). At the same time, the literature was enriched by reports of animal testing carried out between 1976 and 1981 that led us to test the first bioresorbable plates in human surgery in 1982 (Vert *et al.* 1984). Since then, more and more people became interested in LA-based polymers and it has been shown that polymers can be synthesized using a number of initiator and cocatalyst systems. However little attention was paid to the behavior of the polymers resulting from these special synthesis routes. Nowadays, many industrial companies offer LA-based polymers for bone surgery. However the advances that resulted from the contributions of scientists of different disciplines working on polymers of different sources and different processing histories and different properties contributed to generate confusion, especially among clinicians. The remark made in 1981 (Vert *et al.* 1981) that experiments involving a PLAGA polymer must be considered as specific and adoption or generalization of a reported behavior is always something to be considered with caution. This is particularly true for surgical bioresorbable devices that are currently used in ACL reconstruction.

In the following, we are going to make a long story short by emphasizing the general characteristics that govern the *in vivo* behavior of PLAGA polymers for the profit of orthopedic surgeons that are or will be users of PLAGA polymers for osteosynthesis and bone reconstruction.

PLAGA structural characteristics

As already mentioned, PLAGA polymers have rather complex structural characteristics (Vert 2002). On the other hand, they are far from being inert when implanted in a living medium. Insofar as the structural factors are concerned, the chemical composition must be considered first. Table 7.1 shows the formula and the acronyms we proposed in 1981 (Vert *et al.* 1981) to differentiate the main members of the PLAGA family and better reflect their chemical and chiral (configurational) compositions. A fast glance at the literature is sufficient to realize that this recommendation is seldom respected and that experiments and papers dealing with PLAGA polymers do not describe properly the chain composition and other structural characteristics, the acronym PLA being often used as a generic polymer name. The lack of precision at this stage can be critical in the cases of L- or D-LA and GA copolymers and L-LA- and D-LA- containing stereocopolymers and terpolymers because of the influence of the distribution of LA and GA co-unit or of chiral L- and D-LA co-units along the polymer chains. Figure 7.1 exemplifies some of the various structures one can find when dealing with a PLAGA polymer of a defined chemical composition, G, L, and D representing glycolyl, L-lactyl, and D-lactyl units, respectively. A fast glance at the few examples shown in Figure 7.1 is enough to deduce that compounds with the same gross composition can have very different, fine macromolecular structures and thus macroscopic properties.

Combined with the fact that, as for any polymer, most of the properties also depend on the molecular weight (the length of the molecules) and on the distribution of the lengths of these macromolecules (polydispersity), one can easily imagine how important it is to clearly identify the macromolecular structures in order to understand and control the expected mechanical and resorption properties.

(a) Cases with 25% L-lactyl/25% D-lactyl/50%Glycolyl units, the three different units
   being represented by L, D, and G respectively:
   Triblock copolymer: LLLLLLLLLLDDDDDDDDDDGGGGGGGGGGGGGGGGGGGGGGG
   Random copolymer: LLDDGGLLGGLLGGLLDDGGDDGGGGLLDDGGDDGGGGGG
   Blocky copolymer: LLLLLLGGGGGGGGGLLDDGGDDGGGGLLGGDDDDDGGGG

(b) Cases with 50% L-lactyl and 50 glycolyl units:
   Diblock structures: LLLLLLLLLLLLLLLLLLLLGGGGGGGGGGGGGGGGGGGGGG
   Random structures: LLLLGGLLLLGGLLLLGGGGGLLLLGGLLGGGGGLLGGGGGG
   Blocky structures: LLLLLLGGGGGGGGLLLLLLLLLLLGGLLLLGGGGGGGGGGGG

Fig. 7.1

Schematic representation of some of the numerous unit distributions that can be found in
PLAGA polymers composed of 50% lactyl units and 50% glycolyl units.

Glycolic and lactic acid-based polymers are exceptional because
of their chiral chain structures and the pair addition of repeating
units mentioned before. Many other factors contribute to make
members of the family different, c.a. possibility of racemization,
occurrence of transesterification reactions during polymerization
and post-polymerization processing, degradation during processing
to devices, during sterilization and even on the shelf. This is well-
documented in literature (Vert 1990; Li and Vert 1999). However, it
is by considering the degradation mechanism of large devices that
the complexity of PLAGA polymers was largely understood. In particular the understanding of the phenomena that govern the degradation of aliphatic polyesters helped in understanding the *in vivo*
phenomena observed by surgeons postoperatively, in particular,
occasional inflammatory reactions during degradation, too fast or
too slow degradation, and dramatic late inflammatory responses.

PLAGA DEGRADATION

For almost 20 years after the early work on high molecular weight
PLAGA, aliphatic polyesters that led to surgical resorbable sutures,
the hydrolytic degradation in the absence of enzyme was regarded
as homogeneous (bulk erosion) (Pitt *et al.* 1981). From a surgical
viewpoint, this mechanism suggested that degradation by-products
were released progressively along the whole period of degradation.
About 12 years ago, the understanding of the hydrolytic degradation
of PLAGA polymers advanced significantly, thanks to the use of
Size Exclusion Chromatography (SEC) to investigate the hydrolytic
degradation. This technique reflects the molecular weight and the
polydispersity of the macromolecules forming polymeric materials.
Its use revealed the appearance of two populations of partially
degraded macromolecules when PLAGA devices aimed at mimicking bone plates, and screws were allowed to degrade under physiological conditions of pH, temperature, and ionic strength. This
discovery led us to introduce the concept of heterogeneous degradation related to diffusion-reaction-dissolution phenomena (Li *et al.*
1990a).

To summarize, once a device made of a PLAGA polymer is placed in contact with an aqueous medium, water penetrates into the specimen and the hydrolytic cleavage of ester bonds starts. Some authors questioned the contribution of enzymes in the case of *in vivo* degradation. However there has been no convincing evidence that enzymes contribute to the *in vivo* degradation of PLAGA polymers that are implanted parenterally. The absence of sensitivity to enzymes is an interesting feature because it minimizes the risk of immune response, both phenomena relying on comparable specific recognition mechanisms. On the other hand, the fact that GAs and LAs are metabolites minimizes the risk of toxicity due to degradation by-products. The uptake of water triggers off the onset of degradation and also regulates the rate of degradation according to very simple and well-known chemical and kinetic laws. One of them is the breakdown of the polymer by ester hydrolysis catalyzed by acids. It is worth noting that each PLAGA macromolecules is terminated by an acid group that can contribute to the degradation by the catalyzing of the cleavage of the intrachain ester groups. Furthermore, as the polymer is degraded each cleaved ester bond generates a new carboxyl end group that contributes to an increase in the acidity and thus increases the rate of the hydrolytic cleavage of the remaining ester bonds. In other words, the rate of degradation increases exponentially as the reaction advances according to a phenomena named autocatalysis (Scheme 7.1) (Pitt *et al.* 1981).

For a time the partially degraded macromolecules remain insoluble in the surrounding aqueous medium, regardless of its nature, and the degradation proceeds homogeneously. The weight of the dried device stays constant. However, as soon as the molecular weight of some of the partially degraded macromolecules becomes low enough to allow dissolution in the aqueous medium, diffusion starts within the whole bulk, the soluble compounds moving slowly to and off the surface while they continue to degrade. This defines the clinical setting where the mechanical properties diminish progressively, yet macroscopically little degradation of the screw occurs until some time after implantation, and once started rapid disintegration may occur.

It is from this point where the molecular weight of some of the partially degraded macromolecules becomes low enough to allow dissolution in the aqueous medium, that we introduced a fundamental

$$HO\text{-}R\text{-}COO\text{-}R'\text{-}COOH \rightarrow OH\text{-}R\text{-}COOH + HO\text{-}R'\text{-}COOH$$

$$(\ 1\ COOH \rightarrow 2\ COOH \rightarrow 4\ COOH\ .....)$$

(Autocatalysis)

Scheme 7.1

Acid catalyzed hydrolysis of intrachain ester bonds of PLAGA polymers and increase of the number of catalytic acidic end groups at each chain cleavage.

difference from the homogeneous autocatalysis mechanism. Indeed, the release of the soluble small fragments of macromolecules (oligomers) combines diffusion, chemical reaction, and dissolution phenomena that lead to differentiation between the rates of degradation at the surface and in the interior of the matrix. The oligomers that are located close to the surface can escape from the polymer mass before complete degradation and thus eliminate ester bonds that will not be able to contribute to local autocatalysis. In contrast, those oligomers that are located far inside continue to degrade during diffusion toward the surface, and thus they liberate in the bulk all the acid catalytic potential that is stored under the form of ester bonds. Degradation is thus slower at the surface than in the center or bulk of the material, a phenomenon that well explains the formation of a more or less thick layer at the surface of some large-size devices surrounding a hollow interior. This has been occasionally reported from histological preparations of implanted bone screws or plates (Schwach and Vert 1999). This is also the reason why we named this type of degradation 'heterogeneous degradation'.

In an animal body, the release of soluble compounds is detected by the surrounding tissues and initiates a secondary inflammatory response. The primary inflammatory response is observed right after implantation as usual for biomaterial implantation, and lasts for a few weeks only limited by the good biocompatibility properties of PLAGA polymers. GA-rich PLAGA copolymers and PGA being more hydrophilic and degrading faster in aqueous media than PLA and LA-rich PLAGA copolymers, the leaching of the water-soluble oligomers from the surface of large-size devices made of a GA-rich PLAGA occurs relatively earlier than for LA-rich analogs.

The secondary inflammatory response is related to the release of soluble material from degradation and has been reported after various implantation periods of time because of the different rates of degradation. The solubility and the diffusion of PLAGA oligomers depends on the chemical and chiral compositions of these oligomers; the time after which the secondary inflammatory response occurs is also dependent on these characteristics. The formation of the slowly degrading outer layer (skin) and of hollow interior is not always clinically apparent, it is most likely with intrinsically amorphous PLAGA (Li et al. 1990b,c), and depends on the crystalline nature of the polymer chains or on the ability of the material to form crystalline residues (Vert et al. 1994; Li and Vert 1999). If any crystalline material exists initially or is formed during degradation, then the interior remains filled up despite the faster inner degradation. It is known that some PLAGA polymers crystallize spontaneously unless they are quenched during processing. It is the case of the crystalline materials PGA, GA-rich PLAGA, L-LA-rich PLAGA, and PLA_{100} (also named PLLA). Other members of the PLAGA family with more irregular distributions of similar repeating units are not spontaneously crystalline but they can crystallize upon plastification by the water that is absorbed after implantation. Last but not the least, other PLAGA polymers are not able to crystallize after implantation, but they can generate crystalline residues because of selective cleavage of some irregular parts of the macromolecules and crystallization of some of the more stable regular segments. The extent of the crystallinity of the initial material or its breakdown products regulates the degradation and the timing of any observed or delayed secondary inflammatory response.

The heterogeneous degradation mechanism allowed us to explain some unpredictable features of PLAGA polymers too. There are recorded differences between the degradation rates of thin films, tiny particles, or microspheres issued from the same batch of polymer (Grizzi et al. 1995). The work showed conclusively that the smaller the size of a polymer device; the slower the degradation rate, because a small size allows soluble oligomers to be released rapidly. This occurs regardless of their location since the interior is always close to the surface in tiny devices. From the same logic, one could explain why a porous system degrades at a slower rate than a plain one, especially if the dimensions of the considered device are millimetric.

The heterogeneous degradation mechanism was able to account for the behavior of PLAGA polymers in which additives or foreign molecules have been introduced or are present. Indeed any electrostatic interaction between a PLAGA matrix and acidic, basic, or amphoteric molecules can drastically affect the degradation characteristics by changing the natural acid–base equilibrium within the matrix in relation to the presence of chain end carboxylic groups. For acidic compounds, one can expect faster hydrolysis of ester bonds. In contrast, in the case of basic compounds, two effects can be observed: base catalysis of ester bond cleavage when the basic compound is in excess with respect to acid chain ends, and a decrease of the degradation rate in the contrary situation. It is thus important to know the nature of any small molecules or residue that can be present in a PLAGA polymer. The effects of factors like the sterilization process, presence of residual monomer and solvent in the material, uptake of physiological low molecular weight lipophilic compounds, all affect the crystallinity and rate of degradation of any particular material (Li and Vert 1995, 1999; Barber 1998; Brannon-Peppas and Vert 2000; Schwach and Vert 1999).

Recently, attention was paid to the effects of the initiator on the degradation characteristics of some LA-based bioresorbable polymers. It has been shown that dramatic differences in repeating unit distributions can be observed in the case of stereocopolymers obtained via stannous octoate or zinc metal initiation (Schwach et al. 1994). These differences were related to the presence of hydrophobic octanoic residues that contributed to hydrophobize the polymeric mass, thus delaying the onset of degradation, and also to some chain end modifications. Such modifications do not occur in the case of zinc metal or zinc lactate initiations thus explaining the higher hydrophily and the faster rate of degradation of PLAGA polymers synthesized with zinc as compared to other compounds (Schwach and Vert 1999). Whether similar effects can be observed in the case of polymers obtained using other and more sophisticated initiating systems, or through solution polymerization, or in the presence of alcohols is still unknown. In the case of commercial PLAGA compounds and devices, it is rather difficult to obtain precise information because manufacturers are usually rather silent regarding the exact chemical structure and processing history of their products. On the other hand, scientists rarely investigated the effects of chemical and morphology (crystallinity) structures on degradation characteristics and comparison of literature data is seldom feasible significantly, as already pointed out. In the absence of accurate information on structure and processing history, it is rather difficult to predict prior to clinical use how much the various factors mentioned above contribute to the degradation characteristics and the release of oligomers. Clinicians need to be aware that each material, polymer, manufacuring, processing, and sterilization technique, and size of the implant affects the crystallinity and degradation of any given implant and it is incorrect to assume that one generic material or implant behaves in the same way as another of similar but not identical implant.

The features recalled above should allow the surgeon to better understand the various and controversial statements that are present in the literature of bioresorbable devices currently used in bone surgery and especially as interference screws in anterior cruciate ligament (ACL) reconstruction surgery. From a general viewpoint, one can summarize the main characteristics that can be expected from the constituting polymeric molecules, keeping in mind that so many factors contribute to the behavior of such devices that deviations can be observed especially when one takes into account factors like sterilization, storage, and processing conditions.

Application to bioresorbable PLAGA polymers used in ACL reconstruction. Presently, PLAGA polymers have been proposed or are used as bioresorbable matrices to make temporary therapeutic devices aimed at tissue reconstruction and healing in many body sites (Table 7.2). However it is critical to realize that a compound that is good for one of these applications is not necessarily acceptable for another. Therefore, PLAGA polymers that serve as matrices to make ACL interference screws, namely self-reinforced PLA, as-polymerized PLA, PLA_{100}, PLA_{98}, $PLA_{85}GA_{15}$, PLA_{50}, etc., have to be confronted to the specifications typical of that application. The present understanding of the behaviors of PLAGA polymers can be of interest to predict the main characteristics of commercial PLAGA-based interference screws. The self-reinforced PGA and PLA are variants of genuine PGA and PLA matrices and can be

Table 7.2 Bioresorbable polymers and temporary therapeutic applications

Soft tissues	Sutures
	Nerve guides
	Tissue engineering
Hard tissues	Bone fracture fixation
	Bone recontruction
	Tissue guided regeneration
	Tissue engineering
Controlled drug delivery	Implant
	Microparticles
	Nanoparticles
	Micelles
Medicated degradable prostheses	Antitumoral drug
	Antibiotic drug
	Growth factors

regarded as composite materials although they are composed of only one polymer. Indeed they are processed to create aligned tiny crystalline fibrils during cold drawing. This particular structure provides better initial properties. However one can predict a more rapid decrease in the mechanical properties upon hydrolysis than for a more isotropic amorphous matrix. Basically such a structure is beneficial to secure better mechanical properties during the first weeks. The risk of intermediate inflammatory response due to the release of soluble oligomers is rather small because of slow degradation and extension of the release over a rather long period of time. On the other hand, complete elimination of the device is likely to require several years and much more time than for an amorphous matrix. Furthermore, rather degradation-resistant crystalline residues are to be expected. This may result in a marked tertiary inflammatory response at a late stage, dependant on the amount and on the size and shape of the crystallites. Similar features are to be expected in the case of as-polymerized PLLA (PLA_{100}) compounds. Indeed these compounds are highly crystalline, rather porous, and contain monomer and initiator residues since the polymerized mass is used without further purification. This raw polymer mass contains rather large crystalline spherolites that can generate a drastic late particulate inflammatory response when they are eventually released. This may present as a clinical problem (Bersgma *et al.* 1993; Gogolewski *et al.* 1993). This clinical problem cannot be generalized to bioabsorbable interference screws. In particular, screws based on purified and more or less quenched PLA_{100} should be expected to result in a smaller number of smaller residual crystallites and less of a late inflammatory response than the self-reinforced or the as-polymerized ones.

Highly purified PLA_{98} interference screws that are processed by injection molding appear to be transparent and thus highly amorphous. The initial amorphous morphology and the presence of 2 per cent

Table 7.3 Important factors that can condition the *in vivo* fate of interference screws

| Composition | *Type of PLAGA co- and/or stereo-copolymer* | | |
	Molecular weight	MW polydispersity	Co-unit distribution
		Polymerization	
Catalyst—	Residuals—		Treatment—
Tin- or Zinc-based	Monomer, catalyst, oligomers, solvent		Purified or as-polymerized
		Processing	
As-polymerized	Self-reinforced		Injection molded
		Morphology	
Amorphous			Semi-crystalline
		Sterilization	
Ethylene oxide	γ or β rays		Cold plasma
		Requirements	
Stress loading	Degradation rate		Life-time

D-lactyl units within 98 per cent L-lactyl-containing polymer chains are two features that act in favor of slightly faster degradation and formation of less and smaller crystalline residues during degradation. If zinc lactate is used as polymerization initiator, the degradable matrix is likely to be more hydrophylic and thus to be degraded slightly faster as compared with PLA_{100} screws made of PLA_{100} polymerized by stannous octanoate. Amorphous morphology, faster degradation, and a minimum of crystalline residues are to be expected from $PLA_{42.5}GA_{15}$ screws and to a smaller extent from $PLA_{85}GA_{15}$ ones. However, lower glass transition temperature and presence of GA units within the PLA chains should make the matrix more hydrophilic and thus more sensitive to aqueous media. This trend may be counterbalanced by the hydrophoby related to the use of stannous octanoate as intiator of the polymerization. PLA_{50}-based screws are likely to degrade rather fast through polymerization, but the addition of stannous octanoate may have a beneficial stabilizing effect. Table 7.3 presents the main factors one should consider if one wants to compare screws of different compositions and origins.

Conclusion

From this rapid survey of the origins, properties, and degradation characteristics of PLAGA polymers presented in this contribution, one can easily realize that commercial interference screws are likely to present different inflammatory responses, degradation rates, evolution of morphology, and formation of crystalline residues, depending on the synthesis of the polymer, its processing, the sterilization method, protocol, the storage history, and size of the implant. Better technical control of degradable interference screws and better understanding of tissue responses are two major issues for the surgeon. However, one must keep in mind that factors like implantation site or circulation of body fluids can also contribute, making the prediction of the behavior of a screw and the comparison between screws more of an art than a predicable science. The clinician must also be aware of the undesirability of PGA in ACL fixation devices and of the possibility of a late significant inflammatory response and cyst formation in some PLAGA devices.

Acknowledgements

The author thanks very much David Johnson, Consultant Orthopaedic Surgeon, St Mary's Hospital, Bristol, UK, for editing the manuscript and making some additions to the text.

References

Barber AF (1998) Resorbable fixation devices: A product guide, *Orthopaedic Special Edition*, 4, 11–17.

Bersgma EJ, Rozema FRM, Bos RR, and De Bruijn WC (1993) Foreign body reactions to resorbable poly (L-Lactide) bone plates and screws used for the fixation of unstable zygomatic fractures, *J. Oral Maxillofac. Surg.*, 51, 666–670.

Brannon-Peppas L and Vert M (2000) Polylactic and polyglycolic acids as drug delivery carriers, in LR Wise *et al.*, eds, *Handbook of Pharmaceutical Controlled Technology*, pp. 90–130, Marcel Dekkar, New York, NY.

Chabot F, Vert M, Chapelle S, and Granger P (1983) Configurational structires of lactic acid stereocopolymers as determined by 13C-1H-NMR, *Polymer*, 24, 53–59.

Cutright DE, Perez B, Beasley JD, Larson WJ, and Rosey WR (1974) Degradation rates of polymers and copolymer of polylactic and polyglycolic acids, *Oral Surg.*, 37, 142–152.

Frazza EJ and Schmitt EE (1971) A new absorbable suture, *J. Biomed. Mater. Sci.*, 1, 43–58.

Gogolewski S, Jovanovic M, Perren SM, Dillon JG, and Hughes MK (1993) Tissue response and in vivo degradation of selected polyhydroxyacids: Polylactides (PLA), poly(3-hydroxybutyrate-co-3-hydroxyvalerate) (PHB/VA), *J. Biomed. Mater. Res.*, 27, 1135–1148.

Grizzi I, Garreau H, Li S, and Vert M (1995) Biodegradation of devices based on poly(DL-lactic acid): Size dependence, *Biomaterials*, 16, 305–311.

Kleine J and Kleine H (1959) Unber hochmolekulare, insbesondere optische aktive polyester des milchsäure, ein beitrag zur stereochemie makromoilekularer verbindungen, *Makromol. Chem.*, 30, 23–38.

Kronenthal RL (1974) Biodegradable polymers in medicine and surgery, in RL Kronenthal, Z User, and E Martin, eds, '*Polymers in Medicine and Surgery*', pp. 119–137, Plenum Publishing Corp., New York, NY.

Kulkarni RK, Pani KC, Neuman C, and Leonard F (1966) Polylactic acid for surgical implants, *Arch. Surg.*, 93, 839–843.

Kulkarni RK, Moore EG, Hegyeli AF, and Leonard F (1971) Biodegradable poly(lactic acid) polymers, *J. Biomed. Mater. Res.*, 5, 169–181.

Li S and Vert M (1995) Biodegradation of aliphatic polyesters, in G Scott and D Gilead, eds, *Biodegradable Polymers, Principles and Applications*, pp. 43–87, Chapman & Hall, London.

Li S and Vert M (1999) Biodegradable polymers: Polyesters, in A Mathiowitz, ed., *The Encyclopaedia of controlled drug delivery*, pp. 71–93, J. Wiley & Sons, New York, NY.

Li S, Garreau H, and Vert M (1990a) Structure–property relationships in the case of the degradation of massive aliphatic poly-(alpha-hydroxy acids) in aqueous media: Part 1. Poly(DL-lactic acid), *J. Mat. Sci. Mat. In Med.*, 1, 123–130.

Li S, Garreau H, and Vert M (1990b) Structure–property relationships in the case of degradation of solid aliphatic poly (α-hydroxy acids) in aqueous media: 2. $PLA_{37.5}GA_{25}$ and $PLA_{75}GA_{25}$ copolymers, *J. Mat. Sci. Mat. In Med.*, 1, 131–139.

Li S, Garreau H, and Vert M (1990c) Structure–property relationships in the case of degradation of solid aliphatic poly (α-hydroxy acids) in aqueous media: 3. Amorphous and semi-crystalline PLA 100, *J. Mat. Sci. Mat. Med.*, 1, 198–206.

Lillie E and Schultz RC (1975) ^{1}H and ^{13}C–{^{1}H}–NMR spectra of stereopolymers of lactide, makromol. *Chem.*, 176, 1901–1906.

Lowe CH (1954) Preparation of high molecular weight polyhydroxyacetic ester. U.S. patent 2,668,162, Appl. March 24, 1952.

Pitt CG, Gratzel MM, Kimmel GL, Surles J, and Schindler A (1981) Aliphatic polyesters. 2. The degradation of poly(DL-lactide), poly (ϵ-caprolactone) and their complexes in vivo. *Biomaterials*, 2, 215–220.

Reed AM and Guilding DK (1981) Biodegradable polymers for use in surgery—poly(glycolic)/poly(lactic acid) homo and copolymers, *Polymer*, 22, 494–498.

Salthouse TN and Matlaga BF (1976) Polyglactin 910 suture absorption and the role of cellular enzymes, *Surg. Gynecol. Obstet.*, 142, 544–550.

Schwach G and Vert M (1999) In vitro and in vivo degradation of lactic acid-based interference screws used in cruciate ligament reconstruction, *Intern. J. Biol. Macromol.*, 25, 283–291.

Schwach G, Engel R, Coudane J and Vert M (1994) Stannous octoate versus zinc-initiated polymerization of racemic lactide: Effect of configurational structures, *Polym. Bull.*, 32, 617–623.

Sedel L, Chabot F, Christel P, de Charantenay FX, Leray J and Vert M (1978) Les implants biodégradables en chirurgie orthopédique, *Rev. Chir. Orthop.*, 64, 92–101.

Vert M (1990) Degradation of polymeric biomaterials with respect to temporary applications, in JM Anderson *et al.*, eds, *Degradable Materials*, pp. 11–37, CRC Press, Boca Raton, FL.

Vert M (2002) Polyglycolide and copolyesters with lactide in Biopolymers, in A Steinbüchel and Y Doi, eds, *Polyesters III: Applications and Commercial Products*, pp. 179–202, Wiley—VCH, Weinheim.

Vert M, Chabot F, Leray J, and Christel P (1981) Bioresorbable polyesters for bone surgery, *Makromol. Chem. Suppl.*, 5, 30–41.

Vert M, Christel P, Chabot F and Leray J (1984) Bioresorbable plastic materials for bone surgery, in GW Hastings and P Ducheyne, eds, *Macromolecular Biomaterials*, pp. 119–141, CRC Press, New York, NY.

Vert M, Li S, and Garreau H (1994) Attempts to map structure and degradation characteristics of aliphatic polyesters derived from lactic and glycolic acids, *J. Biomat. Sci., Polym. Ed.*, 6, 639–649.

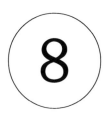

Bio-absorbable interference screws in ACL reconstruction

David P. Johnson and Jason L. Koh

Introduction

The use of bioabsorbable implants in anterior cruciate ligament (ACL) surgery has come about from various perceived advantages of such absorbable implants and the concurrent development of synthetic polymers that can be broken down by the body. These implants have been demonstrated to have initial fixation strength comparable to metallic implants, yet are radiolucent, do not interfere with magnetic resonance imaging (MRI) (Lajtai *et al.* 1999a, b), do not interfere with revision surgery, and consequently have had an expanding role in the fixation of both patellar tendon (BTB) and soft tissue grafts. Early clinical results with BTB grafts demonstrate similar outcomes to metallic implants. Limited data on soft tissue grafts such as quadrupled semitendonosis and gracilis tendons also demonstrate good outcomes, with some caveats. However, as more clinical results become available, it is becoming evident that potential disadvantages related to incomplete or inflammatory degradation may arise. Third generation bioactive implants may reduce some of these disadvantages, and theoretically could enhance early fixation and healing of the graft.

History of bioabsorbable materials

First generation biomedical materials, such as titanium interference screws or polyester suture, are designed to be biologically inert and avoid adverse reactions. Currently, second generation biomaterials are designed to produce a controlled action and reaction in the physiological environment. An example of this is absorbable suture, which is generally a polymer composed of polylactic (PLA) and polyglycolic (PGA) acids which hydrolyzes into carbon dioxide (CO_2) and water (H_2O). The use of this material in fracture fixation surgery had become routine by 1984, and prompted the development of other absorbable implants, such as plates and screws for maxillo-facial reconstruction, and in other orthopaedic applications. Rokkanen *et al.* reported in the Lancet in 1985 on early results of biodegradable fixation of ankle fractures (Rokkanen *et al.* 1985; Strycker 1995). However, the relatively rapid loss of strength of early implants made of polyglycolide (PGA) made them unsuitable for areas exposed to high mechanical stress. In addition, the rapid breakdown of this mate-rial resulted in the creation of sterile cysts in the bone adjacent to the resorbing implant. This lead to the creation of materials with a greater mechanical strength and slower rate of *in vivo* degradation, such as the various forms of polylactic acid (PLA).

Ideal characteristics of an implant

There are several characteristics that are essential for appropriate implant function. The implant must have initial sufficient mechan-ical strength to secure tissue and be able to maintain this strength for a minimum period in order to allow tissue to heal. Ideally, in the ACL reconstruction situation the strength of graft fixation should be sufficient to allow for early mobilization, weight-bearing and rehabilitation. The ideal implant will not interfere with healing process, and would not be an impediment to other procedures, or revision surgery.

Speer and Warren have stated four criteria for a bioabsorbable implant (Speer and Warren 1993):

1   it must have adequate fixation strength;
2   it must maintain strength until tissue heals adequately;
3   it should not degrade too slowly with risk of breakage/migration;
4   it should be made of completely safe materials.

Bioabsorbable implants have several theoretical advantages. The primary advantage of such materials is that after serving their func-tion, the implant would be absorbed and would therefore not be a retained foreign body that could interfere with subsequent surgery or be the cause of chemical reaction to long term retention of metal-lic implants. The graft tunnels would in the ideal situation fill in with cancellous bone over time and the knee would then be closer to a 'virgin knee' if revision tunnels for ACL reconstruction or a total knee replacement is needed. Unfortunately it is apparent that such ideal resorption and replacement does not always take place as envisaged.

Another more distinct advantage of bioabsorbable implants is that most implant materials are radiolucent and do not interfere with x-ray, computed tomography, or magnetic resonance imaging. This advantage becomes particularly important in the evaluation of sub-sequent injuries to the knee, such as meniscal tears or re-ruptures of the ACL or evaluation of degenerative changes.

Bioabsorbable screws are also reportedly less likely than metallic screws to diverge from the drill channel when inserted alongside the graft in an interference fit situation. Metallic, sharp edged screws are able to cut a divergent path through bone easier than softer threaded bioabsorbable screws.

There are also advantages that are particular to the fixation of soft tissue grafts. The threads of the screw maybe less likely to cut the fibers of soft tissue grafts than those of metallic screws. This allows direct compression of the graft against the side of a bone tunnel, which may provide a more direct type of tendon to bone healing than fixation at the end of the tunnels (Weiler *et al.* 2002a). Interference screw fixation allows fixation closer to the joint line than external or cortical fixation such as button, endo-button or staple fixation. This may decrease the 'windshield wiper' effect of cortical fixation and reduce the tunnel expansion over time. The use of such absorbable screws has been shown in clinical experience to reduce tunnel expansion of hamstring grafts (Simonain *et al.* 2001).

Basic science of bioabsorbables

Degradation of current bioabsorbable implants is by hydrolysis of the implant material into water and carbon dioxide through the citric acid cycle. The process of hydrolysis of the polymer releases the individual breakdown products, some of which are acidic and potentially detrimental to the healing process. Several studies have reported adverse reactions to various absorbable implants, including foreign-body reaction, synovitis, sterile cyst formation, osteolysis, and seromas. The adverse reactions may be related to the rate of hydrolysis and rapid breakdown of the material. The crystallinity of the material, and the isomeric composition of the material has a significant effect on reducing the rate of hydrolysis, breakdown and cyst formation. Different chemicals or isomers of the same chemical composition may behave in very different ways. This is utilized to modify the characteristics of each individual type of screw.

Once hydrolysis takes effect degradation and fragmentation may also occur. Degradation results in the fragmentation of the implant into particles that are phagocytosed, primarily by macrophages. The resultant inflammatory response is related to the number of particles released over a period of time. A more rapid degradation may therefore be associated with more inflammation. Crystallinity may play an important role in the reactivity of the body to biodegradable implants. Crystalline breakdown products have been implicated in synovitis similar to that seen in crystalline inflammatory arthropathies such as gout. A foreign body reaction has been noted to occur in response to highly crystalline PLA fragments from plates used in facial reconstruction (Bergsma *et al.* 1995; Menche *et al.* 1999). They suggested that a lower crystallinity may provoke less of a reaction. In addition, it has been suggested that higher crystallinity may result in a more brittle screw that is more easily fractured during insertion (Fink *et al.* 2000). Crystalline particles have been found in lymph nodes distant to the original site of implantation (Stahelin *et al.* 1995), and could trigger a systemic inflammatory response.

Various materials have been used for absorbable screw implants for ACL reconstruction. These include polyglycolide (PGA); poly-L-lactide (PLLA) and poly-D,L-lactide (PDLLA). Additionally, PGA has been used in conjunction with trimethylene carbonate (TMC), and PDLLA with calcium phosphate (hydroxyapatite, or HA). The amount of crystallinity of the implants also varies considerably, from 60 per cent to almost zero (amorphous). The net result is that the degradation characteristics of these screws vary considerably, with some significantly absorbed by 3–6 months (PGA-TMC, PDLLA-co-PGA), and others remaining intact for up to 3–5 years, and potentially longer (PDLLA). The tissue that replaces the screw also is quite variable, ranging from loose granulation tissue or inflammatory tissue, to more organized connective tissue and bone. Bioabsorbable screws therefore must not be assumed to behave in a similar manner and different types have markedly different characteristics on insertion and degradation.

Clinical results of absorbable implants

Polyglycolide acid (PGA) was one of the first bioabsorbable polymers used for orthopaedic implants (Ciccione *et al.* 2001). The most well-known and popular use was in a bioabsorbable tack for shoulder repair (Suretac, Smith and Nephew Endoscopy). This polymer was noted to have a relatively short half-life, losing approximately 50 per cent of its strength in a period of 2–4 weeks. Several authors have noted adverse reactions to this device, including an incidence of synovitis of the shoulder joint, and osteolysis around the implant (Edwards *et al.* 1994; Burkart *et al.* 2000). Several orthopaedic implants for knee reconstruction use PGA, including a PGA-trimethylene carbonate (TMC) implant (Endofix, Smith and Nephew Endoscopy) and PGA-PLA 15/85 copolymer (Bioscrew). These products have a relatively rapid period of hydrolysis of the implant. PGA screws in a rabbit osteotomy model (Bostman 1992a) were shown to have minimal invasion of connective tissue into the polymer at six weeks, and by 12 weeks, had erosion of the thread and replacement by connective tissue. At 36 weeks, the screw had completely degraded, and had been replaced by connective tissue, new bone, or loose granulation tissue. Bostman has variously reported on the clinical and histological use of such PGA fixation devices in clinical ankle proactive fixation (Bostman *et al.* 1990; Bostman *et al.* 1992b; Bostman *et al.* 1995; Bostman 1998). Walton (1999) reported on a PGA-TMC screw (Endofix) that was tested in a sheep model of bone-tendon-bone (BTB) healing. By four weeks, the failure load of the BTB construct was equivalent whether or not the screw was present. The screw did demonstrate significant degeneration. The failure strength of the bioabsorbable screw was lower initially but not statistically different than metallic screws. A mild reaction occurred around the screw, and in specimens sacrificed at 12 months the screw was largely replaced by fibrous tissue. A clinical study of 20 patients (Fink *et al.* 2000) who underwent follow-up CT scanning of the knee found degradation of the implant to be significant from six weeks to three months. Only minimal fragments were seen at six months, and none were detected at a year. No adverse reactions were noted at the screw sites. However, the screw was never replaced by bone in follow-up scans up to three years postoperatively. The replacement tissue had the density of loose granulation tissue. Benedetto *et al.* reported clinical results of this screw with 1 year follow-up in a randomized trial in comparison to metallic screws (Benedetto *et al.* 2000). The clinical results were statistically identical (92 per cent normal/nearly normal in Endo-Fix vs. 90 per cent metallic) at 12 months. There were no instances of screw breakage, which the authors attributed to pre-tapping of the tunnel. In 5 cases out of 67, the tap caused some injury (minor lacerations in three, and medial femoral condyle damage in two), although the metallic screw caused laceration in one case. One patient had a subcutaneous cyst develop at six months at the site of a tibial absorbable screw, but this resolved spontaneously within three months and the patient had an 'A' IKDC score at 12 month follow-up. No tunnel widening was seen on x-ray at 12 months.

Initial reports on a copolymer 85/15 D,L lactide/glycolide composite screw (Biologically Quiet Screw, Instrument Makar, Okemos, MI) were provided by Johnson. He reported good clinical results equal to those seen with a metallic screw (Johnson 1995). Lajtai has reported on this screw at 2.5 and 5 year follow-up (Lajtai *et al.* 2001). The initial report demonstrated breakdown of the screw by 12 months, with some adjacent bone edema and fluid collection in the proximal femoral bone tunnel. The edema was felt to be normal postoperative reaction to the surgery, and resolved without sequelae by the five year follow-up. The fluid collection was described as a 'container phenomenon' related to liquid trapped in the femoral tunnel by walls of compacted bone. Again, these collections resolved without sequelae. There was also some early bone tunnel enlargement, which was felt to be associated with the breakdown of the screw. Bone tunnel enlargement did not appear to have any clinical significance, and in most cases was followed by gradual remodeling and filling in of the tunnel with new tissue. The neoligament soft tissue did not remodel. The OAK, IKDC, and Lysholm scores were greater than 90 per cent good-excellent results, and were felt to be comparable to metallic screws in securing BTB grafts. Of particular interest is that these screws were replaced by bone on follow-up MRI.

Canine studies of this implant had previously demonstrated that the screw retained material properties for three weeks and was dissolved and replaced by bone at six months. The authors stated that the retention of strength for four weeks was sufficient to permit adequate bone-to-bone healing of the graft in the tunnel. It is unclear whether this is sufficient length of time to permit tendon to bone healing if this was used to secure hamstring tendon grafts. There has been one report of spontaneous extrusion of this screw (Stahelin *et al.* 1995). A patient developed a draining sinus two days post-operatively from the tibial screw site and returned to the office three weeks post-op with the screw in an envelope. Arthroscopy showed an intact patella tendon-bone plug graft and no adverse sequelae were noted. Recurrent effusions resolved by three months postoperatively, and may have been related to the implanted femoral screw. These authors felt that the rapid breakdown of the co-polymer screw led to good replacement by bone, but also led to the consequences of rapid hydrolysis, and an inflammatory reaction that resulted in local cyst formation, seroma and eventual extrusion of the material.

Polylactide (PLA) has been a popular material for use in absorbable interference screws, due to its relatively longer half-life than PGA and its superior mechanical properties. This material comes in L and D isomers, which have significantly different degradation characteristics. The D isomer (PDLA) resorbs in a period of several months, whereas the L isomer (PLLA) degrades very slowly and may take years to break down. There have been no reports describing the full degradation of PLLA screws in humans. PLLA interference screws have been demonstrated to remain macroscopically intact in some cases at least up to 2.5 years postoperatively.

PDLA screws have been used in Europe (Sysorb, Synos Medical AG, Niederwangen, Bern, Switzerland) and have been shown to degrade by 10 months postoperatively and be replaced by bone. A recent study by Weiler demonstrated in a sheep model that the screw degraded by 24 weeks and was at least partially replaced by bone (Weiler *et al.* 2002b). The attachment of the tendon graft to bone was similar to the direct insertion that is seen in a normal ACL. However, limited clinical data is available in the English language literature.

PLLA screws (BioScrew, Linvatec, Largo, FL, and Arthrex, Naples, FL) have been used extensively in the United States and elsewhere. Initial reports with the Linvatec Bioscrew demonstrated excellent clinical results equivalent to those seen using metallic screws to fix bone-patella tendon-bone grafts. Specifically, Barber (1995) reported good clinical results; with statistically equivalent outcomes for the absorbable and metal screws. He also noted a 7 per cent incidence of screw breakage, with no adverse sequelae despite need for removal of screw fragments. There were no problems with osteolysis or cyst formation. A control patient with metallic screw fixation experienced tunnel widening, which was not seen in with the PLLA screw. McGuire (McGuire *et al.* 1999) reported excellent clinical results in a follow-up multicenter study, with

Lysholm scores of 95.0 and 97.2 for the Bioscrew and metal screw, respectively. The Tegner activity level score means were Bioscrew, 6.1 and metal, 5.8. Barber also reported in 2000 on this multicenter group with similar results (Barber 2000; Barber *et al.* 2000).

Barber (1999) also reported on the use of the Bioscrew in securing a tripled semitendinosus-autologous tendon graft with additional cancellous bone plug in ACL reconstruction. This population was relatively older (mean age 38) and was followed for a mean of 29 months. The manual maximum KT difference was 2.9 mm, and 2/22 knees had a pivot shift. No complications were noted with respect to the Bioscrew. Warden (Warden *et al.* 1999) found that the screw remained visible on MRI scans in 19/20 cases at two years, with the one screw that dissolved having cracked on insertion. Abnormal signal was noted in two cases (in the tibia and in the graft) but this resolved without adverse sequelae. All knees were clinically stable with a negative Lachman on manual testing.

Kotani and Ishii (2001) also reported equivalent clinical results between metal and PLLA screws in the clinical outcomes of patients treated with a patella tendon graft. No adverse events such as synovitis or abnormal biochemical findings in the blood were seen. Little clinical data is available for the Arthrex bioabsorbable screw.

Limited breakdown data is available on PLLA screws. McGuire (McGuire *et al.* 2001) reported on a four month post-mortem specimen that demonstrated showed no evidence of tunnel widening, lytic bone changes, or inflammatory or foreign body reaction. Several authors have noted that PLLA screws have extended degradation times. Martinek (Martinek *et al.* 2001) reported on screws that retained their normal configuration up to 2.5 years postoperatively. The screw was removed in fragments; there was no evidence of replacement by native tissue. Stahelin *et al.* (1997) reported that a PLLA screw had partially degraded, but that large fragments remained. There are no published reports demonstrating complete degradation of this type of screw.

PLA98 (98 per cent PLLA, 2 per cent PDLA, Phusis, SA) screws have been used in Europe with good clinical results. However, animal studies have demonstrated persistence of these screws for several years in a sheep model, and also evidence of multiple crystalline fragments which may remain long term in the tissues (Therin *et al.* 1996). In vivo evaluation of this bioabsorbable interference screw (98 per cent p1LA, 2 per cent PDLLA) in sheep led the investigators to conclude that the long term presence of these breakdown products was potentially worrisome.

Hamstring graft fixation

Clinical results of hamstring ACL reconstruction with bioabsorbable screws presents a different situation to that of BTB reconstruction. Although a number of biomechanical studies have been conducted with absorbable screw fixation of soft tissue grafts, there have been few published reports on the clinical use of these screws for hamstring graft fixation in ACL reconstruction (Houle and Johnson 1998). The clinical reports have noted generally good results, but have focused on tunnel widening. Conflicting results have been reported on tunnel widening. Simonian (Simonian *et al.* 2001) noted good clinical results and a decrease in tunnel widening with an absorbable screw used to fix a hamstring graft. Beulow (Beulow *et al.* 2000, 2002) reported good results, and that the placement of the screw can cause bone compaction and tunnel widening, followed by eventual stabilization of tunnel size. Both studies have noted that there was no correlation between clinical outcomes and radiographic tunnel widening. More recent studies analyzing the fixation strength of soft tissue hamstring grafts with bioabsorbable screws have raised some concerns (Liew and Johnson 2000; Scheffler *et al.* 2002 and Becker *et al.* 2001).

The initial strength and stiffness of bioabsorbable screw fixation of hamstring grafts was shown to be significantly less than BTB graft fixation or following use of metallic screws (Magen *et al.* 1999). The deterioration in fixation strength and stiffness over the first four weeks in soft tissue tendon graft fixation with bioabsorbable screws was shown to be 63 and 40 per cent. After four weeks the screws only contributed 6 per cent of the fixation strength and 40 per cent of the stiffness (Singhatat *et al.* 2002). As in other studies the authors questioned the use of bioabsorbable screw fixation for hamstring graft fixation. Further, the safety of using a rapid rehabilitation program in such patients has been shown to result in an unacceptable incidence of late laxity by Barber (1999), who reported a clinical study in which there was a 65 per cent incidence of a KT arthrometer measurement greater than 3 mm side to side difference after two years.

Biomechanical evaluation of bioabsorbable screws

Biomechanical evaluation of bioabsorbable interference screws has been conducted with both bone-patella tendon-bone grafts and soft tissue grafts (Laitinen *et al.* 1993; Seil *et al.* 1998). These have generally shown satisfactory initial fixation strength in securing the grafts. In consideration of the numerous reports one must be careful in comparing similar size of screws. Often the same study will compare screws of different types but not standardize the size of screw analysed. Kousa (Kousa *et al.* 1995; Kousa *et al.* 2001b) reported on the fixation strength of a 6.3 mm PLLA screw in securing a bone-patella tendon-bone (BTB) graft in calf bone, and found excellent failure strength (1211 N). Pena (Pena *et al.* 1996) reported that in young and middle-aged human cadaver specimens, metal interference screws had significantly higher insertional torque and pull-out strength compared to bioabsorbable screws. The mean failure load for the metal screws (mean 640 N; SD 201) was significantly higher than for the absorbable screws (mean 418 N; SD 118) in these specimens.

The authors expressed some concern about the potential for failure, since some studies have estimated that the loads on the ACL during activities of daily living in the 500 N range. However, the clinical results from McGuire using an accelerated rehabilitation protocol demonstrated no graft slippage, increased laxity or early failures. Therefore for practical use the forces on the graft-screw construct may not require fixation strength above the 500 N range.

In his experiments Rupp (Rupp *et al.* 1999) found different maximum loads to failure for different screws. The mean load for titanium and the Linvatec screws was 785 N and 844 N, respectively, which was significantly higher ($P < 0.05$) than that of the Acufex (555 N), and Arthrex (592 N) screws. Johnson (Johnson and van Dyke 1996) compared 9 mm metal and bioabsorbable interference screws and found no significant difference, with the mean strength of the metal screw approximately 130 N higher (565 vs. 436 N). Abbate (1998) tested two types of bioabsorbable screw designs in calf bone (standard and wedge) and found that fixation strength of the standard design was equivalent to a metallic screw. In one example, the mean strength of a 9×30 standard design PLA screw was 914.4 N, vs. 733.2 N for a metal screw. Hoffman (1999) demonstrated equivalent fixation strengths of the Sysorb screw compared to a metal screw for securing a flipped patella tendon-bone graft.

Rittmeister and others have commented that soft tissue grafts secured either by bioabsorbable or metallic screws fail by pull-out of the soft tissue adjacent to the screw and tunnel side Rittmeister (Kousa *et al.* 2001b; Rittmeister *et al.* 2002). The screws themselves remained in the tunnel and did not significantly move. Weiler (Weiler *et al.* 1998a, 1998b) found that the Sysorb screw was significantly stronger (roughly 100 N) than the titanium RCI screw in securing hamstring grafts in calf bone. The pull-out strength was further significantly increased (approximately +200 N) if a bone plug was at the end of the harvested graft, preventing the slippage of the tendon graft beyond the screw. A follow-up study by the same group (Weiler *et al.* 2002a) using cyclic loading demonstrated that hamstring ACL fixation was significantly improved by 'anatomic' fixation (i.e. with screws adjacent to the joint line) when compared to external or cortical suspensory fixation with linkage devices such as suture. This also has the benefit of preventing toggling of the graft within the tunnel and may reduce tunnel widening. However, Weiler cautioned that the graft could migrate beyond the screw and again suggested that a bone plug or other supplementary fixation could be used to back up the fixation (Weiler *et al.* 2002b). They have developed a bioabsorbable 'endopearl' to be sewn onto the end of the graft, which significantly improves pull-out in cyclic loading studies (Nagarkatti *et al.* 2001; Weiler *et al.* 2001). Rittmeister (Rittmeister *et al.* 2002; Harding *et al.* 2002) also found that the majority of graft failure (92 per cent) was from slippage of the tendon past the graft. Don Johnson (Personal communication 2002) has in hamstring graft fixation compared the clinical use of the endopearl and a bone plug, and has not noted any significant difference in the early clinical outcomes.

Caborn and Brand demonstrated that bone density and insertional torque are related to the pull-out strength of the screw-graft construct (Caborn et al. 1994; Caborn et al. 1998; Brand et al. 2000a; Brand et al. 2000b; Caborn and Selby 2002). Selby has also found that increased screw length improved pull-out strength (Selby et al. 2001). However, Stadelmaier found that a 7×25 and 7×40 mm screw had similar pull-out strengths (Stadelmaier et al. 1999). Weiler (Weiler et al. 2000) found that increasing the diameter of the screw (graft + 1 mm) improved the pull-out strength by over 30 per cent. They found that increasing the length from 23 to 28 mm increased pull-out by 46 per cent. Rittmeister (Rittmeister et al. 2001) has found that tunnel dilation has increased pull-out strength only minimally (11 per cent).

In summary most of the biomechanical studies have reported a slightly reduced initial fixation strength, insertional torque and pull-out strength with bioabsobable screws as compared to comparable metal screws (Imhoff et al. 1997). However the difference is not thought to result in a significant reduction with the initial strength adequate for a normal rapid rehabilitation protocol. Generally the reports show that the larger the screw used the greater the initial fixation strength. The strength of fixation in the tibia is in general less than that in the oblique femoral tunnel. This is due to the nature of the cancellous bone in the upper tibial and the tunnel alignment along the line of the ACL graft compared with the oblique alignment of the femoral tunnel. Therefore in light of the data available it is recommended that a larger 9 mm bioabsorbable screw is always used for tibial fixation.

Complications

Complications of the use of bioabsorbable fixation devices are related either to the initial screw implantation, to clinical failure of healing/graft security or to the long term sequelae of the degradation of the screw material.

The most commonly noted complication with bioabsorbable screws is of screw breakage during insertion. The material of bioabsorbable implants is weaker than metal, and design of the screws and the screw driver that were developed for metallic implants are not necessarily appropriate for bioabsorbable materials. Failures can occur of the screw (screw fracture, either by splitting radially or transverse fracture), at the driver-screw interface (screw stripping), or of the driver itself (bending of the driver). Any of these types of failure can result in a significant complication intra-operatively. Such failures can result in loose bodies, inadequate graft fixation, and inability to remove or revise the implant.

A number of factors contribute to initial screw strength and security during insertion. These include the material of the screw, width and length of the screw, design of the screw tip, pitch, core diameter, drive system, and insertion instrumentation and technique. Some authors have attributed screw breakage to the crystalline nature of certain polymers used. However, screw design appears to play a significant role in the overall strength of the screw during insertion. In particular the design of the screw driver profile and its engagement in the internal slot in the screw is important. The corners of the screw driver may result in stress risers in the screw material and result in cracks and breakage of the screws. Clinically, it has been noted that tapping and/or notching the screw path has decreased the incidence of screw breakage.

The modes of screw failure has been tested by Weiler and Costi using screws either fully or half imbedded in resin (Weiler *et al.* 2000; Costi *et al.* 2001). The failures have been related to the design of the driver. A driver with a turbine profile produces less stress within the screw, and is less likely to lead to cracks or breakages than a trilobed, trigonal, hexagonal, torx or rectangular designs. The hexagonal and torx screws were found to have mean torque of failure close to mean peak insertional torque, and Weiler stated that this 'may present a risk of drive failure during insertion' (Weiler *et al.* 2000). Costi *et al.*, using half-imbedded screws, have similarly demonstrated that these modes of failure are within the torque levels needed for insertion of the screw (Costi *et al.* 2001).

Particularly with these implants, tapping of the screw channel may be important for the use of bioabsorbable screws, unlike less fragile, self-cutting metallic screws. However, tapping itself may create abnormal channels, damage the medial femoral condyle, or lacerate the graft, as often seen in the clinical situation. Many of these insertional complications can be avoided by two simple modifications in the surgical technique. First, the tunnel is tapped to receive the screw before insertion. This may only be for part of the depth as once the thread engages in the tunnel the insertion usually proceeds without further problems. Second, it is important to ensure that the screw driver is maintained in a position whereby it is fully inserted throughout the length of the screw, and that this position is maintained throughout the insertion of the screw.

Another complication noted in the early postoperative phase is the development of a fluid collection at the end of the tunnel (Lataj *et al.* 1999a). This has been attributed to a 'container phenomenon' associated with the use of dilators to form the femoral tunnel. However the reports suggest that these collections quickly resolve without sequlae.

Tunnel widening has been reported with the use of hamstring grafts and with cortical or suspensory fixation. Tunnel widening has been noted in soft tissue grafts undergoing endpoint fixation, such as with staples or Endobutton. No relationship to clinical outcomes with tunnel widening has ever been noted. However several authors have noted the development of apparent tunnel widening on radiographs following the use of bioabsorbable screws (Loubignac *et al.* 1998). This may be related to the breakdown of the screw prior to replacement with tissue, the 'windshield wiper' effect of the graft in the tunnel, or simply to dilation of the tunnel by the interference screw in soft tibial bone. Other authors such as Simonian have demonstrated that bioabsorbable screws may actually decrease tunnel widening, possibly by decreasing the motion of the graft in the tunnel (Simonian *et al.* 2001).

The longer term complications are related to the hydration, disintegration, and absorption of the screw material. Fragments of the screw material have been noted to create symptomatic loose bodies which may mimic meniscal pathology or cause articular cartilage damage (Bottoni *et al.* 2000). This has been more common with the use of bioabsorbable implants for osteochondral lesions, but has been reported with absorbable interference screws. Several authors have reported the development of sterile cysts around the screw. In some cases the cyst failed to resorb. Alternately a discharging seroma or sterile sinus may form. This has been felt to be a reaction to the breakdown products of the bioabsorbable screw. Rarely, more severe cases of osteolysis (Martinek *et al.* 1999) or reaction have occurred, resulting in the extrusion of the screw. The histology is usually one of a sterile inflammatory reaction. Patients have also developed postoperative effusions following the use of absorbable implants. Typically these spontaneously resolve, but there is a possibility of a mild inflammatory synovitis with the use of such implants (Friden and Rydholm 1992).

Other bioabsorbable materials

Interference screws made of processed cortical bone have been created and are commercially available. Little clinical or animal data is available but it is reasonable to presume that as long as there is not chemical reaction to the processing these screws would function like normal bone grafts. Clinical reports of their use have been confined to a small series that demonstrated satisfactory results, however the brittle nature of the screws resulted in several cases of screw breakage.

Third generation absorbable screws are now commercially available from several companies (Bi-Lok – Atlantech, Harrogate, UK , Alaron; Bio-RCI – Smith and Nephew Endoscopy Andover, MA, USA, Biocryl – Mitek Johnson and Johnson, Norwood, MA, USA) that combine PLA and tri-calcium phosphate. These screws may have several unique advantages. The hydroxyapatite crystals are osteoconductive, which may stimulate bone ingrowth and promote a more rapid rate of healing of tendon to bone or bone to bone, and therefore improve the early fixation strength. This is in contrast to the osteo-neutral or inhibitory effect of many other bioabsorbable screws. The calcium phosphate also acts as a pH buffering agent in decreasing the acidity of the environment (Agrawal *et al.* 1996). The breakdown products of the polylactic acid material are acidic, this may be related to the incidence of cyst formation and osteolysis around the resorbing material. Tri-calcium phosphate acts as a buffer which may reduce the incidence of such complications. The osteoconductive nature of the tri-calcium phosphate crystals may also stimulate replacement of the screw with bone rather than soft tissue and therefore restore the integrity of the tunnel. This may be helpful if a revision of the graft were ever necessary.

The strength and stiffness properties of the Bi-Lok PLA-TCP screw are reported to match those of human bone. The surface of the screw is slightly roughened with a porous texture when compared to the all-PLLA screws. This rougher surface with its relatively higher coefficient of friction may decrease slippage of soft tissue grafts past the screw, and therefore may also increase the pull-out strength.

Tuompo *et al.* have presented biomechanical evidence with respect to a novel bioabsorbable expanding plug made of PLLA (Tuompo *et al.* 1996). This device demonstrates equivalent fixation strength to interference screw fixation in a bovine cadaver model. However, in a clinical study he found that a 'fixation with expansion plug seems technically more challenging, with a tendency to inferior results compared to screw fixation' (Tuompo *et al.* 1999). Sherman has reported on a wedge-shaped PGA-TMC interference device for bone plug fixation. Biomechanical testing demonstrated good pull-out strength, and presented clinical results with the device have been comparable to interference screw fixation (Sherman *et al.* 2001).

Another method of fixation which is particularly applicable to soft tissue grafts is a cross-pin fixation across the tunnel. Absorbable cross-pin implants for bone and soft tissue fixation are currently available from several companies (Rigid-Fix, Mitek Westwood, MA, USA; and Bio-Trans-Fix, Arthrex). These implants seek to obtain the benefits of rigid fixation and circumferential bone growth. Little biomechanical and clinical data is available on these pins (made of PLLA) but histological data from the manufacturer demonstrates good bone ingrowth in a circumferential pattern. The biomechanical properties of the absorbable cross-pin construct may have similar strength and stiffness characteristics to tested metal cross-pins. Our clinical results in over 40 patients with the use of a bioabsorbable cross-pin system to secure a doubled semi-tendinosus/ gracillis graft have demonstrated a restoration of stability and no adverse reactions that can be attributed to this device (JLK). No graft failures or excessive laxity has been found in this cohort of patients with relatively short (one year) follow-up. Further data is being collected.

Future areas of research include the creation of artificial ligaments, and the addition of bioactive substances such as osteoinductive agents or growth factors to existing implants. Several attempts to build absorbable ligaments with woven PLLA and braided swine intestinal submucosa strands have been attempted; however, none of these devices are currently in any clinical trials. An artificial, bioabsorbable ligament replacement or scaffold may eventually be a graft choice that would avoid donor-site morbidity and risk of allograft disease transmission (Lin *et al.* 1999).

Clinical recommendations

The material of a bioabsorbable screw should allow for appropriate degradation and replacement with bone in a reasonable period of time after the graft is securely healed. For bone plug grafts, this is probably some time after four weeks. For soft tissue grafts, the implant should maintain its material properties for at least eight weeks. Eventual degradation and replacement is more important with interference screws than for cross-pins, due to the potential difficulties with revising an enlarged, cystic or osteolytic bone tunnel.

The use of a tap prior to the insertion of an absorbable screw in securing a bone plug is suggested to reduce the chance of screw or driver failure. This is probably not necessary in securing a soft tissue graft. Instead, for soft tissue fixation we would recommend sizing the diameter of the screw to be line to line (same size as the tunnel) on the femoral side due to its relatively dense bone. On the tibial side, the screw diameter should be 1 mm larger than graft/tunnel size, and both screws should be at least 28 mm in length in the fixation of soft tissue grafts. Use of a cortical disk or supplementary suspensory double fixation may be considered to decrease the chance of failure under cyclic load. Alternatively, absorbable cross-pins may provide strong and stiff graft fixation, and is the preferred choice of one of us (JLK) for hamstring ACL reconstruction. In BTB graft fixation tapping is more appropriate to allow the soft absorbable screw to engage its thread. Femoral fixation with a 7 mm screw is adequate and comparable to hamstring fixation strength. On the tibial side a 9 mm screw is advised due to the generally lower tibial fixation strength.

Conclusions

Bioabsorbable implants used in ACL reconstruction have demonstrated excellent clinical results equivalent to non-absorbable implants. These implants, in the form of absorbable screws, wedges, and transfixion devices, have been successfully used in bone-tendon-bone and soft tissue reconstructions with minimal complications. They have distinct advantages compared to non-absorbable implants, particularly in repeat imaging, and avoid some of the complications associated with metal implants in revision situations. There have been several specific complications noted that are unique to bioabsorbable implants, but these have been reported primarily as case reports. However, it is clear that not all bioabsorbable implants have similar degradation and replacement characteristics. This may result in more difficulty in revising these reconstructions. However, newer implants made with osteoconductive and bioactive materials may stimulate appropriate healing and reduce the possibility of long term complications. Eventually, bioabsorbable implants may be used to replace the ACL itself, eliminating donor-site morbidity and risk of allograft disease transmission.

References

Abate JA.III, Fadale PD, Hulstyn MJ, Walsh WR (1998). Initial fixation strength of polylactic acid interference screws in anterior cruciate ligament reconstruction. *Arthroscopy* 14(3):278–84.

Agrawal CM, Fan M, Zhu C, Athanasiou KA (1996). A new technique to control the pH in the vicinity of biodegradeable implants. Fifth World Biomaterials Congress May 29–June 2 1996, Toronto, Canada.

Barber FA, Elrod BF, McGuire DA, Paulos LE (1995). Preliminary results of an absorbable interference screw. *Arthroscopy* 11(5):537–48.

Barber FA (1999). Tripled semitendinosus-cancellous bone anterior cruciate ligament reconstruction with bioscrew fixation. *Arthroscopy* 15(4):360–7.

Barber FA (2000). Flipped patellar tendon autograft anterior cruciate ligament reconstruction. *Arthroscopy* 16(5):483–90.

Barber FA, Elrod BF, McGuire DA, Paulos LE (2000). Bioscrew fixation of patellar tendon autografts. *Biomaterials* 21(24):2623–9.

Becker R, Voigt D, Starke C, Heymann M, Wilson GA, Nebelung W (2001). Biomechanical properties of quadruple tendon and patellar tendon femoral fixation techniques. *Knee Surg Sports Traumatol Arthrosc* 9(6):337–42.

Benedetto KP, Fellinger M, Lim TE, Passler JM, Schoen JL, Willems WJ (2000). A new bioabsorbable interference screw: Preliminary results of a prospective, multicenter, randomized clinical trial. *Arthroscopy* 16(1):41–8.

Bergsma JE, de Bruijn WC, Rozema FR, Bos RRM, Boering G (1995). Late degradation tissue response to poly(L-lactide) bone plates and screws. *Biomaterials* 16:25–31.

Bostman O, Hirvensalo E, Makinen J, Rokkanen P (1990). Foreign body reactions to fracture fixation implants of biodegradable synthetic polymers. *J Bone Joint Surg Br* 72:592–6.

Bostman O, Paivarinta U, Partio E, Vasenius J, Manninen M, Rokkanen P (1992a). Degradation and tissue replacement of an absorbable polyglycolide screw in the fixation of rabbit femoral osteotomies. *J Bone Joint Surg Am* 74(7):1021–31.

Bostman OM (1992b). Intense granulomatous inflammatory lesions associated with absorbable internal fixation devices made of polyglycolide in ankle fractures. *Clinical Orthopaedics & Related Research* May (278):193–9.

Bostman O, Pihalajamaki U, Partio EK, Rokkanen PU (1995). Clinical biocompatibility and degradation of polylevolactide screws in the ankle. *Clin Ortho Rel Res* 320:101–9.

Bostman OM (1998). Osteoarthritis of the ankle after foreign-body reaction to absorbable pins and screws: a three- to nine-year follow-up study. *J Bone Joint Surg Br* 80(2):333–8.

Bottoni CR, DeBerardino TM, Fester EW, Mitchell D, Penrod B (2000). An intra-articular bioabsorbable interference screw mimicking an acute meniscal tear 8 months after an anterior cruciate ligament reconstruction. *Arthroscopy* 16(4):395–8.

Brand JC, Jr., Pienkowski D, Steenlage E, Hamilton D, Johnson DL, Caborn DNM (2000a). Interference screw fixation strength of a quadrupled hamstring tendon graft is directly related to bone mineral density and insertion torque. *Am J Sports Med* 28:705–10.

Brand J Jr., Weiler A, Caborn DNM, Brown CH Jr., Johnson DL (2000b). Graft fixation in cruciate ligament reconstruction. *Am J Sports Med* 28:761–74.

Buelow JU, Siebold R, Ellermann A (2000). A new bicortical tibial fixation technique in anterior cruciate ligament reconstruction with quadruple hamstring graft. *Knee Surg Sports Traumatol Arthrosc* 8(4):218–25.

Buelow JU, Siebold R, Ellermann A (2002). A prospective evaluation of tunnel enlargement in anterior cruciate ligament reconstruction with hamstrings: Extracortical versus anatomical fixation. *Knee Surgery, Sports Traumatology, Arthroscopy* 10(2):80–5.

Burkart A, Imhoff AB, Roscher E (2000). Foreign-body reaction to the bioabsorbable suretac device. *Arthroscopy* 16(1):91–95.

Caborn DNM, Urban WP Jr., Johnson DL, Nyland J, Pienkowski D (1994). Biomechanical comparison between bioscrew and titanium interference screws for bone-patellar tendon-bone graft fixation in anterior cruciate ligament reconstruction. *Arthroscopy* 13:229–32.

Caborn DNM, Coen M, Neef R, Hamilton D, Nyland J, Johnson DL (1998). Quadrupled semitendinosus-gracilis autograft fixation in the femoral tunnel: A comparison between a metal and a bioabsorbable interference screw. *Arthroscopy* 14(3):241–5.

Caborn DNM, Selby JB (2002). Allograft anterior tibialis tendon with bioabsorbable interference screw fixation in anterior cruciate ligament reconstruction. *Arthroscopy* 18(1):102–5.

Ciccione WJ II, Motz C, Bentley C, Tasto JP (2001). Bioabsorbable implants in orthopaedics: new developments and applications. *J Am Acad Orthop Surg* 9(5):280–8.

Costi JJ, Kelly AJ, Hearn TC, Martin DK (2001). Comparison of torsional strengths of bioabsorbable screws for anterior cruciate ligament reconstruction. *Am J Sports Med* 29:575–80.

Edwards DJ, Hay G, Saies AD, Hayes MG (1994). Adverse reactions to an absorbable shoulder fixation device. *J Shoulder Elbow Surg* 3:230–3.

Fink C, Benedetto KP, Hackl W, Hoser C, Freund MC, Rieger M (2000). Bioabsorbable polyglyconate interference screw fixation in anterior cruciate ligament reconstruction: A prospective computed tomography-controlled study. *Arthroscopy* 16(5):491–8.

Friden T, Rydholm U (1992). Severe aseptic synovitis of the knee after biodegradable internal fixation. A case report. *Acta Orthop Scand* 63(1):94–7.

Griffith LG, Naughton G (2002). Tissue engineering – current challenges and expanding opportunities. *Science* 295:1009–13.

Harding N, Barber FA, Herbert MA (2002). The effect of the EndoPearl on soft-tissue graft fixation. *J Knee Surg* 15(3):150–4.

Hoffmann RF, Peine R, Bail HJ, Sudkamp NP, Weiler A (1999). Initial fixation strength of modified patellar tendon grafts for anatomic fixation in anterior cruciate ligament reconstruction. *Arthroscopy* 15(4):392–9.

Houle JB, Johnson DH (1998). Comparison of intra-operative AP translation of two different modes of fixation of the semitendinosis graft used in ACL reconstruction. *J Bone Joint Surg Br* 80-B (Supp II): 137.

Imhoff AB, Marti C, Romero J (1997). Interference fixation in ACL-reconstruction: Metal versus bioabsorbable screws – A prospective study. *J Bone Joint Surg Br* 79-B (Supp II):190.

Johnson LL (1995). Comparison of bioabsorbable and metal interference screws in anterior cruciate ligament reconstruction: A clinical trial. Procs. AAOSM, San Francisco.

Johnson LL, van Dyke GE (1996). Metal and bioabsorbable interference screw: Comparison of failure strength. *Arthroscopy* 12: 452–6.

Johnson DH, Bessette B (2002). ACL reconstruction with hamstring and bio-interference screws. ACL Study Group, Big Sky, Montana.

Kotani A, Ishii Y (2001). Reconstruction of the anterior cruciate ligament using poly-L-lactide interference screws or titanium screws: A comparative study. *Knee* 8(4):311–15.

Kousa P, Jarvinen TL, Pohjonen T, Kannus P, Kotikoski M, Jarvinen M (1995). Fixation strength of a biodegradable screw in anterior cruciate ligament reconstruction. *J Bone Joint Surg Br* 77(6):901–5.

Kousa P, Järvinen TLN, Kannus P, Ahvenjärvi P, Kaikkonen A, Järvinen M (2001a). A bioabsorbable plug in bone-tendon-bone reconstruction of the anterior cruciate ligament. Introduction of a novel fixation technique. *Arthroscopy* 17(2):144–50.

Kousa P, Jarvinen TLN, Kannus P, Jarvinen M (2001b). Initial fixation strength of bioabsorbable and titanium interference screws in anterior cruciate ligament reconstruction: Biomechanical evaluation by single cycle and cyclic loading. *Am J Sports Med* 29:420–5.

Laitinen O, Pohjonen T, Tormala P, Saarelainen K, Vasenius J, Rokkanen P, Vainionpaa S (1993). Mechanical properties of biodegradable poly-L-lactide ligament augmentation device in experimental anterior cruciate ligament reconstruction. *Arch Orthop Trauma Surg* 112(6):270–4.

Lajtai G, Humer K, Aitzetmuller G, Unger F, Noszian I, Orthner E (1999a). Serial magnetic resonance imaging evaluation of a bioabsorbable interference screw and the adjacent bone. *Arthroscopy* 15(5):481–8.

Lajtai G, Noszian I, Humer K, Unger F, Aitzetmuller G, Orthner E (1999b). Serial magnetic resonance imaging evaluation of operative site after fixation of patellar tendon graft with bioabsorbable interference screws in anterior cruciate ligament reconstruction. *Arthroscopy* 15(7):709–18.

Lajtai G, Schmiedhuber G, Unger F, Aitzetmuller G, Klein M, Noszian I, Orthner E (2001). Bone tunnel remodeling at the site of biodegradable interference screws used for anterior cruciate ligament reconstruction: 5-year follow-up. *Arthroscopy* 17(6):597–602.

Liew ASL, Johnson DH (2000). Efficacy of bioabsorbable interference fit screws for hamstring fixation in ACL reconstruction. *J Bone Joint Surg Br* 82-B (Supp 1):7.

Lin VS, Lee MC, O'Neal S, McKean J, Sung KL (1999). Ligament tissue engineering using synthetic biodegradable fiber scaffolds. *Tissue Eng* 5(5):443–52.

Loubignac F, Lecuire F, Rubini J, Basso M (1998). Troublesome radiologic changes after reconstructive fixation of the anterior cruciate ligament with resorbable interference screws. *Acta Orthop Belg* 64(1):47–51. French.

Magen HE, Howell SM, Hull ML (1999). Structural properties of six tibial fixation methods for anterior cruciate ligament soft tissue grafts. *Am J Sports Med* 27:35–43.

Martinek V, Friederich NF (1999). Tibial and pretibial cyst formation after anterior cruciate ligament reconstruction with bioabsorbable interference screw fixation. *Arthroscopy* 15(3):317–20.

Martinek V, Seil R, Lattermann C, Watkins SC, Fu FH (2001). The fate of the poly-L-lactic acid interference screw after anterior cruciate ligament reconstruction. *Arthroscopy* 17(1):73–6.

McGuire DA, Barber FA, Elrod BF, Paulos LE (1999). Bioabsorbable interference screws for graft fixation in anterior cruciate ligament reconstruction. *Arthroscopy* 15(5):463–73.

McGuire DA, Barber FA, Milchgrub S, Wolchok JC (2001). A post-mortem examination of poly-L lactic acid interference screws 4 months after implantation during anterior cruciate ligament reconstruction. *Arthroscopy* 17(9):988–92.

Menche DS, Phillips GI, Pitman MI, Steiner GC (1999). Inflammatory foreign-body reaction to an arthroscopic bioabsorbable meniscal arrow repair. *Arthroscopy* 15(7):770–2.

Nagarkatti DG, McKeon BP, Donahue BS, Fulkerson JP (2001). Mechanical evaluation of a soft tissue interference screw in free tendon anterior cruciate ligament graft fixation. *Am J Sports Med* 29:67–71.

Pena F, Grontvedt T, Brown GA, Aune AK, Engebretsen L (1996). Comparison of failure strength between metallic and absorbable interference screws. Influence of insertion torque, tunnel-bone block gap, bone mineral density, and interference. *Am J Sports Med* 24:329–34.

Rittmeister ME, Noble PC, Bocell JR Jr, Alexander JW, Conditt MA, Kohl HW 3rd (2001). Interactive effects of tunnel dilation on the mechanical properties of hamstring grafts fixed in the tibia with interference screws. *Knee Surg Sports Traumatol Arthrosc* 9(5):267–71.

Rittmeister ME, Noble PC, Bocell JR Jr, Alexander JW, Conditt MA, Kohl HW 3rd (2002). Components of laxity in interference fit fixation of quadrupled hamstring grafts. *Acta Orthop Scand* 73(1):65–71.

Rokkanen P, Bostman O, Vainionpaa S, Vihtonen K, Tormala P, Laiho J, Kilpikari J, Tamminmaki M (1985). Biodegradable implants in fracture fixation: Early results of treatment of fractures of the ankle. *Lancet* 1(8443):1422–4.

Rupp S, Seil R, Schneider A, Kohn DM (1999). Ligament graft initial fixation strength using biodegradable interference screws. *J Biomed Mater Res* 48(1):70–4.

Scheffler SU, Sudkamp NP, Gockenjan A, Hoffmann RF, Weiler A (2002). Biomechanical comparison of hamstring and patellar tendon graft anterior cruciate ligament reconstruction techniques: The impact of fixation level and fixation method under cyclic loading. *Arthroscopy* 18(3):304–15.

Seil R, Rupp S, Krauss PW, Benz A, Kohn DM (1998). Comparison of initial fixation strength between biodegradable and metallic interference screws and a press-fit fixation technique in a porcine model. *Am J Sports Med* 26:815–19.

Selby JB, Johnson DL, Hester P, Caborn DNM (2001). Effect of screw length on bioabsorbable interference screw fixation in a tibial bone tunnel. *Am J Sports Med* 29:614–19.

Sherman MF, Abate JA II, Brown DG, Huddleston JI, Fleming BC, Beynnon B (1999). Introducing wedge fixation: A comparison study of the sherman polylactic acid wedge and metal interference screw as a means of femoral side bone-patella-tendon-bone fixation. aaos scientific exhibit SE066, Anaheim, CA.

Sherman MF, Bonamo JR, Flynn MI (2001). Femoral fixation of a bone-tendon-bone graft in ACL reconstruction using a bioabsorbable wedge: Early clinical results. Eastern Orthopaedic Association, JBJS. Org. Abstracts, 30–31.

Simonian PT, Monson JT, Larson RV (2001). Biodegradable interference screw augmentation reduces tunnel expansion after ACL reconstruction. *Am J Knee Surg* 14(2):104–8.

Singhatat W, Lawhorn KW, Howell SM, Hull ML (2002). How four weeks of implantation affect the strength and stiffness of a tendon graft in a bone tunnel. *Am J Sports Med* 30:506–13.

Speer KP, Warren RF (1993). Arthroscopic shoulder stabilization. A role for biodegradable materials. *Clin Ortho Rel Res* 291:67–74.

Stadelmaier DM, Lowe WR, Ilahi OA, Noble PC, Kohl HW III (1999). Cyclic pull-out strength of hamstring tendon graft fixation with soft tissue interference screws: Influence of screw length. *Am J Sports Med* 27:778–83.

Stähelin AC, Weiler A, Rüfenacht H, Hoffmann R, Geissmann A, Feinstein R (1997). Clinical degradation and biocompatibility of different bioabsorbable interference screws: A report of six cases. *Arthroscopy* 13(2):238–44.

Stahelin AC, Feinstein R, Friederich N (1995). Clinical experience using a bioabsorbable interference screw for ACL reconstruction. Proc. AAOS, Orlando, 1995 and Orthopaedic Transactions. *J Bone Joint Surg* 19(2):287–8.

Strycker ML (1995). Biodegradable internal fixation. [Review] [43 refs] [Journal Article. Review. Review, Tutorial] *Journal of Foot & Ankle Surgery* 34(1): 82–8.

Therin M, Chambat P, Fayar J, Christel P (1996). In vivo evaluation of bioabsorbable interference screw (98%p1LA, 2% PDLLA) in sheep. Proc ESSKA 1996, Budapest, Hungary.

Tuompo P, Partio EK, Jukkala-Partio K, Pohjonen T, Helevirta P, Rokkanen P (1996). Strength of the fixation of patellar tendon bone grafts using a totally absorbable self-reinforced poly-L-lactide expansion plug and screw. An experimental study in a bovine cadaver. *Arthroscopy* 12(4):422–7.

Tuompo P, Partio EK, Jukkala-Partio K, Pohjonen T, Helevirta P, Rokkanen P (1999). Comparison of polylactide screw and expansion bolt in bioabsorbable fixation with patellar tendon bone graft for anterior cruciate ligament rupture of the knee. A preliminary study. *Knee Surg Sports Traumatol Arthrosc* 7(5): 296–302.

Walton M (1999). Absorbable and metal interference screws: Comparison of graft security during healing. *Arthroscopy* 15(8):818–26.

Warden WH, Friedman R, Teresi LM, Jackson DW (1999). Magnetic resonance imaging of bioabsorbable polylactic acid interference screws during the first 2 years after anterior cruciate ligament reconstruction. *Arthroscopy* 15(5):474–80.

Weiler A, Hoffmann RF, Stahelin AC, Bail HJ, Siepe CJ, Sudkamp NP (1998a). Hamstring tendon fixation using interference screws: A biomechanical study in calf tibial bone. *Arthroscopy* 14(1): 29–37.

Weiler A, Windhagen HJ, Raschke MJ, Laumeyer A, Hoffmann RF (1998b). Biodegradable interference screw fixation exhibits pull-out force and stiffness similar to titanium screws. *Am J Sports Med* 26(1):119–26.

Weiler A, Hoffmann RF, Siepe CJ, Kolbeck SF, Sudkamp NP (2000). The influence of screw geometry on hamstring tendon interference fit fixation. *Am J Sports Med* 28(3):356–9.

Weiler A, Richter M, Schmidmaier G, Kandziora F, Sudkamp NP (2001). The EndoPearl device increases fixation strength and eliminates construct slippage of hamstring tendon grafts with interference screw fixation. *Arthroscopy* 17(4):353–9.

Weiler A, Peine R, Pashmineh-Azar A, Abel C, Sudkamp NP, Hoffmann RF (2002a). Tendon healing in a bone tunnel. Part I: Biomechanical results after biodegradable interference fit fixation in a model of anterior cruciate ligament reconstruction in sheep. *Arthroscopy* 18(2): 113–23.

Weiler A, Hoffmann RF, Bail HJ, Rehm O, Sudkamp NP (2002b). Tendon healing in a bone tunnel. Part II: Histologic analysis after biodegradable interference fit fixation in a model of anterior cruciate ligament reconstruction in sheep. *Arthroscopy* 18(2):124–35.

9

The physiology of bone-tendon healing must be considered for successful ACL reconstruction rehabilitation

Deryk G. Jones and J.-K. Francis Suh

Introduction

Over the past three decades (1970–2000) there has been an enormous amount of research and clinical interest in the anterior cruciate ligament (ACL)-deficient knee. The anatomy, physiology and biomechanics of this ligament have been well studied. The information gathered in these studies has led to the development and application of reconstructive procedures and rehabilitation protocols currently used in treating these patients. Anterior cruciate ligament reconstruction methods typically strive for strong graft fixation that will allow for early, 'aggressive' rehabilitation; early motion in the operative limb aids in avoiding the increased stiffness and muscular atrophy associated with prolonged immobilization. This trend towards early, strenuous rehabilitation has led increasing numbers of athletes to attempt a return to their sports-specific activities at a time when the graft may be vulnerable. Studies of soft tissue incorporation following tendon placement within a bone tunnel demonstrate a consistent timeline for graft revascularization, incorporation and remodeling; this process can take up to three years (Arnoczky *et al.* 1982; Rodeo *et al.* 1993a). In light of these facts, the orthopaedist is often placed in a precarious position in counseling the ACL-reconstructed athlete. The athlete feels great, has a functionally sound knee, and wishes to return to sports. Unfortunately, in the case of current ACL reconstruction techniques, the athlete's wishes to return to play occur before the intraarticular remodeling process is complete.

Based on these operative and rehabilitative trends, it is imperative that the surgeon be aware of the physiologic factors in play when a tendon heals within a bone tunnel. This knowledge allows the orthopaedist to take the necessary steps during the reconstruction that will optimize the tendon-bone healing process. In addition, an awareness of this physiologic process allows the surgeon to direct the therapist and patient postoperatively and to avoid early clinical failure.

While it is widely accepted amongst knee surgeons that good bone-tendon healing is necessary for successful ligament reconstructive procedures, there is limited clinical evidence supporting this statement. Review articles discussing revision ACL surgery frequently list the failure of graft incorporation as one of the etiologic factors in primary ACL reconstruction failure. However, even limited clinical or even anecdotal evidence to support the statement is seldom given (Brown and Carson 1999; Carson et al. 1998; Greis et al. 1993; Johnson et al. 1996; Johnson and Coen 1995; Noyes and Barber-Westin 2001; Safran and Harner 1995). A review of the basic science literature demonstrates that there is a renewed interest in this topic as there are numerous *in vivo* animal studies assessing the factors that promote improved tendon healing within a tunnel (Anderson et al. 2001; Greis et al. 2001a; Itoh 1991; Ohtera et al. 2000; Panni et al. 1997; Rodeo et al. 1993a, 1999a; Suh et al. 2002; Yasuda et al. 1999).

This chapter will first discuss the historical perspectives of anterior cruciate ligament reconstructive surgery with an emphasis on the causes of failure that have led to our current operative techniques and choices of tissue grafts. Next, the basic scientific issues concerning healing of the tendon graft to the bone tunnel will be discussed. Finally, a critical discussion of those physiologic factors that should be considered during the early and late postoperative rehabilitation of the reconstructed patient will be undertaken.

Historical perspectives of ACL reconstruction surgery

Early history of ACL reconstruction surgery

In the 1600s Galen first described the ACL as a supportive structure stabilizing the joint against abnormal joint motion (Galen 1968; Snook 1983). The first written description of an ACL rupture is credited to Stark in 1850 (Stark 1850). He treated the pathology with braces but noted persistent disability after treatment. Battle, Mayo Robsin and Goetjes reported on the results of surgical repair of the ligament in the early 1900s (Battle 1900; Goetjes 1913; Mayo Robsin 1903). In 1917 Hey Groves described the use of the fascia lata, which was passed through tibial and femoral tunnels, to reconstruct the ACL. During this same case he reconstructed the posterior cruciate ligament with the semitendinosis tendon. Further demonstrating his remarkable grasp of the condition, he recommended early range of motion and mobilization.

A landmark publication, *On the Injuries to the Ligament of the Knee Joint*, was released in 1938 by Ivar Palmer (Palmer 1938). This book discussed the typical injury mechanisms and associated pathologic patterns, and also reported on a histologic autopsy study of Hey

Groves' procedure demonstrating graft revascularization (Eriksson 1983; Palmer 1938). Between 1930 and 1950 there was a movement away from intraarticular repair or reconstruction of the ligament towards extra-articular reconstructive procedures (Bosworth and Bosworth 1936; Campbell 1939a, 1993b). By reporting on a series of acute ligament tears in young athletes in 1950, O'Donoghue rekindled the appreciation for the anterior cruciate ligament (O'Donoghue 1991). In 1963 he described a modification of Groves' ACL reconstruction using the iliotibial band (O'Donoghue 1963).

Use of bone-patellar tendon-bone (BPTB) graft

In the early 1960s, E.K. Jones reported on the use of the central one third of the patellar tendon to reconstruct the ACL (Ivey *et al.* 1980). His technique was modified by Lam in 1968 (Lam 1968). Lam understood the importance of proper osseous tunnel placement in the intercondylar notch, striving to maintain a constant distance between the tunnel and the tibial tuberosity. He gained more length by removing an inferior tibial bone block with the attached tendon. This block was then placed into a bony trough, and the femoral block was placed on the outer side of the lateral femoral condyle. Both blocks were then fixed with screws. Eriksson using the medial third of the patellar tendon emphasized the importance of anchoring the graft at its normal insertion site within the notch (Eriksson 1976). Alm demonstrated the importance of appropriate femoral tunnel placement. Through a second-look arthrotomy he clearly showed that improper graft placement led to laxity, inflammation and postoperative degenerative changes within the joint (Alm 1973).

Since these initial reports the BPTB has become the 'gold standard' against which other ACL reconstruction techniques are measured. Separate animal studies by Clancy and Alm clearly demonstrated rapid, eight weeks, revascularization of the BPTB graft by endosteal blood supply (Alm and Stromberg 1974b, 1974a; Clancy Jr. *et al.* 1981).

Use of hamstring tendon graft

Concerns about postoperative quadriceps atrophy, patellofemoral problems and patellar fracture pushed the knee surgeon to explore additional graft options. Using the hamstring tendon as an ACL graft was first suggested by Augustine (1956). He left the tissue attached proximally but released the tissue from its distal insertion and routed the graft through the intercondylar notch and into a tibial tunnel. Cho performed the opposite, releasing the tendon proximally; it was then routed through tibial and femoral tunnels (Cho 1975). The graft was then tied over the iliotibial band. Lipscomb reported on a semitendinosis tenodesis technique in 1979 for isolated ACL or ACL and meniscal tears (Lipscomb *et al.* 1979). In this article and a subsequent study two years later he combined the intraarticular procedure with a posteromedial reefing procedure (Lipscomb et al. 1979, 1981). In a more recent prospective study, Lipscomb demonstrated more postoperative contractures, stiffness and patellofemoral symptoms in patients who underwent combined intra- and extra-articular procedures, as compared to those patients who underwent intraarticular BPTB or quadrupled hamstring tendon reconstruction alone (Anderson et al. 2001). As a result of the observed morbidity associated with extra-articular procedures, there has been a trend over the last 15 years towards intraarticular ACL reconstruction. Currently, the quadrupled hamstring tendon has become as popular as the BPTB graft. Initial strength assessments by Noyes and coworkers demonstrated that the hamstring tendon (single-stranded gracilis or semitendinosis) was significantly weaker than the BPTB graft (Noyes et al. 1984). However, Hamner and coworkers demonstrated that the quadrupled hamstring tendon construct was actually stronger than the BPTB (Hamner et al. 1999). Further, it has been demonstrated that the hamstring tendon exhibits more elastic behavior than the BPTB graft making it more similar to the native ACL than the BPTB graft.

Use of other synthetic grafts

The search for alternative reconstructive materials lead in the early 1980s to prosthetic ligament reconstructions (Bejui et al. 1984; Drouin 1986; Makisalo et al. 1989; Mendenhall et al. 1987). These materials promised unlimited supply and lack of donor-site morbidity or risk of disease transmission, raising a great deal of initial enthusiasm about these devices (Tremblay et al. 1980). Two popular prosthetic replacements were released, the Gore-Tex ligament prosthesis (Gore and Company, Flagstaff, AZ) and the Dacron ligament prosthesis (Stryker Endoscopy Company, Sunnyvale, CA). Several scaffold-type augmentation devices were also released, such as the Leed's-Keio ligament, providing a substrate for soft tissue and fibroblastic ingrowth. All three categories of devices were used extensively throughout the world (Bernett et al. 1987; Fujikawa 1985; James et al. 1983; Scharling 1981). However, a minimum four-year follow-up study with the Gore-Tex prosthesis in 188 patients (Paulos et al. 1992) revealed that they had subjective improvement in less than 50 per cent and objective improvement in only 43 per cent of the patients. The complication rate was an astounding 76 per cent. Similar results were also reported with the Dacron prosthesis (Wilk and Richmond 1993). The terrible experience with these devices clearly demonstrates how poor graft incorporation into the surrounding bone can directly affect clinical outcomes. These materials were rejected by the host, and caused osteolysis within the bone tunnels, sterile effusions secondary to the generation of particulate debris and early graft rupture due to poor incorporation, vascularity and bony ingrowth (Friedman 1991; Klein and Jensen 1992; Olson *et al.* 1988; Seemann and Steadman 1993).

Allograft versus autograft

The use of allograft tissues in orthopaedic procedures has grown enormously since the mid 1980s. Like the prosthetic devices, these tissues offered the advantage of shorter operative time, no donor-site morbidity, smaller incisions and and greater supply compared to autograft tissue sources (Olson *et al.* 1992). Unlike the synthetic materials, allografts have the potential advantage of eventual bio-logic incorporation. In a dog model, Arnoczky demonstrated a marked inflammatory and rejection response to fresh patellar tendon allografts; only a minimal host response to deep-frozen allograft patellar tendon tissue was observed in the same study (Arnoczky *et al.* 1986). In a separate study by Jackson, histologic and microangiographic evaluation demonstrated cellular repopulation and near normal collagen fiber orientation with revascularization rivaling that seen with autologous tissues (Jackson *et al.* 1987b, 1987a, 1991). While there have been recent reports of early clostridial infections with the use of allograft tissues, the estimated risk of viral transmission is currently less than 1 per 1,667,000 (Buck *et al.* 1989). Fideler *et al.* assessed 60 BPTB allograft tissues with varying doses of gamma irradiation and demonstrated a dose-dependent reduction in biomechanical parameters at 2.0 or greater Mrad. As a result, current tissue banking facilities are providing fresh-frozen or cryo-preserved allograft tissues for surgical application (Fideler *et al.* 1995).

Graft fixation

Much of the concern about hamstring or other soft tissue grafts over the last decade has centered around the poor fixation of soft tissue to bone, as opposed to the more established bone to bone fixation with the patellar tendon graft fixed by interference screw (Aune *et al.* 1998; Brand *et al.* 2000a; Brown *et al.* 1999; Steiner *et al.* 1994). Brown and coworkers have demonstrated that the use of the continuous loop Endobutton (Smith and Nephew Endoscopy, Inc., Andover, MA) for femoral fixation has a failure load of 1345 N which is higher than the published literature on most femoral fixation methods (Brown *et al.* 1999). A recent report reviewing the numerous fixation methods for both the femoral and tibial sides demonstrated femoral fixation failure loads ranging from 235 N to 640 N for the BPTB grafts and 242 N to 699 N for the soft tissue grafts (Brand *et al.* 2000a).

The critical question is the following: what fixation failure load is sufficient to withstand the forces that occur during activities of daily living and more strenuous activities? Estimates on the forces distributed to the ACL during daily activities range from 67 N (ascending stairs) to 445 N (descending stairs) (Cooper *et al.* 1993; Mundy 1993; Woo *et al.* 1991). The ultimate strength to failure is 2160 N for the native ACL, 2977 N for the central third patellar tendon graft and 4140 N for the quadrupled hamstring tendon graft (Hamner *et al.* 1999; Morrison 1968, 1969). Stiffness for the native ACL is 242 N/mm, 455 N/mm for the patellar tendon and 807 N/mm for the quadrupled hamstring tendon. Based on these figures, our current graft choices and fixation techniques should be sufficient to withstand the loads required during early rehabilitation following ACL reconstruction.

Several basic science studies have recently been published that demonstrate the important interplay between bone tunnel preparation and graft position within the tunnel during soft tissue reconstructive procedures. Brand *et al.* demonstrated that bone mineral density at the host bone site was an important determinant in initial fixation strength when an interference screw was used to fix a hamstring tendon graft (Brand *et al.* 2000b). Similarly, Cain *et al.* demonstrated a much higher mean peak load for tibial specimens wherein the tunnel had been sequentially dilated (616 ± 263 N) compared to reamed tibial specimens (453 ± 197 N) in a hamstring tendon cadaveric model (Cain *et al.* 1999). They also found a correlation between bone density and pull-out strength. Greis *et al.*, using a dog model, demonstrated that both the length of the tendon and the tendon fit within the tunnel were significant determinants of the pull-out strength (Greis *et al.* 2001b). Histologically, they demonstrated a more mature appearing interface between the tendon and bone in the specimens with a tighter fit at the time of surgery.

Basic science of tendon graft-to-bone attachment

Ligament-to-bone insertion: Sharpey's fibers

In many aspects, the ligament-to-bone insertion site shares similar morphological characteristics to the tendon-to-bone insertion. Over approximately 1 mm, the junction between these soft tissues and bone demonstrates a drastic transition from collagen fibers embedded in a soft extracellular matrix environment to those embedded in a highly calcified bone matrix. In general, the soft tissue-to-bone insertion can be classified into two distinctive morphological types – direct and indirect insertions (Woo *et al.* 1988). In direct insertion, the collagen fibers approach the bone at nearly ninety degrees, and the insertion site is histologically well defined as an abrupt, basophilic, transition zone with the presence of the interfacial fibrocartilage and the calcified fibrocartilage (Cooper and Misol 1970; Laros *et al.* 1971). In indirect insertion, the collagen fibers approach the bone at an acute angle. Instead of perforating directly into the bone, the fibers blend with the periosteum, which is in turn attached to the bone via perforating collagen fibers, called Sharpey's fibers (Benjamin *et al.* 1986; Hurov 1986; Woo *et al.* 1988). Using Goldner's trichrome staining on the tibial insertion site of a rabbit's medial collateral ligament, Matyas *et al.* found continuous fibrous bundles that extend from the ligament into the periosteum and then into an underlying calcified layer in the bone (Matyas *et al.* 1990). Unlike direct insertion, indirect insertion has little or no transitional zone of fibrocartilage, yet a basophilic boundary still exists between the noncalcified and calcified tissues (Matyas *et al.* 1990; Woo *et al.* 1988).

The insertion of soft tissue into bone was first described by Sharpey and Ellis in 1856 when they identified distinctive bundles of 'perforating fibers' (or Sharpey's fibers) extending from the periosteum into the underlying bone (Sharpey and Ellis 1856). It is believed that these fibers are the result of subperiosteal bone formation adjacent to the cambium layer of the periosteum. Such perforating fibers are also present in most tendon-bone junctions as a continuous, fibrous anchorage of the tendon into the bone. While the exact definition of these fibers is still controversial, such collagen fibers extending from soft tissues into bone at insertion sites are generally referred to as Sharpey's fibers (Woo *et al.* 1988).

Physiology of tendon graft-to-bone attachment

The firm healing or attachment of a tendon graft to bone has been considered a key factor for the long-term success of many reconstructive operative procedures for damaged tendons and ligaments. A tendon graft firmly anchored to the bone will allow for an earlier 'aggressive' functional rehabilitation of the graft and thus improve the success of the surgery. Gallie and his associates reported that the failure of a tendon transplant was usually attributed to the premature separation of the transplanted tendon graft from its bony anchorage (Gallie 1913; Gallie and Le Mesurier 1921).

It has been observed that a tendon-bone interface undergoes a considerable remodeling process driven by an invasion of mesenchymal cells from bone marrow (Forward and Cowan 1963; Rodeo *et al.* 1993b; Whiston and Walmsley 1960). However, the remodeling and ossification process of a transplanted tendon graft takes place slowly after an initial lag time during which the mechanical strength of the graft-bone construct undergoes some degradation (Amiel *et al.* 1986; Forward and Cowan 1963; Kernwein *et al.* 1938; Kernwein 1942; McFarland *et al.* 1986; Whiston and Walmsley 1960). The remodeling process of the tendon involves the turnover of existing collagen and the synthesis of new collagen at the interface (Jones *et al.* 1987; Klein *et al.* 1972). Using a rabbit model, Liu *et al.* demonstrated a temporal distribution of collagen types I, II, and III during the early healing of a long flexor tendon in a calcaneal bone tunnel

(Liu *et al.* 1997). It was observed that type III collagen is abundant in the region of the tendon-bone interface during the early healing period, but gradually decreases over time with the formation of Sharpey's fibers. It has been suggested that the presence of type III collagen is a precursor to the formation of Sharpey's fibers in a tendon-bone interface (Frank *et al.* 1983; Galatz *et al.* 2002; Liu *et al.* 1995, Liu *et al.* 1997).

With the progressive increase in Sharpey's fiber formation, the mechanical strength of the interface gradually increases over time (Blickenstaff *et al.* 1997; Grana *et al.* 1994; Jones *et al.* 1987; Rodeo *et al.* 1993b). During the course of healing, the failure mode of the tendon-bone construct under tensile loading progresses from a pull-out mechanism at the tendon-bone interface to a mid-substance failure of the tendon (Pinczewski *et al.* 1997; Rodeo *et al.* 1993b). However, the ultimate strength of experimental graft fixation never reaches that of a normal tendon-bone insertion site (Blickenstaff *et al.* 1997; Grana *et al.* 1994; Jones *et al.* 1987; Kennedy *et al.* 1980). This implies that the cause of the mid-substance failure of the tendon at the later stage of the healing process is due to an atrophic degradation of the tendon graft, rather than a strengthening of the tendon-bone interface. By achieving a strong interface between the tendon graft and host bone at an early stage in the healing process, ACL reconstruction patients are able to undergo an early aggressive functional rehabilitation and thus prevent atrophic degradation of the tendon graft.

Tissue engineering approaches for tendon-bone tunnel healing

While tendon-bone tunnel healing has long been a challenging orthopaedic problem, most experimental and clinical studies have focused on the development of mechanical devices to physically attach a tendon in a bone tunnel. Around the turn of the twenty-first century, tissue engineering as a concept has led to major changes in the mindset of tissue repair. That is, a damaged tissue can be repaired via the use of natural materials, instead of synthetic materials. In light of the enormous success of tissue engineering approaches in various medical problems, the use of a natural, biologic constructs to repair a normal tendon-to-bone insertion is appealing. This can be achieved in many ways: (1) *in vitro* cultivation of a tendon-to-bone insertion that can be subsequently implanted into a patient; (2) a biocompatible, biodegradable composite scaffold can be used to replace the tendon-to-bone insertion, which is later naturally replaced by the host tissue *in vivo*; (3) biological stimulant(s) can be used to reconstruct the tendon-to-bone insertion *in vivo*.

Despite the potential of tissue engineering, only a handful of studies have examined the use of exogenous biologic materials to modulate the bone-tendon healing process. Growth factors such as BMP-2 and BMP-7 have been applied to the tendon-bone junction at the time of tendon reconstruction surgery (Nicklin *et al.* 2000; Rodeo *et al.* 1999b). Although the addition of these growth factors resulted in improved the integration at the tendon-bone interface, the results were highly dependent on the dosage of the agent and can were variable. Furthermore, the choice of an optimal exogenous agent(s) suitable for tendon-bone healing, in humans, is uncertain at the present time (Nicklin *et al.* 2000). Orthopedic clinicians and scientists must identify the optimal biological agents that will enhance the attachment of tendon or ligament to bone before such tissue engineering approaches are appropriately applied to these clinical problems.

Periosteal augmentation of tendon-to-bone attachment

In our laboratory, we have recently investigated the efficacy of a free periosteal patch as a tissue engineering vehicle for tendon-bone tunnel healing. Periosteum, a thin membrane covering the outer surface of cortical bone, is responsible for the lateral growth of cortical bone and has been known for its osteogenic potential (Blaisdell 1925; Iwasaki *et al.* 1995; Nakahara *et al.* 1991; Topping *et al.* 1994). Therefore, we have hypothesized that the osteogenic potential of periosteum can provide a means to augment the healing potential of a tendon graft in a bone tunnel. The periosteum consists of two layers – the fibrogenic outer layer and the osteogenic cambium layer. We hypothesized that the periosteal augmentation of a tendon graft presents a better result when the periosteal cambium side is in contact with bone than when the periosteal fibrous side is in contact with bone.

Using a rabbit ankle model with Hallucis longus tendon (HLT), the HLT tendon was wrapped with a fresh autologous periosteum patch and fixed in a bone tunnel made on the calcaneal process. The rabbits were sacrificed at six weeks after the surgery, and the tendon-bone tunnel complexes were evaluated biomechanically and histologically. We found that the pull-out strength of the tendon-bone interface was the highest when a piece of fresh periosteal tissue was wrapped around the tendon with the cambium (inner) layer facing the bone (Figure 9.1). Interestingly, when fresh periosteum was placed around the tendon with the cambium layer facing the tendon, the biomechanical strength of the tendon-bone interface was similar to that of the tendon fixed to the bone without periosteal augmentation. The hematoxilin and eosin staining of the tendon-bone interface from the group in which the cambium layer was facing the bone revealed that newly formed bone penetrated into the graft tendon with an abundant formation of Sharpey's fibers at the tendon-bone interface (Figure 9.2). These results are promising in light of the ready availability of this tissue at the proximal tibial bone. Although

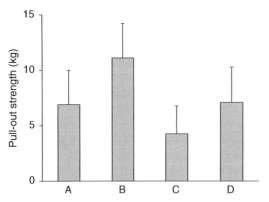

Fig. 9.1

Pull-out strength of the tendon-bone interface complexes from an experimental rabbit model using HLT tendon and the calcaneal bone. (A) Periosteally augmented tendon-bone interface with the cambium layer facing towards the tendon; (B) periosteally augmented tendon-bone interface with the cambium layer facing towards the bone; (C) tendon-bone interface augmented with an inert periosteal patch; (D) tendon-bone interface without periosteal augmentation.

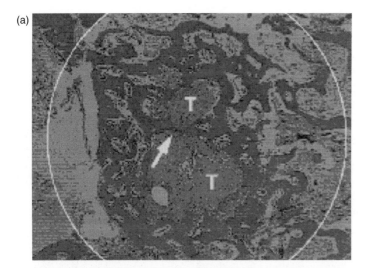

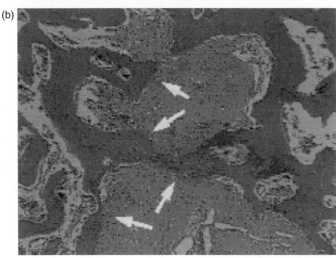

Fig. 9.2

(a) H&E histology (40x) of the tendon-bone interface at 6 weeks after surgery. Significant ossification of the interface is noticed along with penetration of new bony trabeculae into and through the tendon (arrow). The white circle represents an approximated area of the bone tunnel created at the time of surgery. (b) A high power (100x) image of Fig. 9.2(a). Notice the abundant formation of Sharpey's fibers at the tendon-bone interface (arrows).

the study was not in an intraarticular model, one can see the potential application of this technique in soft tissue reconstructive procedures using either autologous or allograft tissues. Further studies will be performed to assess these possibilities.

Current trends in rehabilitation following ACL-reconstructive surgery

It is clear from the historical review of ACL reconstructive techniques that there has been a transition from the nonanatomic, extra-articular reconstruction to the anatomic, intraarticular reconstruction. Further, the failures of the prosthetic ligament devices clearly demonstrated the need to use tissue grafts that promote host incorporation with revascularization, fibroblastic ingrowth and reinnervation. Along with this knowledge, there has been the concomitant development of arthroscopic techniques that decrease the perioperative morbidity and pain leading to shorter postoperative recovery periods. As a result, patients and surgeons have shortened and intensified their rehabilitative protocols, stressing the reconstruction at a much early recovery point than in the past. As pointed out by Joseph Buckwalter, there has been a transition from strict immobilization to controlled resumption of activity in the postoperative patient (Buckwalter 1995, 1996). However, a strong tendon-to-bone attachment at an early stage in the healing process has to be considered a prerequisite to such intensified rehabilitation protocols. As pointed out in the previous discussion on graft fixation methods, most available fixation methods for soft tissue grafts will withstand large forces if performed with the appropriate techniques. As a result, graft incorporation has now become an important determinant in the final outcome following reconstructive surgery.

In the early 1990s Donald Shelbourne retrospectively reviewed the ACL reconstructions performed at his facility focusing on the cause(s) of arthrofibrosis (Shelbourne *et al.* 1991). He demonstrated a clear relationship between the time from injury to surgery and the occurrence of postoperative knee contractures. Surgeries performed within one week of injury had a significantly increased risk for postoperative motion complications compared to those performed three weeks and longer following ACL injury. An equally important contribution to the timing of surgery and rehabilitation was Shelbourne's 'accelerated rehabilitation' protocol that was published at around the same time (Shelbourne and Nitz 1990; Shelbourne and Wilckens 1990). He noticed that patients who were noncompliant with the more established (conservative) rehabilitation protocols developed less postoperative complications and subjective complaints and returned to sporting activities sooner. Further, there was no difference in long-term knee stability between patients who were compliant with the conservative rehabilitation recommendations and those patients who were more noncompliant. Histologic biopsies

139

performed at various time points demonstrated no adverse affects on graft incorporation.

These results did not coincide with the large numbers of basic science studies on the timing and sequence of graft incorporation. As a result, there was a gradual movement away from the strict rehabilitation protocols of the 1980s and early 1990s toward Shelbourne's accelerated ACL program. Surgeons and therapists have 'pushed the envelope' following surgery with little regard for graft type or fixation technique. In Shelbourne's 800 plus cases, all were performed with an autologous bone patellar tendon graft using a mini-arthrotomy. Application of these same accelerated protocols to patients treated with autologous hamstring grafts has produced varying results. Marder prospectively assessed 80 ACL reconstructions using either patellar or hamstring tendon grafts (Marder *et al.* 1991). While he did note significant differences in hamstring strength between the two groups, KT-1000 measurements demonstrated no difference in postoperative laxity. However, he noted that all patients followed the 'standard rehabilitation' protocols that at that time included protected weight-bearing for six weeks and avoidance of active terminal extension for six months. Muneta *et al.* retrospectively reviewed 103 of 110 ACL reconstructions comparing patellar and hamstring tendon grafts (Muneta *et al.* 1998). All patients underwent an 'aggressive, early rehabilitation' protocol. KT measurements revealed a statistically higher number of patients in the hamstring group with greater than 5 mm side to side difference. Recently, Barrett *et al.* published a single surgeon, prospective evaluation of female patients treated with either hamstring or patellar tendon grafts fixed along the femoral side with an EndoButton regardless of graft type (Barrett *et al.* 2002). Follow-up revealed increased rates of knee laxity on clinical examination and larger side to side differences with KT measurements in the hamstring tendon group. These studies demonstrate that both the surgeon and therapist must consider the complex interaction between the physiology and biomechanics of the graft type and fixation techniques used as well as those patient specific characteristics that have demonstrated influence on surgical outcomes. The rehabilitation protocols for patients treated with patellar tendon grafts probably should not be applied to patients treated with soft tissue grafts without considering these issues.

Conclusion and future directions

The orthopaedic surgeon must have a clear understanding of the complex interplay between a soft tissue graft and the bone tunnel during ACL reconstruction. To avoid failures the graft should be placed isometrically into a bone tunnel with minimal size mismatch and maximum tendon to bone contact. Tunnels should be dilated rather than reamed to increase the consistency of the tunnel wall improving graft fixation. If the patient has poor bone density, fixation methods utilizing cortical bone should be performed. Gender differences and sports-specific activities should be taken into account when deciding on graft choice.

The optimal fixation of a tendon into a bone tunnel could be achieved through a biological attachment of the tendon to the bone utilizing tissue engineering techniques. The periosteal study described herein has shown the feasibility of augmentation at the tendon and bone tunnel as a means to accelerate the reformation of Sharpey's fibers. The use of an autogenous periosteum patch would be an optimal choice for biological augmentation of the tendon graft in the bone tunnel, as this autologous tissue is readily available. Nonetheless, an extended tissue engineering approach based on profound physiological perspectives of the naturally occurring tendon-to-bone interface can further accelerate and enhance the tendon-bone healing process. One plausible tissue engineering approach is the use of exogenous growth factors along with periosteal augmentation of the tendon graft.

Once the surgery has been completed patient-specific issues as well as any associated pathology should be taken into account in determining the timing and sequence of the postoperative rehabilitation protocol. Shelbourne's accelerated rehabilitation demonstrates that the patient and specifically the ACL graft can have a positive response to physiologic loads. Although the exact mechanisms that contribute to this response are not known, as with other areas in the body, tissues at the cellular level can respond to mechanical stresses. Indeed, the fibroblast has been shown to respond to mechanical loads (Parsons *et al.* 1999; Prajapati *et al.* 2000; Theilig *et al.* 2001). These forces can stimulate and/or promote cellular proliferation, metabolism and growth factor production. Further, the duration and type of load or force applied to the cell can determine the response (Park *et al.* 1999; Prajapati *et al.* 2000). Finally, fibroblast will interact with their local extracellular matrix further affecting the cellular behavior (Eckes *et al.* 1999). Amiel *et al.* described a process of 'ligamentization' in their basic science study of the natural history of the patellar tendon autograft where extrinsic cells repopulated the graft and began to produce collagen type III and glycosaminoglycan at levels similar to that found in the native ACL (Amiel *et al.* 1986).

The role of proprioception and the neuromuscular system is outside the scope of this chapter but damage to this system has been implicated in the natural history of the ACL-deficient knee (Kennedy *et al.* 1982). Barrack *et al.* demonstrated reinnervation of a free patellar tendon graft in a dog model with mechanoreceptors and free nerve endings seen histologically 6 months after surgery (Barrack *et al.* 1997). Aune *et al.* in a rat model implicated sensory innervation in the healing process using a patellar tendon graft (Aune *et al.* 1996). Certainly, one could see how increased postoperative activity could stimulate the neuromuscular system promoting

141

sensory input and subsequent reinnervation. Once again the surgeon should have a full understanding of the physiology of the tissue–bone interaction as well as all of the other factors discussed in this chapter before recommending a certain rehabilitation protocol. As with all other areas in medicine, tailoring the recommendations to the patient based on that individual's unique characteristics can assure the desired outcome.

References

Alm, A. 1973, 'Survival of part of patellar tendon transposed for reconstruction of anterior cruciate ligament', *Acta Chir Scand.*, vol. 139(5): 443–447.

Alm, A. and Stromberg, B. 1974b, 'Transposed medial third of patellar ligament in reconstruction of the anterior cruciate ligament. A surgical and morphologic study in dogs', *Acta Chir Scand. Suppl*, vol. 445: 37–49.

Alm, A. and Stromberg, B. 1974a, 'Vascular anatomy of the patellar and cruciate ligaments. A microangiographic and histologic investigation in the dog', *Acta Chir Scand. Suppl*, vol. 445: 25–35.

Amiel, D., Kleiner, J. B., Roux, R. D., Harwood, F. L., and Akeson, W. H. 1986, 'The phenomenon of "ligamentization": Anterior cruciate ligament reconstruction with autogenous patellar tendon', *J. Orthop. Res.*, vol. 4: 162–172.

Anderson, A. F., Snyder, R. B., and Lipscomb, A. B., Jr. 2001, 'Anterior cruciate ligament reconstruction. A prospective randomized study of three surgical methods', *Am. J. Sports Med.*, May–June; 29(3): 272–279.

Anderson, K., Seneviratne, A. M., Izawa, K., Atkinson, B. L., Potter, H. G., and Rodeo, S. A. 2001, 'Augmentation of tendon healing in an intra-articular bone tunnel with use of a bone growth factor', *Am. J. Sports Med.*, vol. 29(6): 689–698.

Arnoczky, S. P., Tarvin, G. B., and Marshall, J. L. 1982, 'Anterior cruciate ligament replacement using patellar tendon. An evaluation of graft revascularization in the dog', *J. Bone Joint Surg. Am.*, vol. 64(2): 217–224.

Arnoczky, S. P., Warren, R. F., and Ashlock, M. A. 1986, 'Replacement of the anterior cruciate ligament using a patellar tendon allograft. An experimental study', *J. Bone Joint Surg. Am.*, vol. 68(3): 376–385.

Augustine, R. W. 1956, 'The unstable knee', *J. Surg.*, 92: 380–388.

Aune, A. K., Ekeland, A., and Cawley, P. W. 1998, 'Interference screw fixation of hamstring vs patellar tendon grafts for anterior cruciate ligament reconstruction', *Knee Surg. Sports Traumatol. Arthrosc.*, vol. 6: 99–102.

Aune, A. K., Hukkanen, M., Madsen, J. E., Polak, J. M., and Nordsletten, L. 1996, 'Nerve regeneration during patellar tendon autograft remodelling after anterior cruciate ligament reconstruction: an experimental and clinical study', *J. Orthop. Res.*, vol. 14: 193–199.

Barrack, R. L., Lund, P. J., Munn, B. G., Wink, C., and Happel, L. 1997, 'Evidence of reinnervation of free patellar tendon autograft used for anterior cruciate ligament reconstruction', *Am. J. Sports Med.*, vol. 25(2): 196–202.

Barrett, G. R., Noojin, F. K., Hartzog, C. W., and Nash, C. R. 2002, 'Reconstruction of the anterior cruciate ligament in females: A comparison of hamstring versus patellar tendon autograft', *Arthroscopy* Jan., 18(1): 46–54.

Battle, W. H. 1900, 'A case after open section of the knee joint for irreducible traumatic dislocation.', *Clin. Soc. London Trans.*, vol. 33: 232–232.

Bejui, J., Perot, F., Perault, F., Vignon, E., Bejui-Thivolet, F., and Hartmann, D. 1984, '[Experimental study of intraarticular carbon fibers in the knee of the dog with and without preservation of the anterior cruciate ligament] Etude experimentale des fibres de carbone intraarticulaires dans le genou du chien avec et sans conservation du ligament croise anterieur', *Rev. Chir Orthop. Reparatrice Appar. Mot.*, vol. 70(Suppl 2): 27–29.

Benjamin, M., Evans, E. J., and Copp, L. 1986, 'The histology of tendon attachments to bone in man', *J. Anat.*, vol. 149: 89–100.

Bernett, P., Feldmeier, C., and Pieper, B. 1987, 'Anterior cruciate ligament (ACL) repair by augmentation with the polypropylene braid (Kennedy LAD). Biocompatibility, technique, early clinical results', *Acta Orthop. Belg.*, vol. 53: 356–359.

Blaisdell, F. E. 1925, 'The osteogenetic function of the periosteum', *Arch. Surg.*, vol. 11: 933.

Blickenstaff, K. R., Grana, W. A., and Egle, D. 1997, 'Analysis of a semi-tendinosus autograft in a rabbit model', *Am. J. Sports Med.*, vol. 25(4): 554–559.

Bosworth, D. M. and Bosworth, B. M. 1936, 'Use of fascia lata to stabilize the knee in cases of ruptured crucial ligaments.', *J. Bone Joint Surg. Am.*, vol. 18, 178–179.

Brand, J., Jr., Weiler, A., Caborn, D. N., Brown, C. H., Jr., and Johnson, D. L. 2000a, 'Graft fixation in cruciate ligament reconstruction', *Am. J. Sports Med.*, vol. 28(5): 761–774.

Brand, J., Jr., Weiler, A., Caborn, D. N., Brown, C. H., Jr., and Johnson, D. L. 2000b, 'Graft fixation in cruciate ligament reconstruction', *Am. J. Sports Med.*, vol. 28(5): 761–774.

Brown, C. H., Wilson DPhil, D. R., Hecker Aaron, and Ferragamo, M. 1999, Comparison of Hamstring and Patellar Tendon Femoral Fixation: Cyclic Load. AOSSM 25th Annual Meeting Traverse City, Michigan, 413–414. 6–19.

Brown, C. H., Jr. and Carson, E. W. 1999, 'Revision anterior cruciate ligament surgery', *Clin. Sports Med.*, vol. 18: 109–171.

Buck, B. E., Malinin, T. I., and Brown, M. D. 1989, 'Bone transplantation and human immunodeficiency virus. An estimate of risk of acquired immunodeficiency syndrome (AIDS)', *Clin. Orthop.*, no. 240: 129–136.

Buckwalter, J. A. 1995, 'Activity vs. rest in the treatment of bone, soft tissue and joint injuries', *Iowa Orthop. J.*, vol. 15: 29–42.

Buckwalter, J. A. 1996, 'Effects of early motion on healing of musculo-skeletal tissues', *Hand Clin.*, vol. 12(1): 13–24.

Cain E. Lyle, Phillips, B. B., Charlebois Steven J., Daniels, A. U., and Azar, F. M. 1999, Effect of tibial tunnel dilation on pullout strength of quadrupled semitendinosus/gracilis with bioabsorbable interference screws. AOSSM 25th Annual Meeting Traverse City, Michigan, 415–415. 6–19.

Campbell, W. C. 1939b, 'Reconstruction of the ligaments of the knee', *Am. J. Surg.*, vol. 43: 473–480.

Campbell, W. C. 1939a, 'Repair of the ligaments of the knee', *Surg. Gynec. and Obst.*, vol. 62: 964–968.

Carson, E. W., Simonian, P. T., Wickiewicz, T. L., and Warren, R. F. 1998, 'Revision anterior cruciate ligament reconstruction', *Instr. Course Lect.*, vol. 47: 361–368.

Cho, K. O. 1975, Reconstruction of the anterior cruciate ligament by semi-tendinosis tenodesis. *J. Bone Joint Surg. Am.*, 57(5): 608–612.

Clancy, W. G., Jr., Narechania, R. G., Rosenberg, T. D., Gmeiner, J. G., Wisnefske, D. D., and Lange, T. A. 1981, 'Anterior and posterior cruciate ligament reconstruction in rhesus monkeys', *J. Bone Joint Surg. Am.*, vol. 63(8): 1270–1284.

Cooper, D. E., Deng, X. H., Burstein, A. L., and Warren, R. F. 1993, 'The strength of the central third patellar tendon graft. A biomechanical study', *Am. J Sports Med.*, vol. 21(6): 818–823.

Cooper, R. R. and Misol, S. 1970, 'Tendon and ligament insertion. A light and electron microscopic study', *J. Bone Jt. Surg.*, vol. 52-A(1): 1–20.

Drouin, G. 1986, 'The prosthetic replacement of the cruciate ligament', *Clin. Orthop.*, vol. 208:59–60.

Eckes, B., Kessler, D., Aumailley, M., and Krieg, T. 1999, 'Interactions of fibroblasts with the extracellular matrix: implications for the understanding of fibrosis', *Springer Semin. Immunopathol.*, vol. 21(4): 415–429.

Eriksson, E. 1976, 'Reconstruction of the anterior cruciate ligament', *Orthop. Clin. North Am.*, vol. 7(1): 167–179.

Eriksson, E. 1983, 'Ivar Palmer, a great name in the history of cruciate ligament surgery', *Clin. Orthop.*, 172: 3–10.

Fideler, B. M., Vangsness, C. T., Jr., Lu, B., Orlando, C., and Moore, T. 1995, 'Gamma irradiation: effects on biomechanical properties of human bone-patellar tendon-bone allografts', *Am. J Sports Med.*, vol. 23(5): 643–646.

Forward, A. D. and Cowan, R. J. 1963, 'Tendon suture to bone. An experimental investigation in rabbits', *J. Bone Jt. Surg.*, vol. 45-A: 807–823.

Frank, C., Schachar, N., and Dittrich, D. 1983, 'The natural history of healing in the repaired medical collateral ligament', *J. Orthop. Res.*, vol. 1: 179–188.

Friedman, M. J. 1991, 'Prosthetic anterior cruciate ligament', *Clin. Sports Med.*, vol. 10: 499–513.

Fujikawa, K. 1985, '[Reconstruction of the cruciate ligament of the knee using an artificial ligament]', *Kango. Gijutsu*, vol. 31: 99–101.

Galatz, L. M., Ditsios, K., Burns, M., Zhu, Y., Carlisle, J. C., Sandell, L., and Silva, M. J. 2002, 'Tendon to bone healing: Correlation between collagen levels and biomechanical properties', Trans. 48th Orthop. Res. Society (2002 Orthopedic Research Society) Dallas, TX, p. 146.

Galen, C. 1968, On the usefulness of the parts of the body, (Translated by May, M.T.) Cornell University Press, Ithaca.

Gallie, W. E. 1913, 'Tendon fixation: An operation for the prevention of deformity in infantile paralysis', *Am. J. Orthop. Surg.*, vol. 11: 151–155.

Gallie, W. E. and Le Mesurier, A. B. 1921, 'The use of living sutures in operative surgery', *Canadian Med. Assoc. Journal*, vol. 11: 504.

Goetjes, H. 1913, 'Uber verletzungen der ligamenta cruciata des kniegelenks.', *Dtsch. Z. Chir.*, vol. 123: 221–221.

Grana, W. A., Egle, D. M., Mahnken, R., and Goodhart, C. W. 1994, 'An analysis of autograft fixation after anterior cruciate ligament reconstruction in a rabbit model', *Am. J. Sports Med.*, vol. 22(3): 344–351.

Greis, P. E., Burks, R. T., Bachus, K., and Luker, M. G. 2001a, 'The influence of tendon length and fit on the strength of a tendon-bone tunnel complex. A biomechanical and histologic study in the dog', *Am. J. Sports Med.*, vol. 29(4): 493–497.

Greis, P. E., Burks, R. T., Bachus, K., and Luker, M. G. 2001b, 'The influence of tendon length and fit on the strength of a tendon-bone tunnel complex. A biomechanical and histologic study in the dog', *Am. J. Sports Med.*, vol. 29(4): 493–497.

Greis, P. E., Johnson, D. L., and Fu, F. H. 1993, 'Revision anterior cruciate ligament surgery: causes of graft failure and technical considerations of revision surgery', *Clin. Sports Med.*, vol. 12: 839–852.

Hamner, D. L., Brown, C. H., Jr., Steiner, M. E., Hecker, A. T., and Hayes, W. C. 1999, 'Hamstring tendon grafts for reconstruction of the anterior cruciate ligament: biomechanical evaluation of the use of multiple strands and tensioning techniques', *J. Bone Joint Surg. Am.*, vol. 81(4): 549–557.

Hurov, J. R. 1986, 'Soft tissue bone interface: How do attachments of muscles, tendons, and ligaments change during growth?: A light microscopic study', *J. Morphol.*, vol. 189: 313–325.

Itoh, O. 1991, '[An experimental study on effect of bone morphogenetic protein and fibrin sealant in tendon implantation into bone]', *Nippon Seikeigeka Gakkai Zasshi*, vol. 65(8): 580–590.

Ivey, F. M., Blazina, M. E., Fox, J. M., and Del Pizzo, W. 1980, 'Intraarticular substitution for anterior cruciate insufficiency. A clinical comparison between patellar tendon and meniscus', *Am. J. Sports Med.*, vol. 8(6): 405–410.

Iwasaki, M., Nakahara, H., Nakata, K., Nakase, T., Kimura, T., and Ono, K. 1995, 'Regulation of proliferation and osteochondrogenic differentiation of periosteum-derived cells by transforming growth factor-beta and basic fibroblast growth factor', *J. Bone Jt. Surg.*, vol. 77-A(4): 543–554.

Jackson, D. W., Grood, E. S., Arnoczky, S. P., Butler, D. L., and Simon, T. M. 1987a, 'Cruciate reconstruction using freeze dried anterior cruciate ligament allograft and a ligament augmentation device (LAD). An experimental study in a goat model', *Am. J. Sports Med.*, vol. 15(6): 528–538.

Jackson, D. W., Grood, E. S., Arnoczky, S. P., Butler, D. L., and Simon, T. M. 1987b, 'Freeze dried anterior cruciate ligament allografts. Preliminary studies in a goat model', *Am. J. Sports Med.*, vol. 15(4): 295–303.

Jackson, D. W., Grood, E. S., Cohn, B. T., Arnoczky, S. P., Simon, T. M., and Cummings, J. F. 1991, 'The effects of in situ freezing on the anterior cruciate ligament. An experimental study in goats', *J. Bone Joint Surg. Am.*, vol. 73(2): 201–213.

James, S. L., Kellam, J. F., Slocum, D. B., and Larsen, R. L. 1983, 'The proplast prosthetic ligament stent as a replacement for the cruciate ligaments of the knee', *Aktuelle Probl. Chir Orthop.*, vol. 26: 116–120.

Johnson, D. L. and Coen, M. J. 1995, 'Revision ACL surgery. Etiology, indications, techniques, and results', *Am. J. Knee Surg.*, vol. 8: 155–167.

Johnson, D. L., Swenson, T. M., Irrgang, J. J., Fu, F. H., and Harner, C. D. 1996, 'Revision anterior cruciate ligament surgery: experience from Pittsburgh', *Clin. Orthop.*, vol. 325:100–109.

Jones, J. R., Smibert, J. G., McCullough, C. J., Price, A. B., and Hutton, W. C. 1987, 'Tendon implantation into bone: An experimental study', *J. Hand Surg.*, vol. 12-B(3): 306–312.

Kennedy, J. C., Alexander, I. J., and Hayes, K. C. 1982, 'Nerve supply of the human knee and its functional importance', *Am. J. Sports Med.*, vol. 10(6): 329–335.

Kennedy, J. C., Roth, J. H., Mendenhall, H. V., and Sanford, J. B. 1980, 'Presidential address. Intraarticular replacement in the anterior cruciate ligament-deficient knee', *Am. J. Sports Med.*, vol. 8: 1–8.

Kernwein, G., Fahey, J., and Garrison, M. 1938, 'The fate of tendon, fascia and elastic connective tissue transplanted into bone', *Ann. Surg.*, vol. 108: 285–290.

Kernwein, G. A. 1942, 'A study of tendon implantation into bone', *Surg. Genec and Obstet.*, vol. 75: 794–796.

Klein, L., Junseth, P. A., and Aadalen, R. J. 1972, 'Comparison of functional and non-functional tendon grafts: Isotopic measurement of collagen turnover and mass', *J. Bone Jt. Surg.*, vol. 54-A(8): 1745–1753.

Klein, W. and Jensen, K. U. 1992, 'Synovitis and artificial ligaments', *Arthroscopy*, vol. 8(1): 116–124.

Lam, S. J. S. 1968, 'Reconstruction of the anterior cruciate ligament using the Jones procedure and its Guy Hospital modification.', *J. Bone Joint Surg. Am.*, vol. 50(6): 1213–1224.

Laros, G. S., Tipton, C. M., and Cooper, R. C. 1971, 'Influence of physical activity on ligament insertions in dogs', *J. Bone Jt. Surg.*, vol. 53-A: 275–286.

Lipscomb, A. B., Johnston, R. K., and Snyder, R. B. 1981, 'The technique of cruciate ligament reconstruction', *Am. J Sports Med.*, vol. 9: 77–81.

Lipscomb, A. B., Johnston, R. K., Synder, R. B., and Brothers, J. C. 1979, 'Secondary reconstruction of anterior cruciate ligament in athletes by using the semitendinosus tendon. Preliminary report of 78 cases', *Am. J Sports Med.*, vol. 7: 81–84.

Liu, S. H., Panossian, V., al-Shaikh, R., Tomin, E., Shepherd, E., Finerman, G. A., and Lane, J. M. 1997, 'Morphology and matrix composition during early tendon to bone healing', *Clin. Orthop. Rel. Res.*, vol. 339: 253–260.

Liu, S. H., Yang, R. S., al-Shaikh, R., and Lane, J. M. 1995, 'Collagen in tendon, ligament, and bone healing. A current review', *Clin. Orthop. Rel. Res.*, vol. 318: 265–278.

Makisalo, S., Paavolainen, P., Holmstrom, T., and Skutnabb, K. 1989, 'Carbon fiber as a prosthetic anterior cruciate ligament. A biochemical and histological analysis in pigs', *Am. J Sports Med.*, vol. 17: 459–462.

Marder, R. A., Raskind, J. R., and Carroll, M. 1991, 'Prospective evaluation of arthroscopically assisted anterior cruciate ligament reconstruction. Patellar tendon versus semitendinosus and gracilis tendons', *Am. J Sports Med.*, vol. 19: 478–484.

Matyas, J. R., Bodie, D., Anderson, M., and Frank, C. B. 1990, 'The developmental mophology of a 'periosteal' ligament insertion: Growth and maturation of the tibial insertion of the rabbit medial collateral ligament', *J. Orthop. Res.*, vol. 8: 412–424.

Mayo Robsin, A. W. 1903, 'Ruptured crucial ligaments and their repair by operation.', *Am. Surg.*, vol. 37: 716–718.

McFarland, E. G., Morrey, B. F., An, K. N., and Wood, M. B. 1986, 'The relationship of vascularity and water content to tensile strength in a patellar tendon replacement of the anterior cruciate in dogs', *Am. J. Sports Med.*, vol. 14(6): 436–448.

Mendenhall, H. V., Roth, J. H., Kennedy, J. C., Winter, G. D., and Lumb, W. V. 1987, 'Evaluation of the polypropylene braid as a prosthetic anterior cruciate ligament replacement in the dog', *Am. J Sports Med.*, vol. 15: 543–546.

Morrison JB 1968, 'Bioengineering analysis of force actions transmitted by the knee joint', *Biomed Eng*, April, 164.

Morrison JB 1969, 'Function of the knee joint in various activities', *Biomed Eng*, vol. 4: 573–580.

Mundy, G. R. 1993, 'Cytokines and growth factors in the regulation of bone remodeling', *J Bone Mineral Res*, vol. 8(S2): S505–S510.

Muneta, T., Sekiya, I., Ogiuchi, T., Yagishita, K., Yamamoto, H., and Shinomiya, K. 1998, 'Effects of aggressive early rehabilitation on the outcome of anterior cruciate ligament reconstruction with multistrand semitendinosus tendon', *Int. Orthop.*, vol. 22(6): 352–356.

Nakahara, H., Dennis, J. E., Bruder, S. P., Haynesworth, S. E., Lennon, D. P., and Caplan, A. I. 1991, 'In vitro differentiation of bone and hypertrophic cartilage from periosteal-derived cells', *Exp. Cell Res.*, vol. 195(2): 492–503.

Nicklin, S., Morris, H., Yu, Y., Harrison, J., and Walsh, W. R. 2000, 'OP-1 augmentation of tendon-bone healing in an ovine ACL reconstruction', Trans. 46th Orthop. Res. Society, Orlando, FL, p. 155.

Noyes, F. R. and Barber-Westin, S. D. 2001, 'Revision anterior cruciate surgery with use of bone-patellar tendon-bone autogenous grafts', J. Bone Joint Surg. Am., August, 83-A(8): 1131–1143.

Noyes, F. R., Butler, D. L., Grood, E. S., Zernicke, R. F., and Hefzy, M. S. 1984, 'Biomechanical analysis of human ligament grafts used in knee-ligament repairs and reconstructions', J. Bone Joint Surg. Am., vol. 66(3): 344–352.

O'Donoghue, D.H. 1963, 'A method for replacement of the anterior cruciate ligament of the knee.', J. Bone Joint Surg. Am., vol. 45(5): 905–924.

O'Donoghue, D.H. 1991, 'Surgical treatment of fresh injuries to the major ligaments of the knee 1950', Clin. Orthop., vol. 271: 3–8.

Ohtera, K., Yamada, Y., Aoki, M., Sasaki, T., and Yamakoshi, K. 2000, 'Effects of periosteum wrapped around tendon in a bone tunnel: A biomechanical and histological study in rabbits', Crit Rev.Biomed.Eng, vol. 28(1–2): 115–118.

Olson, E. J., Harner, C. D., Fu, F. H., and Silbey, M. B. 1992, 'Clinical use of fresh, frozen soft tissue allografts', Orthopedics, vol. 15: 1225–1232.

Olson, E. J., Kang, J. D., Fu, F. H., Georgescu, H. I., Mason, G. C., and Evans, C. H. 1988, 'The biochemical and histological effects of artificial ligament wear particles: in vitro and in vivo studies', Am. J. Sports Med., vol. 16(6): 558–570.

Palmer, I. 1938, 'On injuries to the ligaments of the knee joint.', Acta. Chir. Scand. (Suppl.), vol. 53: 1–282.

Panni, A. S., Milano, G., Lucania, L., and Fabbriciani, C. 1997, 'Graft healing after anterior cruciate ligament reconstruction in rabbits', Clin. Orthop., no. 343: 203–212.

Park, J. M., Adam, R. M., Peters, C. A., Guthrie, P. D., Sun, Z., Klagsbrun, M., and Freeman, M. R. 1999, 'AP-1 mediates stretch-induced expression of HB-EGF in bladder smooth muscle cells', Am. J. Physiol., vol. 277(2 Pt 1): C294–C301.

Parsons, M., Kessler, E., Laurent, G. J., Brown, R. A., and Bishop, J. E. 1999, 'Mechanical load enhances procollagen processing in dermal fibroblasts by regulating levels of procollagen C-proteinase', Exp. Cell Res., vol. 252(2): 319–331.

Paulos, L. E., Rosenberg, T. D., Grewe, S. R., Tearse, D. S., and Beck, C. L. 1992, 'The GORE-TEX anterior cruciate ligament prosthesis. A long-term followup', Am. J. Sports Med., vol. 20(3): 246–252.

Pinczewski, L. A., Clingeleffer, A. J., Otto, D. D., Bonar, S. F., and Corry, I. S. 1997, 'Integration of hamstring tendon graft with bone in reconstruction of the anterior cruciate ligament', Arthroscopy: J. Arthro. Rel. Surg., vol. 13(5): 641–643.

Prajapati, R. T., Chavally-Mis, B., Herbage, D., Eastwood, M., and Brown, R. A. 2000, 'Mechanical loading regulates protease production by fibroblasts in three-dimensional collagen substrates', Wound. Repair Regen., vol. 8(3): 226–237.

Prajapati, R. T., Eastwood, M., and Brown, R. A. 2000, 'Duration and orientation of mechanical loads determine fibroblast cyto-mechanical activation: monitored by protease release', Wound. Repair Regen., vol. 8(3): 238–246.

Rodeo, S. A., Arnoczky, S. P., Torzilli, P. A., Hidaka, C., and Warren, R. 1993b, 'Tendon-healing in a bone tunnel', J. Bone Jt. Surg., vol. 75-A(12): 1795–1803.

Rodeo, S. A., Arnoczky, S. P., Torzilli, P. A., Hidaka, C., and Warren, R. F. 1993a, 'Tendon-healing in a bone tunnel. A biomechanical and histo-logical study in the dog', *J. Bone Joint Surg. Am.*, vol. 75(12): 1795–1803.

Rodeo, S. A., Suzuki, K., Deng, X., Wozney, J., and Warren, R. 1999b, 'Use of recombinant human bone morphogenetic protein-2 to enhance ten-don healing in a bone tunnel', *Am. J. Sports Med.*, vol. 27(4): 476–488.

Rodeo, S. A., Suzuki, K., Deng, X. H., Wozney, J., and Warren, R. F. 1999a, 'Use of recombinant human bone morphogenetic protein-2 to enhance tendon healing in a bone tunnel', *Am. J. Sports Med.*, vol. 27(4): 476–488.

Safran, M. R. and Harner, C. D. 1995, 'Revision ACL surgery: technique and results utilizing allografts', *Instr. Course Lect.*, vol. 44: 407–415.

Scharling, M. 1981, 'Replacement of the anterior cruciate ligament with a polyethylene prosthetic ligament', *Acta Orthop. Scand.*, vol. 52: 575–578.

Seemann, M. D. and Steadman, J. R. 1993, 'Tibial osteolysis associated with Gore-Tex grafts.', *Am. J. Knee Surg.*, vol. 6: 31–38.

Sharpey, W. and Ellis, G. V. 1856, *Elements of Anatomy by Jones Quain*, Walton and Moberly, London.

Shelbourne, K. D. and Nitz, P. 1990, 'Accelerated rehabilitation after anterior cruciate ligament reconstruction', *Am. J. Sports Med.*, vol. 18(3): 292–299.

Shelbourne, K. D. and Wilckens, J. H. 1990, 'Current concepts in anterior cruciate ligament rehabilitation', *Orthop., Rev.*, vol. 19(11): 957–964.

Shelbourne, K. D., Wilckens, J. H., Mollabashy, A., and DeCarlo, M. 1991, 'Arthrofibrosis in acute anterior cruciate ligament reconstruction. The effect of timing of reconstruction and rehabilitation', *Am. J. Sports Med.*, vol. 19(4): 332–336.

Snook, G. A. 1983, 'A short history of the anterior cruciate ligament and the treatment of tears', *Clin. Orthop.* no. 172: 11–13.

Stark J. 1850, 'Two cases of rupture of the crucial ligaments of the knee joint.', *Edinb. Med. Surg.*, vol. 74: 267.

Steiner, M. E., Hecker, A. T., Brown, C. H., Jr., and Hayes, W. C. 1994, 'Anterior cruciate ligament graft fixation. Comparison of hamstring and patellar tendon grafts', *Am. J. Sports Med.*, vol. 22(2): 240–246.

Suh, J.-K., Youn, I., Andrews, P., Cook, M., Cohen Sarah, J., and Jones Deryk, G. 2002, Periosteal augmentation of tendon graft improves the tendon healing within the bone tunnel. 69th Annual Meeting Proceedings 3, 600–600. 2–13.

Theilig, C., Bernd, A., Leyhausen, G., Kaufmann, R., and Geurtsen, W. 2001, 'Effects of mechanical force on primary human fibroblasts derived from the gingiva and the periodontal ligament', *J. Dent. Res.*, vol. 80(8): 1777–1780.

Topping, R. E., Anderson, P. C., and Balian, G. 1994, 'Type X collagen expression by incubated periosteum', Trans. 40th Orthop. Res. Society, New Orleans, LA, p. 390.

Tremblay, G. R., Laurin, C. A., and Drovin, G. 1980, 'The challenge of prosthetic cruciate ligament replacement', *Clin. Orthop.*, vol. 147:88–92.

Whiston, T. B. and Walmsley, R. 1960, 'Some observations on the reaction of bone and tendon after tunnelling of bone and insertion of tendon', *J. Bone Jt. Surg.*, vol. 42-B(2): 377–386.

Wilk, R. M. and Richmond, J. C. 1993, 'Dacron ligament reconstruction for chronic anterior cruciate ligament insufficiency', *Am. J. Sports Med.*, vol. 21(3): 374–379.

Woo, S. L.-Y., Maynard, J., Butler, D., Lyon, R., Torzilli, P., Akeson, W., Cooper, R., and Oakes, B. 1988, 'Ligament, tendon, and joint capsule insertions to bone,' in S. L.-Y. Woo and J. Buckwalter (eds), *Injury and*

Repair of the Musculoskeletal Soft Tissues, AAOS, Park Ridge, IL, 133–166.

Woo, S. L., Hollis, J. M., Adams, D. J., Lyon, R. M., and Takai, S. 1991, 'Tensile properties of the human femur-anterior cruciate ligament-tibia complex. The effects of specimen age and orientation', *Am. J Sports Med.*, vol. 19(3): 217–225.

Yasuda, K., Yamakazi, S., Tomita, F., Tohyama, H., and Kaneda, K. 1999, The effect of graft-tunnel diameter disparity on intraosseous healing of the flexor tendon graft in anterior cruciate ligament reconstruction. AOSSM 25th Annual Meeting Traverse City, Michigan, 417–418. 6–19.

10

The evolution of rehabilitation for ACL reconstruction

K. Donald Shelbourne and Michael D. Dersam

Introduction

The development of an anterior cruciate ligament (ACL) rehabilitation program involves an understanding of the normal knee and its functions. Conventional ACL rehabilitation programs have been associated with complications related to an inadequate understanding of normal knee function and of basic science research regarding the ACL. Attention to detail is required to reach maximal functional benefit following ACL reconstruction. A continuous review of patient follow-up must be done to minimize morbidity and to ensure the success of the rehabilitation program. By identifying potential complications and striving to eliminate them, the senior author has established a progressive and logical evolution in the ACL rehabilitative program. This chapter outlines the evolution of changes that have been implemented cautiously and gradually from 1982 through the present day. During that period we have followed the clinical outcomes of patients treated for ACL insufficiency to determine whether there were any ill-effects associated with these rehabilitation regimens. Moreover, by questioning and evaluating non-compliant patients and those patients who were willing to return to high level activities at an 'early' interval, we have progressed to our current perioperative rehabilitative program with great success.

Current surgical procedure

Our current surgical procedure is felt to be the most predictable aspect of our treatment for ACL injuries. Our surgical reconstruction stresses avoiding repetitive fat pad trauma, placing the graft appropriately and obtaining full range of motion intraoperatively to limit postoperative complications and to assist with obtaining postoperative rehabilitation goals.

A thorough knee examination is performed with the patient under anesthesia. An arthroscopic examination is used to assess and address associated meniscus injuries. The ACL reconstruction is performed through a mini-arthrotomy, as described by Shelbourne and Klootwyk (1993). The arthrotomy allows for precise and reproducible intercondylar notch measurements, notchplasty, and tunnel placement. A ten millimeter patellar tendon graft with 25 mm bone plugs from the patella and tibia are harvested. Graft fixation is secured with 19 mm polyethylene buttons on the tibia and femur. Bone grafting of the patella and the tibial graft site is done before closure. Before and after closure, the knee is taken through a full range of motion, including hyperextension and flexion that should be equal to the contralateral limb. Currently, we use either ipsilateral or contralateral bone patellar bone autogenous grafts, depending on the patient's preference.

Conventional ACL rehabilitation

Conventional rehabilitation following anterior cruciate ligament reconstruction was based on earlier surgical procedures, animal studies and achieving stability. This approach was applied early in the development of ACL reconstruction techniques and often resulted in knee motion loss. These rehabilitation programs relied on protection of the reconstructed ligament by limiting knee extension, weight-bearing, and the return to activities after surgery to achieve stability (Akeson 1990; Arnoczky et al. 1982; Arms et al. 1984; Bilko et al. 1986; Clancy et al. 1981; Fulkerson et al. 1990; Grood et al. 1984; Kleiner et al. 1989; Paulos et al. 1981). Acute surgical treatment for ACL and multi-ligamentous injuries was considered to be ideal. In addition, the intraarticular ACL reconstructions performed before 1985 were commonly augmented with extra-articular reconstructions to alleviate secondary restraint laxity (Clancy et al. 1982). Postoperatively, patients were immobilized in 30° of knee flexion to protect the extra-articular procedure and to avoid excessive ACL graft loading. Weight-bearing without a brace was not allowed for six to eight weeks after surgery; patients were restricted from full activities for one year. Although stability could be achieved, it was generally at the expense of postoperative complications, most notably flexion contractures, and anterior knee problems. Moreover, there was a low predictability to high-level sports following ACL repair (Fullerton and Andrews 1984; Harner et al. 1992; Mohtadi et al. 1991; Paulos et al. 1987; Sachs et al. 1989).

Evolution of accelerated rehabilitation

Data collection and review

Our early goals were to assess the postoperative complications following ACL repair and identify methods to eliminate them. We believe that surgical complications are best avoiding by a clear understanding of their etiology. As such, this goal remains the focus of our data collection and patient follow-up. We have maintained an extensive prospective database, which is constantly reviewed by a full-time research staff. Review of this data and long-term follow-up of patients has allowed us to learn, update and make changes to the rehabilitation regimen.

Early rehabilitation changes – regaining motion

In the early 1980s, a review of our results showed that our patients obtained good stability after ACL reconstruction, but 19 per cent of patients had difficulty obtaining full range of motion of the operated knee. Without full range of motion, patients frequently complained of chronic knee soreness and a slow functional recovery. In an attempt to decrease postoperative knee stiffness problems, casting was eliminated and a removable 30° flexion splint was used postoperatively. The use of the removable splint allowed the use of a continuous passive motion machine; CPM was used to encourage knee motion in the early postoperative period. While knee motion improved following this change, flexion contractures remained a clinical problem. As a means to address this problem, the knee splint angle was decreased to 20°, to 10° and subsequently to 0°. As the knee flexion angle was decreased, a positive effect on knee extension was served. We soon questioned the stabilizing effect of the extra-articular procedure. Ultimately, during the mid 1980s the extra-articular procedure along with the splint was eliminated.

Acute versus chronic reconstructions

Collectively, the institution of these seemingly minor changes had a noticeable positive effect on knee motion, especially in patients treated for chronic ACL insufficiency. However, patients who underwent acute ACL reconstruction continued to struggle with reestablishing knee motion and often required further surgical intervention for scar resection or manipulation. As we became more aware of the differences between acute reconstruction (improved stability) and chronic reconstructions (decreased likelihood of knee motion problems), we reasoned the optimal situation would combine the benefits of both acute and chronic ACL reconstruction. Clearly one of the most common problem was knee motion loss, thus we sought to identify these patients and soon discovered that those patients with combined ACL/MCL injury were particularly predisposed to motion problems. It had been demonstrated that isolated MCL injuries usually heal nonoperatively (Indelicato *et al.* 1983); this observation lead us to begin to treating combined ACL/MCL injured knees with a short interval of cast immobilization. The cast was changed weekly for evaluation of healing. Once the MCL began to exhibit stability (usually after one to two weeks of immobilization),

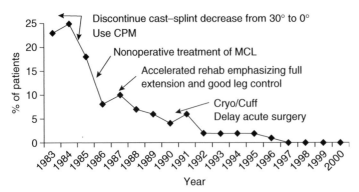

Fig. 10.1
The percentage of patients who required a scar resection to obtain full symmetrical range of motion after ACL reconstruction for an acute injury.

the ACL reconstruction was performed. This new approach decreased the incidence of scar resections and manipulations to 9 per cent following acute reconstructions and to 6 per cent following chronic reconstructions (Shelbourne and Porter 1992) (Figure 10.1).

Patient 'non-compliance'

During this same time period, a study was conducted to determine the compliance of our patients to the prescribed rehabilitation program. After discontinuing the use of rigid postoperative protection, many patients had admitted to being non-compliant with regard to weight-bearing restrictions. Surprisingly, those patients that had not complied had fewer long-term knee motion problems, fewer subjective complaints, and no difference in long-term knee stability (Shelbourne *et al.* 1992; Shelbourne and Wilckens 1990). As a result of these findings we learned that (1) early loss of extension led to long-term extension loss and subjective symptoms, (2) patients who failed to gain leg control (functional quadriceps strength) early after surgery often lacked quadriceps muscle strength later, and (3) patients who participated in high level activities before the protocol called for such activities had equal stability testing to patients who were compliant to our restrictions. Overall we soon began to realize that conventional rehabilitation programs may have been more restrictive than necessary.

Accelerated rehabilitation

A culmination of these observations led to the advent of the 'accelerated rehabilitation program' (Shelbourne and Nitz 1990). The program included the following: immediate full knee extension, early weight-bearing, and gradual increases in strengthening and functional activities to tolerance. With the evolution of the accelerated rehabilitation program we have decreased the incidence of postoperative problems. However, as patients progressed more reliably and quickly, we were concerned that that incidence of knee stiffness was still too high and looked to evaluate other factors that contribute to complications.

Pre-operative knee condition

In 1988, a retrospective look at the timing of surgery and the incidence of postoperative stiffness was conducted to determine if there was an optimal time to perform ACL reconstruction surgery. We discovered that patients who had surgery greater than three weeks after the injury had a lower incidence of knee stiffness and improved knee extension compared to those patients who had surgery less than three weeks after injury (Shelbourne *et al.* 1991). While it first appeared that the time from injury was important, we soon determined that it was the condition of the knee that was critical in surgical timing. Essentially once knee swelling has subsided, full hyperextension and flexion has been achieved and quadriceps control has been established, ACL reconstruction can be performed.

Two-staged meniscus repair and ACL reconstruction

Another group of patients who were noted to have a higher incidence of postoperative stiffness were patients who underwent ACL reconstruction for chronic ACL instability combined with treatment of a displaced, bucket-handle meniscus tear. Often times these patients presented with a significant knee flexion contracture. In an attempt to decrease complications and salvage a greater number of torn menisci, a two-staged approach was adopted. We began performing knee arthroscopy for meniscus repair or removal first, and then, when the patient regained full range of motion, an ACL reconstruction was performed (Shelbourne and Johnson 1993). This approach gave us a chance to evaluate our meniscal repair at the time of ACL reconstruction; this approach reduced our postoperative incidence of scar resections for loss of extension to 1 per cent (Figure 10.2).

Fig. 10.2

The percentage of patients who required a scar resection to obtain full symmetrical range of motion after an ACL reconstruction for chronic instability.

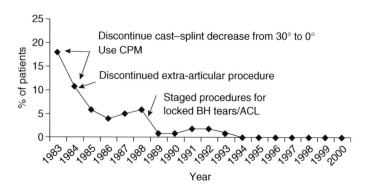

Preoperative rehabilitation

We believe that successful rehabilitation begins not after the surgery but more importantly immediately after the injury. There is a normal psychological process that a patient must go through after the injury and during the rehabilitation process. It has been shown that there are periods of depression, denial and anger prior to the final acceptance period of an injury (Smith *et al.* 1990). By utilizing this psychological process, patients are prepared for surgery and have time to organize their school and work schedules and the needed assistance they require after surgery. This process also allows time for patients to understand what is involved with the surgery and rehabilitation and their responsibilities in the postoperative period. In addition, this pre-operative time is used to reduce knee swelling and reestablish knee motion that is equal to the contralateral limb. It has been shown that patients who gain full range of motion before surgery are less likely to experience motion problems after surgery (Shelbourne and Patel 1997). The final stage of the preoperative rehabilitation process is a discussion with the patient and the person who will provide assistive care. Each patient is instructed on the goals of the surgical procedure and expectations of taking an active role in the postoperative course.

Early wound healing

As we continued to evaluate patients, we were able to make improvements in our rehabilitation program. Emphasis has been placed on factors that we believe patients would not actively do if not instructed to do so and that, if not done, would lead to complications. These factors included (1) allowing early wound healing, (2) regaining full hyperextension equal to the contralateral knee, and (3) regaining leg and quadriceps muscle control.

The key to early wound healing and early work on range of motion is eliminating the knee effusion and/or knee hemarthrosis. In 1987, patients were allowed to get up and move around on the first postoperative day. This activity led to increased swelling and limited motion. This problem was addressed by implementing the use of a continuous passive motion machine that was used not only to aid knee range of motion but also to serve as a means to consistently elevate the operated limb above the heart. Limitation of out of bed activities for the first seven days after surgery combined with the use of a cold compressive device (Cryo/Cuff, Aircast, Inc., Summit NJ) reduced the amount of swelling in the short-term and long-term. The cold compression device also helped to decrease potential wound problems, decrease pain and assist with obtaining the other early goals.

Full hyperextension

The goal of early full hyperextension equal to the opposite knee was not fully appreciated until the early 1990s. We were frustrated by the incidence of motion problems in acute reconstructions compared to those patients who had waited for surgery for reasons of convenience. Although we had started to wait to perform ACL reconstructions on a semi-acute basis, it was not until the realization that obtaining full hyperextension before surgery was the key variable that we started to use this fact in determining surgical timing.

Two studies were initiated in order to take a closer look at the role of restoring full early extension and its effects on knee stability. In the first study, Shelbourne *et al.* (1995) evaluated the manual-maximum KT-1000 arthrometer results in the same group of patients immediately after full range of motion was regained and then again at two years after surgery. No statistically significant changes in knee laxity were seen through time (Shelbourne *et al.* 1995). The second study by Rubenstein *et al.* (1995), compared patients who had normal but extreme hyperextension (greater than 8°) with a group of patients who had less than 5° of hyperextension. The KT-1000 arthrometer measurements confirmed that there was no difference in stability between these two groups. These two studies confirmed our suspicions that, with a properly placed and tensioned graft, stability would not be compromised by obtaining full extension equal to the contralateral side. In fact, the mean KT-1000 manual-maximum difference between knees has improved for these patients through the years (Table 10.1).

In an additional study, Shelbourne *et al.* evaluated 592 patients one year or more after they had followed our ACL rehabilitation protocol of obtaining full hyperextension (Shelbourne and Trumper 1997). The study patients had similar subjective scores to that of a control group in terms of activities and patellofemoral scores. In addition, we believe that full hyperextension must be achieved postoperatively so that the properly placed graft fits and develops perfectly into the intercondylar notch to prevent notch-graft mismatch. By optimizing preoperative factors and controlling postoperative

Table 10.1 KT-1000 arthrometer results

Years	Mean ± SD	Distribution of measurements – percentage of patients		
		<3 mm	4–5 mm	>5 mm
(N)				
1982–1986 (213)	2.4 ± 2.2	71	21	8
1987–1990 (473)	2.1 ± 1.5	88	10	2
1991–1994 (502)	1.9 ± 1.4	91	8	1
1995–1997 (465)	2.0 ± 1.3	91	7	2
1998–2000 (519)	1.7 ± 1.4	91	8	1

variables that directly influence the patients' abilities to achieve full hyperextension, we rarely encounter complications related to range of motion and yet long-term stability is achieved reliably.

Regaining leg control

The final variable that we emphasize is the idea of early leg and quadriceps control. These goals are accomplished with straight leg raises and short-arc quadriceps muscle contractions. These exercises prevent shut-down of the quadriceps muscles, assist with regaining full motion, and help with mobilization of the patella to prevent a patella contracture. These measures help obtain an early return to higher levels of quadriceps muscle strengthening.

Shelbourne and Gray reported the results of ACL reconstructions at 2 to 9 years after surgery (Shelbourne and Gray 1997). Patients had objective measurements that showed a mean range of motion of 5° of hyperextension to 140° of flexion. The mean KT-1000 arthrometer manual-maximum difference between knees was 2.0 ± 1.5 mm. Isokinetic quadriceps muscle strength testing showed a mean strength of 94 per cent after acute ACL reconstruction and 91 per cent after chronic ACL reconstructions. The mean time for patients to return to sport-specific activities was 6.2 weeks, and the mean time to return time to full competition was 6.2 months postoperatively.

Contralateral graft choice

In 1994, Rubenstien *et al.* (1994) reported the results of using patellar tendon grafts from the contralateral knee for ACL revision surgery. The observation that these patients easily regained full range of motion and quadriceps muscle strength led to the idea of using the contralateral patellar tendon for primary ACL reconstructions. As others have noted, one of the obstacles in ipsilateral autogenous graft reconstructions is the return of strength to the patellar tendon donor site and the already weakened extensor mechanism (Rosenberg *et al.* 1992; Wilk *et al.* 1993). We have also observed that when aggressive strengthening exercises are performed before the patient has 120° of flexion, many patients experience swelling and a loss of extension and flexion. By using a contralateral autogenous graft, the traumatic effects of the surgery are divided between knees so that patients can focus on independent goals for each knee. Patients can concentrate on regaining full range of motion and limiting swelling in the ACL-reconstructed knee. Full range of motion is obtained in the graft-donor knee on the day of surgery, so regaining strength can be the focus immediately after surgery without concern for developing swelling. The results of using contralateral graft for primary ACL reconstructions have been previously reported (Shelbourne and Urch 2000). The results showed that compared to the ipsilateral group, the contralateral group had statistically significant increases in flexion at one week (105° versus 86°) and at two weeks (117° versus 101°) postoperatively. In addition, patients in the contralateral group obtained higher quadriceps muscle strength at one, two, and four months postoperatively in the ACL-reconstructed knee and at one and two months postoperatively in the graft-donor knee. The mean KT-1000 arthrometer manual-maximum difference between knees was 1.9 ± 1.3 mm for the contralateral group and 2.2 ± 1.1 mm for the ipsilateral group. As far returning to sports and activity, the average for all patients returning to preinjury levels was 4.9 ± 2.1 for the contralateral group and 6.1 ± 2.2 mm in the ipsilateral group. In a subgroup of patients participating in competitive sports, the mean time to return to sports at full capacity was 4.1 months for the contralateral group and 5.5 months for the ipsilateral group.

Current rehabilitation program

The current rehabilitation program is based on a series of events through which each patient must progress (Figure 10.3). There are no specific time periods required before the patient advances to the next step. Each event is comprised of goals we feel are paramount for avoiding complications. The perioperative rehabilitation program for ACL reconstruction using a graft from the contralateral knee is summarized in Table 10.2. The goals of rehabilitation for ACL reconstruction with a graft from the ipsilateral knee are the same, except that there is a delay in the introduction of aggressive strengthening exercises until the patient has 120° of flexion. A patient progresses through the cascade of events, meeting the goals of each stage before moving on to the next stage.

The keystones of the rehabilitation process are obtaining and maintaining full hyperextension, minimizing a postoperative

Fig. 10.3

The cascade of events that patients progress through with rehabilitation after ACL reconstruction.

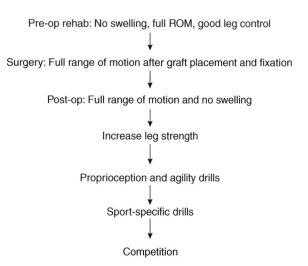

Pre-op rehab: No swelling, full ROM, good leg control

↓

Surgery: Full range of motion after graft placement and fixation

↓

Post-op: Full range of motion and no swelling

↓

Increase leg strength

↓

Proprioception and agility drills

↓

Sport-specific drills

↓

Competition

Table 10.2 Perioperative rehabilitation program after ACL reconstruction with contralateral patellar tendon graft

Time	ACL-reconstructed knee Goals	Exercises	Graft-donor knee Goals	Exercises
Preoperative	Obtain full range of motion Reduce swelling Good leg control Achieve a normal gait Good mental attitude; understand post-op program	Hyperextension device 3 ×/day Prone hangs Heel slides Cold/compression; elevation Active terminal extension Gait training Patient education of program and goals	Maintain leg strength	Practice using the step box
Surgery	Maintain full range of motion Prevent pain and swelling	Move knee from full hypertension to full flexion (heel touches buttocks) Intravenous ketorolac pain prevention program	Close patellar tendon defect Bone graft the defects in the patella and tibia	
Day of surgery to 1 week post-op	Minimize hemarthrosis Full passive hyperextension Flexion to 110° Independent leg raise Weightbearing as tolerated for bathroom privileges only Normal gait	Cold/compression; to remain on the knee except during exercises; elevation Heel props, 10 min, 6 ×/day CPM set at highest flexion; leave leg in maximal flexion 6 ×/day Flexion in shuttle machine with no resistance; place leg in machine and use straps to pull heel toward buttocks	Minimize swelling Full passive hyperextension Full flexion Donor site strengthening	Cold pack; leg elevated on pillow Heel props; maintaining extension is easy; graft-donor knee is used as a comparison for the ACL-reconstructed knee Heel slides; pull heel to buttocks; use measuring

Week 2 (7 to 14 days)	Maintain full extension Flexion to 125° Minimal swelling Normal gait Be able to lock knee straight with bearing full weight	Heel slides; use measuring stick to monitor progress Active quadriceps contractions; straight leg raises; active terminal extension Gait training Heel props; prone hangs Heel slides Cold/compression Gait training in front of a mirror Single leg stance; locking knee in extension	Maintain full extension and flexion No swelling Donor site strengthening	stick to monitor progress Shuttle machine; set resistance so able to do 50 repetitions, 6 ×/day; progressively increase resistance Heel slide Ice after exercise Shuttle exercise: 50 repetitions 6 ×/day Step-box exercise at a height to allow at least 25 and up to 50 repetitions; perform 6 ×/day
Weeks 3 to 4	Maintain full extension Increase flexion equal to opposite knee Maintain minimal swelling Light strengthening	Heel props or prone hang as needed Heel slides; sit on heels Cold/compression after exercise Active terminal extension; Stationary bicycling Stairmaster, 5 to 10 min.	Maintain full range of motion Donor site strengthening	Exercises if needed Stationary bicycle Stairmaster, 5 to 10 min Continue step-box exercise 6 × day Single-leg weight training exercises (still high repetition/low resistance): leg press, leg extension

Table 10.2 (Continued)

Time	ACL-reconstructed knee Goals Exercises		Graft-donor knee Goals Exercises	
Weeks 4 to 8	Maintain full range of motion Control swelling	Heel props or prone hang as needed; sit on heels Cold/compression; adjust activities to keep swelling to a minimum Bicycle; Stairmaster; leg press; leg extension	Donor site strengthening	Increase weight and decrease repetitions for weight training exercises
	Quadriceps strengthening Return to light sports	Functional progression from agility drills, sport-specific agility drills, to controlled practice drills		
From 8 weeks after surgery	Maintain full range of motion	Exercises as needed; range of motion can decrease when activities are increased; monitor daily	Return donor-site functional strength	Continue with weight training 3 ×/week Increase functional strength through sport-specific activities; Alternate intensity with hard and easy days
	Control swelling	Adjust activities to keep swelling to a minimum; Continue using cold compression		
	Return to full sports	Continue sport-specific and controlled practice drills and progress first to part-time competition and then full-time competition		

hemarthrosis, and strengthening the donor site. Limitation of ambulation (except for bathroom use) during the first week after surgery is strictly enforced. The control of hemarthrosis is enhanced by placing the patient's ACL-reconstructed knee in a continuous passive motion machine for knee elevation. Prior to discharge on postoperative day one, full passive extension, independent straight leg raises and 100 to 110 degrees of flexion are required. At the first clinic visit (1 week), full terminal extension, flexion to 110°, minimal swelling, and normal gait are expected.

When terminal extension and knee flexion to 130° are present, strengthening with the use of a stair machine and leg press exercises is initiated. Early return to sport-specific drills such shooting basketballs and kicking a ball as can be started. Finally, prior to advancing to increased activities, patients should have full hyperextension and be able to sit on their heels comfortably. When the return of strength to 70 per cent is seen, a functional progression of sports agility activities can be initiated.

If at any time swelling occurs in the ACL-reconstructed knee or range of motion decreases, activity should be curtailed so that it can be done without causing symptoms. After activities, one measure to check this is to make sure the patient has maintained their extension and the ability to sit on their heels. We continue to update the program based on small changes that are observed in our patient follow-up.

Return to sports

All of the changes made to the rehabilitation have been in an effort to decrease the complications associated with ACL reconstruction; however, as a secondary benefit we have observed that patients are able to return to sports earlier than with conventional rehabilitation. Patients have regained full range of motion and quadriceps muscle control at earlier periods after surgery, which has facilitated the return to sport-related activities and sports competition earlier. These patients have not had any changes in long-term stability, nor have they had a higher graft tear rate compared with those patients who wait extended periods of time before returning to activities. These findings are contrary to what earlier research on cadaveric and animal models would recommend (Akeson 1990; Arnoczky et al. 1982; Clancy et al. 1981). However, our review of graft biopsies undergoing arthroscopic procedures for other reasons showed that, at three weeks after ACL reconstruction, the patellar tendon graft is viable. This finding is also supported by Kliener et al. (1989) who found that at three weeks following reconstruction, living fibroblasts that repopulated the graft had high synthetic capacity. As with other biologic materials it also appears that stressing the graft is beneficial to the organization of the fibroblasts.

The evaluations of our non-compliant patients showed us that by gradually relaxing the restrictions placed on the patients, they could progress at their own desired pace as their confidence increased. However, the two factors of no swelling and knee range of motion equal to the contralateral side are important for preventing postoperative range of motion complications. The key to returning to sports-specific activities and lastly competing at preinjury levels is dependent on equal motion and equal leg strength. We have seen that patients returning to activities with less than 65 per cent strength often had problems with activity related swelling and soreness. In addition, return to competitive sports requires regaining approximately 75 per cent of strength. It should also be noted, however, that this earlier return to sports agility programs does not cause a change in graft stability. Patients return to activities anywhere from two to six months after surgery, depending on personal goals and the ability to regain strength and confidence in the knee. In addition, despite being able to return at two months after surgery, most patients report that it takes an additional there to four months before to totally feeling fully comfortable in game situations.

Summary

The perioperative rehabilitation program represents slowly occurring changes and improvements to the previous rehabilitation protocols. Since 1984, the clinic has continued to employ research staff to record and analyze results and assist with clinical changes. Through analysis of data and observations, we believe that a successful outcome in ACL reconstruction is based on avoidance of complications. Preoperatively, this begins with obtaining a 'normal knee' prior to surgery and preparing mentally for the surgical process. Postoperatively, the goals are to achieve early wound healing, to restore full motion that is equal to the contralateral side and to regain quadriceps control. Once these are acquired, precise placement of the patellar graft allows faster and safer stressing of the graft as the patient proceeds in their comfort and confidence. Our previously reported data on contralateral autogenous grafts indicate that this process can proceed at an even faster more reliable manner. Regardless of the graft site chosen, the ultimate goal with all patients should be to reconstruct the ACL-deficient knee with one surgery at the appropriate time and rehabilitate the knee so that it is symmetrical in motion, strength and stability as the opposite knee.

References

Akeson WH (1990). The response of ligaments to stress modulation and overview of the ligament healing response. In Daniel DM, Akeson WH, O'Connor JJ, eds. *Knee Ligaments:Structure, Function, Injury and Repair*, pp 315–327. Raven Press, New York.

Arms SW, Pope MH, Johnson RJ, Fischer RA, Arvidsson I, Eriksson E (1984). The biomechanics of anterior cruciate ligament rehabilitation and reconstruction. *Am J Sports Med*, 12, 8–18.

Arnoczky SP, Tarvin GB, Marshall JL (1982). Anterior cruciate ligament replacement using patellar tendon. An evaluation of graft revascularization in the dog. *J Bone Joint Surg* Am, 64, 217–224.

Bilko TE, Paulos LE, Feagin JA, Lambert KL, Cunningham HR (1986). Current trends in repair and rehabilitation of complete (acute) anterior cruciate ligament injuries. *Am J Sports Med*, 14, 143–146.

Clancy WG, Narechania RG, Rosenberg TD, Gmeiner JG, Wisnefske DD, Lange TA (1981). Anterior and posterior cruciate ligament reconstruction in rhesus monkeys: A histological microangiographic and biochemical analysis. *J Bone Joint Surg Am*, 63, 1270–1284.

Clancy WG, Nelson DA, Reider B, Narechania RG (1982). Anterior cruciate ligament reconstruction using one third of the patellar ligament, augmented by extra-articular tendon transfers. *J Bone Joint Surg Am*, 64, 352–359.

Fulkerson JP, Berke A, Parthasarathy N (1990). Collagen biosynthesis in rabbit intraarticular patellar tendon transplants. *Am J Sports Med*, 18, 249–253.

Fullerton LR, Andrews JR (1984). Mechanical block to extension following augmentation of the anterior cruciate ligament reconstruction: A case report. *Am J Sports Med*, 12, 166–168.

Grood ES, Suntay WJ, Noyes FR, Butler, DL (1984). Biomechanics of knee extension exercises: Effect of cutting the anterior cruciate ligament. *J Bone Joint Surg Am*, 66, 725–734.

Harner CD, Irrgang JJ, Paul J, Dearwater S, Fu FH (1992). Loss of motion after anterior cruciate ligament reconstruction. *Am J Sports Med*, 20, 499–506.

Indelicato PA (1983). Non-operative treatment of the medial collateral ligament of the knee. *J Bone Joint Surg Am*, 65, 323–329.

Kleiner JB, Amiel D, Harwood FL, Akeson WH (1989). Early histologic, metabolic and vascular assessment of anterior cruciate autografts. *J Ortho Res*, 7, 235–242.

Mohtadi, NH, Webster-Bogaert S, Fowler PJ (1991). Limitation of motion following anterior cruciate ligament reconstruction: A case control study. *Am J Sports Med*, 19, 620–625.

Paulos LE, Noyes FR, Grood ES, Butler DL (1981). Knee rehabilitation after anterior cruciate ligament reconstruction and repair. *Am J Sports Med*, 9, 140–149.

Paulos LE, Rosenberg TD, Drawbert J, Manning J, Abbott P (1987). Infrapatellar contracture syndrome: An unrecognized cause of knee stiffness with patella entrapment and patella infera. *Am J Sports Med*, 15, 331–341.

Rosenberg TD, Franklin JL, Baldwin GN (1992). Extensor mechanism function after patellar tendon graft harvest for anterior cruciate ligament reconstruction. *Am J Sports Med*, 20, 519–526.

Rubenstien RA, Jr, Shelbourne KD, Van Meter CD, McCarroll JR, Rettig AC (1994). Isolated autogenous bone-patellar-bone graft site morbidity. *Am J Sports Med*, 22, 324–327.

Rubenstien RA, Shelbourne KD, Van Meter CD, McCarroll JR, Rettig AC, Gloyeske RL (1995). Effect of knee stability if full hyperextension is restored immediately after anterior cruciate reconstruction. *Am J Sports Med*, 23, 365–368.

Sachs RA, Daniel DM, Stone ML, Garfein RF (1989). Patellofemoral problems after anterior cruciate ligament reconstruction. *Am J Sports Med*, 17, 760–765.

Shelbourne KD, Gray T (1997). Anterior cruciate ligament reconstruction with autogenous patellar tendon graft followed by accelerated rehabilitation. A two- to nine-year followup. *Am J Sports Med*, 25, 786–795.

Shelbourne KD, Johnson GE (1993). Locked bucket-handle meniscal tears in knees with chronic anterior cruciate ligament deficiency. *Am J Sports Med*, 21, 779–782.

Shelbourne KD, Klootwyk TE (1993). The miniarthrotomy technique for anterior cruciate ligament reconstruction. *Operative Tech Sports Medicine*, 1, 26–39.

Shelbourne KD, Klootwyk TE, DeCarlo MS (1992). Update on accelerated rehabilitation after anterior cruciate ligament reconstruction. *J Orthop Sports Phys Ther*, 15, 303–308.

Shelbourne KD, Klootwyk TE, Wilckens JH, DeCarlo MS (1995). Ligament stability two to six years after ACL reconstruction with autogenous patellar tendon graft and participation in accelerated rehabilitation program. *Am J Sports Med*, 23, 575–579.

Shelbourne KD, Nitz P (1990). Accelerated rehabilitation after anterior cruciate ligament reconstruction. *Am J Sports Med*, 18, 292 –299.

Shelbourne KD, Patel DV (1995). Timing of surgery in anterior cruciate ligament-injured knees. *Knee Surgery Sports Trauma Arthroscopy*, 3, 148–156.

Shelbourne KD, Porter DA (1992). Anterior cruciate ligament-medial collateral ligament injury: Non-operative management of the medial collateral ligament tears with anterior cruciate ligament reconstruction. *Am J Sports Med*, 20, 283–286.

Shelbourne KD, Trumper RV (1997). Preventing anterior knee pain after anterior cruciate reconstruction. *Am J Sports Med*, 25, 41–47.

Shelbourne KD, Urch SE (2000). Primary anterior cruciate ligament reconstruction using the contralateral patellar tendon. *Am J Sports Med*, 28, 651–658.

Shelbourne KD, Wilckens JH (1990). Current concepts in anterior cruciate ligament rehabilitation. *Orthopedic Review*, 19, 957–964.

Shelbourne KD, Wilckens JH, Mollabashy A, DeCarlo MS (1991). Arthrofibrosis in anterior cruciate ligament reconstruction: The effect of timing of reconstruction and rehabilitation. *Am J Sports Med*, 19, 332–336.

Smith A, Scott SG, O'Fallon WM, Young ML (1990). Emotional responses of athletes to injury. *Mayo Clinic Proc*, 65, 35–50.

Wilk KE, Andrews JR, Clancy WG (1993). Quadriceps muscular strength after removal of the central third patellar tendon for contralateral anterior cruciate ligament reconstruction surgery. *J Ortho Sports Phys Ther*, 18, 692–697.

11

ACL reconstruction in the skeletally immature: indications, methodology and concerns

George A. Paletta

Introduction

Although initially thought to be rare, isolated tears of the anterior cruciate ligament (ACL) in skeletally immature individuals are being more frequently recognized and reported (Aichroth *et al.* 2002, Andrews *et al.* 1994, Andrish 2001, Angel and Hall 1989, Aronowitz *et al.* 1997, Barrack *et al.* 1990, Baxter and Wiley 1988, Bisson *et al.* 1998, Buckley *et al.* 1989, DeLee and Curtis 1983, Edwards and Grana 2001, Engebresten *et al.* 1988, Fehnel and Johnson 2000, Graf *et al.* 1992, Hofmeister *et al.* 2001, Janarv *et al.* 1996, Kannus and Jarvinen 1988, Lee *et al.* 1999, Lipscomb and Anderson 1986, Lo *et al.* 1998, 1997, Matava and Siegel 1997, McCarroll *et al.* 1988, McCarroll *et al.* 1994, McCarroll *et al.* 1995, Mizuta *et al.* 1995, Nottage and Matsuura 1994, Paletta 2001, Parker *et al.* 1994, Schaefer *et al.* 1993, Simonian *et al.* 1999, Skak *et al.* 1987, Stadelmaier *et al.* 1995, Stanitski 1994, 1995, 1999, Sullivan 1990, Williams *et al.* 1996). Schaefer *et al.* (1993) have reported ACL injury in a four-year-old patient. This increased frequency is the result of increased participation of children in sports, enhanced awareness of ligamentous injuries in the children, and increased proficiency in physical diagnosis of such injuries. An effective and reliable management plan for the care of these injuries has been lacking. This chapter will review the relevant epidemiology, anatomy and pathogenesis, natural history, physical examination, imaging studies, non-operative treatment alternatives, indications for surgery, and options for operative treatment of ACL injuries in the skeletally immature individual.

Epidemiology

Previously published studies of the 'skeletally immature patient' with ACL injury have suffered from design flaws including lack of documentation of skeletal maturity and lack of specificity of diagnosis, making it impossible to determine the true incidence and prevalence of such injuries. Most early studies reported tibial eminence avulsion injuries to be much more common than midsubstance ACL ruptures, Baxter and Wiley (1988), Skak (1987), Zaricznyj (1977). More recent reports have documented significant numbers of skeletally immature individuals who sustained ACL injuries independent of tibial eminence fractures (Aichroth *et al.* 2002, Andrews *et al.* 1994, Andrish 2001, Angel and Hall 1989, Aronowitz *et al.* 1997, Barrack *et al.* 1990, Bisson *et al.* 1998, Buckley *et al.* 1989, DeLee and Curtis 1983, Edwards and Grana 2001, Engebresten *et al.* 1988, Fehnel and Johnson 2000, Graf *et al.* 1992, Hofmeister *et al.* 2001, Janarv *et al.* 1996, Kannus and Jarvinen 1988, Lee *et al.* 1999, Lipscomb and Anderson 1986, Lo *et al.* 1997, 1998, Matava and Siegel 1997, McCarroll *et al.* 1988, McCarroll *et al.* 1994, McCarroll *et al.* 1995, Mizuta *et al.* 1995, Nottage and Matsuura 1994, Paletta 2001, Parker *et al.* 1994, Schaefer *et al.* 1993, Simonian *et al.* 1999, Stadelmaier *et al.* 1995, Stanitski 1999, Sullivan 1990, Williams *et al.* 1996). In 1983 DeLee and Curtis reported 3 of 338 (1 per cent) adolescents of less than 14 years of age with knee injuries had an ACL tear. More recently Lipscomb and Anderson (1986) and McCarroll *et al.* (1995) have reported incidences of 3.4 and 3.3 per cent of skeletally immature ACL injuries. It is now thought that midsubstance ACL tears occur more frequently than tibial eminence fractures. Bony avulsion of the ACL at its femoral insertion is extremely rare.

Partial tears of the ACL are reported to be common in skeletally immature individuals. Stanitski *et al.* (1993) reported on the arthroscopic findings in 70 children with hemarthrosis. Of the preadolescents (aged 7 to 12 years), 47 per cent had ACL tears and 58 per cent of these were partial. Of the adolescents (equally divided between aged 13–15 and aged 16–18), 65 per cent had ACL tears of which 60 per cent were partial. Tibial eminence fractures are a special type of injury to the ACL complex. The classification system described by Zaricznyj (1977) is based on the morphology and amount of displacement of the fracture fragment (Figure 11.1).

Anatomy and pathogenesis

In the skeletally immature individual the tibial attachment of the anterior cruciate ligament is a perichondral epiphyseal cuff that, with skeletal development, progresses to the fibrocartilage-bone attachment seen in adults. Prior to closure of the proximal tibial physis, the intercondylar eminence is less resistant to traction forces than the ligament. This relative strength disparity was believed to be the explanation for the preponderance of tibial eminence avulsions in children rather than intrasubstance ACL ruptures. Knee ligaments in children are now recognized to undergo the same

Fig. 11.1

The Zaricznyj classification of tibial eminence fractures. Type I = non-displaced; Type II = hinged with partial displacement; Type IIIA = complete displacement; Type IIIB = complete displacement + rotation; Type IV = displaced + comminuted.

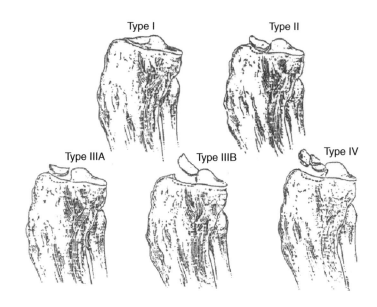

pathodynamics of disruption as adult ligaments. Skak *et al.* (1987) demonstrated that midsubstance ligament injuries occur with low-energy, rapid-loading events while ligament-bone junction injuries occur with high-energy, slow-loading events. Despite such a 'weak link', the ACL does undergo irreversible plastic deformation, elongation, and attenuation prior to chondro-epiphyseal failure.

Natural history

There have been few natural history studies of isolated ACL injury in skeletally immature patients. Most previous reports have suffered from a multitude of deficiencies in study design, including small patient numbers, mixed ages and genders, varied athletic demands and treatment protocols, inadequate definition of mechanism of injury and duration of ligament insufficiency, varied evaluation criteria, and poorly defined control group. It appears that the natural history of ACL deficiency in the skeletally immature patient is similar to that in the adult. Extrapolating from the young adult data, children who fail to modify their activities and continue to participate in demanding acceleration/deceleration athletic activity are likely to experience recurrent giving way episodes with increased risk for meniscal tears and premature degenerative oseoarthritis (Barrack *et al.* 1990). A number of small short-term follow-up series lend support to this conclusion. Kannus and Jarvinen (1988) reported on a small group skeletally immature patients with ACL injuries treated non-operatively and followed for an average of 8.3 years. Most had fair to poor functional outcome scores with gross instabilities and 4/12 developed degenerative radiographic changes. Graf *et al.* (1992) reported on 12 ACL injured patients with average age of 14 years. Of the eight treated with rehabilitation and bracing all developed recurrent instability by seven months post-injury and 7/8 demonstrated new meniscal tears. Mizuta *et al.* (1995) have also reported poor results with only 7/18 patients returning to pre-injury levels of activity and 11/18 developing radiographic evidence of Fairbank's degenerative changes.

The natural history of fractures of the tibial eminence is more clearly understood. A displaced tibial eminence fracture that remains unreduced can act as a mechanical block to knee extension. Most patients with eminence fractures demonstrate some residual ACL laxity in the sagittal plane as indicated by either Lachman or anterior drawer testing. Baxter and Wiley (1988) reviewed 45 patients with history of tibial eminence avulsion fractures. Fractures that had been partially or completely displaced were associated with ACL laxity. Overall, 51 per cent of patients had clinical and arthrometric evidence of positive Lachman or anterior drawer tests. No patient complained of instability and none had positive pivot shift tests.

The fate of the adolescent knee with a partial tear of the ACL is less clear. Buckley *et al.* (1989) reviewed a series of 35 young adults with arthroscopically documented partial ACL tears. All were treated with a program of protected weight-bearing, early range of motion, and strengthening exercises to restore quadriceps to hamstrings strength ration. At mean follow-up of 41 months, 86 per cent were minimally symptomatic and 40 per cent had returned to their preinjury level of performance. The authors concluded that patients with minimal anterior translation, no rotatory instability, and low demand or performance expectations after partial ACL injury appear to do well at three to four years after injury.

History and physical examination

Studies of children with acute knee injuries have shown that clinical diagnosis by careful history and thorough physical exam correlate poorly with the correct diagnosis documented by arthroscopy. Nonetheless, the importance of a careful history and physical exam cannot be overemphasized. As in the adult, the history will usually relate an acute injury (contact or non-contact), the experience of a 'pop' in the knee, and an inability to return to play. Statistics emphasize characterization of the mechanism of injury and its severity based on the history of contact or non-contact deceleration or rotation. Injuries without contact, deceleration, or rotation are less likely to be associated with an ACL injury. Acute patellar instability can also be produced by deceleration/rotation mechanisms. Varus or valgus stress on the knee may suggest collateral ligament of femoral or, less likely, tibial physeal injury. Knee effusion from hemarthrosis occurs rapidly, usually within several hours of acute injury, and is a herald of major intraarticular injury in the pediatric and adolescent athlete.

In a chronically ACL insufficient knee, the patient may complain of functional instability and recurrent giving way with activities requiring pivoting. Recurrent effusion with each giving way episode is common. Recurrent instability episodes may result in meniscal tears and produce meniscal symptoms of joint line pain, locking or catching. Physical examination of the acutely injured knee in the pediatric patient is often difficult due to patient fear, apprehension and limited cooperation. The exam is usually easier in patients with chronic ACL insufficiency. Examination of the whole extremity, especially the hip, as well as the unaffected limb is essential. Knee pain in the skeletally immature patient is assumed to be hip pain until proven otherwise. The presence of an effusion should be noted and range of active and passive motion documented. The presence or absence of tenderness at the collateral ligaments joint line, and femoral and tibial physes should be noted. Examination of the patellofemoral joint is done, including the patellar retinaculum to rule out an acute patella dislocation, which can present with a history similar to acute ACL rupture. Physiologic laxity, which may be significant in children, must be assessed in all planes. The motion and laxity of the opposite knee are used as a baseline for comparison if there has not been previous injury to that knee. Anterior drawer and Lachman tests will usually be positive in an ACL deficient knee. Both the magnitude of translation and quality of endpoint are considered. The child with physiologic laxity may have abnormal anterior translation but has a distinct, firm endpoint. In the acute setting the pivot shift may be difficult to perform because of muscle spasm and pain. The pivot shift sign is usually easily detected in the chronic ACL insufficient knee. Use of instrumented arthrometers may provide baseline sagittal plane laxity information and side-to-side comparison but age-adjusted normal values are not available. Limb length and girth constraints may also invalidate arthrometer testing in small statured patients.

Imaging studies

Radiographic evaluation should include a routine radiographic four-view knee series: AP, lateral, tunnel and skyline views. Comparison and stress views may be required if tibial and/or femoral physeal fractures are suspected. Stress radiographs can be used to distinguish physeal separation from ligament disruption (Sullivan 1990). Malformation of the tibial spine and/or femoral notch suggests congenital absence of the ACL. The extent of physeal closure can also be assessed on routine radiographs. Computed tomographic (CT) scans or MRI can be used to assess the degree of epiphyseal closure if skeletal maturity is in question.

Magnetic resonance imaging can provide valuable information about the location of ACL tear, presence of associated meniscal or bony injury, and status of maturity of the femoral and tibial

171

epiphyses (Lee *et al.* 1999). A common secondary MRI sign of acute ACL tear is the so-called 'bone bruise' most commonly seen involving the subchondral bone of the lateral femoral condyle and/or lateral tibial plateau. These secondary findings are reported to occur in a majority of patients with acute ACL injury and contribute to the sensitivity and specificity of MRI as a diagnostic tool in the skeletally immature patient with ACL injury. MR imaging has made a significant impact on knee injury diagnosis but false positive and false negative studies are not uncommon, especially in the setting of radiologic inexperience with pediatric musculoskeletal MR assessment (Lee *et al.* 1999). Patient history and physical exam findings must still be correlated with the MR images. MR imaging is recommended in all patients in whom ACL injury is suspected but is not a substitute for a complete history and physical examination.

Treatment of tibial eminence avulsion

Treatment of tibial eminence avulsion injuries is dependent upon the displacement of the fracture. Type I and II injuries are treated with closed reduction and immobilization with the knee in extension for four to six weeks. Closed reduction is best achieved by maximally extending the knee. As the final 5–10° of extension is reached, the femoral condyles impinge upon the fragment and reduce it. Type II fractures that cannot be anatomically reduced by closed means and all Type IIIA, IIIB, and IV fractures are treated with surgical reduction and internal fixation (Figure 11.2). This can usually be done arthroscopically through standard portals. The fracture is reduced anatomically and fixed with sutures, pins, or screws. Regardless of the choice of fixation, the fixation should be confined to the proximal tibial epiphysis without violation of the tibial physeal plate. Postoperative rehabilitation is similar to that for ACL reconstruction, but the time course to full activity participation is usually shorter because of rapid osseous union.

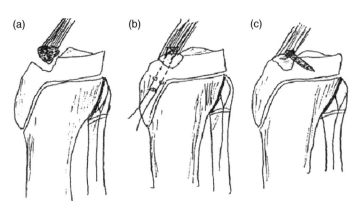

(a) (b) (c)

Fig. 11.2

Fixation options for displaced tibial eminence fractures. (a) Type IIIA fracture; (b) suture fixation – note sutures remain proximal to physis; (c) screw fixation – note screw does not cross physis.

Treatment approach to intrasubstance ACL injuries

Treatment of intrasubstance ACL injuries in the child and young adolescent remains controversial. No consensus has been reached because of the paucity of accurate, objective date of sufficient follow-up length. An ACL injury is not a surgical emergency. An accurate initial diagnosis is imperative to institution of proper treatment and the assurance of a predictable successful outcome. Data from the history, physical exam, and imaging studies is usually sufficient however if the diagnosis is in doubt, arthroscopy may be necessary. Once a specific diagnosis is made, a specific treatment program can be outlined. The patient and his or her family must understand the rehabilitation effort and time necessary for any treatment option, be it operative or nonoperative. Any treatment plan must take into consideration assessment of the patient's physical maturity, level of functional instability, and the vocational and avocational demands on his/her knee.

Assessment of maturity

Skeletal maturity has important implications for potential treatment. The adolescent nearing physeal closure with limited skeletal growth remaining differs markedly from the prepubescent juvenile with wide-open physes and significant skeletal growth remaining. Physical maturity is a dynamic process. Onset, duration, rate, and magnitude of skeletal growth vary from individual to individual. Maturity must be evaluated on chronologic, physiologic, and radiologic bases. In 1985, Tanner and Davies reported the normal growth curves for North American children. They observed that, on average, the adolescent growth spurt begins, at age 10.5 years in girls and 12.5 years in boys. Peak height velocity was reported to occur at age 11.5 years in girls and 13.5 years in boys. Cessation of changes in shoe size has been reported to be a useful indicator of growth deceleration since feet reach approximately 95 per cent of their adult size by age 12.5 years in girls and 14 years in boys.

Menarche is an excellent predictor of growth deceleration. Onset of menses is preceded by peak velocity of longitudinal growth. Following menarche there is a rapid diminution of skeletal growth. The Tanner grading scale of development of secondary sexual characteristics should be used to assess physical maturity. Development of pigmented pubic and axillary hair in boys is approximately equivalent physiologically to the onset of menarche in girls.

The use of imaging techniques to establish maturity suffers from potential inaccuracies because of the wide range of normal values. This is especially true of bone age determination, in which standards are based on the fairly uniform genetic pool used for estimation almost 50 years ago. It is unknown if those standards hold true for today's multicultural American society.

Functional instability

Functional instability is defined as repeated giving way episodes with activities of daily living and/or sports participation. Children with complete ACL insufficiency typically fall into one of two groups based on the significance of their functional instability. One group of children will demonstrate no functional instability. Such patients will be able to carry out activities of daily living and participate in sports without giving way episodes. The second group will have varying degrees of instability with such activities. Functional instability does not imply functional limitation. Children with functional instability may continue to participate fully in athletics.

Although classification of functional instability is important when formulating a treatment plan, at the time of initial acute injury accurate prediction of which child will have such instability is impossible. In an effort to determine the level of functional instability, a trial of non-operative treatment may be warranted in the prepubescent child with an acute ACL injury. It is essential to inform the patient and parents that each giving way episode puts the menisci and articular cartilage at risk for injury. In the prepubescent child with chronic ACL insufficiency and functional instability, treatment should be instituted to limit the risk of damage to the menisci and articular cartilage. In the post-pubescent adolescent with limited skeletal growth remaining, determination of functional instability is less crucial to formulating a treatment plan because the treatment options are less constrained. Such children can essentially be treated as adults.

Non-operative treatment

The natural history of the unreconstructed isolated ACL-deficient knee in children is one of recurrent episodes of instability and development of meniscal tears. Several authors (Kannus and Jarvinen 1988, Mizuta *et al.* 1995) have reported poor results of non-surgical treatment. However, such a history should not serve as condemnation of non-operative treatment of ACL insufficiency in the skeletally immature. A trial of non-operative treatment may be indicated in children with isolated acute ACL injuries who are determined to be truly skeletally immature with significant growth remaining. This includes premenarchal females and Tanner stage 1 and 2 males. Non-operative treatment is also indicated in those individuals who have contraindications to or refuse consideration of surgery.

The goal of non-operative treatment of ACL insufficiency is to prevent recurrent episodes of giving way with the sequelae of meniscal injury, intraarticular damage, and premature degenerative arthritis. Non-operative management of acute tears consists of a three-phase program. Phase I includes early crutch protected walking with progressive weight-bearing as tolerated; early, active-assisted and passive range of motion exercises, and use of a knee immobilizer for comfort. The emphasis of this phase is regaining full, pain-free knee motion.

This phase usually lasts 7–10 days. During this phase, the patient and parents are counseled about the treatment options including the need for activity modification with reduction or elimination of sports that place high demands on ACL function. Progression to Phase II occurs when the goal of full, pain-free knee motion has been achieved.

Phase II is a supervised rehabilitation effort to restore normal muscle balance to the lower extremity. Emphasis is on regaining and maintaining quadriceps strength as well as normalizing the quadriceps-hamstring strength ratio. This phase usually lasts up to six weeks.

Phase III is a graduated return to functional activities. Return to low and moderate-demand sports is allowed when lower extremity strength approaches that of the uninjured side. Progression to high-demand sports and competitive levels of participation are allowed only if the patient demonstrates no functional instability at lower levels of activity.

The role of functional braces to control instability following ACL injury is controversial. There is no unanimity of opinion on the timing or use of functional braces. The mechanism of brace efficacy is unknown. Improved proprioceptive feedback has been suggested. Proper fit of a functional brace is often difficult in children as a result of smaller leg length and girth. Customized braces may be required, but the high cost may make their use prohibitive. Use of a functional brace in conjunction with a comprehensive rehabilitation program may allow temporization until the patient reaches skeletal maturity. If, at that time, functional instability remains, a surgical reconstruction is considered. Understanding that no current consensus for its use exists, functional bracing during sports participation is recommended in those patients undergoing a trial of non-surgical treatment.

Indications for surgery

Surgery is indicated in any patient who demonstrates functional instability with activities of daily living or refuses to comply with activity modification to prevent recurrent giving way episodes. Surgical reconstruction of the ACL is also indicated in those patients with associated knee injuries requiring surgical treatment, especially meniscal tears. In patients who are physically immature and have associated meniscal injury, arthroscopy allows accurate assessment of intraarticular pathology, especially characterization of meniscal pathology. If the tear pattern is amenable to repair all reasonable attempts should be made to preserve the menisci. If the meniscus is repairable simultaneous surgical stabilization of the knee is recommended.

Operative treatment

A number of surgical procedures have been attempted to stabilize the skeletally immature ACL-deficient knee. Operative management options include primary repair, intraarticular reconstruction, intraarticular plus an extraarticular procedure, or extraarticular procedures alone. Both primary repair of intrasubstance tears and extraarticular reconstructions have resulted in poor long-term functional stability. Primary repair of a midsubstance rupture or isolated extra-articular reconstruction is not recommended. Engebretsen *et al.* (1988) reported on eight adolescent patients who underwent primary repair of the ACL. All patients 'dropped a level of sports activity' and 5/8 patients demonstrated instability. The mean side-to-side KT-1000 laxity difference was 5 mm. The exception to primary repair is the case of a bony avulsion injury with a large bone fragment, which may be fixed.

Intraarticular reconstructions include physis-sparing and partial or complete transphyseal procedures. The choice of graft tissue is, in part, determined by the reconstructive procedure itself. The primary choices include bone-patellar tendon bone autograft, hamstrings (semitendinosis/gracilis) autograft, and allograft. The use allograft tissue for routine cases is not recommended in the pediatric population. The use of synthetic grafts and ligament augmentation devices (LAD) remain controversial and are not recommended for pediatric knee reconstruction.

Many surgeons have been reluctant to attempt intraarticular, isometric ACL reconstruction (such as that achieved in adults using bone-patella tendon-bone) in the skeletally immature patient because of the risk of premature growth arrest and angular deformity associated with violation of the tibial and femoral physes. The surgical procedure of choice has classically been determined by the physical maturity of the patient. Complete physeal-sparing or partial (tibia only) transphyseal techniques have been historically recommended for Tanner stage 1 patients who fail non-operative treatment and have persistent functional instability with activities of daily living. Complete transphyseal reconstructions have historically been recommended for all other patients. Patients at any Tanner stage who have associated meniscal pathology with the ACL tear undergo surgical treatment for both lesions. Meniscal treatment depends on tear morphology, location, and stability.

Questions about tolerance of the lack of isometry with a variety of non-anatomic reconstruction procedures will only be answered with longer follow-up. Whether youth and diminished graft size allow more rapid maturation of the transferred neoligament is unknown. A 6 or 7 mm graft may be appropriate and proportional for the patient's size at the time of the reconstruction. It is unknown whether such a graft will, with growth, hypertrophy in its intraarticular segment to assume the size and mechanical properties of an adult ACL and withstand long-term vocational and avocational demands.

Physeal sparing reconstruction

Nontransphyseal or physeal sparing reconstruction can be accomplished using an arthroscopic-assisted technique with autograft

Fig. 11.3

Non-transphyseal
reconstruction – hamstring
tendons placed 'over the front'
of the tibia and 'over the top'
on the femur.

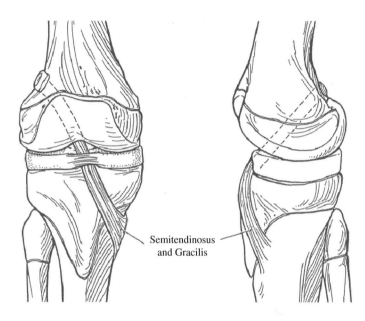

Semitendinosus
and Gracilis

tendon augmentation. Autograft patella tendon or hamstrings may
be selected as a graft tissue. After standard arthroscopic preparation
of the intercondylar notch, including notchplasty if necessary, an
anteromedial incision is used to harvest the selected autograft tissue
and provide access to the anterior tibial epiphysis. The graft tissue
may be left attached to the proximal tibia (tibial tubercle for patella
tendon, pes anserinus for hamstrings). A second incision is made
laterally at the level of the femoral metaphyseal flair. The graft is
passed in continuity over the front of the tibia, beneath the transverse meniscal ligament, through the intercondylar notch, and over-
the-top position of the femur (Figure 11.3). This eliminates physeal
violations. The graft can be fixed to the lateral femur by direct suture
to the periosteum, screw and washer, or tying the suture around a
screw post. Disadvantages of these physis-sparing procedures
include non-anatomic, non-isometric graft position and the
unknown effect of continued skeletal growth on the biologic maturation of the neo-ligament.

Parker *et al.* (1994) have reported good results in a group of six
adolescent patients using this technique. Five of six patients
returned to their pre-operative level of activity. All had excellent
functional outcome scores and no recurrent instability. No patient
had a leg length abnormality or physeal arrest.

Partial transphyseal reconstruction

Partial transphyseal reconstruction is accomplished using an
arthroscopic-assisted technique. Autograft hamstring tendons are
the preferred graft tissue. Use of autograft patella tendon is

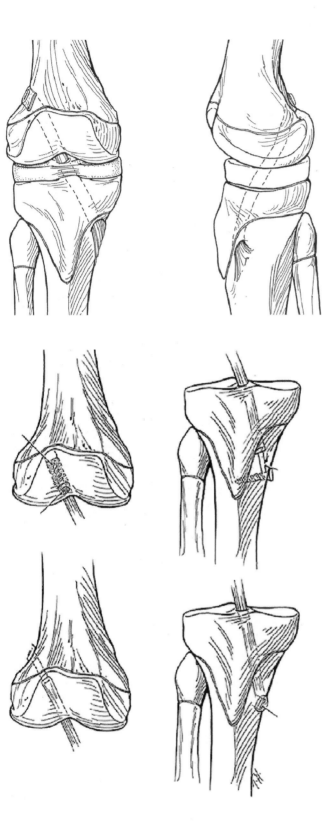

Fig. 11.4

Partial-transphyseal reconstruction – hamstring tendons placed transphyseal through tibia and 'over the top' on the femur.

Fig. 11.5

Complete transphyseal reconstruction – tibial and femoral fixation options; use of interference screws has also been described on the tibial side.

contraindicated because of risk of injury to the anterior tibial physis at the tibial tubercle. Premature closure of this area of the physis will result in a recurvatum deformity. Allograft tissue should be reserved for cases with a contraindication to autograft tissue use. After standard arthroscopic preparation of the intercondylar notch, an antero-medial incision is used to harvest the selected autograft tissue and provide access to the anterior tibial metaphysis. Autograft hamstring graft tissue may be left attached to the pes anserinus at the proximal tibia or harvested as a free graft. The graft should be prepared using large, non-absorbable suture at the free ends. In partial transphyseal reconstructions, the tendon graft is passed through a drill hole in the center of the tibial physis and placed in an over-the-top femoral position. A 6–8 mm tibial bone tunnel is drilled depending on the size of the graft tissue. A second incision is made at the lateral femur at the level of the metaphyseal flair. The graft is passed through the tibial drill hole and intercondylar notch and over-the-top position of the femur (Figure 11.4). This eliminates eccentric violation of the femoral physis. The graft is fixed to the lateral femur by direct suture to the periosteum, screw and washer, or tying the suture around a screw post. If the graft is harvested as free tissue and not left attached at its insertion on the proximal tibia, fixation to the tibia can be accomplished using staples or sutures tied to a screw post (Figure 11.5). Disadvantages of the partial transphyseal procedure are similar to those listed for the nontransphyseal technique.

Paletta recently reported on a series of Tanner stage 1, 2, and 3 adolescents comparing partial transphyseal and complete transphyseal reconstructions. The complete transphyseal reconstruction group had better knee stability as documented by pivot shift and KT-1000. The complete transphyseal group had mean side-to-side difference of 1.25 mm vs. 3 mm in the partial transphyseal group. There were no physeal arrests, angular deformities, or leg length discrepancies in any of the patients.

Complete transphyseal reconstruction

More recent basic science and clinical data suggest that complete transphyseal reconstruction may be safe. Guzzanti *et al.* (1994) presented experimental data on the effects of intra-articular ACL reconstruction on physeal growth in a rabbit model. The lapine model used a semitendinosus tendon placed through 2 mm tibial and femoral tunnels in skeletally immature rabbits. The mean involvement of the femoral physis was 11 per cent in the frontal plane and 3 per cent of its cross-sectional area. There was no alteration of longitudinal growth or angular deviation. On the tibial side the mean physeal involvement was 12 per cent in the frontal plane and 4 per cent of the cross-sectional area. Two tibia developed varus angulation and one was shortened. Histologic examination of the physeal specimens up to six months post-op showed no epiphysiodeses Stadelmaier *et al.* (1995)

179

published results on the effects of transphyseal drilling on physeal growth in a dog model. The canine model utilized a fascia lata graft for ACL reconstruction placed across transphyseal tibial and femoral bone tunnels. Histologic and radiographic follow-up demonstrated no evidence of bony bridge formation, epiphysiodesis, longitudinal growth disturbance, or angular deformity. Clinical results from small clinical series with limited follow-up do not clarify the treatment of choice in the truly skeletally immature individual with ACL insufficiency (Buckley *et al.* 1989; De Lee and Curtis 1983; Edwards and Grana 2001; Engebresten *et al.* 1988). Surgical options remain constricted in such patients because of concern about physeal violation. The threshold ratio of physeal area to graft tunnel size that is safe is currently unknown.

Complete transphyseal reconstructions require placement of graft tissue through tibial and femoral bone tunnels and can be performed using an arthroscopic-assisted technique with autograft or allograft tendon augmentation. Autograft patella tendon or hamstrings may be selected as graft tissue. Allograft tissue should be reserved for cases with a contraindication to autograft tissue use. After standard arthroscopic preparation of the intercondylar notch, including notchplasty if necessary, an anteromedial incision is used to harvest the selected tissue as a free graft and provide access to the anteromedial tibial metaphysis. The graft should be prepared using a large, non-absorbable suture at both ends. Hamstring tendons may be doubled or even quadrupled. Depending on the size of the graft tissue, an 8–10 mm tibial bone tunnel is drilled. A matched size femoral drill hole is made using an endoscopic technique or an outside-in technique, which requires a second incision at the lateral femur (as described above). The tibial and femoral drill holes should be placed in the anatomic positions to optimize graft isometricity. The graft is passed through the tibial tunnel, intercondylar notch, and femoral tunnel. The graft can be fixed to the lateral femur by direct suture to the periosteum, screw and washer, or tying the suture around a screw post. Fixation at the femur can be accomplished using an interference screw placed either endoscopically or from outside-in. Newer femoral fixation techniques include extracortical devices such as the endobutton, which eliminates the risk of transecting the graft when placing an interference screw. Fixation at the tibia is best accomplished using an interference screw. Staples or sutures tied to a screw post can also be used. The complete transphyseal reconstruction allows for anatomic, isometric placement of the graft. Disadvantages include technical demand of procedure (especially femoral tunnel placement), risk of pain at tibial screw site, and risk of partial or complete transection of graft with endoscopic interference screw placement.

Since the mid-1990s an increasing number of studies have reported the successful use of soft tissue grafts such as hamstrings being placed through drill holes across open tibial and femoral physes. Andrews *et al.* (1994) reported on a group of eight patients with a mean age 13 years, 6 months who underwent transphyseal reconstruction using hamstrings. At a mean follow-up of 58 months 7/8 had a good or excellent outcome with return to pre-operative levels of activity. No patient had a significant leg length or physeal abnormality. Lipscomb and Anderson (1986) reported on 24 patients ranging in age from 12 to 15 years of age. All underwent transphyseal reconstruction but with a femoral drill hole placed transversely distal to the level of the femoral physis. At a mean follow-up of 35 months 23 of 24 patients reported good to excellent results. One patient developed a leg length discrepancy of 2 cm but this was thought to be the result of direct stapling of the hamstring graft at the level of the femoral physis. Aronowitz *et al.* (1997) have reported on 19 adolescent ranging in age from 11–14 years, with a bone age of 14 years or less, and open physes. At mean follow-up of 25 months all knees were stable, mean Lysholm score was 97, and there were no leg length or physeal abnormalities.

Postoperative rehabilitation

Current rehabilitation programs after ACL reconstruction incorporate the biologic principle of progressive, physiologically tolerable stress by allowing early motion, weight-bearing, and muscle strengthening to prevent the sequelae of disuse, misuse, and abuse. Emphasis on rehabilitation of entire lower extremity strength and endurance through the use of isometric, isotonic, and closed and open chain isokinetic exercises (both concentric and eccentric) contributes to rapid rehabilitation. The rehabilitation program is customized to accommodate the patient's size and their available rehabilitation equipment. The graduated rehabilitation program places early emphasis on regaining full knee motion and quadriceps control. Early strengthening emphasizes co-contraction of the hamstrings and quadriceps as well as limited arcs of motion with avoidance of active resisted knee extension beyond 30 degrees. Progression of the rehabilitation program with gradual return to full activity is allowed only as full motion is achieved and restoration of normal hamstring-quadriceps strength ratios occurs. The pre-participation phase incorporates sport-specific tasks performed at full speed before return to full sports participation is allowed.

Complications

As seen post-operatively in ACL reconstruction in the adult patient, complications may include motion loss (especially extension), arthrofibrosis, infrapatellar fat pad contractures, anterior knee pain, infection, and graft harvest site morbidity. Complications unique to the skeletally immature patient are those of potential limb length inequality and/or angular and rotational deformities. Too few truly skeletally immature patients have been followed for sufficient time to have adequate data about the prevalence of these complications.

Summary

Anterior cruciate ligament injury in children is being recognized with greater frequency because of improved diagnostic techniques as well as heightened awareness of the condition. Unfortunately, the diagnosis is still missed because the contention that children to not suffer ligament injuries persists. Hemarthrosis must be considered an indication of a significant intraarticular injury. During the past decade, ACL reconstruction has evolved to a reproducible technique with low morbidity. Aggressive rehabilitation programs allow accelerated return to activity while allowing the biology of graft maturation to progress.

The basic principle of diagnosis and the treatment goals in the skeletally immature patient are the same as those in the adult patient. However, the diagnosis approach to ACL injury in the scholastic-age patient must also include evaluation of the patient's skeletal maturity since it plays a major role in treatment decisions. Maturity is evaluated on the basis of the patient's chronologic age; various physiologic factors, such as family height, patient's projected height, and estimation of sexual development; and radiographic findings in the knee, pelvis (Risser sign), or hand and wrist (bone-age study). Because of the special characteristics of the skeletally immature patient, the orthopaedic surgeon must act as 'knee counselor' by attempting to identify at-risk patients, particularly those who abuse their knees for any of a variety of reasons. The non-operative treatment principles are the same as those in an adult. Consideration of surgical treatment must take into account assessment of skeletal maturity. If questions remain about the status of the femoral and tibial physes, polytomography or MR imaging is used to assess the extent of physeal closure. The surgical reconstruction used reflects the patient's skeletal maturity. As the skeletal maturity threshold is reached, transphyseal reconstructions may be done with diminished reservation about causing sequelae of physeal arrest.

References

Aichroth PM, Patel DV, Zorrilla P (2002) The natural history and treatment of rupture of the anterior cruciate ligament in children and adolescents: A prospective review. *J Bone Joint Surge [Br]* Jan. 84(1):38–41.

Andrews M, Noyes FR, Barber-Westin SD (1994) Anterior cruciate ligament allograft reconstruction in the skeletally immature athlete. *Am J Sports Med* 22:48–54.

Andrish JT (2001) Anterior cruciate ligament injuries in the skeletally immature patient. *Am J Orthop* 30(2):103–110.

Angel KR, Hall DJ (1989) Anterior cruciate ligament injury in children and adolescents. *Arthroscopy* 5(3):197–200.

Aronowitz ER, Ganley TJ, Goode JR, *et al.* (1997) Anterior cruciate ligament reconstruction in adolescents with open physes (Abstract #14). *Pediatrics* 100 (3 Pt 2):477.

Barrack RL, Bruckner JD, Kneisl J, Inman WS, Alexander AH (1990) The outcome of nonoperatively treated complete tears of the anterior cruciate ligament in active young adults. *Clin Orthop* 259:192–199.

Baxter MP, Wiley JJ (1988) Fractures of the tibial spine in children: An evaluation of knee stability. *J Bone Joint Surg* 70-B:228–230.

Bisson LJ, Wickiewicz T, Levinson M, Warren R (1998) ACL reconstruction in children with open physes. *Orthopedics* 21(6):659–663.

Buckley SL, Barrack RL, Alexander AH, *et al.* (1989) The natural history of conservatively treated anterior cruciate ligament tears. *Am J Sports Med* 17:221–225.

DeLee JC, Curtis R (1983) Anterior cruciate ligament insufficiency in children. *Clin Orthop* 172:112–118.

Edwards PH, Grana WA (2001) Anterior cruciate ligament reconstruction in the immature athlete: Long-term results of intra-articular reconstruction. *Am J Knee Surg* 14(4):232–237.

Engebresten L, Svennginsen S, Benum P (1988) Poor results of anterior cruciate ligament repair in adolescents. *Acta Orthop Scand* 59:684–686.

Fehnel DJ, Johnson R (2000) Anterior cruciate injuries in the skeletally immature athlete: A review of treatment outcomes. *Sports Med* Jan. 29(1):51–63.

Graf BK, Lange RH, Fujisaki CK, *et al.* (1992) Anterior cruciate ligament tears in skeletally immature patients: Meniscal pathology at the time of presentation and after attempted conservative treatment. *Arthroscopy* 8:229–233.

Guzzanti V, Falciglia F, Gigante A, *et al.* (1994) The effect of intra-articular ACL reconstruction on the growth plates of rabbits. *J Bone Joint Surg* 76-B:960–963.

Hofmeister EP, Gillingham BL, Bathgate MB, Mills WJ (2001) Results of anterior cruciate ligament reconstruction in the adolescent female. *J Pediatr Orthop* 21(3):302–306.

Janarv PM, Nyström A, Werner S, Hirsch G (1996) Anterior cruciate ligament injuries in skeletally immature patients. *J of Pediatr Orthop* 16(5):673–677.

Kannus P, Jarvinen M (1988) Knee ligament injuries in adolescents. Eight year follow-up of conservative treatment. *J Bone Joint Surg* 70-B:772–776.

Lee K, Siegel MJ, Lau DM, Hildebolt CF, Matava MJ (1999) Anterior cruciate ligament tears: MR imaging-based diagnosis in a pediatric population. *Radiology* 213(3):697–704.

Lipscomb AB, Anderson AF (1986) Tears of the anterior cruciate ligament in adolescents. *J Bone Joint Surg* 68:19–28.

Lo IK, Bell DM, Fowler PJ (1998) Anterior cruciate ligament injuries in the skeletally immature patient. *Instr Course Lec* 47:351–359.

Lo IK, Kirkley A, Folwer PJ, Miniaci A (1997) The outcome of operatively treated anterior cruciate ligament disruptions in the skeletally immature child. *Arthroscopy* 13(5):627–634.

Matava MJ, Siegel MG (1997) Arthroscopic reconstruction of the ACL with semitendinous-gracilis autograft in skeletally immature adolescent patients. *Am J Knee Surg* 10(2):60–69.

McCarroll JR, Shelbourne KD, Patel DV (1995) Anterior cruciate ligament injuries in young athletes: Recommendations for treatment and rehabilitation. *Sports Med* 20(2):117–127.

McCarroll JR, Shelbourne KD, Porter DA, *et al.* (1994) Patella tendon graft reconstruction for midsubstance anterior cruciate ligament rupture in junior high school athletes: An algorithm for management. *Am J Sports Med* 22:478–484.

McCarroll JR, Rettig AC, Shelbourne KD (1988) Anterior cruciate ligament injuries in the young athlete with open physes. *Am J Sports Med* 16:44–47.

Mizuta H, Kubota K, Shiraishi M, Otsuka Y, Nagamoto N, Takagi K (1995) The conservative treatment of complete tears of the anterior cruciate ligament in skeletally immature patients. *J Bone Joint Surg [Br]* 77(6):890–894.

Nottage WM, Matsuura PA (1994) Management of complete traumatic anterior cruciate ligament tears in the skeletally immature patient: current concepts and review of the literature. *Arthroscopy* 10(5):569–573.

Paletta, GA (2002) ACL Reconstruction in the skeletally immature: A comparison of two techniques. Abstract ACL Study Group, Big Sky, MT, February 2002.

Parker AW, Drez D, Jr., Cooper, JL (1994) Anterior cruciate ligament injuries in patients with open physes. *Am J Sports Med* 22:44–47.

Schaefer RA, Eilert RE, Gillogly SD (1993) Disruption of the anterior cruciate ligament in a 4-year old child. *Orthop Rev* 22(6):725–727.

Simonian PT, Metcalf MH, Larson RV (1999) Anterior cruciate ligament injuries in the skeletally immature patient. *Am J Orthop* 28(11): 624–628.

Skak SV, Jensen TT, Poulsen TD, *et al.* (1987) Epidemiology of knee injuries in children. *Acta Orthop Scand* 58:78–81.

Stadelmaier DM, Arnoczky SP, Dodds J, *et al.* (1995) The effect of drilling and soft tissue grafting across open growth plates. A histologic study. *Am J Sports Med* 23:431–435.

Stanitski CL (1999) ACL surgery in children. *Orthopedics* 22(2):190.

Stanitski CL (1995) Anterior cruciate ligament injury in the skeletally immature patient: Diagnosis and treatment. *J Am Acad Orthop Surg* 3:146–158.

Stanitski CL (1994) Surgical reconstruction for symptomatic ACL insufficiency in skeletally immature athletes. *Am J Sports Med* 22(3):433.

Stanitski CL, Harvell JC, Fu FH (1993) Observations on acute hemarthrosis in children and adolescents. *J Pediatr Orthop* 13:506–510.

Sullivan JA (1990) Ligamentous injuries of the knee in children. *Clin Orthop* 255:44–50.

Tanner JM, Davies PSW (1985) Clinical longitudinal standards for height and weight velocity for American children. *J Pediatr* 107:317–329.

Williams JS, Abate JA, Fadale PD, Tung GA (1996) Meniscal and nonosseous ACL injuries in children and adolescents. *Am J Knee Surg* 9(1):22–26.

Zaricznyj B (1977) Avulsion fracture of the tibial eminence: Treatment by open reduction and pinning. *J Bone Joint Surg* 59-A:1111–1114.

12

Indications for ACL reconstruction in the over-forty age group

John Bartlett

Introduction

Indications for anterior cruciate ligament (ACL) reconstruction in younger patients may be summarized as a surgical solution for the treatment of symptoms. These symptoms may be current as in giving way episodes and restriction of function after conservative care; or they may be anticipated symptoms such as the acute injury in an athlete participating in jumping and twisting sports. However:

1   Why should these indications be any different in the 40-year-old or the 60-year-old?
2   What are the aging changes in the ACL; the donor tendons selected as graft; and the muscles necessary for strength and proprioception?
3   What are the activity levels and potential performance standards of the 40 to 70 year age groups?

Aging changes in ligament and tendon

Vogrin et al.[1] tested kinematics of intact knees in response to a 110N antero-posterior tibial load and in situ forces in the ACL and PCL using cadavers from two age groups – less than 50 years old and more than 50 years old.

Anterior tibial translation of the intact knee was significantly larger in the older donors by an average of 1.4 mm at 90° of flexion. Internal rotation under the anterior tibial load decreased from a mean 8.2° in the younger donors to 4.3° in the older donors at 30° of flexion.

The in situ forces in the ACL under the 110N antero-posterior tibial load at 30° of flexion were found to be 12 per cent lower in the older donors. However the detectable effects of donor age were relatively small.

With regard to the structural properties of the ACL, Woo[2] reported that younger specimens (22–35 years) had a higher linear stiffness and ultimate load than the older specimens (60–97 years). He concluded that the ultimate load of the ACL decreases rapidly with increasing age – being at 45 years about half that at 22 years.

The patellar tendon is the most commonly used graft for ACL reconstructions. In testing a young group (29–50 years) against an old group (64–93 years) Woo[2] found that aging has little or no effect on the tensile and visco–elastic properties of the bone-patellar tendon-bone complex. It would appear that the older ACL is significantly weaker and presumably more easily torn and yet the patellar tendon does not deteriorate with age.

Activity levels with increasing age

What then of the activity levels in middle age which may place the ACL at risk? The community encourages more physical activity in this age group. The 1995 Australian National Nutrition Survey revealed that 18 per cent of adults were obese with a Body Mass Index greater than 30. This appears more related to sloth than gluttony.[3] Kenneth Cooper[4] has stated that 'it is better to be fat and fit than thin and unfit'.

There are positive affects of exercise on cardiovascular health, diabetes etc., but also musculoskeletal health with less osteopenia, improved strength and neuro-muscular coordination.

The American College of Sports Medicine reports that muscle strength in sedentary persons declines by 15 per cent per decade between the ages of 50 and 70 years. Age-associated muscle atrophy differs from disuse atrophy in that it involves loss of muscle fibres as well as a reduction in cross-sectional area of fibres.

Different sports have different rates of age related decline in performance. In Masters athletic events 100 metre sprint records decline at 10 per cent per decade between 35 and 65 years of age; 400 metre records remain under one minute until 65 years with only a four per cent decline per decade. Javelin throwers decline at 20 per cent per decade whilst marathon runners of 50 years of age are only 10 per cent slower than their younger colleagues.[5]

Aging population

Middle-age people have the potential to be athletic; are advised to increase activity levels; have strong muscles and tendons but weak ACLs. There is little doubt that the proportion of the population in this age group is rising – the USA Census Bureau has predicted that by 2010, 25 per cent of Americans will be aged more than 55 years.

ACL injuries

ACL tears do occur in this older age group and can lead to symptomatic instability – the most frequent injury occurs with skiing.

Concerns in undertaking ACL reconstruction in patients more than 40 years of age have been:

1   It is unnecessary because of low activity levels;
2   Arthrofibrosis may result;
3   Osteoarthritis may be accelerated;
4   Autografts may be of poor tensile strength.

Cicotti[6] reported non operative treatment of 40–60 year old patients having ACL instability with an 83 per cent satisfaction rate – however 60 per cent were lost to follow-up and 37 per cent suffered reinjury. There is growing evidence that the results of ACL reconstruction are comparable to those in younger patients, both in patients over the age of 40 years[7–10] and in patients with articular cartilage damage.[11, 12] Plancher[10] reported reinjuries in five knees out of 75 (7 per cent) in patients more than 40 years of age following ACL reconstruction.

Blyth[13] reported results of 30 consecutive patients of more than 50 years old undergoing 31 ACL reconstructions. No patients were lost to follow-up at mean time of 46 months (24–95). There were 15 males, 15 females, average age 54.5 years. The single most common injury related to skiing – 12 cases. Evaluation was performed by clinical examination, KT-1000, isokinetic strength, Lysholm, Cincinnati, Tegner and IKDC scores. The results are as follows:

- Range of movement: Seven knees had less than five degrees loss of extension; 13 knees had less than 15° loss of flexion – none had greater loss. Positive correlations were shown with loss of motion, osteoarthritis and previous meniscectomy.
- KT-1000: Average side to side difference was 2.7 mm at manual maximum KT-1000 – there was no difference between patellar tendon and hamstring grafts.
- Isokinetic strength: Mean torque ratio compared to the opposite normal limb was 95 per cent extension strength and 102 per cent flexion strength. It is interesting to note that there was no difference between patellar tendon and hamstring graft.
- Scoring systems: Lysholm improved from pre-operatively 63 to 93 at review; Cincinnati from 49 to 89; and Tegner activity level from 3.7 to 5.2. International Knee Documentation Committee (IKDC) Scores revealed twelve category C abnormal and 19 category D severely abnormal knees pre-operatively. This improved at about four year mean follow-up to five category A normal, 20 category B nearly normal, six category C abnormal with no category D severely abnormal knees ($P < 0.001$). Amongst the six knees with abnormal grades, there were three knees with grade 4 and one with grade 3 articular changes at time of their reconstruction. The mean time to surgery from injury in these patients was increased with a mean of 130 months compared with 85 months for the group as a whole.

Summary

Poor results of ACL reconstruction in patients over 50 years old correlated with osteoarthritis, which in turn correlated with an increased time from injury to surgery and an increased number of pre-operative giving way episodes. All patients reported functional improvement.

Conclusion

Anterior cruciate ligament injuries do occur in the over-40 age group and may result in symptomatic instability. This may persist with functional restriction despite modification of activity levels and thorough conservative treatment – it may lead to meniscus tears and degenerative changes.

The ACL does weaken with increasing age, but commonly used grafts such as patellar tendon show minimal changes. The results of reconstructive surgery match those of younger counterparts with in most respects. Our own results however, as reported by Blyth,[13] have shown more laxity with KT-1000 2.7 mm side-to-side difference. This may relate to graft fixation techniques in slightly osteopenic bone.

In considering indications for surgery, age is only one of many variables – the prime consideration is treatment of symptoms and the older patients should be excluded from treatment which may be able to provide functional and symptomatic improvement.

References

1. Vogrin TM, Zeminski JA, Rudy TW, Harner CD, Fischer J, Woo SL-Y (2000). Function of the anterior and posterior cruciate ligaments: Effects of age and gender. *The Pittsburgh Orthopaedic Journal* 11: 210–11.
2. Woo SL-Y (2001). Basic science and properties of tissue as a function of aging. Instructional Course Lecture, ISAKOS, Montreux, Switzerland.
3. Prentice A, Jebb S (1995). Obesity in Britain: Gluttony or sloth? *British Medical Journal* 311: 437–9.
4. Cooper K (1999). An evening of sports medicine and humour. AAOS Anaheim USA.
5. Menard D (1996). The aging athlete. In M Harries, C Williams, WD Standish, LJ Micheli (eds) *Oxford Textbook of Sports Medicine*. Oxford University Press, pp. 596–620.
6. Cicotti MG, Lombardo SJ, Nonweiler B, Pink M (1994). Non-operative treatment of ruptures of the anterior cruciate ligament in middle-aged patients. *Journal Bone Joint Surgery* 76-A: 1315–21.
7. Barber FA, Burton FE, McGuire DA, Paulos LE (1996). Is anterior cruciate ligament reconstruction age dependent? *Arthroscopy* 12: 720–5.
8. Brandsson S, Kartus J, Larsson J, Eriksson BI, Karlsson J (2000). A comparison of results in middle-aged and young patients after anterior cruciate ligament reconstruction. *Arthroscopy* 16(2): 178–82.

9. Heier KA, Mack DR, Mosey JR, Paine R, Bocell JR (1997). An analysis of anterior cruciate ligament reconstruction in middle-aged patients. *American Journal Sports Medicine* 25: 527–32.

10. Plancher KD, Steadman JR, Briggs KK, Hutton KS (1998). Reconstruction of the anterior cruciate ligament in patients who are at least forty years old. *Journal Bone Joint Surgery* 80A: 184–97.

11. Noyes FR, Barber-Westin SD (1997). Anterior cruciate ligament reconstruction with autogenous patellar tendon graft in patients with articular cartilage damage. *American Journal Sports Medicine* 25: 626–34.

12. Shelbourne KD, Wilckens JH (1993). Intra articular anterior cruciate ligament reconstruction in the symptomatic arthritic knee. *American Journal Sports Medicine* 21: 685–9

13. Blyth MJG, Gosal HS, Peake WM, Bartlett RJ (2003). Anterior cruciate ligament reconstruction in patients over the age of fifty years. Two to eight year follow-up. *Knee Surg., Sports Traumatol., Arthrosc.* 11: 204–211.

Part 2. Revision ACl Reconstruction

13

Graft options for revision ACL surgery – which is the most effective?

Eric W. Carson, Alonzo Sexton, and Deryk G. Jones

Introduction

Reconstruction of the anterior cruciate ligament (ACL) is one of the most commonly performed orthopedic operations. According to the National Center of Health Statistics, in 1991 approximately 63,000 ACL reconstructions were performed in the United States. Current industry estimates suggest that over 100,000 ACL reconstructions are performed annually in the United States. The importance of the ACL in the maintenance of normal knee function is now well accepted. An untreated ACL tear can lead to recurrent giving-way episodes as well as damage to the menisci and articular cartilage with potential progression to osteoarthritis (Jones *et al.* 1999; O'Donoghue 1950; O'Donoghue 1963; Snook 1983). Within the literature, poor long-term results of non-operative treatment, primary repair, and extraarticular reconstruction, has led to intraarticular ACL reconstruction becoming the surgical procedure of choice. The success rate of primary intraarticular ACL reconstruction has been reported to range from 75 to 93 per cent good to excellent results relieving episodes of giving way, restoring functional stability, and allowing a return to normal or near normal activity levels (Barber *et al.* 1996; Friedman *et al.* 1985; Johnson *et al.* 1984; Yunes *et al.* 2001). Given the reported success rates, this leaves a significant number of patients with less than satisfactory clinical outcomes. However, what qualifies as an unsatisfactory clinical result or 'failure' after ACL reconstruction has not been well defined. Johnson and Fu defined a failed ACL reconstruction as a knee that demonstrates recurrent pathological laxity or a stable knee that has a range of motion from 10° to 120° (Johnson and Fu 1995). This lack of motion is often painful and creates a functional deficit with activities of daily living. This chapter will focus on those patients who have undergone an ACL reconstruction but have recurrent instability and our personal recommendations with regards to graft selection for these difficult cases.

Many factors are considered in revision ACL graft selection. Preoperatively, the surgeon must critically review the previous ACL reconstruction operation and subsequent post-operative course. This analysis provides crucial information. The type of graft used for the index ACL procedure, the method of graft fixation and specifics about the surgical technique may elucidate the mode of graft failure. This enables the surgeon to better approach the potential revision ACL surgery, and enhance the likelihood of clinical success. It is of paramount importance that the surgeon be versed in the pros and cons concerning graft choices and techniques available, thus allowing the surgeon to adapt to the unique nature of each case.

Graft selection for the revision procedure will depend on the type of graft used for the primary reconstruction, the placement of previous incisions, the presence of enlarged bone tunnels, surgeon's preference and the presence of associated ligamentous laxity (Tables 13.1, 13.2, 13.3, 13.4, 13.5, 13.6). All these variables must be considered when approaching revision ACL surgery (Brown and Carson 1999). It is very difficult to present a simple cookbook recipe for graft selection in revision ACL surgery. Each revision case is unique. Discussion with regards to scenarios gives a better perspective on graft selection for revision ACL surgery. Some surgeons recommend autologous hamstring tendons while others feel just as strongly about autologous patellar tendon tissue; some will never use an allograft while others always use allografts. We feel it is imperative that the surgeon be well versed in the use of all graft sources and surgical techniques to offer the patient the best clinical outcome. Rigid rules have no place in revision ACL surgery. Surgeons who perform these complex procedures must be flexibile and able to adapt to any difficult situation that may be encountered. Many factors must be taken into consideration prior to selection of a graft. The purpose of this chapter is to dispel myths associated with specific grafts and present the basic science for each of the various graft sources. After considering these variables a decision should be made as to the most appropriate graft; three categories of graft choices exist – autograft, allograft and synthetic materials.

Table 13.1 Failed patellar tendon ACL: Graft selection options

Reharvest patellar tendon
Contralateral patellar tendon
Semitendonsus/gracilis tendon
Quadriceps tendon
Allograft tissue

Table 13.2 Failed semitendonsus/gracilis tendon: Graft selection options

Patellar tendon
Quadriceps tendon
Contralateral semitendonsus/gracilis tendon
Allograft tissue

Table 13.3 Failed allograft: Graft selection options

Autogenous graft source
Allograft tissue

Table 13.4 Failed synthetic graft: Management options

Staged revision ACL reconstruction
Removal/debridement/bone graft
ACL reconstruction with graft of choice

Table 13.5 Enlarged tunnels: Management options

Staged reconstruction with bone graft sequentially followed with
  reconstruction
Allograft with large bone plugs
Quadriceps tendon bone complex

Table 13.6 ACL failure associated with injured secondary restraints

Meniscal deficient knee
- meniscal transplant
- knee osteotomy
- revision ACL

Injured ligamentous restraints
- reconstruction of injured structures with allograft patellar tendon/Achilles
  tendon or quadriceps tendon bone complex
- consider knee osteotomy for chronic cases (+/− ACL reconstruction)

Synthetic ACL grafts

Synthetic ligaments have been associated with consistently poor
clinical outcomes and complications such as sterile effusions, chronic
synovitis, and tunnel enlargement related to osteolysis and breakage
(Andersen *et al.* 1992; Marcacci *et al.* 1996; Richmond *et al.* 1992;
Seitz *et al.* 1998). Based on the poor track record associated with
these materials we do not recommend their use in primary or
revision ACL surgery. These grafts are no longer commonly used in
the United States but within the international orthopedic community, synthetic ligaments continue to be utilized. As a result, the
surgeon should have a solid understanding of what can be expected
while revising a synthetically reconstructed patient.

In most of these cases there is extensive bone loss around the
tibial tunnel. As a result, revision surgery in this patient population
should be staged with an initial debridement of the failed synthetic
ligament and damaged bone followed by concomitant bone grafting.
Once the bony defect has healed, usually after 4 to 6 months, the

second stage of the reconstruction should be performed (Greis and Steadman 1996).

Autografts

Autograft tissues have been the mainstay for primary ACL surgery and considering all factors these tissue sources are still an excellent option in revision ACL surgery. However, there are circumstances in which autograft is not indicated with revision ACL surgery. If the surgeon elects to use autogenous tissue many sources are available including:

1   Hamstring tendons: ipsilateral or contralateral
2   Quadriceps tendon: ipsilateral or contralateral
3   Patellar tendon: ipsilateral (reharvested)
4   Patellar tendon: contralateral.

Use of autogenous tissue eliminates potential disease transmission (hepatitis, HIV), bacterial contamination or immunological reaction associated with allograft tissues. However, autogenous tissues pose other potential problems such as donor-site morbidity, increased operative time, skin compromise related to multiple previous incisions or lack of availability if previously utilized (Johnson *et al.* 1996a; Safran and Harner 1995).

Ipsilateral patellar tendon autograft

The patellar tendon complex has a high ultimate strength and stiffness, making its ability to restore stability in the knee more predictable (Noyes *et al.* 1984). The advantage of bone-to-bone fixation allows for rapid healing and revascularization (Arnoczky 1996; Falconiero *et al.* 1998; Ishibashi *et al.* 2001; Paulos *et al.* 1983). Furthermore, interference screw fixation allows for solid fixation and stiffness as well as an accelerated rehabilitation program that is difficult to match with other graft/fixation choices (Aune *et al.* 1998; Brown *et al.* 1999; Shelbourne and Nitz 1990). Ipsilateral patellar tendon is often the preferred graft when it is available; however due to its popularity as a graft source for primary ACL reconstruction, it is often not available (Table 13.1). Reharvest of the patellar tendon from the ipsilateral knee is another potential option for revision of a failed primary patellar tendon reconstruction (Kartus *et al.* 1998). An MRI study supported reharvesting of the patellar tendon by demonstrating high signal intensity consistent with edema and scar in the early postoperative period; this phenomena was followed by a decrease in signal intensity over time (Coupens *et al.* 1992). At 18 months, the donor graft site appeared normal using by MRI inspection. The authors believed these findings revealed the ability of the patellar tendon to remodel and regenerate. Alternatively, Liu and associates reported morphologic changes in the harvested patellar tendon that lasted up to seven years after surgery (Liu *et al.* 1996). Bernicker noted patellar tendon defects were found in 10 of 12 knees evaluated 12 months postoperatively by MRI (Bernicker *et al.* 1998). Proctor *et al.*, using a goat model, demonstrated that the patellar tendon donor site fills with scar repair tissue, and that the tensile properties of this new tissue are significantly reduced compared to the normal contralateral patellar tendon at 21 months postoperatively (Proctor *et al.* 1997). Similar findings have been reported in a dog model by LaPrade *et al.* (1997). As a result of these findings, both authors have recommended that alternative grafts be used for revision ACL surgery. Kartus *et al.* reported the clinical results using the reharvested patellar tendon to perform revision ACL surgery in 20 patients (Kartus *et al.* 1998). The ipsilateral patellar tendon was reharvested and used as the revision ACL graft source in ten patients, and the contralateral patellar tendon was used in another ten as a control. The Lysholm score, IKDC rating, and Tegner activity levels were reported to be significantly lower in the patients with reharvest of the ipsilateral patellar tendon. One patellar fracture and one patellar tendon rupture were reported to have occurred in the reharvest group. Because of the significantly lower functional scores and 20 per cent incidence of major donor site complications in the reharvest group, the authors did not recommend the use of the reharvested ipsilateral patellar tendon for revision ACL surgery.

Contralateral patellar tendon autograft

Use of the contralateral patellar tendon provides the same advantages as the primary patellar tendon with the additional advantage of being available for revision ACL cases. However, use of the contralateral patellar tendon carries the risk of creating extensor mechanism problems in a knee that was previously 'normal'. Another argument against the use of the contralateral patellar tendon is the observation that patients with ACL injured knees have an increased risk of injuring the intact contralateral ACL, particularly in female athletes (Harmon and Ireland 2000; Messina *et al.* 1999; Powell and Barber-Foss 2000). Use of the contralateral patellar tendon as graft source would then likely preclude its use for a subsequent ACL reconstruction. Rubinstein *et al.* reported on the use of the contralateral patellar tendon as a graft source in 20 patients (Rubinstein *et al.* 1994). They found that all patients had regained full range of motion by three weeks, and that quadriceps strength had returned to 93 per cent at one year and 95 per cent at two years postoperatively in the donor knee. No patient complained of patellofemoral pain in the donor knee; however, patellar tendonitis occurred in 55 per cent of the patients during the first year. The authors did add the caveat that the observed patellar tendinopathy rarely limited patients, and often resolved after the first year. The authors felt that the donor-site morbidity from harvesting the contralateral patellar tendon was minimal and its use was viewed as a good option for revision ACL surgery.

Semitendinosus/gracilis autograft

Semitendinosus and gracilis hamstring tendons are readily available in many revision ACL patients. Use of these tendons for ACL surgery carries no risk of disease transmission, usually experience timely graft incorporation, and do not result in a host versus graft immunological reaction as can occur with the use of allograft tissues. Several other potential advantages in using the hamstring tendons versus the patellar tendon include the following (Brown et al. 1993; Kleipool et al. 1994; Muller et al. 2000):

1   decreased donor site morbidity
2   lesser incidence of anterior knee pain postoperatively
3   a decreased risk of postoperative flexion contracture in the operated knee
4   better maintenance of quadriceps strength.

Early studies voiced concern about the use suitability of hamstring tendons for ACL reconstruction on the basis of the tensile and biomechanical properties of hamstring tendon grafts (Noyes et al. 1984). Subsequent biomechanical studies have demonstrated that hamstring tendon grafts are stronger and stiffer than a 10 mm patellar tendon graft (Hamner et al. 1999). Similarly with an increasing number of quadrupled hamstring ACL reconstructions being performed in recent years, long-term clinical results have matched those reported in patients treated with the patellar tendon grafts (Marcacci et al. 2003; Scranton et al. 2002). The tensile properties of hamstring tendon grafts from donors between 23 to 43 years of age, a group typically undergoing ACL reconstruction, have recently been investigated by Hamner et al. This study reported a mean failure load of 3560 ± 742 N, and a stiffness of 855 ± 156 N/m for quadrupled semitendinosus grafts, and a mean failure load of 4140 ± 969 N, and stiffness of 807 ± 164 N/m for combined doubled semitendinosus and gracilis grafts (Hamner et al. 1999). These values are significantly higher than those observed for 10 mm patellar tendon grafts from similar aged donors.

Potential disadvantages of hamstring tendon grafts in revision ACL surgery include a smaller diameter compared to patellar tendon grafts, and the lack of bone blocks at the ends of the graft that might improve initial graft fixation. The typical tunnel size for patellar tendon reconstruction is between 9 and 11 mm, compared to 7 to 9 mm for four-stranded hamstring tendon grafts. Because of the smaller diameter of the hamstring tendon graft, it is not possible to overdrill the existing patellar tendon bone tunnel and fill these tunnels adequately. If the surgeon desires to use a hamstring tendon graft in a knee in which the placement of the existing tibial bone tunnels are satisfactory, either the extraarticular position of the new bone tunnels must be diverged from the path of the preexisting bone tunnels, or the preexisting bone tunnels over drilled, bone grafted, with the ACL reconstruction performed at a later date as the second stage of the overall procedure.

Femoral tunnels that are significantly malpositioned anteriorly in the intercondylar notch at 'residents' ridge' are easy to handle as the surgeon can simply drill the revision femoral tunnel in the appropriate position posterior to the tunnel made at the index ACL reconstruction. When there is tunnel overlap between revision and index ACL reconstruction, though interference screws may be used, it may be necessary to employ more distal fixation to bypass an area of tunnel enlargement on compromised bone quality. In such circumstances the Endobutton (Smith and Nephew Endoscopy, Inc., Andover, MA), cross-pin type fixation, or positioning of the graft in the 'over the top' position represent viable options for revision femoral graft fixation. These fixation techniques are of great use in those cases where there has been a 'blow out' of the posterior cortex of the femoral tunnel.

A third potential disadvantage of hamstring tendon grafts is the longer elongation to failure and lower stiffness of many hamstring graft fixation techniques (Brown *et al.* 1993; Hamner *et al.* 1999). This can be of significance in those patients that are ligamentously lax, or in cases where there is an associated ligamentous injury to the knee (collateral ligament, posterolateral corner or PCL). A stiffer construct such as autogenous patellar tendon tissue fixed with interference screw fixation may be more appropriate under these circumstances; all ligament injuries should be addressed to avoid ACL graft failure. However, recent biomechanical testing has demonstrated improved stiffness and elongation to failure of doubled gracilis and semitendinosus grafts fixed in the femur with any of several different devices. The Bone Mulch Screw (Arthrotek, Ontario, CA), the TransFix (Arthrex, Naples, FL), the LinX-HT (Innovasive Devices, Inc., Marlborough, MA), the EndoButton with continuous polyester loop (Smith and Nephew Endoscopy, Inc., Andover, MA), the Rigid-fix (Mitek Products, Westwood, MA) or bioabsorbable interference screws placed with appropriate bone density and insertion torque all have ultimate failure strengths similar to those previously reported for patellar tendon grafts fixed with interference screws (Brand *et al.* 2000a, 2000b; Steenlage *et al.* 2002).

The tibial tunnel remains the 'weak link' in ACL graft fixation. As such, there is concern about tibial tunnel fixation during the use of soft-tissue grafts such as the hamstring tendons. There are several fixation methods that have been developed for the tibial tunnel that may improve tibial fixation for these types of grafts, including the Intra-fix device (Mitek Products, Westwood, MA). Newer generation tibial fixation devices may allow for better control of graft tension at fixation and more definitive fixation at the proximal aspect of the tunnel. It is the authors' feeling that lower stiffness hamstring fixation techniques require a longer period of cyclical loading prior to graft fixation, a higher initial graft tension at fixation, and fixation of the graft at 10–30° of knee flexion lowering postoperative laxity and failure rates (Fleming *et al.* 2001; Simonian *et al.* 2000). As with the femoral tunnel, any bony deficit along the tibial tunnel may limit the graft fixation strength and limit the type of fixation methods that can be utilized. Cortical fixation at the tibial surface, with a spiked staple or post-washer construct could be utilized in these situations. At the present time there are few published studies that have analyzed the use of hamstring tendons for revision ACL surgery. While hamstring tendons can be utilized for revision ACL surgery, one can see there are limitations to the use of this type of graft in revision cases.

Quadriceps tendon autograft

Staubli has recently refocused attention on the use of the quadriceps tendon as an alternative graft source for primary and revision cruciate ligament surgery (Staubli *et al.* 1996, 1999). Potential advantages of the quadriceps tendon construct include the ability to create large bone blocks to fill an enlarged tunnel and the large cross-sectional area of the quadriceps tendon (Staubli *et al.* 1996). Disadvantages and potential complications are similar to those reported when using the bone-patellar tendon-bone complex. Most the potential difficulties associated with use of quadriceps tendon grafts center around extensor mechanism dysfunction or the occurrence of patellar fractures (Kornblatt *et al.* 1988; Yasuda *et al.* 1991). However, recent reports have documented a significantly lower incidence of patellofemoral problems (Chen *et al.* 1999; Noronha 2002; Scranton *et al.* 2002). Biomechanical testing has shown that the quadriceps tendon is about the same strength as the patellar tendon, but has lower initial stiffness. However, the cross-sectional area of the quadriceps tendon is significantly greater than that of the patellar tendon based on described methods of graft harvest (quadriceps tendon = 65 mm^2, patellar tendon = 36.8 mm^2) (Staubli *et al.* 1999). The large cross-sectional area of this graft and the presence of a bone block at one end make it possible to fill enlarged bone tunnels. One area of potential concern about this graft source is that harvest of a second bone block from the superior pole of the patella may place the patella at risk for fracture following these revision cases. Another potential limitation with the quadriceps tendon graft is that there is bone to bone fixation on one side while there is tendon to bone fixation on the other side. Clinically, Purnell has reported good results in 14 patients with an average follow-up of 3.5 years using a 9–11 mm width quadriceps tendon graft to revise failed primary ACL reconstructions (Harris and Smith 1997). All knees were reported to have less than 2 mm side-to-side difference using the KT-1000 arthrometer, the hop test averaged 94 per cent, and the isokinetic strength testing at 240°/sec and 60°/sec averaged 82 per cent. Complications included one non-displaced patellar fracture one year after surgery. Although the clinical use of this graft has been limited to date, it does represent a viable autograft option for revision ACL cases.

Allografts

The use of allograft tissue offers many obvious advantages compared to autograft tissue. These advantages include decreased surgical time, smaller incisions, less surgical dissection, the ability to customize bone block size and shape to accommodate enlarged bone tunnels, increased graft diameter, and no donor-site morbidity (Safran and Harner 1995). However, there are also a number of disadvantages related to allograft tissue utilized in revision ACL surgery. The disadvanatages include potential disease transmission (HIV or hepatitis) and potential bacterial or fungal infections, and variability in graft incorporation. The reported risk of viral transmission per the American Academy of Orthopedic Surgeons is 1 in 3–4 million with no reportable cases since the advent of testing techniques such as PCR analysis (Gala *et al.* 1997; Roder *et al.* 1994). Most frozen allograft tissue used for ACL reconstruction undergoes gamma irradiation for sterilization purposes. This method neutralizes viruses and bacterial spores, but weakens the allograft biomechanically. Radiation dosing that is greater than 3 Mrad is required to thoroughly deactivate both the hepatitis and AIDS viruses. This same dosage has unfortunately been shown to alter graft collagen structure and ultimately weaken the graft by approximately 27 per cent (Fideler *et al.* 1995a). Moreover, allograft tissues have been shown to undergo a slower graft incorporation process compared to autograft tissues (Fideler *et al.* 1995b; Jackson *et al.* 1987, 1991, 1996). The secondary effects of irradiation and delayed biological incorporation may place allograft ACL reconstructions at increased risk for failure.

Recently, there has been a greater concern over bacterial infections, particularly clostridium species, when using allograft tissues (2002a). In an attempt to avoid this complication, the current graft processing protocols use aseptic harvesting technique, multiple antibiotic soaks, multiple graft cultures and low dose radiation (dosage: 1.5–2.5 Mrad). Freezing techniques (Cryolife Atlanta, GA) and Biocleanse solutions (Regeneration Technology Inc., Naples Florida) have also been applied to better create a 'sterile graft'. The most likely cause of these clostridial infections is often poor procurement procedure and/or packaging techniques by the organ bank or distributor. Martinez documented an exponential increase in the incidence of clostridium infections in allograft tissue that is harvested greater than 12 hours post-mortem (Malinin *et al.* 1985). New regulations and guidelines are currently being proposed by the Federal Drug Administration (United States) and the American Association of Tissue Banks for the harvest of fresh tissues that will later be used in orthopedic procedures (Centers for Disease Control U.S.A. 2002b).

As noted previously, graft incorporation is a concern when using allograft tissue sources for ACL reconstruction. Studies have shown that both autograft and allograft tissues undergo the same biological process of graft incorporation: graft necrosis, revascularization, cellular repopulation with cells of extrinsic origin, collagen deposition, graft maturation and remodeling (Arnoczky 1996, Arnoczky *et al.* 1986). This complex biological healing response has been called *ligamentization* since it results in a replacement structure that grossly resembles the normal ACL (Amiel *et al.* 1986). Jackson *et al.*, using a goat model, demonstrated that the time course and extent of graft remodeling is slower and less complete in allografts compared to autografts (Jackson *et al.* 1987, 1991). In this study, the allografts were also found to be biomechanically inferior to autografts. The biological factors responsible for delayed incorporation of allografts have not been completely identified at the present time but immunologic factors are sure to play an important role (Friedlaender *et al.* 1999). Recent work by Resnick and colleagues looking at the incorporation of osteochondral allografts by MRI found a direct correlation between poor graft incorporation and serum levels of anti-human leukocyte antigens, suggesting a rejection phenomenon was involved in clinical failures (Sirlin *et al.* 2001). A similar phenomenon has been implicated in the poor incorporation rates of allograft tissues used in ACL reconstructions (Pinkowski *et al.* 1989).

Traditionally, the patellar and Achilles tendon have been the most commonly used allografts (Johnson *et al.* 1996a; Johnson and Coen 1995a; Noyes and Barber-Westin 1996a; Noyes *et al.* 1994). Newer allograft tissue sources include the use of allograft anterior tibialis tendon and hamstring tendons (Caborn and Selby 2002). The recent increase in the use of these allografts tendons has resulted from the relative shortage of patellar tendon and Achilles tendon allografts available for ACL reconstruction. Tibialis and hamstring allografts are commonly available, and their use in ACL reconstruction has been described (Caborn and Selby 2002). The tibialis anterior tendon allograft in particular has increased in popularity and utilization. This is directly related to its excellent biomechanical properties, strength and large cross-sectional area allowing better fill of enlarged tunnels compared to other soft tissue allograft sources (Haut Donahue *et al.* 2002).

Clinical results of primary ACL reconstructions performed with irradiated allograft tissue, and chronic ACL reconstructions performed with non-irradiated allograft tissues have been favorable.

202

In 1996, Johnson and associates reported on the experience from the University of Pittsburgh wherein fresh frozen patellar and Achilles tendon allograft tissues were employed for revision ACL reconstruction. Twenty-five consecutive revision patients received fresh frozen irradiated allograft tissue. The authors reported that the results were unfavorable with 24 to 36 month follow-up revealing nine patients (36 per cent) had failed revision surgery with more than 5 mm increased translation on KT 1000 testing (Johnson *et al.* 1996a). Noyes *et al.* presented a study of 66 consecutive patients who underwent ACL reconstruction utilizing fresh frozen allograft patellar tendon with an average follow up of 42 months (range 23 to 78 months) postoperatively (Noyes and Barber-Westin 1996a). Concomitant procedures were common including 19 meniscal repairs, 10 meniscal allograft reconstructions, 7 lateral collateral ligament reconstructions, 11 posterolateral corner repairs, 4 medial collateral ligament reconstructions and 4 posterior cruciate ligament reconstructions. Once again results were variable with a 33 per cent (25 of 75 knees) overall failure rate using pivot shift and KT 2000 testing. However, significant improvement was found for the symptoms of pain, swelling and giving away.

Several studies comparing allograft with autograft for revision ACL reconstruction demonstrated no significant difference between the two groups from either a functional or an objective standpoint. Uribe *et al.* reported on 54 patients with 2 to 6.5 years postoperative follow-up (Uribe *et al.* 1996). Nineteen received patellar tendon allografts and 35 autogenous grafts (ipsilateral or contralateral patellar tendon or quadrupled hamstring tendon). The autograft group had a significantly greater objective stability when compared to the allograft group, with average KT 1000· arthrometer (Medmetric, San Diego, CA) measurements for the autograft group of 2.2 mm compared to 3.3 mm for the allograft group. Interestingly, there was no functional difference based on graft source as measured by Tegner and Lysholm scores. Getelman and associates compared the clinical results of 12 patients treated with ipsilateral autogenous patellar tendon grafts and 14 patients treated with allograft patellar tendon tissue (Getelman and Friedman 1999). Follow-up was between 20 to 34 months postoperatively. The allograft group had poorer IKDC scores with 29 per cent normal or nearly normal as compared to 67 per cent in the autograft group.

Comparison allograft and autograft studies in an animal model have demonstrated that autograft and allograft tissues undergo the same healing process following implantation. However, the time course for allografts appears to be prolonged, and the biological response is less robust than seen with autograft tissue (Arnoczky *et al.* 1982, 1986; Drez *et al.* 1991; Jackson *et al.* 1987). Because of the delayed biological incorporation, the use of allografts in these revision cases should be carefully considered and these tissues used only if no other autograft tissue is available.

Conclusion

An increasing number of revision ACL reconstructions are being performed each year. In general the results of revision ACL reconstruction do not appear to be as favorable as those of primary reconstructions (Harilainen and Sandelin 2001; Johnson et al. 1996b; Johnson and Coen 1995b; Noyes and Barber-Westin 1996b). The success rate of revision ACL reconstruction is determined by many factors including the etiology of the primary failure, the preoperative laxity of the knee, the status of the secondary restraints, menisci and articular cartilage, and patient motivation and compliance. In order to maximize the success of revision ACL surgery, a methodical and organized approach is required. Graft selection in no less important in these often difficult cases. Each ACL revision is unique. Many factors are taken into account when considering revision ACL graft selection. Graft selection for the revision procedure will depend on the type of graft used for the primary reconstruction, prior tunnel placement, tunnel enlargement, surgeon's preference and associated ligamentous injuries. All these variables must be considered when considering revision ACL surgery. The authors' first choice of graft is the autogenous tissue, especially the bone-patellar tendon-bone graft. We strongly recommend the use of this tissue source and we urge surgeons to consider using the contralateral tendon if the ipsilateral tendon was previously harvested. If this graft is not available, we would then consider using the autogenous quadriceps tendon bone graft especially in cases with bony deficits. Alternatively, the surgeon may consider a two-staged procedure wherein hardware removal and bone grafting could be performed initially followed by the definitive ACL reconstruction using either a bony-ended graft or soft tissue graft. If there is no bony defect, hamstring tendons are appealing in cases of failed patellar tendon grafts. Finally, allograft tissues should be considered in all revision cases but only if there is no viable autograft alternative, for example, in the multiply operated knee where further donor-site morbidity is not desired. Traditionally, bone-patellar tendon-bone or Achilles tendon allograft tissues have been used and to reiterate, these grafts are particularly appealing in cases with bony deficits. However, the tibialis anterior tendon allograft is another excellent tissue source based on recent studies. Special situations that must be considered include cases in which failure was related to loss of secondary restraints (i.e. posterolateral corner or posterior cruciate ligament) or ligamentous laxity where a stiffer graft construct such as autogenous or allograft bone-patellar tendon-bone would be desirable compared to a soft tissue graft source. In addition, patients that are predisposed to postoperative contracture would benefit from the use of a soft tissue graft where there is more elasticity in the graft. Concomitant post-meniscectomy changes, articular cartilage damage or malalignment issues should push the surgeon towards the use of allograft tissue as this could avoid further trauma to the knee due to donor site morbidity. It is clear that the knee surgeon must be familiar with the advantages and disadvantages of the graft choices that are available for ACL surgery. This knowledge should be used in conjunction with the special circumstances that are unique to each case. In the coming years with the increasing number of revision ACL surgeries being performed, there will be additional data to better support the algorithm for graft selection.

References

2002a, 'Update: allograft-associated bacterial infections–United States, 2002', *Morb. Mortal. Wkly. Rep.* 51(10): 207–210.

2002b, 'From the Centers for Disease Control and Prevention. Update: allograft-associated bacterial infections – United States, 2002', *JAMA* 287(13): 1642–1644.

Amiel, D., Kleiner, J. B., Roux, R. D., Harwood, F. L., and Akeson, W. H. 1986, 'The phenomenon of "ligamentization": Anterior cruciate ligament reconstruction with autogenous patellar tendon', *J. Orthop. Res.*, vol. 4: 162–172.

Andersen, H. N., Bruun, C., and Sondergard-Petersen, P. E. 1992, 'Reconstruction of chronic insufficient anterior cruciate ligament in the knee using a synthetic Dacron prosthesis. A prospective study of 57 cases', *Am. J. Sports Med.*, vol. 20: 20–23.

Arnoczky, S. P. 1996, 'Biology of ACL reconstructions: what happens to the graft?', *Instr. Course Lect.*, vol. 45: 229–233.

Arnoczky, S. P., Tarvin, G. B., and Marshall, J. L. 1982, 'Anterior cruciate ligament replacement using patellar tendon. An evaluation of graft revascularization in the dog', *J. Bone Joint Surg. Am.*, vol. 64(2): 217–224.

Arnoczky, S. P., Warren, R. F., and Ashlock, M. A. 1986, 'Replacement of the anterior cruciate ligament using a patellar tendon allograft. An experimental study', *J. Bone Joint Surg. Am.*, vol. 68(3): 376–385.

Aune, A. K., Ekeland, A., and Cawley, P. W. 1998, 'Interference screw fixation of hamstring vs patellar tendon grafts for anterior cruciate ligament reconstruction', *Knee. Surg. Sports Traumatol. Arthrosc.*, vol. 6: 99–102.

Barber, F. A., Elrod, B. F., McGuire, D. A., and Paulos, L. E. 1996, 'Is an anterior cruciate ligament reconstruction outcome age dependent?', *Arthroscopy*, vol. 12: 720–725.

Bernicker, J. P., Haddad, J. L., Lintner, D. M., DiLiberti, T. C., and Bocell, J. R. 1998, 'Patellar tendon defect during the first year after anterior cruciate ligament reconstruction: appearance on serial magnetic resonance imaging', *Arthroscopy*, vol. 14: 804–809.

Brand, J., Jr., Weiler, A., Caborn, D. N., Brown, C. H., Jr., and Johnson, D. L. 2000a, 'Graft fixation in cruciate ligament reconstruction', *Am. J. Sports Med.*, 28(5): 761–774.

Brand, J. C., Jr., Pienkowski, D., Steenlage, E., Hamilton, D., Johnson, D. L., and Caborn, D. N. 2000b, 'Interference screw fixation strength of a quadrupled hamstring tendon graft is directly related to bone mineral density and insertion torque', *Am. J. Sports Med.*, 28(5): 705–710.

Brown, C. H., Wilson DPhil, D. R., Hecker Aaron, and Ferragamo, M. 1999, Comparison of hamstring and patellar tendon femoral fixation: Cyclic load. Transactions of the 25th Annual Meeting of the American Orthopedic Society for Sports Medicine Traverse City Michigan 1999.

Brown, C. H., Jr. and Carson, E. W. 1999, 'Revision anterior cruciate ligament surgery', *Clin. Sports Med.*, vol. 18: 109–171.

Brown, C. H., Jr., Steiner, M. E., and Carson, E. W. 1993, 'The use of hamstring tendons for anterior cruciate ligament reconstruction. Technique and results', *Clin. Sports Med.*, vol. 12: 723–756.

Caborn, D. N. and Selby, J. B. 2002, 'Allograft anterior tibialis tendon with bioabsorbable interference screw fixation in anterior cruciate ligament reconstruction', *Arthroscopy*, 18(1):102–105.

Chen, C. H., Chen, W. J., and Shih, C. H. 1999, 'Arthroscopic anterior cruciate ligament reconstruction with quadriceps tendon-patellar bone autograft', *J. Trauma*, vol. 46: 678–682.

Coupens, S. D., Yates, C. K., Sheldon, C., and Ward, C. 1992, 'Magnetic resonance imaging evaluation of the patellar tendon after use of its central one-third for anterior cruciate ligament reconstruction', *Am. J. Sports Med.*, vol. 20: 332–335.

Drez, D. J., Jr., DeLee, J., Holden, J. P., Arnoczky, S., Noyes, F. R., and Roberts, T. S. 1991, 'Anterior cruciate ligament reconstruction using bone-patellar tendon-bone allografts. A biological and biomechanical evaluation in goats', *Am. J. Sports Med.*, vol. 19(3): 256–263.

Falconiero, R. P., DiStefano, V. J., and Cook, T. M. 1998, 'Revascularization and ligamentization of autogenous anterior cruciate ligament grafts in humans', *Arthroscopy*, vol. 14: 197–205.

Fideler, B. M., Vangsness, C. T., Jr., Lu, B., Orlando, C., and Moore, T. 1995b, 'Gamma irradiation: effects on biomechanical properties of human bone-patellar tendon-bone allografts', *Am. J. Sports Med.*, vol. 23(5): 643–646.

Fideler, B. M., Vangsness, C. T., Jr., Lu, B., Orlando, C., and Moore, T. 1995a, 'Gamma irradiation: effects on biomechanical properties of human bone-patellar tendon-bone allografts', *Am. J. Sports Med.*, vol. 23: 643–646.

Fleming, B. C., Abate, J. A., Peura, G. D., and Beynnon, B. D. 2001, 'The relationship between graft tensioning and the anterior-posterior laxity in the anterior cruciate ligament reconstructed goat knee', *J. Orthop. Res.*, 19(5):841–844.

Friedlaender, G. E., Strong, D. M., Tomford, W. W., and Mankin, H. J. 1999, 'Long-term follow-up of patients with osteochondral allografts. A correlation between immunologic responses and clinical outcome', *Orthop. Clin. North Am.*, vol. 30: 583–588.

Friedman, M. J., Sherman, O. H., Fox, J. M., Del Pizzo, W., Snyder, S. J., and Ferkel, R. J. 1985, 'Autogeneic anterior cruciate ligament (ACL) anterior reconstruction of the knee. A review', *Clin. Orthop.*, 9–14.

Gala, J. L., Vandenbroucke, A. T., Vandercam, B., Pirnay, J. P., Delferriere, N., and Burtonboy, G. 1997, 'HIV-1 detection by nested PCR and viral culture in fresh or cryopreserved postmortem skin: potential implications for skin handling and allografting', *J. Clin. Pathol.*, vol. 50: 481–484.

Getelman, M. H. and Friedman, M. J. 1999, 'Revision anterior cruciate ligament reconstruction surgery', *J. Am. Acad. Orthop. Surg.*, vol. 7: 189–198.

Greis, P. E. and Steadman, J. R. 1996, 'Revision of failed prosthetic anterior cruciate ligament reconstruction', *Clin. Orthop.*, pp. 78–90.

Hamner, D. L., Brown, C. H., Jr., Steiner, M. E., Hecker, A. T., and Hayes, W. C. 1999, 'Hamstring tendon grafts for reconstruction of the anterior cruciate ligament: biomechanical evaluation of the use of multiple strands and tensioning techniques', *J. Bone Joint Surg. Am.*, vol. 81: 549–557.

Harilainen, A. and Sandelin, J. 2001, 'Revision anterior cruciate ligament surgery. A review of the literature and results of our own revisions', *Scand. J. Med. Sci. Sports,* 11(3): 163–169.

Harris NL, Smith DA, Lamoreaux L, Purnell M Central quadriceps tendon for anterior cruciate ligament reconstruction. Part I: Morphometric and biomechanical evaluation. *Am J Sports Med.,* Jan-Feb, 25(1): 23–28.

Harmon, K. G. and Ireland, M. L. 2000, 'Gender differences in noncontact anterior cruciate ligament injuries', *Clin. Sports Med.,* 19(2): 287–302.

Haut Donahue, T. L., Howell, S. M., Hull, M. L., and Gregersen, C. 2002, 'A biomechanical evaluation of anterior and posterior tibialis tendons as suitable single-loop anterior cruciate ligament grafts', *Arthroscopy,* Jul.–Aug., vol. 18(6.): 589–597.

Ishibashi, Y., Toh, S., Okamura, Y., Sasaki, T., and Kusumi, T. 2001, 'Graft incorporation within the tibial bone tunnel after anterior cruciate ligament reconstruction with bone-patellar tendon-bone autograft', *Am. J. Sports Med.,* vol. 29(4): 473–479.

Jackson, D. W., Corsetti, J., and Simon, T. M. 1996, 'Biologic incorporation of allograft anterior cruciate ligament replacements', *Clin. Orthop.,* vol. 324: 126–133.

Jackson, D. W., Grood, E. S., Arnoczky, S. P., Butler, D. L., and Simon, T. M. 1987, 'Freeze dried anterior cruciate ligament allografts. Preliminary studies in a goat model', *Am. J. Sports Med.,* vol. 15(4): 295–303.

Jackson, D. W., Grood, E. S., Cohn, B. T., Arnoczky, S. P., Simon, T. M., and Cummings, J. F. 1991, 'The effects of in situ freezing on the anterior cruciate ligament. An experimental study in goats', *J. Bone Joint Surg. Am.,* vol. 73(2): 201–213.

Johnson, D. L. and Coen, M. J. 1995a, 'Revision ACL surgery. Etiology, indications, techniques, and results', *Am. J. Knee. Surg.,* vol. 8: 155–167.

Johnson, D. L. and Coen, M. J. 1995b, 'Revision ACL surgery. Etiology, indications, techniques, and results', *Am. J. Knee. Surg.,* vol. 8: 155–167.

Johnson, D. L. and Fu, F. H. 1995, 'Anterior cruciate ligament reconstruction: why do failures occur?', *Instr. Course Lect.,* vol. 44: 391–406.

Johnson, D. L., Swenson, T. M., Irrgang, J. J., Fu, F. H., and Harner, C. D. 1996, 'Revision anterior cruciate ligament surgery: experience from Pittsburgh', *Clin. Orthop.,* 100–109.

Johnson, R. J., Eriksson, E., Haggmark, T., and Pope, M. H. 1984, 'Five- to ten-year follow-up evaluation after reconstruction of the anterior cruciate ligament', *Clin. Orthop.,* 122–140.

Jones, D. G., Lee, M., Irrgang, J. J., Harner, C. D., and Fu, F. H. 'Patient characteristics, surgical findings and procedures which determine functional status in patients following ACL reconstruction', (Personal Communication).

Kartus, J., Stener, S., Lindahl, S., Eriksson, B. I., and Karlsson, J. 1998, 'Ipsi- or contralateral patellar tendon graft in anterior cruciate ligament revision surgery. A comparison of two methods', *Am. J. Sports Med.,* vol. 26: 499–504.

Kleipool, A. E., van Loon, T., and Marti, R. K. 1994, 'Pain after use of the central third of the patellar tendon for cruciate ligament reconstruction. 33 patients followed 2–3 years', *Acta Orthop. Scand.,* vol. 65: 62–66.

Kornblatt, I., Warren, R. F., and Wickiewicz, T. L. 1988, 'Long-term follow-up of anterior cruciate ligament reconstruction using the quadriceps tendon substitution for chronic anterior cruciate ligament insufficiency', *Am. J. Sports Med.,* vol. 16: 444–448.

LaPrade, R. F., Hamilton, C. D., Montgomery, R. D., Wentorf, F., and Hawkins, H. D. 1997, 'The reharvested central third of the patellar tendon. A histologic and biomechanical analysis', *Am. J. Sports Med.*, vol. 25: 779–785.

Liu, S. H., Hang, D. W., Gentili, A., and Finerman, G. A. 1996, 'MRI and morphology of the insertion of the patellar tendon after graft harvesting', *J. Bone Joint Surg. Br.*, vol. 78: 823–826.

Malinin, T. I., Martinez, O. V., and Brown, M. D. 1985, 'Banking of massive osteoarticular and intercalary bone allografts – 12 years' experience', *Clin. Orthop.*, pp. 44–57.

Marcacci, M., Zaffagnini, S., Iacono, F., Vascellari, A., Loreti, I., Kon, E., and Presti, M. L. 2003, 'Intra- and extra-articular anterior cruciate ligament reconstruction utilizing autogeneous semitendinosus and gracilis tendons: 5-year clinical results', *Knee. Surg. Sports Traumatol. Arthrosc.*, 11(1): 2–8.

Marcacci, M., Zaffagnini, S., Visani, A., Iacono, F., Neri, M. P., and Petitto, A. 1996, 'Arthroscopic reconstruction of the anterior cruciate ligament with Leeds-Keio ligament in non-professional athletes. Results after a minimum 5 years' follow-up', *Knee. Surg. Sports Traumatol. Arthrosc.*, vol. 4: 9–13.

Messina, D. F., Farney, W. C., and DeLee, J. C. 1999, 'The incidence of injury in Texas high school basketball. A prospective study among male and female athletes', *Am. J. Sports Med.*, vol. 27: 294–299.

Muller, B., Rupp, S., Kohn, D., and Seil, R. 2000, '[Donor site problems after anterior cruciate ligament reconstruction with the middle third of the patellar ligament] Entnahmestellenproblematik nach vorderer Kreuzbandplastik mit dem mittleren Drittel der Patellarsehne', *Unfallchirurg*, 103(8): 662–667.

Noronha, J. C. 2002, 'Reconstruction of the anterior cruciate ligament with quadriceps tendon', *Arthroscopy*, 18(7): E37.

Noyes, F. R. and Barber-Westin, S. D. 1996a, 'Revision anterior cruciate ligament surgery: experience from Cincinnati', *Clin. Orthop.*, 116–129.

Noyes, F. R. and Barber-Westin, S. D. 1996b, 'Revision anterior cruciate ligament surgery: experience from Cincinnati', *Clin. Orthop.*, 116–129.

Noyes, F. R., Barber-Westin, S. D., and Roberts, C. S. 1994, 'Use of allografts after failed treatment of rupture of the anterior cruciate ligament', *J. Bone Joint Surg. Am.*, vol. 76: 1019–1031.

Noyes, F. R., Butler, D. L., Grood, E. S., Zernicke, R. F., and Hefzy, M. S. 1984, 'Biomechanical analysis of human ligament grafts used in knee-ligament repairs and reconstructions', *J. Bone Joint Surg. Am.*, vol. 66: 344–352.

O'Donoghue 1950, 'Surgical treatment of fresh injuries to the ligaments of the knee.', *J. Bone Joint Surg. Am.*, vol. 32: 721–738.

O'Donoghue 1963, 'A method for replacement of the anterior cruciate ligament of the knee.', *J. Bone Joint Surg. Am.*, vol. 45(5): 905–924.

Paulos, L. E., Butler, D. L., Noyes, F. R., and Grood, E. S. 1983, 'Intra-articular cruciate reconstruction. II: Replacement with vascularized patellar tendon', *Clin. Orthop.*, 172: 78–84.

Pinkowski, J. L., Reiman, P. R., and Chen, S. L. 1989, 'Human lymphocyte reaction to freeze-dried allograft and xenograft ligamentous tissue', *Am. J. Sports Med.*, vol. 17: 595–600.

Powell, J. W. and Barber-Foss, K. D. 2000, 'Sex-related injury patterns among selected high school sports', *Am. J. Sports Med.*, 28(3): 385–391.

Proctor, C. S., Jackson, D. W., and Simon, T. M. 1997, 'Characterization of the repair tissue after removal of the central one-third of the patellar ligament. An experimental study in a goat model', *J. Bone Joint Surg. Am.*, vol. 79: 997–1006.

Richmond, J. C., Manseau, C. J., Patz, R., and McConville, O. 1992, 'Anterior cruciate reconstruction using a Dacron ligament prosthesis. A long-term study', *Am. J. Sports Med.*, vol. 20: 24–28.

Roder, W., Kruse, M., Runkel, M., Muller, W. E., and Isemer, F. E. 1994, '[Possibility for detecting HIV-1 in bone transplant by PCR using the HIV-1 microtiter plate assay] Nachweismoglichkeit von HIV-1 im Knochentransplantat durch PCR mittels HIV-1-Microtiter-Plate-Assay', *Unfallchirurg*, vol. 97: 629–632.

Rubinstein, R. A., Jr., Shelbourne, K. D., VanMeter, C. D., McCarroll, J. C., and Rettig, A. C. 1994, 'Isolated autogenous bone-patellar tendon-bone graft site morbidity', *Am. J. Sports Med.*, vol. 22: 324–327.

Safran, M. R. and Harner, C. D. 1995, 'Revision ACL surgery: technique and results utilizing allografts', *Instr. Course Lect.*, vol. 44: 407–415.

Scranton, P. E., Jr., Bagenstose, J. E., Lantz, B. A., Friedman, M. J., Khalfayan, E. E., and Auld, M. K. 2002, 'Quadruple hamstring anterior cruciate ligament reconstruction: a multicenter study', *Arthroscopy*, 18(7): 715–724.

Seitz, H., Marlovits, S., Schwendenwein, I., Muller, E., and Vecsei, V. 1998, 'Biocompatibility of polyethylene terephthalate (Trevira hochfest) augmentation device in repair of the anterior cruciate ligament', *Biomaterials*, vol. 19: 189–196.

Shelbourne, K. D. and Nitz, P. 1990, 'Accelerated rehabilitation after anterior cruciate ligament reconstruction', *Am. J. Sports Med.*, vol. 18(3): 292–299.

Simonian, P. T., Levine, R. E., Wright, T. M., Wickiewicz, T. L., and Warren, R. F. 2000, 'Response of hamstring and patellar tendon grafts for anterior cruciate ligament reconstruction during cyclic tensile loading', *Am. J. Knee. Surg.*, 13(1): 8–12.

Sirlin, C. B., Brossmann, J., Boutin, R. D., Pathria, M. N., Convery, F. R., Bugbee, W., Deutsch, R., Lebeck, L. K., and Resnick, D. 2001, 'Shell osteochondral allografts of the knee: comparison of mr imaging findings and immunologic responses', *Radiology*, 219(1): 35–43.

Snook, G. A. 1983, 'A short history of the anterior cruciate ligament and the treatment of tears', *Clin. Orthop.*, 172: 11–13.

Staubli, H. U., Schatzmann, L., Brunner, P., Rincon, L., and Nolte, L. P. 1996, 'Quadriceps tendon and patellar ligament: cryosectional anatomy and structural properties in young adults', *Knee. Surg. Sports Traumatol. Arthrosc.*, vol. 4: 100–110.

Staubli, H. U., Schatzmann, L., Brunner, P., Rincon, L., and Nolte, L. P. 1999, 'Mechanical tensile properties of the quadriceps tendon and patellar ligament in young adults', *Am. J. Sports Med.*, vol. 27: 27–34.

Steenlage, E., Brand, J. C., Jr., Johnson, D. L., and Caborn, D. N. 2002, 'Correlation of bone tunnel diameter with quadrupled hamstring graft fixation strength using a biodegradable interference screw', *Arthroscopy*, 18(8): 901–907.

Uribe, J. W., Hechtman, K. S., Zvijac, J. E., and Tjin, A. T. E. 1996, 'Revision anterior cruciate ligament surgery: experience from Miami', *Clin. Orthop.*, 91–99.

Yasuda, K., Ohkoshi, Y., Tanabe, Y., and Kaneda, K. 1991, 'Muscle weakness after anterior cruciate ligament reconstruction using patellar and quadriceps tendons', *Bull. Hosp. Jt. Dis. Orthop. Inst.*, vol. 51: 175–185.

Yunes, M., Richmond, J. C., Engels, E. A., and Pinczewski, L. A. 2001, 'Patellar versus hamstring tendons in anterior cruciate ligament reconstruction: A meta-analysis', *Arthroscopy*, 17(3): 248–257.

14

One stage versus two stage revision ACL reconstruction: indications and techniques

Giancarlo Puddu and Guglielmo Cerullo

Introduction

Anterior cruciate ligament (ACL) reconstruction is today the treatment of choice for the functional unstable knee and it is widely performed. Good or excellent results have been reported to be obtained in up to 90 per cent of cases (Bach *et al.* 1998; Harter *et al.* 1992; Holmes *et al.* 1991; Shelbourne and Gray 1997). This means, however, that fair or poor results are possible and there are several causes for these failures. It is not unusual for ACL revision surgery to be required as a result of symptomatic failed ligament reconstruction, but the patient and the surgeon too must recognize that the results of revision ACL reconstruction surgery are less successful as compared to primary reconstruction (Eberhardt *et al.* 2000; Johnson *et al.* 1996; Noyes and Barber-Westin 1996; Safran and Harner 1995; Uribe *et al.* 1996; Wirth and Kohn 1996).

This chapter analyzes the main causes of failure of ACL reconstruction, discusses the indications for revision surgery and tries to give operative guidelines to surmount the difficulties that often arise during revision surgery.

Aetiology of failure

Johnson and Coen classified the reasons for the failure of ACL reconstruction into four categories (Johnson and Coen 1995):

1 Arthrofibrosis;
2 Extensor mechanism disfunction;
3 Arthritis or recurrent pain;
4 Recurrent patholaxity.

Arthrofibrosis

Arthrofibrosis is the most common cause of loss of motion following ACL reconstruction (Graf and Uhr 1998; Harner *et al.* 1992; Paulos *et al.* 1987; Shelbourne *et al.* 1991). Today the incidence of arthrofibrosis is not very frequent compared to the severe degree of arthrofibrosis experienced in those patients treated in the 80 years before using continuous passive motion and rapid rehabilitation after ACL reconstruction; but a cyclop's lesion (Jackson and Schaefer 1990), or hypertrophy of the neoligament, remains a common problem (Fisher and Shelbourne 1993; Reider *et al.* 1996). These conditions give a loss of only a few degrees of extension, but are very troublesome for the patient because of the resulting anterior knee pain, intraarticular clicks, muscle hypotrophy and limping. In these cases arthroscopic debridement of the scar tissue is a relatively simple procedure, the results of which are very good. In other cases loss of motion is due to a surgical error (malpositioned or too tight ACL) (Echigo *et al.* 1999; Hooglan and Hillen 1984; Tanzer and Lenzer 1990; Yoshiya *et al.* 1987) or an inadequate notchplasty (Howell *et al.* 1991; Tanzer and Lenzer 1990). It is often the case that if the impingement and loss of knee extension is not too severe, an arthroscopic notchplasty, excision of the Cyclops lesion and if necessary a partial reduction of the neoligament can be undertaken to achieve full knee extension. This often avoids the need for a revision ACL reconstruction. However if the ACL is very malpositioned, its ablation is recommended and a staged ACL reconstruction is undertaken. One stage revision ACL reconstruction is not indicated in the presence of a loss of motion ($>5°$ of extension and $>20°$ of flexion), because of a high risk of a recurrence of the arthrofibrosis, a restricted postoperative range of motion (ROM). If necessary reconstruction is delayed until the knee has regained a complete range of motion either by intensive rehabilitation and splintage or arthroscopic intervention (Tredinnick and Friedman 2001).

Other causes of arthrofibrosis are a reflex sympathetic dystrophy and infection. Algodystrophy often responds to specific treatment and intensive rehabilitation. This condition should not be made by default without excluding any other underlying pathology. Infection may require urgent antibiotics and surgical intervention to debride and wash out the infective material. Infection often results in a long term restriction of the range of motion and in these situations prolonged rehabilitation maybe necessary.

Extensor mechanism dysfunction

Extensor mechanism dysfunction and the related anterior knee pain is common after ACL reconstruction (Navarro and Fu 1998; Sachs *et al.* 1989) but we think that this is a problem often limited to the period of rehabilitation and not a real cause of long term loss of function and failure. The early symptoms of anterior knee pain often settle after a period of 8–10 months following surgery and do not require any surgical intervention (Cerullo *et al.* 1995), but it is very important that this is recognized at an early stage and then proper control of rehabilitation can be managed.

Arthritis

The onset of arthritis after ACL reconstruction is seen many years after surgery. Meniscectomy, bad preoperative cartilage status, mechanical axis malalignment and delayed surgery are predisposing conditions. The literature does not identify whether the ACL reconstruction itself is the causal agent of arthrosis or whether it is the initial articular damage, meniscal pathology, abnormal knee mechanics, over-constraint or persistent laxity. Treatment of any arthritic or degenerative changes depends on the stage of arthrosis present. The treatment varies from conservative management to various different surgical options. These surgical options include: debridement, smoothing of the articular cartilage irregularity, Priddy or Steadman microfractures, osteochondral autografts, allographs chondrocyte transplantation or realignment osteotomy. Minor additional procedures to manage the degeneration can often by undertaken in conjunction with ACL revision, however, more significant procedures often need to be performed as a separate procedure. Careful consideration must be given to operative planning. Procedures such as a valgus opening wedge high tibial osteotomy may present a problem for revision ACL reconstruction because of the poor quality of cancellous bone in the upper tibia.

Recurrent knee laxity

The University of Pittsburgh classification divided the mechanism or aetiology of primary intraarticular ACL failure leading to recurrent laxity into three categories (Johnson and Coen 1995; Johnson *et al.* 1996):

1 Errors in surgical techniques,
2 Failure of graft incorporation,
3 Traumatic causes.

Surgical error involves the femoral and/or tibial tunnel position, the graft tension and fixation.

A femoral tunnel too anterior leads to graft lengthening with knee flexion; if the position is very anterior, there is increased tension in both flexion and extension. Posterior insertions result in decreased length and increased laxity of the graft as the knee is flexed. If the graft is placed in too vertical a position, decreased resistance to anterior tibial translation results, while medial or lateral positioning results in notch impingement and potential early graft rupture.

Placement of the tibial tunnel too anterior results in roof impingement and a Cyclops lesion, while posterior placement results in a lack of knee extension and increased tension in the graft. Medial positioning of the tibial tunnel damages the weight bearing area of the medial tibial plateau; too lateral a tunnel results in graft impingement against the medial side of the lateral femoral condyle (Carson *et al.* 1998; Henning *et al.* 1985; Jackson and Gasser 1994; Johnson and Coen 1995; Jones *et al.* 2001; Safran and Harner 1996). It is inevitable that a malpositioned tunnel results in a degree of restricted range of knee motion, graft impingement, increased graft tension or a recurrence of knee laxity. Graft impingement, abrasion or overload often results in early failure (Howell *et al.* 1992; Howell and Taylor 1993).

Graft tensioning is also another factor to be considered in recurrent laxity. Excessive tensioning leads to restriction of motion and stiffness, but with time results in graft elongation or failure, probably due to excessive tension which results in delayed vascularization, myxoid degeneration and failure (Yoshiya *et al.* 1987). Inadequate ligament tensioning results in a persistent knee instability because the graft is not functional. The optimal intra-operative tension still remains to be determined and in practice probably varies to some extent in each knee (Burks and Leland 1988; Bylski-Austrow *et al.* 1990; Livesay *et al.* 1997; Nabors *et al.* 1995; Yohsiya *et al.* 1987).

The modern advanced rapid rehabilitation protocols require stable fixation that permits immediate knee motion without compromising graft tension or position. Many metallic or biodegradable screws and other devices give the possibility of a strong fixation, but other factors interfere with the final stabilization, such as type and quality of the graft, quality of the bone, dimensions of the graft, tunnels and fixation device and so when recurrence of laxity occurs in absence of trauma, is very difficult to determine the real cause of failure (Kurosaka *et al.* 1987; Robertson *et al.* 1986).

Biological graft selection whether an autograft bone-patellar tendon-bone, quadrupled hamstring or quadriceps graft probably play very little part in influencing the quality of the results of ACL surgery compared to the effect of using other grafts such as autogenous or prosthetic grafts (Aglietti *et al.* 1994; Anderson *et al.* 2001; Bach *et al.* 1998; Harter *et al.* 1988; Holmes *et al.* 1991; Howe *et al.* 1991; Kaplan *et al.* 1991; Kornblatt *et al.* 1988; Marder *et al.* 1991; O'Brien *et al.* 1991; Otero and Hutcheson 1993; Shelbourne and Gray 1997). It is well known that prosthetic ligaments, even if technically well implanted, are subjected to a fatigue failure with time, causing graft breakage. We avoid the use of such implants (DiGiovine and Shields 1991; Woods *et al.* 1991).

The graft remodelling and incorporation process includes ischaemic necrosis, revascularization, cellular repopulation and proliferation and collagen remodelling and replacement is influenced by vascular, immunological and hormonal factors (Amiel *et al.* 1986;

Arnoczky *et al.* 1982; Corsetti and Jackson 1996; Fahey and Indelicato 1994; Jackson *et al.* 1991; Jaureguito and Paulos 1996; Oakes 1993; Shino *et al.* 1990). Thus the causes of failure of graft incorporation are sometimes very difficult to determine if the procedure is technically correct.

The incidence of reinjury for a new traumatic event in the patients that were returned to sports after ACL reconstruction has been reported to be approximately 5–25 per cent (Harner 2000 unpublished communication; Johnson *et al.* 1996; Paessler 2000 unpublished communication). In these cases the knee presents with a history of a new injury, a hemarthrosis and increased laxity that was not present at the previous postoperative examination. This should be distinguished from other cases in which a too aggressive or wrong rehabilitation program, a failure of the patient to adhere to the rehabilitation program, or a minor traumatic event during the early postoperative period can cause elongation of the immature and weak reconstructed ACL that has not already completed the process of incorporation.

Indications – one stage versus two stage

The main indication for revision ACL reconstruction is a symptomatic failed primary reconstruction; a symptomatic knee with objective laxity and subjective instability whether in daily life activities or sports. In general if there are no technical problems with tunnel placement or the existing fixation devices then the revision operation can usually be performed in one stage. If other symptoms, conditions or complications are present (pain, loss of motion, malalignment, osteolysis, tunnel enlargement, fixation devices, degeneration, malalignment or meniscal pathology), two stage revision surgery should be considered.

The patient and the surgeon have to recognize that revision ACL reconstruction gives satisfactory results in a low-demand knee, but the results are less successful in returning high-demand patients to meet their sporting aspirations and are poor in the so-called knee abusers (Johnson *et al.* 1996; Noyes and Barber-Westin 1996; Safran and Harner 1995; Uribe *et al.* 1996; Wirth and Kohn 1996). Other post reconstruction symptoms or complications such as pain, swelling, minimal loss of motion without subjective instability, even if in presence of laxity, are not sufficient to warrant revision ACL reconstruction but these complaints should be specifically addressed. The patient with pain during the activities of daily life is very different from the patient who complains of knee instability during vigorous sports activity. In the first situation the appropriate intervention should be to address the pathology by meniscal surgery, microfracture, osteochondral grafting, meniscal reconstruction, or osteotomy. Secondary staged ACL reconstruction can be considered if knee instability subsequently presents as a problem. In the presence of malalignment with recurrent instability or degeneration some surgeons advise a corrective osteotomy in conjunction with ACL reconstruction. Once again a staged reconstruction is recommended in knees with significant loss of motion (i.e. extension loss >5° and flexion loss >20°) (Tredinnick and Friedman 2001) in which the first goal must be the restoration of a full ROM with a secondary staged revision ACL reconstruction. Staged reconstructions are also recommended if osteolysis of the articular cartilage is present or if tunnel enlargement which requires bone grafting is present. In this situation initial removal of any ACL remnant (biological or prosthetic), debridement and bone grafting of the graft tunnels is undertaken first stage, whilst revision of the ACL reconstruction is undertaken as a second stage 3–6 months later, once the bone graft has incorporated. At the second stage the tunnels can be fashioned in the correct site for isometric placement without being compromised by bone defects, previous tunnels or metalwork.

Preoperative evaluation

An accurate history, physical examination and radiographic and MRI evaluation are very important to establish the appropriate indication for surgery and planning it. It is also advisable to discuss with the patient a realistic approach to the expectations and functional results following surgery, the risks, goals, complications and risks in these technically demanding cases in order to avoid false expectations and disappointment. It is also advisable to make the patient conscious of the possibility of a staged procedure being required.

History

The history should detail the exact nature and mechanism of the original injury, identify the extent and nature of the damage, the previous procedures undertaken, the ligament and fixation devices implanted, and the current symptomatic complaints of the patient. Further information as the rehabilitation was undertaken, functional level achieved, aspirations and expectations of the patients and practical functional restrictions of the patient should be identified and documented.

Physical examination

An accurate and extensive knee examination should evaluate: skin incisions, swelling, origin of pain (menisci, tendons, bone), direction and extent of any knee laxity (anterior, posterior, medial, lateral or rotatory), range of motion and limb alignment. We also recommend static stance and dynamic gait evaluation, in particular the determination of any varus thrust on weight-bearing. Objective laxity measurement such as the KT-1000 arthrometer completes the examination.

Radiographic evaluation

Radiographic evaluation should include antero-posterior (AP) weight bearing, lateral, merchant and posteroanterior (PA) 45° flexion weight-bearing views (Rosenberg *et al.* 1988). It is important to evaluate the position of the bone tunnels both on radiographs and MRI scans and to determine the presence and type of fixation devices. For absorbable devices the state of the resorption and any associated cyst formation should be determined. The patellar height, status of the notch, arthritic changes, joint space narrowing, osteolysis and alignment should also be determined. Varus-valgus deformity is better studied on full limbs standing X-rays.

Computed tomography (CT) is useful in evaluating the bone defects (Seeman and Steadman 1993), while MRI can give good information about the previous reconstruction, meniscal and chondral pathology, but sometimes signal intensity changes are misinterpreted (Echigo *et al.* 1999; Maywood *et al.* 1993) and the identification and detail of articular cartilage lesions may not be reliable from MRI scanning even when specific articular cartilage imaging sequences are used. We currently believe that it is better to plan surgery on clinical and standard radiographic examination.

Surgical techniques

Skin incisions

Usually during ACL revision surgery is possible to reuse the previous incisions, especially if an allograft is used. If other exposures are required, to reduce risks for necrosis or infections we must avoid incisions that cross old incisions and leave skin bridges less than 5–7 cm wide. When multiple anterior incisions are present, the most laterally sited one is generally selected; transverse incision can be crossed and prior tissue expansion may be indicated (Manifold and Scott 2000; Tredinnick and Friedman 2001).

Hardware and prosthetic ligament removal

The appropriate instrumentation for hardware removal should be available. Specialized instrumentation for removal of cannulated fixation screws is available as is equipment to remove staples. Most arthroscopic instrument companies offer a specialized revision ACL set. Sometimes intra-operative use of the fluoroscope is necessary to localize interference screws, especially in the tibia. If the hardware does not interfere with the tunnel, it can be left in place and a new tibial tunnel drilled. If revision is to be performed endoscopically but the primary femoral fixation is via a two-incisions technique, the femoral screw is often inaccessible but can on many occasions be left alone (Navarro and Fu 1998). If the internal thread of the screw has been stripped, then it can be removed by a self-tapping awl or drilled out, but sometimes this leads to an excessive bone loss which requires bone grafting and a staged reconstruction. Experienced operative surgeons should be involved with the management of these cases because the surgeon must be prepared to readily alter the approach, changing from an endoscopic to a two-incision technique or vice versa. In some cases of revision cruciate ligament surgery the femoral fixation device can be ignored (Nabors *et al.* 1995).

Sometimes the removal of the existing hardware is difficult and takes time. For this reason we prefer to begin the operation without inflating the tourniquet. However intraarticular haemorrhage can interfere with visualization and make the procedure more difficult.

If a prosthetic ligament is present, it has to be removed making all efforts to do it en bloc, avoiding drills and arthroscopic knives and punches, minimizing potential creation of inflammatory synthetic particles. This is particularly important for grafts which incorporate carbon fibre or Dacron. Grasp the ligament with a Kocher clamp whilst using instruments to divide fibrous tissue around the ligament in the tunnel and allow its removal. The tunnel is then submitted to curettage in order to remove all debris and present fresh cancellous bone for the incorporation of the new revision graft. Use of a drill is discouraged in order to avoid tunnel enlargement. A tunnel larger than 12 mm demands an allograft bone-patellar tendon-bone (BPTB) or a staged reconstruction after having bone grafted the expanded tunnels.

Graft selection

There are two options in graft selection: autografts and allografts, while synthetic replacement which has a high complication rates and breakage has largely been abandoned (Di Giovine and Shields 1991; Klein and Jenson 1989 unpublished communication; Will and Collins 1989; Woods *et al.* 1991). Selection of a graft depends on many factors: availability, previous surgery, size of tunnels, choice of patient and preference of surgeon. Various types of graft are available but commonly in revision surgery autograft BPTB (Eberhardt *et al.* 2000; Kartus *et al.* 1998; LaPrade *et al.* 1997; Rubinstein *et al.* 1993), quadruple hamstring tendon (Aglietti *et al.* 1994) and quadriceps tendon (Fulkerson and Langeland 1996) are used and BPTB and Achilles tendon as allograft tissue. Autogenous tissue has the advantage of eliminating the potential risk of disease transmission, immunologic reaction and delayed graft incorporation (Jackson *et al.* 1993). Potential disadvantages of the use of autograft tissue include donor-site morbidity, longer surgery time, and extensor mechanism dysfunction (when BPTB or quadriceps are used).

Allograft tissue has several advantages. Its availability, no donor-site morbidity, smaller incisions, shorter surgery time and possibility of large dimensions of bone block (up to 15 mm) (Noyes and Barber 1992; Shino *et al.* 1990). Potential disadvantages include decreased graft strength, risk of disease transmission (< in 1 million) (Buck *et al.* 1989; Shelton *et al.* 1998), delayed incorporation (Jackson *et al.* 1993), a higher failure rate and poorer clinical results comparing autograft for revision ACL reconstruction (Alexander *et al.* 1996; Peterson *et al.* 2001). For all these reasons many orthopaedic surgeons, especially in North America, prefer to use allografts in revision ACL reconstructions.

Autografts are indicated for failed allograft primary reconstructions without gross technical failures and in which recurrence of laxity is probably due to failure of graft incorporation or adverse immunological reaction. These are also indicated if the patient refuses allograft. Allografts are indicated for failed autograft primary reconstructions, in the presence of large bone tunnels less than 15 mm, otherwise bone grafting and staged reconstruction is recommended as in complex revision cases (Fu and Martinek 2000 unpublished communication). At our Institute in Rome, allograft is not available so we always use autograft. If the patellar tendon has been utilized in previous reconstruction, we recommend ipsilateral doubled gracilis and semitendinosus for tunnels up to 8 mm, and contralateral BPTB for tunnels up to 10–11 mm. In the presence of larger tunnels we perform bone grafting and staged reconstruction. If the previous graft was a hamstring then we recommend using ipsilateral BPTB autograft.

Reharvesting BPTB is not a reliable nor reasonable procedure. Various animal studies have documented inferior biomechanical properties in these grafts. A recent study comparing autogenous reharvested ipsilateral BPTB with autogenous contralateral BPTB in ACL revision surgery demonstrated inferior clinical results with lower functional scores and higher rate of complications with ipsilateral BPTB grafts (Kartus *et al.* 1998; LaPrade *et al.* 1997; Proctor *et al.* 1997).

Tunnel management

In technically demanding surgery such as that involved in revision ACL reconstruction it is better to have preoperatively planned the different surgical steps, in order to save time, have the correct tools and equipment available and so that time is not lost taking decisions during the operation. For this reason an accurate evaluation of radiographic examination or MRI of the tunnels usually gives the solution for what is often the prinicpal factor in determining the surgical approach (Howell *et al.* 1991, 1992, 1993).

A preliminary notchplasty is performed before tunnel drilling, to remove soft tissue and osteophytes. In addition avoidance of notch-graft impingement is necessary by use of the impingement test after placement of the tibial tunnel. Often in ACL revision the normal landmarks are missing and it is important not to remove too much bone from the notch and to carefully site the tunnels. We find it useful to expose the posterior arch of the intercondylar notch to locate the femoral tunnel. After the definitive tibial tunnel has drilled, the impingement test is performed with a tunnel expander coming out from the tibial tunnel and then removing more bone from the notch if necessary.

FILLING THE TUNNEL DEFECTS

In revision ACL surgery it is not unusual to have large bony defects due to the previous tunnels. As discussed in these cases it is reasonable to stage the reconstruction with an initial autologous bone graft from the iliac crest. An alternative could be an artificial bone substitute (which is expensive) or in minor defects, obtaining bone graft from the tibia within the scope of the surgical exposure or using the swarf from the coring drill reamers (Tredinnick and Friedman 2001).

FEMORAL TUNNEL

The femoral tunnel in revision ACL reconstruction has sometimes been correctly placed. In this situation it is simple to redrill the tunnel after removal of the fixation device. However, if the quality of the tunnel margins is poor or defective then a tunnel can be fashioned at a different angle and alignment. This can most readily be achieved by using a two-incisions technique or vice versa. Alternately if the anterior tunnel is only slightly too anterior, the overlapping tunnel can be drilled posteriorly and or enlarged. The BPTB graft can then be placed with a bone block of the needed size orientated to the anterior side of the tunnel (Navarro and Fu 1998; Tredinnick and Friedman 2001). Similar solutions are used if a slight vertical or horizontal tunnel is present.

If the femoral tunnel is far too anterior, then often a completely new tunnel can be fitted posteriorly without any overlap. If the femoral tunnel is too posteriorly placed or the posterior wall of the tunnel is deficient an over the top placement can be utilized with fixation through a lateral approach.

Where there is a large expanded tunnel with a deficient rim it is preferable to fill the defect with bone graft and to stage the ACL reconstruction 3 to 6 months later.

TIBIAL TUNNEL

If the previous tibial tunnel is in the good or quite good position, the options illustrated for the femoral tunnel are applied. If a wrong position is present (distant more than one tunnel diameter), a new tunnel can be drilled in the correct position, filling the old defect if necessary with bone graft or an oversized bone block. The most frequent situation is that after drilling a new tunnel in a slightly posterior position, this typically leaves a bony defect anteriorly which can be filled with either a separate block of bone graft or impacted with bone graft. The graft is then placed in the desired position (Jones *et al.* 2001, Navarro and Fu 1998, and Tredinnick and Friedman 2001) by orientation of the graft and bone block within the tunnel. One alternative is to fill the defect with a stacked bioabsorbable screw (Tredinnick and Friedman 2001), however this may present further problems with cyst formation during absorption of the screws.

In the presence of a large bone defect it is reasonable to fill the defect with autologous bone and to stage the reconstruction, otherwise another technique consists of identifying the right intra-articular tibial position and drilling a new tunnel, divergent to the previous, over a guide pin from a different starting point (Brown and Carson 1990).

Graft fixation

Many different fixation devices are available today to fix a graft in ACL reconstruction. Surgeons must use those they are familiar with. In revision surgery if the bone quality and tunnel rim is satisfactory a routine interference fit screw can be used. However, if the tunnel bone is poor or deficient it is preferable utilize extrarticular fixation (staple, spiked washer, Endobutton, etc.) in conjunction with an intratunnel device so as to achieve double fixation at the cortex for strength and at the tunnel margin to avoid excessive movement in the tunnel and tunnel widening. Clearly all the different options of graft fixation must be considered in advance so that the correct equipment is readily available.

As secure fixation is critical to the outcome and the process of graft incorporation and maturation will probably be slower than in a primary case, a slow non-agressive rehabilitation program is undertaken, often protected within a brace. The regimen has to be personally tuned, in relation to the knee status, fixation and stability achieved and particular procedure performed.

Conclusions

Revision ACL reconstruction is a high technically demanding procedure that sometimes requires a two-stage surgery. Subjective instability is the main indication, but it is very important to address the whole knee and to ensure that the patient understands the goals, limitations and functional expectations as commonly the results of revision ACL reconstruction do not match those of primary surgery.

Preoperative planning is critical and the surgeon must be familiar with many different techniques for graft selection, tunnel management and graft fixation. Different hardware removal and fixation devices should be available during surgery to meet every possible eventuality.

References

Aglietti P, Buzzi R, Zaccherotti G, De Biase P (1994). Patellar tendon versus doubled semitendinosus and gracilis tendons for anterior ligament reconstructions. *American Journal of Sports Medicine*, 22, 211–8.

Alexander A, Garcia E, Bynum B, Sitler D (1996). Allograft versus autograft patellar tendon anterior cruciate ligament reconstruction: a prospective randomised study (early results). *Orthopaedic Transactions*, 24, 193–7.

Amiel D, Kleiner JB, Roux RD, Harwood FL, Akeson WH (1986). The phenomen of 'ligamentization': anterior cruciate ligament reconstruction with autogenous patellar tendon. *Journal of Orthopaedic Research*, 4, 162–72.

Anderson AF, Snyder RB, Lipscomb AB Jr (2001). Anterior ligament reconstruction: a prospective randomised study of three surgical methods. *American Journal of Sports Medicine*, 29, 272–9.

Arnoczky SP, Tarvin GB, Marshall JL (1982). Anterior cruciate ligament replacement using patellar tendon: an evaluation of graft revascularization in the dog. *Journal of Bone and Joint Surgery*, 64A, 217–24.

Bach BR Jr, Tradonsky S, Bojchuck J, Levy ME, Bush-Joseph CA, Khan NA (1998). Arthroscopically assisted anterior cruciate ligament reconstruction using patellar tendon autograft: 5- to 9-year follow-up evaluation. *American Journal of Sports Medicine*, 26, 20–9.

Brown CH Jr, Carson EW (1990). Revision anterior cruciate ligament surgery. *Clinics in Sports Medicine*, 18, 109–71.

Buck BE, Malinin TI, Brown M (1989). Bone transplantation and human immunodeficiency virus. *Clinical Orthopaedics and Related Research*, 40, 129–36.

Burks RT, Leland R (1988). Determination of graft tension before fixation in anterior cruciate ligament reconstruction. *Arthroscopy*, 4, 260–6.

Bylski-Austrow DI, Grood ES, Hefzey MS, Holden JP, Butler DL (1990). Anterior cruciate ligament replacements: a mechanical study of femoral attachment location, flexion angle at tensioning and initial tension. *Journal of Orthopaedic Research*, 8, 522–31.

Carson EW, Simonian PT, Wickiewicz TL, Warren RF (1998). Revision anterior ligament reconstruction. *Instructional Course Lectures*, 47, 361–8.

Cerullo G, Puddu G, Gianni E, Damiani A, Pigozzi F (1995). Anterior cruciate ligament reconstruction: it is probably better to leave the the tendon defect open! *Knee Surgery Sports Traumatology and Arthroscopy*, 3, 14–7.

Corsetti JR, Jackson DW (1996). Failure of anterior ligament reconstruction: the bilogic basis. *Clinical Orthopaedics and Related Research*, 325, 42–9.

Coupens SD, Yates CK, Sheldon C, Ward C (1992). MRI evaluation of the patellar tendon after use of its central one-third for ACL reconstruction. *American Journal of Sports Medicine*, 20, 332–5.

Di Giovine NM, Shields CL (1991). Ligaments in ACL reconstruction: a review. *American Journal of Knee Surgery*, 4, 42–8.

Eberhardt C, Kurth AH, Hailer N, Jäger A (2000). Revision ACL reconstruction using autogenous patellar tendon graft. *Knee Surgery Sports Traumatolgy and Arthroscopy*, 8, 290–5.

Echigo J, Yoshioka H, Takahashi H, Nitsu M, Fukubayashi T, Iai Y (1999). Signal intensity changes in anterior cruciate ligament autografts: relation to magnetic field orientation. *Acta Radiologica*, 6, 206–10.

Fahey M, Indelicato PA (1994). Bone tunnel enlargement after anterior cruciate ligament replacement. *American Journal of Sports Medicine*, 22, 410–4.

Fisher SE, Shelbourne KD (1993). Arthroscopic treatment of symptomatic extension block complicating anterior cruciate ligament reconstruction. *American Journal of Sports Medicine*, 21, 558–64.

Fu FH, Martinek V (2000). Revision ACL reconstruction. Book of Abstracts. Presented at AOSSM, Sun Valley, Idaho. Unpublished Communication.

Fulkerson JP, Langeland R (1996). The central quadriceps tendon for cruciate ligament reconstruction. Presented at the Specialty Day Meeting of the Arthroscopy Association of North America. Atlanta, Georgia.

Graf B, Uhr F (1998). Complications of intraarticular anterior cruciate ligament reconstruction. *Clinics in Sports Medicine*, 17, 835–48.

Harner CD, Irrgang JJ, Paul J, Dearwater S, Fu FH (1992). Loss of motion after anterior cruciate ligament reconstruction. *American Journal of Sports Medicine*, 20, 499–506.

Harner CD (2000). Failed ACL Surgery: evaluation and management. Book of Abstracts. Presented at ACL at the beginning of the third millennium. Montecatini Terme Italy. Unpublished Communication.

Harter RA, Osternig LR, Singer KM, James SL, Larson RL, Jones DC (1988). Long-term evaluation of knee stability and function following surgical reconstruction for anterior cruciate ligament insufficiency. *American Journal of Sports Medicine*, 16, 434–43.

Henning CE, Lynch MA, Glick KRJ (1985). An *in vivo* strain gauge study of elongation of the anterior cruciate ligament. *American Journal of Sports Medicine*, 13, 22–6.

Holmes PF, James SL, Larson RL, Singer KM, Jones DC (1991). Retrospective direct comparison of three intraarticular anterior cruciate ligament reconstruction. *American Journal of Sports Medicine*, 19, 596–600.

Hoogland T, Hillen B (1984). Intraarticular reconstruction of the anterior cruciate ligament: an experimental study of length changes in different ligament reconstructions. *Clinical Orthopaedic and Related Research*, 185, 197–202.

Howe JG, Johnson RJ, Kaplan MJ, Fleming B, Jarvinen M (1991). Anterior cruciate ligament reconstruction using quadriceps patellar tendon graft, I: long-term follow-up. *American Journal of Sports Medicine*, 19, 447–57.

Howell SM, Clark JA, Farley TE (1991). A rationale for predicting anterior cruciate graft impingement by the intercondylar roof. *American Journal of Sports Medicine*, 19, 276–82.

Howell SM, Clark JA, Farley TE (1992). Serial magnetic resonance study assessing the effects of impingement on the MR image of the patellar tendon graft. *Arthroscopy*, 8, 350–8.

Howell SM, Taylor MA (1993). Failure of reconstruction of the anterior cruciate ligament due to impingement by the intercondylar roof. *Journal of Bone and Joint Surgery*, 75A, 1044–55.

Jackson DW, Gasser SI (1994). Tibial tunnel placement in ACL reconstruction. *Arthroscopy*, 10, 124–31.

Jackson DW, Grood ES, Cohn BT, Arnoczky SP, Simon TM, Cunning JF (1991).The effects of *in situ* freezing on anterior cruciate ligament: an experimental study in goats. *Journal of Bone and Joint Surgery*, 73A, 201–13.

Jackson DW, Grood ES, Goldstein JD, *et al.* (1993). A comparison of patellar tendon autograft and allograft used for anterior cruciate ligament reconstruction in the goat model. *American Journal of Sports Medicine*, 21, 176–85.

Jackson DW, Schaefer RK (1990). Cyclops syindrome: loss of extension following intraarticular ACL reconstruction. *Arthroscopy*, 6, 171–8.

Jaureguito JW, Paulos LE (1996). Why grafts fail. *Clinical Orthopaedics and Related Research*, 325, 25–41.

Johnson DL, Coen MJ (1995). Revision ACL surgery. Etiologies, indications, techniques, and results. *American Journal of Knee Surgery*, 8, 155–67.

Johnson DL, Swenson TM, Irrgang JJ, Fu FH, Harner CD (1996). Revision anterior cruciate ligament surgery: experience from Pittsburgh. *Clinical Orthopaedics and Related Research*, 325, 100–9.

Jones DG, Galland M, Fu FH (2001). Complications and pitfalls in anterior cruciate ligament revision reconstruction. In MM Malek (ed.) *Knee Surgery: complications, pitfalls and salvage*, pp. 138–58. Springer-Verlag, New York.

Kaplan MJ, Howe JG, Fleming B, Johnson JR, Jarvinen M (1991). Anterior cruciate ligament reconstruction using quadriceps patellar tendon graft, II: a specific sport review. *American Journal of Sports Medicine*, 19, 458–62.

Kartus J, Stener S, Lindahl S, Eriksson B, Karlsson J (1998). Ipsi- or contralateral patellar tendon graft in anterior cruciate ligament revision surgery. A comparison of two methods. *American Journal of Sports Medicine*, 26, 499–504.

Klein W, Jenson K (1989). Arthritis in artificial anterior cruciate ligaments. Presented at the 6th Congress of the ISK, Rome. Unpublished Communication.

Kornblatt I, Warren RF, Wickiewicz TL (1988). Long-term follow-up of anterior cruciate ligament reconstruction using the quadriceps substitution for chronic anterior ligament insufficiency. *American Journal of Sports Medicine*, 16, 444–8.

Kurosaka M, Yoshiya S, Andrish JT (1987). A biomechanical comparison of different surgical techniques of graft fixation in anterior cruciate ligament reconstruction. *American Journal of Sports Medicine*, 15, 225–9.

LaPrade RF, Hamilton CD, Montgomery RD, Wentorf F, Hawkins HD (1997). The reharvested central third of the patellar tendon. A histologic and biomechanical analysis. *American Journal of Sports Medicine*, 25, 779–85.

Livesay GA, Rudy TW, Woo SL (1997). Evaluation of the effect of joint constraints on the in situ force distribution in the anterior cruciate ligament. *Journal of Orthopaedic Research*, 15, 278–84.

Manifold S, Scott W. Revision ACL surgery: how I do it (2000). In J Insall (ed.) *Surgery of the Knee*, 3rd edn, pp. 835–40. WB Saunders, Philadelphia.

Marder RA, Raskind JR, Carroll M (1991). Prospective evaluation of arthroscopically assisted anterior cruciate ligament reconstruction. Patellar tendon versus semitendinosus and gracilis tendons. *American Journal of Sports Medicine*, 19, 478–84.

Maywood RM, Murphy BJ, Uribe JW, Hechtman KS (1993). Evaluation of arthroscopic anterior cruciate ligament reconstruction using magnetic resonance imaging. *American Journal of Sports Medicine*, 21, 523–7.

Miller MD (1998). Revision cruciate ligament surgery with retention of femoral interference screws. Technical note. *Arthroscopy*, 14, 111–14.

Nabors ED, Richmond JC, Vannah WM, Mc Conville OR (1995). Anterior cruciate ligament graft tensioning in full extension. *American Journal of Sports Medicine*, 23, 488–92.

Navarro RA, Fu FH (1998). Anterior cruciate ligament revision surgery: an overview. In: KM Chan, N Maffulli, M Kurosaka, FH Fu, CG Rolf, SH Liu (eds) *Controversies in Orthopedic Sports Medicine*, pp. 74–89. Williams and Wilkins, Hong Kong.

Noyes FR, Barber SD (1992). The effect of a ligament-augmentation device on allograft reconstructions for chronic ruptures of the anterior cruciate ligament. *Journal of Bone and Joint Surgery*, 74A, 960–73.

Noyes FR, Barber-Westin SD (1996). Revision anterior cruciate ligament surgery: experience from Cincinnati. *Clinical Orthopaedics and Related Research*, 325, 116–29.

Oakes BW (1993). Collagen structure in the normal ACL and in ACL graft. In DW Jackson, SP Arnoczky (eds) *The Anterior Cruciate Ligament: Current and future concepts*, p. 209. Raven Press, New York.

O' Brien SJ, Warren RF, Pavlov H, Panariello R, Wickiewicz TL (1991). Reconstruction of the chronically insufficient anterior cruciate ligament with the central third of the patellar ligament. *Journal of Bone and Joint Surgery*, 73A, 278–86.

Otero AL, Hutcheson L (1993). A comparison of the doubled semitendinosus/gracilis and central third of the patellar tendon autografts in arthroscopic anterior cruciate ligament reconstruction. *Arthroscopy*, 9, 143–8.

Paessler HH (2000). ACL revision surgery: analysis of failure of 300 reconstructions and surgical solutions for reconstruction. Book of Abstract Presented at ACL at the beginning of the third millennium. Montecatini Terme, Italy. Unpublished Communication.

Paulos LE, Rosenberg TD, Drawbert J, Manning J, Abbott P (1987). Infrapatellar contracture syndrome: an unrecognized cause of knee stiffness with patella entrapment and patella infera. *American Journal of Sports Medicine*, 15, 331–41.

Peterson RK, Shelton WR, Bombay AL (2001). Allograft versus autograft patellar tendon anterior cruciate ligament reconstruction: a 5-year follow-up. *Arthroscopy*, 17, 9–13.

Proctor CS, Jackson DW, Simon TM (1997). Characterization of the repair tissue after removal of the central one-third of the patellar ligament. An experimental study in a goat model. *Journal of Bone and Joint Surgery*, 79A, 997–1006.

Reider B, Belniak RM, Preiskorn DO (1996). Arthroscopic arthrolysis for flexion contractur following intra-articular reconstruction of the anterior cruciate ligament. *Arthroscopy*, 12, 165–73.

Robertson DB, Daniel DM, Biden E (1986). Soft tissue fixation to bone. *American Journal of Sports Medicine*, 14, 398–403.

Rosenberg TD, Paulos LE, Parker RD, Coward DB, Scott SM (1988). The 45° posteroanterior flexion weight-bearing radiograph of the knee. *Journal of Bone and Joint Surgery*, 70A, 1479–83.

Rubinstein RA Jr, Shelbourne KD, McCarroll JR, *et al.* (1993). The results of a second autogenous bone-patellar tendon-bone ACL reconstruction after failure of the first reconstruction. Presented at the 19th Annual American Orthopedic Society for Sports Medicine Meeting. San Francisco, California.

Sachs RA, Daniel DM, Stone ML, Garfein RF (1989). Patellofemoral problems after anterior cruciate ligament reconstruction. *American Journal of Sports Medicine*, 17, 760–5.

Safran MR, Harner CD (1995). Revision ACL surgery: technique and results utilizing allografts. *Instructional Course Lectures*, 44, 407–15.

Safran MR, Harner CD (1996). Technical considerations of revision anterior cruciate ligament surgery. *Clinical Orthopaedics and Related Research*, 325, 50–64.

Seeman MD, Steadman JR (1993). Tibial osteolysis associated with Gore-tex grafts. *American Journal of Knee Surgery*, 6, 31–8.

Shelbourne KD, Gray T (1997). Anterior cruciate reconstruction with autogenous patellar tendon graft followed by accelerated rehabilitation: a 2- to 9-year follow-up. *American Journal of Sports Medicine*, 25, 786–95.

Shelbourne KD, Wilckens JH, Mollabashy A, De Carlo M (1991). Arthrofibrosis in acute cruciate ligament reconstruction. The effect of timing reconstruction and rehabilitation. *American Journal of Sports Medicine*, 19, 332–6.

Shelton WR, Treacy SH, Dukes AD, Bomboy AL (1998). Use of allografts in knee reconstruction, I: basic science aspects and current status. *Journal of American Academy of Orthopaedic Surgeons*, 6, 165–68.

Shino K, Inoue M, Horibe S, Hamada M, Ono K (1990). Reconstruction of the anterior cruciate ligament using allogenic tendon: long-term follow-up. *American Journal of Sports Medicine*, 18, 457–65.

Shino K, Inoue M, Horibe S, Nakata K, Maeda A, Ono K (1991). Surface blood flow and histology of human anterior cruciate ligament allografts. *Arthroscopy*, 7, 171–6.

Tanzer M, Lenzer E (1990). The relationship of intercondylar notch size and content in notchplasty requirement in anterior cruciate ligament surgery. *Arthroscopy*, 6, 89–93.

Tredinnick TJ, Friedman MJ (2001). Revision anterior cruciate ligament reconstruction: Technical considerations. *American Journal of Knee Surgery*, 14, 193–200.

Uribe JW, Hectman KS, Zvijac JE, Tjin-A-Tsoi EW (1996). Revision anterior cruciate ligament surgery: experience from Miami. *Clinical Orthopaedics and Related Research*, 325, 91–9.

Will PD, Collins MR (1989). Intraarticular Gore-Tex ACL reconstruction, 2 to 6 year follow-up. Presented at the Interim Meeting of the AOSSM, Traverse City MI.

Wirth CJ, Kohn D (1996). Revision anterior cruciate ligament surgery: experience from Germany. *Clinical Orthopaedics and Related Research*, 325, 110–5.

Woods GA, Indelicato PA, Prevot TJ (1991). The Gore-Tex anterior cruciate ligament prosthesis – 2 versus 3 year results. *American Journal of Sports Medicine*, 19, 48–55.

Yoshiya S, Andrish JY, Manley MT, Bauer TW (1987). Graft tension in anterior cruciate ligament reconstruction. *American Journal of Sports Medicine*, 15, 464–70.

Part 3. Medial Collateral Ligament

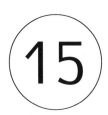

Medial collateral ligament repair at the time of primary ACL reconstruction: when and why

Joseph H. Guettler and Laurence D. Higgins

Indications for medial collateral ligament repair or reconstruction

Structure and function of the medial collateral ligament in medial knee stability

The structures of the medial side of the knee can be divided into dynamic and static stabilizers. The superficial medial collateral ligament (MCL) and the posterior oblique ligament are the main static stabilizers (Warren and Marshall 1979). The superficial MCL attaches proximally to the medial femoral epicondyle and distally to the tibial metaphysis four to five centimeters distal to the joint line. Deep to the superficial MCL is the medial capsular ligament, or deep MCL. The superficial MCL is separated from the deep MCL by a bursa anteriorly (Brantigan and Voshell 1941, 1943). Failure to recreate this anterior separation, or failure to place the MCL insertion distal enough on the tibial metaphysis, can tether the knee joint preventing full range of motion (Muller 1983, Wilson *et al.* 1998, 2000). The posterior third of the deep MCL blends with the oblique fibers of the superficial MCL and the posteromedial capsule. This confluence of structures is referred to as the posterior oblique ligament (Hughston and Eilers 1973, Slocum *et al.* 1974, Warren and Marshall 1979). The vastus medialis, sartorius, gracilis, semitendinosis, and semimembranosis dynamically stabilize these ligaments (Abbott *et al.* 1944, Bosworth 1952, Pope *et al.* 1979, Muller *et al.* 1983). Medial knee stability depends on the interaction between the dynamic and static stabilizers, as well as joint congruity, alignment, and load (Figure 15.1).

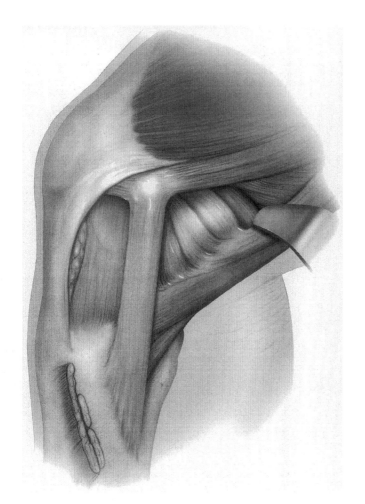

Fig. 15.1
The structures of the medial knee including the superficial medial collateral ligament.

Interaction of the anterior cruciate ligament and MCL in providing knee stability

The medial structures of the knee predominately resist valgus moment and tibial torque, as well as anterior-posterior translation secondarily (Brantigan and Voshell 1941, Kennedy and Fowler 1971, Warren *et al.* 1974, Markolf *et al.* 1976, Mains *et al.* 1977, Piziali *et al.* 1980*b*, Seering *et al.* 1980, Grood *et al.* 1981, Nielsen *et al.* 1984*a*, Nielsen *et al.* 1984*b*). It has been shown that the MCL contributes 78 per cent to the restraining force on the medial side of the knee and is the primary stabilizer to valgus stress at 30 degrees of flexion (Grood *et al.* 1981). A five degree of freedom model suggests, however, that the MCL may be the primary restraint to valgus stress only when knee motion is restricted, such as when the foot is planted, and other studies have challenged traditional biomechanical models of medial knee stability (Fukubayashi *et al.* 1982, Sullivan *et al.* 1984, Inoue *et al.* 1987, Shapiro *et al.* 1991). As the knee flexes, the MCL contribution to medial stability increases (Monahan *et al.* 1984, Markolf *et al.* 1990, Shapiro *et al.* 1991). When the knee is more fully extended, the posteromedial capsule, the posterior oblique ligament, and the anterior cruciate ligament (ACL) assume greater responsibility in preventing valgus opening (Shapiro *et al.* 1991). Therefore, when evaluating the medial side of the knee, increased valgus opening in full extension indicates damage to the posterior oblique ligament, while increased valgus opening at 30° of flexion indicates damage to the superficial MCL (Indelicato 1995, Shelbourne and Patel 1995).

The primary restraint to anterior displacement of the tibia is the ACL (Piziali *et al.* 1980*b*, Butler *et al.* 1980), with the medial structures acting as secondary restraints (Sullivan *et al.* 1984, Inoue *et al.* 1987, Shapiro *et al.* 1991). However, transection of the MCL in an ACL-deficient knee results in increased anterior tibial translation, especially at 30° of flexion (Sullivan *et al.* 1984). In neutral tibial rotation, the ACL bears nearly all the applied anterior translation force (Piziali *et al.* 1980*a*, Butler *et al.* 1980, Fukubayashi *et al.* 1982, Sullivan *et al.* 1984, Inoue *et al.* 1987, Shapiro *et al.* 1991). However, when the tibia is externally rotated, the MCL is also strained when an anterior force is applied (Shapiro *et al.* 1991). If the MCL is then sectioned with the tibia in external rotation, the ACL is subjected to dramatically increased forces although anterior translation of the tibia does not increase significantly (Fukubayashi *et al.* 1982, Sullivan *et al.* 1984, Inoue *et al.* 1987, Shapiro *et al.* 1991). Several authors have also shown that the MCL and posterior oblique ligament provide restraint to external rotation, with the ACL being a secondary restraint (Brantigan and Voshell 1941, Slocum and Larson 1968, Warren *et al.* 1974, Grood *et al.* 1981, Muller 1983). The MCL becomes more active in resisting external rotation torque as the knee is flexed (Shapiro *et al.* 1991). In the MCL-deficient knee, the force generated in the ACL during applied external torque is greater and increases with increasing knee flexion, while in the intact knee, the force generated in the ACL decreases progressively as the knee is flexed (Markolf *et al.* 1990). The degree of external rotation laxity is small in MCL-deficient knees compared to the anteromedial rotatory instability that occurs with combined ACL/MCL injuries (Indelicato 1995).

Animal models have also demonstrated the load sharing that exists between the ACL and MCL, as well as the importance of the ACL in providing a stable environment for the MCL to heal. Inoue *et al.*, in a biomechanical study using canine knees, found that in the case of an isolated MCL injury, its functional deficit was compensated for by the presence of a functional ACL. They concluded that the initial healing process of the injured MCL could take place without much mechanical disturbance because of the existence of an intact ACL preventing excessive valgus stress (Inoue *et al.* 1987). Other authors evaluated the effect of concurrent injury to the ACL on MCL healing in a canine model. They concluded that the healing of the transected MCL ligament is adversely affected by concomitant transection of the ACL. Accordingly, they suggested that the outcome after non-operative management of combined ACL/MCL injuries may be less than ideal (Woo *et al.* 1990c, Anderson *et al.* 1992).

Ohno *et al.* found that for combined ACL/MCL injuries in rabbits, repair of the MCL and ACL led to significantly less varus/valgus rotation of the knee than did repair of the ACL only. At 12 weeks postoperatively, the cross-sectional area of the MCL was 60 per cent greater and the ultimate load in the MCL was 53 per cent greater than in the non-repair group (Ohno *et al.* 1995). However, a later study of rabbits out of the same laboratory by Yamaji *et al.* showed that the early benefits of surgical repair of the MCL seen in the previous study were no longer evident at one year. No difference was demonstrated in varus–valgus rotation or ultimate load at 52 weeks between that repaired and conservatively treated MCLs. Based on this study, the authors recommended reconstruction of the ACL and conservative treatment of the MCL (Yamaji *et al.* 1996). Engle *et al.* demonstrated that reconstruction of the ACL in O'Donoghue triad injuries (ACL, MCL, medial meniscus tear) in rabbits helps to stabilize the joint, improves healing of the medial collateral ligament, and may decrease the incidence of early-onset arthritis seen with such injuries (Engle *et al.* 1994).

Injury mechanisms

Valgus moments and external rotation torques produce MCL tears. The most common mechanism for medial-sided knee injury is a valgus load with the tibia fixed, as with a planted foot, and the femur internally rotated. Valgus load with active external tibial rotation is another common injury mechanism. Several authors have suggested a specific order of injury when the knee is subjected to these forces: the deep MCL is injured first, then the superficial MCL, and finally the ACL (Brantigan and Voshell 1941, Slocum and Larson 1968, Kennedy and Fowler 1971). Pure valgus forces will predominately damage the MCL, whereas valgus forces combined with external rotation forces can damage the posterior oblique ligament and even the ACL before the MCL is ruptured. Strain rate may affect the mode of failure (Crowninshield and Pope 1976), and cyclic loading of the MCL may also play a role in injury (Weisman *et al.* 1980).

The frequent association of ACL and MCL injuries suggests that a significant amount of load sharing exists between the two structures. Miyasaka *et al.* reported on the incidence of knee ligament injuries in the general population. They found that sports accounted for 65 per cent of injuries, with MCL single ligament injury being the most common, followed by ACL single ligament injury, and ACL/MCL combined injury. The ACL was, however, the most frequently injured knee ligament resulting in pathologic knee motion (Miyasaka *et al.* 1991). Fetto and Marshall reported a direct correlation between the severity of the MCL injury and the chance of having a concomitant ACL injury (95 per cent chance with a grade III MCL) (Fetto and Marshall 1978).

Healing capacity: ACL versus MCL

Clinical experience has shown that isolated MCL ruptures can heal with nonoperative care, while midsubstance tears of the ACL do not (Nagineni *et al.* 1992, Amiel *et al.* 1995, Schreck *et al.* 1995). The vast majority of MCL injuries heal within four to six weeks. Variations in healing ability may be attributable to differences in blood supply, intrinsic structural variations (Hart *et al.* 1992), and the articular environment (intra- vs. extraarticular). The hostile synovial environment around the ACL may deter healing (Indelicato 1995), although Nickerson *et al.* demonstrated positive effects of synovial fluid on knee ligament healing in a rabbit model (Nickerson *et al.* 1992). Biomechanical factors may also play a role in the ability to heal. The function of the ligament may also affect its ability to heal (Indelicato 1995). The ACL for example, contributes to knee stability in multiple directions (anterior, internal, valgus). The MCL, on the other hand, primarily restrains valgus knee rotation. The ruptured MCL receives some protection from other structures such as the ACL and joint capsule, and thus it is not subjected to the same forces that may theoretically impede healing in the ACL. The soft tissue structures surrounding the ACL may simply not be able to counteract the multidirectional demands to allow for healing of the ACL (Woo *et al.* 1982).

Effect of immobilization on ligament healing

In the past, immobilization after ligament injury has been advocated to protect the ligament from stress and allow it to heal satisfactorily. It has, however, been shown in the laboratory that immobilization has detrimental effects on ligament healing including disorganization of the collagen fibrils, decreased structural properties of the bone–ligament–bone complex, and resorption of bone at the ligament insertion site (Woo *et al.* 1982, Amiel *et al.* 1983, Akeson *et al.* 1987, Hart and Dahners 1987, Woo *et al.* 1987, Woo *et al.* 1990a, Woo *et al.* 1990b, Gomez *et al.* 1989, 1991, Anderson *et al.* 1992). In contrast, controlled motion has been shown to be beneficial to the healing ligament (Walsh *et al.* 1993). Woo *et al.* showed that passive motion may increase the ultimate load of the femur–MCL–tibia complex by as many as four times (Woo *et al.* 1987a, Woo *et al.* 1987b). Tipton *et al.* showed that exercise positively affected ligament healing in dog and rabbit models (Tipton *et al.* 1970). Reider *et al.* reported favorable clinical results five years after the treatment of isolated MCL injuries with early motion and functional rehabilitation (Reider *et al.* 1994). However, it is generally accepted that motion applied too early or aggressively may be detrimental to the healing process. Lechner and Dahners found that exercise increased the ultimate load to failure but also increased the laxity of the MCL (Lechner and Dahners 1991).

The controversy

The treatment of combined injuries of the anterior cruciate ligament and medial collateral ligament remains controversial. There are advocates for surgical reconstruction of all ligamentous structures (Campbell 1936, Campbell 1939, O'Donoghue 1955, 1959, Ellsasser *et al.* 1974, Fetto and Marshall 1978, Warren and Marshall 1978, Hastings 1980, Anderson 1992), reconstruction of the ACL only (Shelbourne and Baele 1988, Shelbourne and Nitz 1991, Aglietti 1991, Ballmer *et al.* 1991, Shelbourne and Porter 1992), repair of the MCL only (Hughston and Eilers 1973, Hughston and Barrett 1983), and finally, nonoperative treatment of both ligamentous structures (Jokl *et al.* 1984). Previous studies present a myriad of options, and display wide discrepancies in their results. This is due to several factors including the variety of surgical procedures used to repair or reconstruct these ligaments, different rehabilitation protocols, dissimilar outcomes measures, differences in defining injury severity, and disparity in treatment populations (Noyes and Barber-Westin 1995). The objectives of this chapter are to provide a thorough review of the basic science and clinical research relating to combined ACL/MCL injuries, and based on the literature, provide the reader with the most plausible indications for MCL repair at the time of primary ACL reconstruction. In addition, this chapter will review the techniques available for MCL repair, augmentation, or reconstruction and provide the reader with a treatment protocol based on the injury pattern.

Clinical experience and answers to questions

Does repair of the MCL in combined ACL/MCL injuries lead to a better result with less postoperative stiffness? Prior to the 1990s, most authors advocated repair of all damaged structures in combined ligamentous injuries of the knee to restore stability and function to the knee. O'Donoghue, as well as Larson, suggested that the treatment of acute ACL/MCL injuries should include acute repair of all damaged structures (O'Donoghue 1950, 1955, 1959, Larson 1980). Larson recommended extensive reconstruction and repair, including correction of all planes of instability and replacement or repair of all static stabilizers backed by dynamic muscle transfers. O'Donoghue proposed that all ligaments of the knee that have been torn should be sutured. Other authors advocated repair, even with isolated MCL injury. Godshall and Hansen recommended surgical treatment of the medial collateral ligament whenever the joint space could be opened more than 4 millimeters (Godshall and Hansen 1974). Kannus and Jarvinen reported that isolated grade III sprains of the MCL had unacceptable long-term results with nonoperative treatment and therefore recommended surgical repair of isolated grade III MCL injuries (Kannus and Jarvinen 1987, Kannus 1988). However, critical review of this study indicates that the majority of knee injuries were not isolated to the medial ligaments, with moderate to severe anterior instability occurring in almost all of the knees. Hughston, on the other hand, reported on combined ruptures of the ACL and medial ligaments and recommended conservative treatment of the ACL with repair of the medial ligaments, posterior oblique ligaments, and semimembranosis complex (Hughston and Barrett 1983, Hughston and Eilers 1973). He felt that the medial operative repair converted the injury to an isolated ACL injury, which in his opinion led to few functional limitations, instability, or joint degeneration.

Clinical experience, however, showed that this aggressive surgical approach can lead to an unacceptably high incidence of postoperative stiffness of the knee, and other authors advocated conservative management of both ligaments in combined ACL/MCL injuries. Jokl et al. reported on 28 patients followed for an average of three years with combined ACL/MCL injuries treated nonoperatively. Patients were treated with early quadriceps strengthening, range of motion, and weight-bearing. Twenty patients had a good or excellent result, with 11 of 15 returning to contact sports and six of nine returning to non-contact sports at their pre-injury level of athletic activity. However, four of these athletes sustained subsequent meniscal injuries (Jokl et al. 1984). McDaniel and Dameron also reported on the long-term follow-up of patients who had conservative treatment for this combined ACL/MCL injuries. Their results were comparable to studies in which these injuries had been treated operatively (McDaniel and Dameron 1980). Ogata noted that the MCL healed in combined ACL/MCL injuries treated conservatively, but used only a manual stress test to assess healing (Ogata et al. 1980). In the early 1980s, authors also began advocating conservative management of isolated MCL injuries. Mok and Good recommended nonoperative treatment of MCL injuries and rehabilitation in a hinged cast (Mok and Good 1989). Ellsasser et al. reported success when treating professional athletes with isolated MCL tears with a similar rehabilitation program (Ellsasser et al. 1974). Similarly, Sandberg et al. could not demonstrate any benefit to surgically treating MCL injuries (Sandberg et al. 1987). Hart and Dahners showed that repair of tears of the MCL did not significantly affect laxity or ultimate load to failure of the ligament (Hart and Dahners 1987). Bray et al. found that immobilization of the knee prevented increased laxity of the MCL, but the stiffness and ultimate load of the MCL did not return to normal (Bray *et al.* 1991).

Thus whether surgical repair of the MCL in combined ACL/MCL injuries improves MCL healing remained an open question. Indelicato helped pave the way for our current understanding of combined ACL/MCL injuries (Indelicato 1983, Indelicato *et al.* 1990). He advocated conservative treatment of most complete MCL tears with an initial period of immobilization followed by protected early motion, and that the key to successful healing was to exclude associated damage to other structures such as the ACL and menisci. Indelicato also pointed out that whether treated operatively or nonoperatively, most knees had mild laxity at follow-up compared to the contralateral knee (Indelicato 1995). Fetto and Marshall found that with a combined injury, a good or excellent result correlated more closely with recovery of ACL stability than with recovery of MCL stability. According to the authors, when the knee must undergo normal daily stress without the binding of a good, firm anterior cruciate ligament – and especially when the MCL is also deficient – the knee deteriorates unless surgery is done to tighten and repair the ligaments. In their study, nearly all of the 176 patients who did not undergo reconstruction of the anterior cruciate ligament showed clinical instability as well as pain and discomfort (Fetto and Marshall 1978).

In the 1990s, the pendulum swung toward nonoperative treatment of the MCL in combined ACL/MCL injuries. Shelbourne and Baele performed a retrospective study followed out 33 months comparing a group of 13 patients who underwent reconstruction of the ACL and repair of the MCL (group 1) to a group of 14 patients in whom only the ACL was reconstructed (group 2) (Shelbourne and Baele 1988). Six of the patients in group 1 were kept in a long leg cast for approximately six weeks, while all of the patients in group 2 were treated with a more aggressive range of motion program emphasizing early full extension and early weight-bearing. They concluded that the patients in whom only the ACL had been reconstructed had less postoperative stiffness and a more rapid return of motion. Delays in reconstruction up to three months did not affect their results. In addition, patients with isolated ACL reconstruction and conservative treatment of the MCL had equal or better range of motion, stability, and function than the patients who had ACL reconstruction combined with MCL repair.

Shelbourne and Porter reported on a series of 68 patients with combined ACL/MCL injuries (Shelbourne and Porter 1992). They underwent ACL reconstruction with conservative management of the MCL injuries and were followed out an average of 3.1 years. The authors concluded that proper reconstruction of the ACL, in conjunction with nonoperative management of the MCL, can give excellent stability and good to excellent functional outcome.

Shelbourne and Patel advocated nonoperative treatment of the MCL and delayed ACL reconstruction (Shelbourne and Patel 1996). They sited the unacceptably high rate of arthrofibrosis when the ACL reconstruction is done acutely. In a recent series, they retrospectively examined 27 patients who had combined ACL/Grade III MCL injuries. Patients underwent ACL reconstruction only or ACL reconstruction plus MCL repair. They found that the patients who underwent medial ligament repair in addition to ACL reconstruction had more postoperative stiffness and more difficulty regaining full range of motion. None of the patients in either group had any functional or objective laxity at follow-up.

Noyes and Barber-Westin reported a prospective study looking at 46 patients with combined ruptures of the anterior cruciate ligament and medial ligamentous structures (Noyes and Barber-Westin 1995). Medial ligamentous injuries were defined anatomically based on whether the parallel fibers of the superficial MCL were ruptured in isolation, or whether a more severe injury had been sustained to the both the parallel and oblique fibers of the superficial MCL as well as the posteromedial capsule. Classification was based on whether medial opening occurred to valgus stress at 0° of extension indicating a more severe injury. Combined ACL/MCL injuries with disruption of the parallel fibers of the superficial MCL only were treated nonoperatively, while combined injuries with more significant disruption of the medial ligamentous structures were treated operatively. Direct operative repair of the MCL and posteromedial capsule was performed using suture (midsubstance rupture) or staple-suture fixation tied over a post (rupture at femoral insertion) when possible, and autogenous semitendinosus was incorporated into the repair when tissue was not amenable to direct repair. Despite immediate motion and rehabilitation in both nonoperative and operative groups, the operative group had more knee stiffness and patellofemoral complications. Using the Cincinnati Knee Rating system, there were 91 per cent excellent of good results in the nonoperative group, but only 58 per cent excellent of good results in the operative group. Based on their results, they recommended nonoperative treatment of the medial ligamentous structures, regardless of the severity of injury, followed by arthroscopically assisted ACL reconstruction when knee motion and function have returned. A symptomatic meniscal tear is an exception where the ACL reconstruction is performed at an earlier time. They now reserve MCL repair for highly competitive athletes with gross MCL rupture and wide medial opening with associated ACL rupture.

These studies clearly indicate that patients undergoing operative treatment of both ligamentous injuries suffer more postoperative stiffness and difficulty regaining full motion, especially if done acutely and subjected to prolonged postoperative immobilization. They also show that the MCL can heal acceptably with conservative treatment in combined ACL/MCL injuries when the ACL is reconstructed. The authors favor an initial approach emphasizing range of motion while protecting the MCL to allow for early healing. ACL reconstruction is carried out when motion has been regained and the acute inflammatory phase has passed.

Criticisms of these studies include the fact the Shelbourne treated his conservatively managed MCL groups with a much more aggressive early range of motion protocol than his operative MCL groups. It would have been interesting to see how patients in the operative MCL groups did with the same early range of motion protocol. In the Noyes/Barber-Westin study, only the more severe MCL injuries were repaired, while the less significant MCL injuries were treated conservatively. Although there were clearly more stiffness problems in the operative MCL group, these were more severe injuries. No comparison was made between the operative and conservative management of combined ACL/MCL injuries with more significant medial-sided injury.

Other questions

Does the timing of the ACL reconstruction affect the final outcome in combined ACL/MCL injuries? Ballmer *et al.* reported on 14 patients who had complete ruptures of the ACL and MCL treated by early ACL reconstruction alone followed by postoperative protection to allow for healing of the MCL (Ballmer *et al.* 1991). Patients were treated postoperatively with early range of motion and protected weight-bearing for six to eight weeks. They concluded that although there was no initial protection of the ACL reconstruction by an intact MCL, reconstruction of the ACL alone with postoperative protection to allow for healing of the MCL was sufficient to restore stability and motion to the majority of the knees. Of note, the typical patient in their study did not have gross medial disruption and wide medial opening indicative of a severe injury to the medial ligamentous structures. Peterson and Laprell evaluated the effect of early vs. late reconstruction in combined ACL/MCL injuries (Peterson and Laprell 1999). Reconstruction of the ACL was carried out either within the first three weeks following injury or at a minimum of 10 weeks out. All MCL injuries were treated nonoperatively. The authors found similar stability in the two groups, but less motion complications in the group treated late. They recommended ACL reconstruction after a minimum interval of 10 weeks. Other authors including Shelbourne and Noyes favor this approach, emphasizing early range of motion and protection of the MCL to allow for healing, followed by delayed reconstruction of the ACL when full motion of the knee has returned and the acute inflammatory reaction has subsided.

Does the location of the MCL injury influence the final functional outcome in combined ACL/MCL injuries? Robins *et al.*, in a retrospective review of 20 patients, looked at knee motion complications associated with the operative treatment of combined ACL/MCL injuries (Robbins *et al.* 1993). All patients were treated by ACL reconstruction with autogenous patellar tendon and primary MCL repair. A significant correlation was found between the location of the MCL tear and both the rate at which motion was regained as well as the final motion achieved. Patients with rupture of the MCL at or above the joint line had a slower return of flexion and extension and achieved less over-all motion than ruptures distal to the joint line.

Does the operative or nonoperative treatment of the MCL in combined ACL/MCL injuries influence the prevalence of late valgus instability? Hillard-Sembell *et al.* performed a retrospective study of 66 patients who had sustained combined ACL/MCL injuries to determine the prevalence of late valgus instability of the knee (Hillard-Sembell *et al.* 1996). Patients had undergone either reconstruction of the ACL and repair of the MCL, reconstruction of the ACL alone, or nonoperative treatment. They found no difference in late valgus instability regardless of the treatment regimen. They also compared combined ACL/MCL injuries that had been treated with ACL reconstruction alone to isolated ACL injuries that were reconstructed and found no significant outcome difference. Based on their findings, they recommended repair of the ACL within 90 days in combined ACL/MCL injuries where there was only mild to moderate initial valgus instability. Although healed MCL tears tested one year out from injury have been shown to regain normal ultimate load and stiffness, the MCL regains only 50–70 per cent of its normal elasticity and strength. Most athletes, regardless of the treatment for their MCL injury, have some degree of valgus laxity. Most authors have found that this small degree of valgus laxity is of little clinical consequence, however, Shapiro *et al.* showed that sectioning of the MCL increases strain on the ACL in response to valgus loading, suggesting that patients with residual valgus laxity of the MCL may be predisposed to ACL injury (Shapiro *et al.* 1991).

Does the presence of a concomitant meniscal injury influence MCL healing? Noyes and Barber-Westin and Shelbourne and Nitz found a high rate of lateral meniscal tears compared to medial meniscal tears in combined ACL/MCL injuries (Noyes and Barber-Westin 2000, Shelbourne and Nitz 1991). Noyes found the rates to be 61 per cent and 33 per cent respectively, while Shelbourne found the rates to be 55 per cent and 10 per cent. Shelbourne also noted that grade III tears of the MCL in association with ACL tears usually have no intraarticular injury. He postulated that this finding can be explained based on a distractive rather than compressive mechanism of injury. Anderson *et al.* studied the effect of partial medial meniscectomy and ACL transection on MCL healing in rabbits (Anderson *et al.* 1992). They compared the effect of an isolated MCL injury to an MCL injury with concomitant ACL transection and partial medial meniscectomy on MCL healing. They found that the varus-valgus rotation was significantly elevated for triad injury, and the biomechanical properties of the healed MCL were substantially inferior. They concluded that an untreated triad injury has deleterious effects on the healing of the MCL substance and its insertions. Furthermore, they showed that the varus-valgus rotation in the triad-injured knees could be restored to levels seen with isolated MCL injury following ACL reconstruction.

Current recommendation

The trend, therefore, has moved toward treating the MCL nonoperatively and performing a delayed reconstruction of the ACL. The question then arises: 'When, if ever, should primary repair of the MCL be undertaken?' Noyes reserved MCL repair for highly competitive athletes with gross MCL rupture and wide medial opening with associated ACL rupture. Noyes *et al.* advocated operative repair of the MCL and posteromedial capsule if there was disruption of the parallel and oblique fibers of the MCL. The decision to repair or not to repair was based clinically on whether there was greater of less than 2 to 3 mm of opening at 0° (Noyes and Barber-Westin 1995).

Indelicato advocated intraoperative assessment of the MCL when treating combined ACL/MCL injuries. If after ACL reconstruction, the knee was still unstable to valgus stress in full extension or slight flexion, indicating a grade II to III MCL injury, the MCL and posterior oblique ligament were exposed and repaired primarily (Indelicato 1995).

We prefer a similar approach to that advocated by Indelicato (1995). This involves an intra-operative decision when treating knees with combined ACL/MCL injuries. If after ACL reconstruction, the knee remains unstable in full extension or demonstrates grade II to III opening at 20°, the MCL and posterior oblique ligament are repaired or reconstructed. The outcome of the medial-sided repair is, of course, dependent on several factors including the location and grade of the MCL tear, the timing of the repair, the presence of associated injuries, and the postoperative rehabilitation.

Techniques for MCL repair/reconstruction

Although most medial-sided knee injuries in combined ACL/MCL injuries are treated conservatively, there remain some indications for operative repair or reconstruction of the medial collateral ligament/posterior oblique ligament complex. In general, these indications include multiligament knee injury and chronic isolated MCL injury with symptomatic instability. Since we are focusing on indications for repair or reconstruction when combined with ACL injury, there is really only one true indication: persistent valgus or rotational instability following ACL reconstruction. The most prudent approach seems to follow the recommendation of Indelicato and Warren. This involves an intra-operative decision when treating knees with combined ACL/MCL injuries. If after ACL reconstruction, the knee remains unstable in full extension or demonstrates grade II to III opening at 20°, the MCL is repaired or reconstructed. If there is a component of anteromedial rotatory instability, plication of the posteromedial capsule, as described by Hughston (Hughston *et al.* 1976), can be carried out.

There are essentially three surgical options: primary repair, primary repair with autograft augmentation, and allograft reconstruction. The final decision is based on surgeon preference and experience, the timing of surgery in relation to injury, the amount of trauma to the knee, and the quality of the tissue at the time of surgery.

Primary repair

A narrow window of time exists for primary repair of the MCL, and primary repair is really only possible in the first seven to ten days following injury. Although early surgical intervention is advocated in the setting of an acute multi-ligament knee injury, the literature suggests that early repair is not applicable in the setting of combined ACL/MCL injuries. If primary repair is undertaken, the location of the injury dictates whether primary repair will suffice, or whether reconstruction or augmentation must accompany such an attempt. A proximal avulsion is the only injury pattern that is easily repaired. Proximal repair can be accomplished by tacking the proximal ligament back to the medial epicondyle using suture anchors, tunnels, staples, or screws if the bony avulsion is large enough. Mid-substance or distal injuries are usually not amenable to repair alone and require augmentation.

Autograft augmentation

The current approach to the treatment of combined ACL/MCL injuries involves an initial period of bracing during which motion is restored. Surgery is performed following the resolution of acute swelling and inflammation, only after full motion has been regained. The vast majority of MCL injuries demonstrate healing during this time period, usually between four and six weeks. Since primary repair is only possible within the first seven to ten days following injury, primary repair is not generally applicable in the treatment of acute, isolated ACL/MCL injuries. Therefore, augmentation of the MCL with hamstring autograft is generally undertaken if repair is necessitated at the time of surgery. As mentioned previously, the MCL and posterior oblique ligament can be assessed intra-operatively following ACL reconstruction. If the knee is unstable to valgus stress in full extension, demonstrates grade II to III medial opening with valgus stress at 20°, or demonstrates anteromedial rotatory instability, then the medial side is addressed surgically.

The Bosworth technique for augmentation of the MCL works well in this setting (Bosworth 1952). Phillips, in 1914, first reported the anterior transposition of the gracilis tendon to augment the torn MCL (Phillips 1914). The Bosworth procedure, first reported in 1952, is still commonly utilized today. The procedure utilizes the semitendinosis or gracilis, tenodesed to the medial epicondyle of the femur, to stabilize the medial aspect of the knee. The description of the procedure is as follows: Layer I is incised in an L-shaped manor, and elevated as a flap. The MCL is next identified and split down to the capsule. The sartorius is retracted medially, and the gracilis and semitendinosis tendons are identified. The semitendinosis is then mobilized anteriorly to the femoral epicondyle, leaving it in continuity with its insertion on the tibia undisturbed. To properly reconstruct the MCL, the isometric point on the medial epicondyle must be located. This can be done using the pin technique. A k-wire or small Steinman pin is drilled into the medial epicondyle, parallel with the joint line. A piece of suture is next looped over the wire or pin, and the suture is distally placed over the insertion site of the native MCL. Appropriate, isometric placement on the medial epicondyle is confirmed if the suture undergoes minimal excursion (0 to 2 mm) as the knee is flexed and extended. Upon confirmation of the isometric point, a 3.2 mm drill bit is used to drill a hole, and a 6.5 mm cancellous screw with soft-tissue washer is placed. Alternatively, this can all be done with a cannulated drill bit and screw over a guide pin. Finally, a bony bed is prepared anterior to the screw using a burr, and the semitendinosis tendon is brought anterior to the screw. The screw and soft tissue washer are next tightened to secure the tendon, effectively tenodesing it to the medial epicondyle (Figure 15.2).

In 1989, Veldhuizen et al. published the results of their treatment of 15 patients with acute, complete MCL ruptures with resultant medial or anteromedial laxity of the knee treated with the Bosworth technique (Veldhuizen et al. 1989). Seven of these patients had concomitant ACL tears. Evaluation at one to three years after surgery revealed excellent results in 14 cases and good results in 1 case using the Marshall score.

If after the ACL reconstruction anteromedial rotatory instability persists, the technique described by Hughston can be utilized to plicate the posteromedial capsule (Hughston et al. 1976). This technique begins with a vertical incision behind and inline with the fibers of the MCL, just anterior to the posterior oblique ligament. The tibia is held at 60 degrees of knee flexion and 10 to 20 degrees of internal rotation. Superiorly, the posterior oblique ligament (POL) can be advanced superiorly and anteriorly onto the femur in the region of the medial epicondyle and adductor tubercle. The

(a) (b)

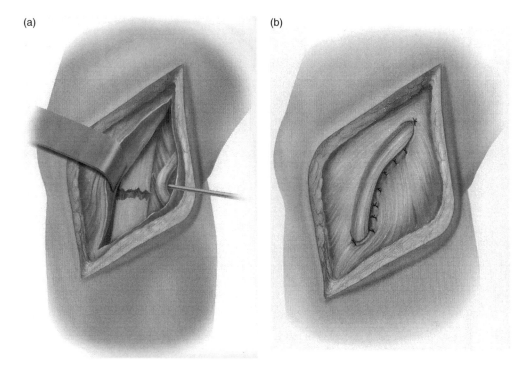

Fig. 15.2
The Bosworth technique for augmentation of a disrupted medial collateral ligament.
(a) Identification and anterior mobilization of the semitendinosus tendon.
(b) Tenodesis of the semitendinosis to the medial femoral epicondyle to augment the disrupted medial collateral ligament.

tissue can be sutured to the periosteum under moderate tension, or suture anchors can be utilized. The posterior oblique ligament is then advanced inferiorly and distally, anchoring it to tissue, through drill holes, or using suture anchors. The mid-portion of the ligament is reinforced by advancing it over the MCL using mattress sutures in a pants-over-vest fashion. In the final step of the reconstruction, the status of the capsular arm of the semimembrinosis is determined. If it is lax, the tendon is advanced distally and superiorly onto the site of the POL advancement using mattress sutures. This restores the direct line of pull of the semimembranosis, and adds dynamic stability to the reconstruction. It is important to avoid over-plication of the POL, which can lead to the development of a flexion contracture (Figure 15.3). Pes anserinus transfer and medial gastrocnemius transfer have also been described (Kennedy *et al.* 1977, Hughston and Barrett 1983). However, we recommend the procedures described by Bosworth and Hughston, as they effectively address both valgus and anteromedial rotatory instability when combined with ACL reconstruction.

Allograft reconstruction

The indications for allograft reconstruction include the acute multi-ligament knee injury that has concomitant damage to the hamstring tendons, or when the addition of further trauma by way

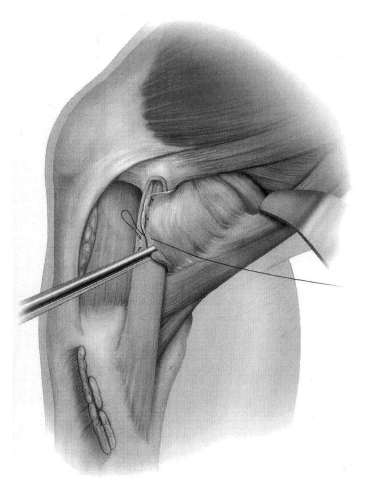

Fig. 15.3
Hughston technique for plication of the posteromedial capsule to address anteromedial rotatory instability.

of graft harvest is not desirable due to the complexity and severity of the injury. Another indication is in the treatment of a chronic MCL injury with a Pelligrini–Steida lesion. Debridement of the lesion must often be extensive, leaving a void of tissue, thus making reconstruction, as opposed to augmentation, a necessity. The last indication is to reconstruct the medial aspect of the knee following failed primary repair of augmentation. Therefore, this technique would seldom, if ever, be necessary in the treatment of an acute, isolated ACL/MCL injury. Nonetheless, this technique has led to good results in rabbit and canine models (Sabiston *et al.* 1990*a*, Sabiston *et al.* 1990*b*, Shino and Horibe 1991), and knowledge of this option is a useful weapon in the surgeon's armamentarium.

The technique for allograft reconstruction is as follows (Toth and Warren, personal communication 2000): Following the approach, the interval, or soft spot, just behind the superficial MCL is incised inline with the fibers of the MCL, anterior to the posterior oblique ligament. The isometric point on the medial epicondyle is identified using the previously described technique. An Achilles tendon/calcaneal allograft is next prepared. A rectangular bone plug is fashioned, and a rectangular trough of similar dimensions is created in the medial femoral condyle, centered at the isometric point. The bone plug is then fixed in the trough to the femur with a cancellous screw and washer. The graft is next cycled and tension is maintained at approximately 30 degrees of flexion with slight varus position of the knee. The distal soft tissue portion of the allograft is fixed distally at the insertion site of the native MCL with soft tissue staples, screw and soft tissue washer, or into a bone tunnel with interference fixation or using a button. If anteromedial rotatory instability or any valgus instability in full extension exists following the allograft reconstruction, the posteromedial corner can be advanced as previously described (Figure 15.4).

Fig. 15.4
Allograft reconstruction of the medial collateral ligament.

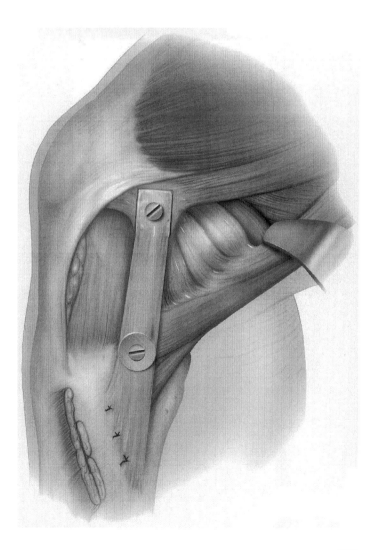

Future directions

Following injury, the biomechanical and constitutional properties of the MCL never return to a normal preinjury state. As previously discussed, if the MCL is incompetent, there is increased strain placed on the ACL with valgus and rotational loads. Theoretically, this may place the ACL at increased risk for injury. Recently, attention has focused on devising methods for improving the rate of MCL healing, as well as improving the quality of the healed tissue. One such method utilizes growth factors to augment healing of the MCL. Because the expressions of various growth factors and their receptors have been demonstrated during various stages of the healing process, it would stand to reason that the understanding of their significance is essential. To date, studies have shown that transforming growth factor-beta is a good promoter of matrix synthesis, while platelet-derived growth factor (PDGF), basic fibroblast growth factor, and epidermal growth factor are positive mitogens on fibroblasts of the ACL and MCL (Woo et al. 2000). Hildebrand et al. and Woo et al. recently showed that growth factors can stimulate matrix synthesis and fibroblast proliferation (Hildebrand et al. 1998, Woo et al. 1998). These studies also showed that PDGF can improve the ultimate elongation values, ultimate load, and energy absorbed to failure when delivered to the injured MCL in a rabbit model. Several problems with the use of growth factors exist including their short half-lives and the difficulty in localizing them accurately. Future study should focus on defining the variables that affect the specificity of growth factors.

Another method with promise is gene therapy. Using gene therapy, host cells in the injured MCL could theoretically be manipulated to produce the desired proteins to enhance ligament healing. Nakamura et al. and Hildebrand et al. have recently demonstrated the ability to transfer genes to host MCL cells in a rabbit model using viral vectors (Nakamura et al. 1998, Hildebrand et al. 1999). Nakamura additionally noted improved ligament healing, with the restoration of biomechanical and constitutional properties, following the successful transfer of genes. One problem with this treatment modality is that it necessitates repetitive application in order to maintain potency. Future research should focus on the ability to control the expression and regulation of proteins in host cells so that treatment can be administered over an extended period of time without the need for repetitive applications (Woo et al. 2000).

A final method under investigation is cell-based therapy. Using this technique, tissue scaffolds and mesenchymal stem cells could theoretically be implanted into the native injured MCL to augment healing. In a recent study involving the transplantation of mesenchymal stem cells around a transected MCL in a rat model, donor cells could be identified in the midsubstance of the ligament after seven days, demonstrating the potential for migration of transplanted cells (Watanabe et al. 1998). The idea of using this technology to augment or accelerate the healing of the human MCL is certainly intriguing, but future research will need to identify the pathways controlling the differentiation and proliferation of transplanted stem cells.

Acknowledgements

We would like to thank Allison P. Toth, MD and Russell F. Warren, MD for their contributions to this chapter.

References

Abbott LC, Saunders JB, Bost FC, *et al.* (1944). Injuries to the ligaments of the knee. *J Bone Joint Surg*, 26, 503–521.

Aglietti P, Buzzi R, Zaccherotti G, *et al.* (1991). Operative treatment of acute complete lesions of the anterior cruciate and medial collateral ligaments. A 4- to 7-year follow-up. *Am J Knee Surg*, 4, 186–94.

Akeson WH, Amiel D, Abel MF, *et al.* (1987). Effects of immobilization on joints. *Clin Orthop*, 219, 28–37.

Amiel D, Nagineni CN, Choi SH, *et al.* (1995). Intrinsic properties of ACL and MCL cells and their responses to growth factors. *Med Sci Sports Exerc*, 27(6), 844–51.

Amiel D, Akeson WH, Harwood FL, *et al.* (1983). Stress deprivation effect on metabolic turnover of the medial collateral ligament collagen. A comparison between nine- and 12-week immobilization. *Clin Orthop*, (172), 265–70.

Anderson DR, Weiss JA, Takai S, *et al.* (1992). Healing of the medial collateral ligament following a triad injury: a biomechanical and histological study of the knee in rabbits. *J Orthop Res*, 10(4), 485–95.

Anderson C and Gillquist J (1992). Treatment of acute isolated and combined ruptures of the anterior cruciate ligament. A long-term follow-up study. *Am J Sports Med*, 20, 7–12. Following a triad injury: a biomechanical and histological study of the knee in rabbits. *J Orthop Res*, 10(4), 485–95.

Ballmer PM and Jakob RP (1988). The non-operative treatment of isolated complete tears of the medial collateral ligament of the knee. A prospective study. *Arch Orthop Trauma Surg*, 107(5), 273–6.

Bosworth DM (1952). Transplantation of the semitendinosus for repair of laceration of the medial collateral ligament of the knee. *J Bone Joint Surg Am*, 34, 196–202.

Brantigan OC and Voshell AF (1941). The mechanics of the ligaments and menisci of the knee joint. *J Bone Joint Surg*, 23A, 44–66.

Brantigan OC and Voshell AF (1943). The tibial collateral ligament: Its function, its bursae, and its relation to the medial meniscus. *J Bone Joint Surg Am*, 25, 121–31.

Bray RC, Frank CB, Shrive NG, *et al.* (1991). Effects of joint instability and joint mobilization on ACL-deficient MCL healing in the adult rabbit model. *Trans Orthop Res Soc*, 16, 135.

Butler DL, Noyes FR and Grood ES (1980). Ligamentous restraints to anterior-posterior drawer in the human knee. A biomechanical study. *J Bone Joint Surg Am*, 62(2), 259–70.

Campbell WC (1936). Repair of the ligaments of the knee. Report of a new operation for repair of the anterior cruciate ligament. *Surg Gynecol Obstet*, 62, 964–68.

Campbell WC (1939). Reconstruction of the ligaments of the knee. *Am J Surg*, 43, 473–80.

Crowninshield RD and Pope MH (1976). The strength and failure characteristics of rat medial collateral ligaments. *J Trauma*, 16(2), 99–105.

Ellsasser JC, Reynolds FC and Omohundro JR (1974). The non-operative treatment of collateral ligament injuries of the knee in professional football players. An analysis of seventy-four injuries treated non-operatively and twenty-four injuries treated surgically. *J Bone Joint Surg Am*, 56(6), 1185–90.

Engle CP, Noguchi M, Ohland K, et al. (1994). Healing of the rabbit collateral ligament following an O'Donoghue triad injury: Effects of anterior cruciate ligament reconstruction. *J Orthop Res*, 12, 357–64.

Fetto JF and Marshall JL (1978). Medial collateral ligament injuries of the knee: a rationale for treatment. *Clin Orthop*, 78(132), 206–18.

Fukubayashi T, Torzilli PA, Sherman MF, et al. (1982). An *in vitro* biomechanical evaluation of anterior-posterior motion of the knee. Tibial displacement, rotation, and torque. *J Bone Joint Surg Am*, 64(2), 258–64.

Godshall RW and Hansen CA (1974). The classification, treatment, and follow-up evaluation of medial collateral ligament injuries of the knee. In *Proceedings of the American Academy of Orthopedic Surgeons. J Bone Joint Surg Am*, 56, 1316.

Gomez MA, Woo SL, Inoue M, et al. (1989). Medical collateral ligament healing subsequent to different treatment regimens. *J Appl Physiol*, 66(1), 245–52.

Gomez MA, Woo SL, Amiel D, et al. (1991). The effects of increased tension on healing medical collateral ligaments. *Am J Sports Med*, 19(4), 347–54.

Grood ES, Noyes FR, Butler DL, et al. (1981). Ligamentous and capsular restraints preventing straight medial and lateral laxity in intact human cadaver knees. *J Bone Joint Surg Am*, 63(8), 1257–69.

Hart DP and Dahners LE (1987). Healing of the medial collateral ligament in rats. The effects of repair, motion, and secondary stabilizing ligaments. *J Bone Joint Surg Am*, 69(8), 1194–99.

Hart RA, Woo SL, Newton PO (1992). Ultrastructural morphometry of anterior cruciate and medical collateral ligaments: An experimental study in rabbits. *J Orthop Res*, 10, 96–103.

Hastings DE (1980). The non-operative management of collateral ligament injuries of the knee joint. *Clin Orthop*, (147), 22–8.

Hildebrand KA, Woo SL, Smith DW, et al. (1998). The effects of platelet-derived growth factor-BB on healing of the rabbit medial collateral ligament. An *in vivo* study. *Am J Sports Med*, 26(4), 549–54.

Hillard-Sembell D, Daniel DM, Stone ML, et al. (1996). Combined injuries of the anterior cruciate and medial collateral ligaments of the knee. Effect of treatment on stability and function of the joint. *J Bone Joint Surg Am*, 78(2), 169–76.

Hughston JC, Andrews JR, Cross MJ, et al. (1976). Classification of knee ligament instabilities. Part I. The medial compartment and cruciate ligaments. *J Bone Joint Surg Am*, 58(2), 159–72.

Hughston JC and Barrett GR (1983). Acute anteromedial rotatory instability. Long-term results of surgical repair. *J Bone Joint Surg Am*, 65(2), 145–53.

Hughston JC and Eilers AF (1973). The role of the posterior oblique ligament in repairs of acute medial (collateral) ligament tears of the knee. *J Bone Joint Surg Am*, 55(5), 923–40.

Indelicato PA (1995). Isolated medial collateral ligament injuries in the knee. *J Am Acad Orthop Surg*, 3(1), 9–14.

Indelicato PA (1983). Non-operative treatment of complete tears of the medial collateral ligament of the knee. *J Bone Joint Surg Am*, 65(3), 323–9.

Indelicato PA, Hermansdorfer J and Huegel M (1990). Nonoperative management of complete tears of the medial collateral ligament of the knee in intercollegiate football players. *Clin Orthop*, (256), 174–7.

Inoue M, McGurk-Burleson E, Hollis JM, *et al.* (1987). Treatment of the medial collateral ligament injury. I: The importance of anterior cruciate ligament on the varus-valgus knee laxity. *Am J Sports Med*, 15(1), 15–21.

Jokl P, Kaplan N, Stovell P, *et al.* (1984). Non-operative treatment of severe injuries to the medial and anterior cruciate ligaments of the knee. *J Bone Joint Surg Am*, 66(5), 741–44.

Kannus P (1988). Long-term results of conservatively treated medial collateral ligament injuries in the knee joint. *Clin Orthop*, 226, 103–12.

Kannus P and Jarvinen M (1987) Conservatively treated tears of the anterior cruciate ligament Long Term Results. *J Bone Joint Surg*, 74A, 1007–12

Kennedy JC and Fowler PJ (1971). Medial and anterior instability of the knee. An anatomical and clinical study using stress machines. *J Bone Joint Surg Am*, 53(7), 1257–70.

Kennedy JC, Hawkins RJ, Willis RB (1977). Strain gauge analysis of knee ligaments. *Clin Orthop*, 6(129), 225–29.

Larson RL (1980). Combined instabilities of the knee. *Clin Orthop*, 147, 68–75.

Lechner CT and Dahners LE (1991). Healing of the medial collateral ligament in unstable rat knees. *Am J Sports Med*, 19, 508–12.

Mains DB, Andrews JG, Stonesipher T (1977). Medial and anterior-posterior ligament instability of the human knee, measured with a stress apparatus. *Am J Sports Med*, 5(4), 144–53.

Markolf KL, Gorek JF, Kabo JM, *et al.* (1990). Direct measurement of resultant forces in the anterior cruciate ligament. An *in vitro* study performed with a new experimental technique. *J Bone Joint Surg Am*, 72(4), 557–67.

Markolf KL, Mensch JS, Amstutz HC (1976). Stiffness and laxity of the knee – the contributions of supporting structures. A quantitative *in vitro* study. *J Bone Joint Surg Am*, 58(5), 583–94.

McDaniel WJ and Dameron TB (1980). Untreated ruptures of the anterior cruciate ligaments. A follow-up study. *J Bone Joint Surg Am*, 62, 696–705.

Miyasaka KC, Daniel DM, Stone ML, *et al.* (1991). The incidence of knee ligament injuries in the general population. *Am J Knee Surg*, 4(1), 3–8.

Muller W (1983). *The Knee: Form, function, and ligament reconstruction*. New York, Springer-Verlag.

Mok DW and Good C (1989). Non-operative management of acute grade III medial collateral ligament injury of the knee: a prospective study. *Injury*, 20(5), 277–80.

Monahan JJ, Grigg P, Pappas AM, *et al.* (1984). *In vivo* stain patterns in the four major canine knee ligaments. *J Orthop Res*, 2(4), 408–18.

Nagineni CN, Amiel D, Green MH, *et al.* (1992). Characterization of the intrinsic properties of the anterior cruciate ligament and medial collateral ligament cells: an *in vitro* cell culture study. *J Orthop Res*, 10(4), 465–475.

Nakamura N, Timmermann SA, Hart DA, *et al.* (1998). A comparison of *in vivo* gene delivery methods for antisense therapy in ligament healing. *Gene Ther*, 5(11), 1455–61.

Nielsen S, Kromann-Anderson C, Rasmussen O, *et al.* (1984*a*). Instability of cadaver knees after transection of capsule and ligaments. *Acta Orthop Scand*, 55(1), 30–34.

Nielsen S, Rasmussen O, Ovesen J, *et al.* (1984*b*). Rotatory instability in cadaver knees after transection of collateral ligaments and capsule. *Arch Orthop Trauma Surg*, 103(3), 165–69.

Nickerson DA, Joshi R, Williams S, *et al.* (1992). Synovial fluid stimulates the proliferation of rabbit ligaments: Fibroblasts *in vivo*. *Clin Orthop*, 274, 294–99.

Noyes FR and Barber-Westin SD (1995). The treatment of acute combined ruptures of the anterior cruciate and medial ligaments of the knee. *Am J Sports Med*, 23(4), 380–9.

Noyes FR and Barber-Westin SD (2000). Arthroscopic repair of meniscus tears extending into the avascular zone with or without anterior cruciate ligament reconstruction in patients 40 years of age and older. *Arthroscopy*, 16(8), 822–29.

O'Donoghue DH (1950). Surgical treatment of fresh injuries to the major ligaments of the knee. *J Bone Joint Surg Am*, 32, 721–38.

O'Donoghue DH (1955). An analysis of end results of surgical treatment of major injuries to the ligaments of the knee. *J Bone Joint Surg Am*, 37, 1–13.

O'Donoghue DH (1959). Surgical treatment of injuries to ligaments of the knee. *J Am Med Assoc*, 169, 1423–31.

Ohno K, Pomaybo AS, Schmidt CC, *et al.* (1995). Healing of the medial collateral ligament after a combined medial collateral and anterior cruciate ligament injury and reconstruction of the anterior cruciate ligament: Comparison of repair and nonrepair of medial collateral ligament tears in rabbits. *J Orthop Res*, 13(3), 442–49.

Ogata K, Whiteside LA, Anderson DA (1980). The intra-articular effect of various postoperative managements following knee ligament repair. An experimental study in dogs. *Clin Orthop*, 150, 271–76.

Peterson W and Laprell H (1999). Combined injuries of the medial collateral ligament and the anterior cruciate ligament. Early ACL reconstruction versus late ACL reconstruction. *Arch Orthop Trauma Surg*, 119(5–6), 258–62.

Phillips CE (1914). Syndesmorraphy and syndesmoplasty: The operative treatment of ruptured ligaments. *Surg Gynecol Obstet*, 19, 729–733.

Piziali RL, Rastegar J, Nagel DA, *et al.* (1980*a*). The contribution of the cruciate ligaments to the load-displacement characteristics of the human knee joint. *J Biomech Eng*, 102(4), 277–83.

Piziali RL, Seering WP, Nagel DA, *et al.* (1980*b*). The function of the primary ligaments of the knee in anterior-posterior and medial-lateral motions. *J Biomech*, 13(9), 777–84.

Pope MH, Johnson RJ, Brown DW, *et al.* (1979). The role of the musculature in injuries to the medial collateral ligament. *J Bone Joint Surg Am*, 61(3), 398–402.

Reider B, Sathy MR, Talkington J, *et al.* (1994). Treatment of isolated medial collateral ligament injuries in athletes with early functional rehabilitation. A five-year follow-up study. *Am J Sports Med*, 22(4), 470–77.

Robbins AJ, Newman AP and Burks RT (1993). Postoperative return of motion in anterior cruciate ligament and medial collateral ligament injuries. The effect of medial collateral ligament rupture location. *Am J Sports Med*, 21(1), 20–25.

Sabiston P, Frank C, Lam T, *et al.* (1990*a*). Allograft ligament transplantation. A morphological and biochemical evaluation of a medial collateral ligament complex in a rabbit model. *Am J Sports Med*, 18(2), 160–68.

Sabiston P, Frank C, Lam T, et al. (1990b). Transplantation of the rabbit medial collateral ligament. II, Biomechanical evaluation of frozen/thawed allografts. *J Orthop Res*, 9(1), 46–56.

Sandberg R, Balkfors B, Nilsson B, et al. (1987). Operative versus non-operative treatment of recent injuries to the ligaments of the knee. A prospective randomized study. *J Bone Joint Surg Am*, 69(8), 1120–26.

Schreck PJ, Kitabayashi LR, Amiel D, et al. (1995). Integrin display increases in the wounded rabbit medial collateral ligament bur not the wounded anterior cruciate ligament. *J Orthop Res*, 13(2), 174–83.

Seering WP, Piziali RL, Nagel DA, et al. (1980). The function of the primary ligaments of the knee in varus-valgus and axial rotation. *J Biomech*, 13(9), 785–94.

Shapiro MS, Markolf KL, Finerman GA, et al. (1991). The effect of sectioning the medial collateral ligament on force generated in the anterior cruciate ligament. *J Bone Joint Surg Am*, 73(2), 248–56.

Shelbourne KD and Nitz PA (1991). The O'Donoghue triad revisited. Combine knee knuuries involving anterior cruciate and medial collateral ligament tears. *Am J Sports Med*, 19(5), 474–77.

Shelbourne KD and Patel DV (1996). Management of combined injuries of the anterior cruciate and medial collateral ligaments. *Instr Course Lect*, 45, 275–80.

Shelbourne KD and Porter DA (1992). Anterior cruciate ligament-medial collateral ligament injury: Nonoperative management of medial collateral ligament tears with anterior cruciate ligament reconstruction. A preliminary report. *Am J Sports Med*, 20, 283–86.

Shino K and Horibe S (1991). Experimental ligament reconstruction by allogenic tendon graft in a canine model. *Acta Orthop Belg*, 57(Suppl 2), 44–53.

Shoemaker SC and Markolf KL (1985). Effects of joint load on the stiffness and laxity of ligament-deficient knees. An *in vitro* study of the anterior cruciate and medial collateral ligaments. *J Bone Joint Surg Am*, 67(1), 136–46.

Slocum DB and Larson RL (1968). Rotatory instability of the knee. Its pathogenesis and a clinical test to demonstrate its presence. *J Bone Joint Surg Am*, 50(2), 211–25.

Slocum DB, Larson RL, James SL (1974). Late reconstruction of ligamentous injuries of the medial compartment of the knee. *Clin Orthop*, 100, 23–55.

Sullivan D, Levy IM, Sheskier S, et al. (1984). Medial restraints to anterior-posterior motion of the knee. *J Bone Joint Surg Am*, 66(6), 930–36.

Tipton CM, James SL, Mergner W, et al. (1970). Influence of exercise on strength of medial collateral knee ligaments of dogs. *Am J Physiol*, 218, 894–902.

Veldhuizen JW, Stapert JW, Oostvogel HJ, et al. (1989). Transposition of the semitendinosus tendon for early repair of medial and anteromedial laxity of the knee. *Injury*, 20, 29–31.

Walsh S, Frank C, Shrive N, et al. (1993). Knee immobilization inhibits biomechanical maturation of the rabbit medial collateral ligament. *Clin Orthop*, 297, 253–61.

Warren LF and Marshall JL (1979). The supporting structures and layers on the medial side of the knee: an anatomical analysis. *J Bone Joint Surg Am*, 61(1), 56–62.

Warren LF, Marshall JL, Girgis F (1974). The prime static stabilizer of the medial side of the knee. *J Bone Joint Surg Am*, 56(4), 665–74.

Warren RF and Marshall JL (1978). Injuries of the anterior cruciate and medial collateral ligaments of the knee. A long-term follow-up of 86 cases – Part II. *Clin Orthop*, 136, 198–211.

Watanabe N, Takai S, Morita N, *et al.* (1998). A new method of distinguishing between intrinsic cells *in situ* and extrinsic cells supplied by auto-geneic transplantation employing transgeneic rats. *Trans Orthop Res Soc*, 23, 1035.

Weisman G, Pope MH, Johnson RJ (1980). Cyclic loading in knee ligament injuries. *Am J Sports Med*, 8(1), 24–30.

Weiss JA, Woo SL, Ohland KJ, *et al.* (1991). Evaluation of a new injury model to study medial collateral ligament healing: primary repair versus nonoperative treatment. *J Orthop Res*, 9(4), 516–28.

Wilson DR, Feikes JD, Zavatsky AB, *et al.* (2000). The components of passive knee movement are coupled to flexion angle. *J Biomech*, 33(4), 465–73.

Wilson DR, Feikes JD, O'Conner JJ (1998). Ligaments and articular contact guide passive knee flexion. *J Biomech*, 31(12), 1127–36.

Woo SL, Gomez MA, Inoue M, *et al.* (1987). New experimental procedures to evaluate the biomechanical properties of healing canine medial collateral ligaments. *J Orthop Res*, 5(3), 425–32.

Woo SL, Gomez MA, Sites TJ, *et al.* (1987a). The biomechanical and morphological changes in the medial collateral ligament of the rabbit after immobilization and remobilization. *J Bone Joint Surg Am*, 69(8), 1200–11.

Woo SL, Gomez MA, Woo YK, *et al.* (1982). Biomechanical properties of tendons and ligaments II: The relationships of immobilization and exercise on tissue remodeling. *Biorhealogy*, 19(3), 397–408.

Woo SL, Inoue M, McGurk-Burleson E, *et al.* (1987b). Treatment of the medial collateral ligament injury II: Structure and function of canine knees in response to differing treatment regimens. *Am J Sports Med*, 15(1), 22–29.

Woo SL, Peterson RH, Ohland KJ, *et al.* (1990a). The effects of strain rate on the properties of the medial collateral ligament in skeletally immature and mature rabbits: a biomechanical and histological study. *J Othop Res*, 8(5), 712–21.

Woo SL, Smith DW, Hildebrand KA, *et al.* (1998). Engineering the healing of the rabbit medial collateral ligament. *Med Biol Eng Comput*, 36(3), 359–64.

Woo SL, Weiss JA, Gomez MA, *et al.* (1990b). Measurement in changes in ligament tension with knee motion and skeletal maturation. *J Biomech Eng*, 112(1), 46–51.

Woo SL, Young EP, Ohland KJ, *et al.* (1990c). The effects of transection of the anterior cruciate ligament on healing of the medial collateral ligament. A biomechanical study of the knee in dogs. *J Bone Joint Surg Am*, 72(3), 382–92.

Woo SLY, An KY, Arnoczky SP, *et al.* (1994). Anatomy, biology, and biomechanics of tendon, ligament, *and meniscus*. In: SR Simon (ed.) *Orthopaedic Basic Science*, American Academy of Orthopaedic Surgeons: Rosemont, IL. pp. 45–87.

Woo S, Vogrin T, Abramowitch S (2000) Healing and Repair of ligament injuries of the knee. *J Am Acad Orthop Surg*, 8(6), 364–72.

Yamaji T, Levine RE, Woo SL, *et al.* (1996). Medial collateral ligament healing one year after a concurrent medial collateral and anterior cruciate ligament injury: An interdisciplinary study in rabbits. *J Orthop Res*, 14, 223–27.

Part 4. Lateral Collateral Ligament/Posterolateral Corner

Acute repair of the posterolateral structures of the knee results in superior clinical outcomes compared to the current methods of reconstruction

Answorth A. Allen and Victor Lopez Jr

Introduction

Although our knowledge of the posterior lateral corner (PLC) of the knee continues to evolve, the anatomic and biomechanical complexity of this region of the knee is unparalleled. It consists of both static and dynamic stabilizers that provide lateral, posterior, and rotatory stability throughout the range of motion of the knee joint. Hughston *et al.* (1976), initially described the concept of a posterolateral corner rotatory instability of the knee, however this manuscript did not describe the injury patterns in great anatomic detail. Baker *et al.* (1983), described the surgical findings in 17 patients with acute posterolateral rotatory instability and provided a more detailed description of specific anatomic injury patterns. Isolated injuries to the posterolateral corner are relatively rare. DeLee *et al.* (1983) reported that of 735 knees that were treated for ligament injuries, only 12 (1.6 per cent) had acute isolated posterolateral instability. Acute and chronic PLC injuries (PLCI) are complex and often associated with injuries to the central pivoting structures of the knee: the anterior cruciate ligament (ACL) (Baker *et al.* 1983) and/or posterior cruciate ligament (PCL) (Baker *et al.* 1984, Cooper *et al.* 1991, Noyes and Barber-Westin 1996). Unless there is a high index of clinical suspicion, an injury to the posterolateral corner can often be missed at the time of the initial evaluation.

Chronic posterolateral corner injuries can cause severe disability due to instability, gait abnormalities and the eventual development of post-traumatic osteoarthritis. O'Brien *et al.* (1991) found that unrecognized and untreated PLC injuries maybe a cause of clinical failure after ACL reconstruction. Harner *et al.* (2000) and LaPrade *et al.* (1999) have demonstrated increased *in situ* graft forces after ACL and PCL reconstructions respectively in cadaveric models.

These findings suggests that failure to reconstruct the PLC in combined ligament injuries may lead to clinical ACL and PCL graft failure.

Injuries of the ligamentous structures of the posterolateral corner are classified according to severity: Grade I (minimal to no abnormal knee joint kinetics), II moderately abnormal knee joint kinetics), or III (severe abnormality) (Kannus 1989, Noyes *et al.* 1989, Covey 2001). Little has been written about non-operative management of PLC injuries. However, most knee surgeons agree that Grade I and II injuries can be managed non-operatively with little residual laxity and minimal risk for post-traumatic arthritis. Grade III injuries that are managed non-operatively have poor functional results. These patients develop chronic posterolateral instability and often present with varus alignment, knee hyperextension, quadriceps atrophy, and a markedly abnormal gait (Noyes 1989). The chronic residual instability in this group of patients may lead to articular surface damage and post-traumatic arthritis (Kannus 1989, Krukhaug *et al.* 1998).

This chapter will focus upon the patient with complete (Grade III) posterolateral corner injury. Furthermore, for the purpose of this discussion, we refer to 'acute injuries' as those diagnosed and treated surgically within three weeks of the injury. It is the opinion of the authors that acute repair of the posterolateral corner of the knee results in superior clinical outcomes compared to current methods of reconstruction. We will review the anatomy and present a clinical overview, with relevant literature that supports our position.

Anatomy of the posterolateral corner

The anatomy of the posterolateral corner is noted for its variability. The principal anatomic structures of the posterolateral corner include: the iliotibial tract, the biceps femoris, the lateral collateral ligament (LCL), the arcuate ligament, the popliteus tendon, the popliteofibular ligament, the fabello-fibular ligament, the short lateral ligament, and the posterolateral part of the joint capsule (Maynard *et al.* 1996, Terry and LaPrade 1996, Seebacher *et al.* 1982, Laprade and Terry 1997).

In an attempt to organize and clarify the anatomy for the clinician Seebacher *et al.* (1982), described the lateral structures of the knee in terms of three distinct layers (Figure 16.1). The first and most superficial layer is comprised of the iliotibial tract with its expansion anteriorly and the portion of the biceps with its expansion posteriorly. At the distal femur, the peroneal nerve lies posterior to the biceps tendon on the deep side of the superficial layer.

The second layer is formed anteriorly by the quadriceps retinaculum adjacent to the patella. The posterior aspect of the second layer is complex and is made up of the two patellofemoral ligaments. Proximally the patellofemoral ligament joins the terminal fibers of

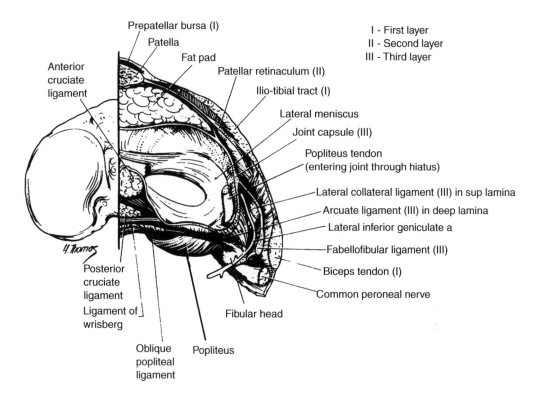

Prepatellar bursa (I)

Patella

Fat pad

Patellar retinaculum (II)

Ilio-tibial tract (I)

Anterior
cruciate
ligament

Lateral meniscus

Joint capsule (III)

Popliteus tendon
(entering joint through hiatus)

Lateral collateral ligament (III) in sup lamina

Arcuate ligament (III) in deep lamina

Lateral inferior geniculate a

Fabellofibular ligament (III)

Biceps tendon (I)

Common peroneal nerve

Posterior
cruciate
ligament

Ligament of
wrisberg

Fibular head

Oblique
popliteal
ligament

Popliteus

I - First layer
II - Second layer
III - Third layer

Fig. 16.1

Drawing of an axial section of the posterolateral corner of the knee showing the three-layer anatomy. Reprinted with permission, Seebacher JR, Inglis AE, Marshall JL, and Warren RF (1982). The structure of the posterolateral aspect of the knee. *Journal Bone and Joint Surgery*, 64A, 536–541.

the lateral intermuscular septum. The distal patellofemoral ligament ends posteriorly at the fabella, when it is present, or at the femoral insertion of the posterolateral part of the capsule and the lateral head of the gastrocnemius.

The third and deepest layer consists of the lateral collateral ligament and the lateral capsule. Seebacher *et al.* (1982) considers the lateral collateral ligament (LCL) to be a discrete thickening of the deepest capsular layer. The LCL runs from the lateral epicondyle to insert on the fibula head distally, posterior to the axis of rotation of the femur. On the LCL is the capsular attachment to the periphery of the lateral meniscus, i.e. the coronary ligament. The popliteus tendon passes through a hiatus in the coronary ligament to attach to the femur, anterior to the femoral origin of the LCL. Posterior to the overlying iliotibial tract, the capsule divides into two laminae: the superficial and deep. The superficial laminae encompass the LCL. It ends posteriorly at the fabellofibular ligament or the short lateral ligament. When a fabella is present, the fabellofibular ligament will be found extending from the LCL to the fibula, to insert posterior to the insertion of the biceps tendon. The inferolateral geniculate vessels lie between the superficial and deep laminae of the posterolateral part of the capsule. The inferolateral geniculate vessels also separate the fabellofibular ligament from the arcuate ligament (Figure 16.2). The deep laminae of the posterolateral part of the capsule pass along the edge of the lateral meniscus to form the coronary ligament

257

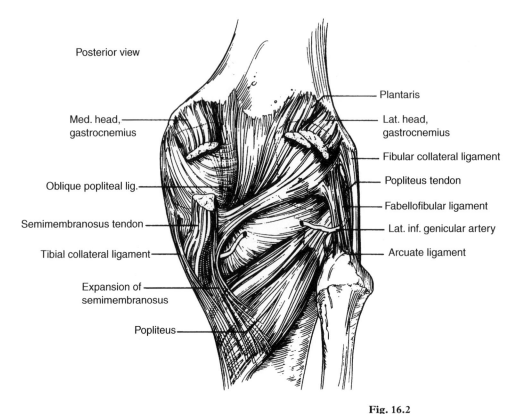

Posterior view

Med. head,
gastrocnemius

Oblique popliteal lig.

Semimembranosus tendon

Tibial collateral ligament

Expansion of
semimembranosus

Popliteus

Plantaris

Lat. head,
gastrocnemius

Fibular collateral ligament

Popliteus tendon

Fabellofibular ligament

Lat. inf. genicular artery

Arcuate ligament

Fig. 16.2

Drawing of the posterior and postero-lateral anatomy of the knee. Note the course of the lateral inferior geniculate artery. Reprinted, with permission, Greenleaf JE (1996). The anatomy and biomechanics of the lateral aspect of the knee. *Operative Techniques in Sports Medicine,* 4(3) 141–147.

and the hiatus of the popliteus tendon. These deep laminae terminate posteriorly at the 'Y-shaped' arcuate ligament. When present, the arcuate ligament consists of a medial limb that arises from the posterolateral part of the capsule at the distal femur and crosses medially over the popliteus muscle to the oblique popliteal ligament. The lateral limb arises from the posterior part of the capsule and courses laterally over the popliteus muscle and tendon deep to the lateral inferior geniculate vessels to insert on the styloid process of the posterior fibula head. The popliteofibular ligament is also called the popliteofibular fascicle. It represents the fibular origin of the popliteus muscle (DeLee *et al.* 1983, Staubli and Birrer 1990, Veltri *et al.* 1996) (Figure 16.3). It lies deep to the lateral limb of the arcuate ligament and arises from the posterior part of the fibula, posterior to the biceps insertion, and courses toward the popliteus musculotendinous junction. The popliteofibular ligament joins the popliteus tendon just proximal to its musculotendinous junction. The popliteofibular ligament has a unique function in that it connects the fibula to the femur through the popliteus tendon. Therefore, the popliteus muscle-tendon unit is a unique 'Y-shaped' structure with a muscle origin from the posterior part of the tibia, a ligamentous origin from the fibular and a common insertion on the femur (Figure 16.4).

As the posterolateral corner remains a complex anatomic area, surgical exposure of this region should be done in a manner that allows

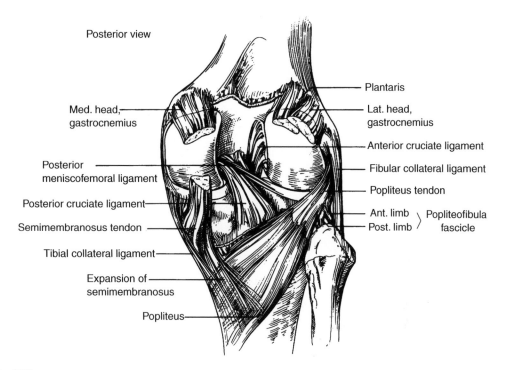

Posterior view

Plantaris

Med. head, gastrocnemius

Lat. head, gastrocnemius

Anterior cruciate ligament

Posterior meniscofemoral ligament

Fibular collateral ligament

Popliteus tendon

Posterior cruciate ligament

Semimembranosus tendon

Ant. limb ⟩ Popliteofibula
Post. limb ⟩ fascicle

Tibial collateral ligament

Expansion of semimembranosus

Popliteus

Fig. 16.3

Drawing of the deep structures of the posterior aspect of the knee. The individual anatomic structures are clearly labeled. Reprinted, with permission, Greenleaf JE (1996). The anatomy and biomechanics of the lateral aspect of the knee. *Operative Techniques in Sports Medicine*, 4(3) 141–147.

for both the evaluation and possible repair/reconstruction of injured structures. As such, Terry and La Prade (1996) have described an anatomic and surgical approach to the posterolateral aspect of the knee that allows evaluation of the components of the posterolateral corner. The first fascial incision they describe is oriented parallel to the fibers of the iliotibial tract. It originates from the mid-point of Gerdy's tubercle and then extends proximally, splitting the proximal portion of the iliotibial tract. This allows retraction of the posterior portion of the iliotibial tract to gain exposure of the deeper structures of the lateral side. A vertical capsular incision parallel to the LCL allows evaluation of the mid-third of the lateral capsule, the popliteal attachments, and the lateral meniscus. The superior lateral geniculate artery runs in this region and must be ligated to prevent a postoperative hematoma.

The second fascial incision is made in the interval between the posterior aspect of the iliotibial tract and the long head of the biceps femoris muscle. This incision usually starts approximately 6 to 7 cm proximal to the lateral epicondyle and extends distally parallel to the femur but posterior to the lateral intramuscular septum. This incision allows evaluation of the attachment of the short head of the biceps onto the tendon of the long head of the biceps, and the biceps attachment to the capsule and the osseous structures. Retraction of the injured biceps complex allows access to the direct head of the short biceps, the capsular attachments to the short head of the biceps femoris muscle, and the fabellofibular ligament (Terry and LaPrade 1996).

The third fascial incision is posterior to the long head of the biceps femoris muscle and parallel to the peroneal nerve. The nerve is usually dissected and protected. Anterior retraction of the biceps femoris muscle and posterior retraction of the peroneal nerve and lateral gastrocnemius muscle allows access to the lateral and medial limbs of the posterior arcuate ligament, the fabellofibular ligament, the popliteofibular ligament, and the popliteus muscle. At this level the inferolateral geniculate artery is just medial to the fibular styloid process.

Clinical overview

Isolated injuries to the PLC are relatively rare. Frequently, there is often associated injury to the cruciate ligament (DeLee *et al.* 1983). These injuries usually result from motor vehicular accidents, industrial accidents, falls, and athletic injuries to the knee. An isolated posterolateral corner injury can result when a posterolateral force is directed against the proximal part of the tibia with the knee at, or near full extension (Hughston *et al.* 1976, DeLee *et al.* 1983) A severe varus force to the flexed knee can also cause an isolated injury to the LCL.

Common mechanisms of injury to the posterior cruciate ligament (PCL) can also result in to injuries to the PLC, such as combined hyperextension and external rotation, contact or non-contact hyperextension, or a severe twisting injury to the knee. A knee dislocation will often include injuries to the PLC (Baker *et al.* 1984, DeLee *et al.* 1983, Fleming *et al.* 1981).

The index of suspicion for PLC injury is based upon a careful history. In an acute situation there is often a history of trauma and the patient will often complain of global knee pain, swelling, and an inability to walk normally. In cases of high energy trauma, the patient may not be able to communicate due to altered mental status or medical treatment. Thus, at the time of the initial presentation, the consulting orthopedic surgeon should thoroughly evaluate all limbs, including the knee joints, to rule out injury. Neurological symptoms from peroneal nerve injury are not uncommon. Krukhaug *et al.* (1998) reported a 16 per cent incidence of peroneal injury in their series of patients with lateral ligament injuries.

Examination of the acutely injured knee will often demonstrate edema, ecchymosis, induration, and tenderness at the lateral side. Abrasion or contusion to the anteromedial aspect of the tibia may imply a PCL and possible PLC injury. If there is any suspicion of a knee dislocation, a thorough evaluation of the patient's neurovascular status should be performed. Patients with chronic injuries often have alignment and gait abnormalities including a varus alignment, and a varus thrust. The physical examination should include a posterior drawer test at 30° and 90° degrees of flexion. Veltri and Warren (1994)

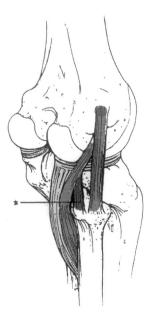

Fig. 16.4
Magnified drawing of the popliteus musculotendinous structure and the politeo-fibular ligament. Arising from the posterior part of the fibula (asterisk), the popliteofibular ligament joins the popliteus tendon just superior to the musculotendinous junction. Reprinted, with permission, Veltri DM and Warren RF (1994). Operative treatment of posterolateral instability of the knee. *Clinics Sports Medicine*, 13, 615–27.

have reported the most useful tests for the diagnosis of PLC injury were the prone external rotation test at 30° and 90° of flexion and varus stress test at 0° and 30° of knee flexion (Veltri *et al.* 1995).

Radiographic evaluation of a knee with an acute PLC injury may demonstrate an increase in the lateral joint space, a fracture of the fibula head, avulsion of Gerdy's tubercle, and or a Segond fracture (bony avulsion of the lateral capsule from the lateral tibial plateau). In chronic cases the radiographs may show evidence of post-traumatic arthritis and varus alignment.

Magnetic resonance imaging can provide detailed information on the specific components of the PLC that may be injured (LaPrade *et al.* 2000, Potter 2000). This can be invaluable for preoperative planning. The images should be obtained to the level of the fibular head and styloid process to allow complete evaluation of the posterolateral corner (Figures 16.5 and 16.6). It is the author's contention that preoperative MRI is absolutely vital in developing a preoperative plan and should always be obtained in those cases where the patient's condition allows for it.

Fig. 16.5

MRI appearance (coronal view, right knee) of an acute posterolateral corner injury. The arrow depicts the popliteofibular ligament (PFL). A thin-slice coronal oblique T1-weighted fat suppression image through the fibular head was used to identify the posterolateral structures.

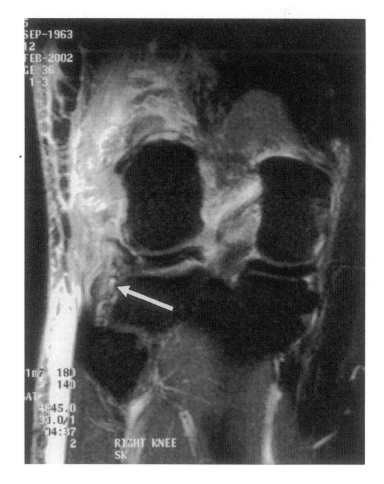

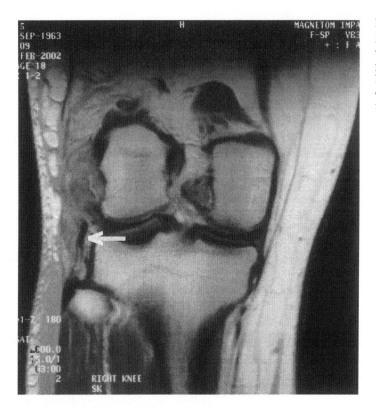

Fig. 16.6

MRI appearance (coronal view, right knee) of an acute posterolateral corner injury. Note the waviness and disruption of the fibers of the lateral ligaments.

Literature review

Operative management of PLC injuries includes primary repair, advancement, and reconstruction. Primary repair and augmentation are usually reserved for acute injuries, while advancement and reconstruction are usually performed in chronic situations. There appears to be an overwhelming consensus in the literature that supports our position that acute primary repairs are more successful than chronic reconstruction of the posterolateral corner (Albright 1994, Baker *et al.* 1983, 1984, Cooper *et al.* 1991, Grana and Janssen 1987, Harner *et al.* 2000, Hughston and Jacobson 1985, Krukhaug *et al.* 1998, Shahane *et al.* 1999, Towne *et al.* 1971, Veltri and Warren 1994). Thus, we again stress the point that suspected patients should be diagnosed aggressively at the outset, so as to optimize the eventual clinical outcome. There are several advantages to operating in the acute situation. These advantages include the following:

1 The ability to easily identify the individual anatomic structures that are compromised at the time of surgery.
2 The ability to fix avulsion-type injuries with suture and suture anchors. Assuming that there is good tissue, this is easier than a reconstructive procedure.
3 If significant tissue damage precludes direct repair and augmentation with autogenous or allograft tissue is necessary,

262

there is a greater healing potential with acute injuries compared to the chronic setting.

4 By intervening early the complications of a chronic posterolateral corner injury of the knee such as quadriceps atrophy, limb malalignment, secondary changes to other structures, and post-traumatic osteoarthritis of the knee are avoided.

O'Donoghue (1950, 1955) was one of the first authors to stress the importance of early surgical repair for acute ligament injuries. In his classic study that analyzed the results of surgical treatment of the major injuries to ligaments of the knee, he concluded that the timing of the repair is more important than the severity of the injury. Essentially, the more severe the injury the more urgent is the need for early repair. He also stated that in all types of ligament injuries, *early* surgical repair (under two weeks) will lead to better results than late repair or reconstruction.

Towne *et al.* (1971) reported on eighteen knees with injuries to the PLC (lateral compartment syndrome of the knee), with special attention to the mechanism of injury, clinical findings, radiographic findings, operative pathology, and the prognosis for recovery. He noted that a favorable outcome could be expected if *early* ligamentous repair is performed. Fifty-six percent of the cases had peroneal nerve injury. The clinical results were best in those patients who did not require nerve repair. DeLee *et al.* (1983) reported on 11 cases of acute posterolateral rotatory instability of the knee, with an average follow-up of 7.5 years. The indications for operative repair included a 2+ or greater varus instability of the knee at 30° flexion in association with a positive external rotation recurvatum or posterolateral drawer test, on examination under anesthesia. All repairs were done *acutely* (within two weeks of injury). The goal of surgery was to advance the complex back to its approximate anatomic location, into a bony bed proximally or distally. Intra-substance tears were repaired primarily in a 'pants over vest' technique. Subjectively, there were eight good, three fair, and no poor results. Objectively there were eight good, two fair and one poor result. The two fair results were so graded because of residual 1+ posterolateral drawer test (neither patient had instability episodes) and one poor result because of symptomatic 2+ posterolateral drawer and 2+ varus laxity at 30° flexion. This patient had a post-surgical infection that required subsequent incision and drainage. Three patients had minimal evidence of arthritic changes on follow-up radiographs. The authors conclusions were as follows: Acute posterolateral instability usually results from a blow to the anteromedial tibia with the knee in extension. Also tenderness and swelling posterolaterally combined with a positive varus stress test with the knee in 30° of flexion strongly suggest a PLC injury. The posterolateral drawer test, while accurate under anesthesia, may be difficult to elicit in the awake due to pain or local muscle spasm. Roentgenographic evidence of fibular head avulsion should suggest the presence of lateral ligament injury. Indications for operative repair include 2+ or greater varus instability at 30° knee flexion in association with a positive external rotation recurvatum or posterolateral drawer test.

Baker *et al.* (1983) evaluated 31 patients with acute posterolateral rotatory instability of the knee over a ten-year period. Thirteen patients who had acute primary repair were available for follow-up evaluation at 53.3 months. Eighty-five percent were rated as good subjectively and 77 per cent were rated as good objectively. Eighty-five percent of these patients returned to preinjury level of athletic activities. The authors concluded posterolateral rotatory instability results from injury to the arcuate ligament complex, caused either by a blow to the anteromedial aspect of the proximal part of the tibia while the knee is hyperextended or by a non-contact, external-rotation hyperextension injury. Furthermore, a positive posterolateral drawer test or external-rotation recurvatum test is diagnostic of posterolateral rotatory instability. A positive adduction-stress test performed with the knee at 30° of flexion is suggestive of this instability, but is not diagnostic. A peroneal nerve palsy may be associated with posterolateral rotatory instability. With correct diagnosis and treatment of *acute* posterolateral rotatory instability, the result should be subjectively acceptable knee function. Subsequently Baker *et al.* (1984) reported on 13 consecutive patients who had acute surgical repair for combined posterior cruciate and posterolateral instability. Eleven patients were available for follow-up evaluation at an average of 56 months. In ten patients (90 per cent) the results were rated as good subjectively and in eight patients (73 per cent) as good objectively. All patients returned to their pre-injury occupation and level of activity. The authors pointed out that injuries to the posterolateral corner are often associated with injuries to the posterior cruciate ligament, and a complete careful examination was necessary to make the appropriate diagnosis. They also concluded that an acute tear of the PCL is often associated with injury to the arcuate ligament complex, resulting in acute combined posterior cruciate and posterolateral instability. Injury to both the PCL and the arcuate ligament complex results from rotational forces associated with a blow to the anteromedial aspect of the knee. In a knee with concomitant injury to the PCL and the arcuate ligament complex that requires surgical repair, all injured structures should be explored and repaired/reconstructed to restore the local knee anatomy and to increase the likelihood of a satisfactory outcome.

Grana and Janssen (1987) evaluated 19 patients with twenty lateral ligament injuries of the knee. The authors note that patients with lateral ligament injuries tend to have worse outcomes than medial collateral or anterior cruciate ligament injury. These authors suggested that the different mechanisms of injury (PLC-high velocity versus ACL/MCL-low velocity) likely played a role in the divergent outcomes noted in these two groups of patients. Lateral ligament tears can be associated with ACL tears. Furthermore, in the operative group the outcomes were better in those patients who had an acute lateral repair (85 per cent satisfactory) while in those patients who had a late reconstruction no satisfactory results were observed.

Krukhaug *et al.* (1998) reported on a group of 25 patients with acute lateral ligament injuries of the knee. Seven patients had isolated injury of the LCL and the lateral capsular structures. The remaining patients had concomitant ligament injuries. Seven of the eighteen patients who had surgery were done acutely, within the first three weeks following injury. At 7.5 years, the functional score (Lysholm) was good in 64 per cent and excellent in 28 per cent. The authors concluded that significant injuries to the lateral ligament complex usually occur in the context of combined ligament injuries. Moreover, the authors also stated that high grade injuries should be managed by acute surgical repair and that low grade injuries to the posterolateral corner should be managed non-surgically.

Authors' preferred approach

In acute posterolateral corner injuries the technique for surgical repair is based on identifying the specific anatomic structures that are compromised and verifying that there is adequate tissue to facilitate primary repair of these structures. The posterior draw test at 30° and 90° and the prone external rotation test at 30° and 90° of flexion and the varus stress test at 0° and 30° of flexion, are applied in the diagnosis of posterior cruciate and posterolateral instability. A careful neurological evaluation is performed with particular attention to the peroneal nerve. Radiographs of the affected knee are obtained. Magnetic resonance imaging is used routinely as this test enables the clinician to thoroughly evaluate the entire knee for injury, which aids the preoperative plan.

In cases where an MRI examination is not possible, a diagnostic arthroscopy can performed. In combination with the examination under anesthesia, diagnostic arthroscopy can complete the work-up by allowing for direct visualization of the cruciate ligaments, the popliteus tendon, the popliteo-meniscal fascicles, articular surfaces, and menisci. If there is cruciate ligament involvement the ACL and PCL can be reconstructed using standard techniques. If there is a PCL avulsion injury it can be repaired primarily using arthroscopic and/or open techniques.

The lateral aspect of the knee is exposed through a 'hockey-stick' incision centered distally between Gerdy's tubercle and the anterior fibular head crossing the lateral epicondyle and extending distally parallel to the femur. The fascial incisions previously described by

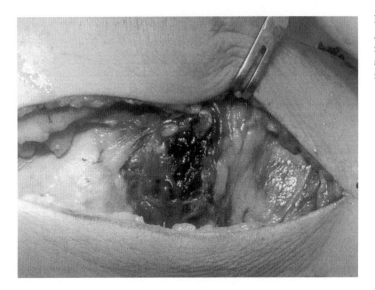

Fig. 16.7
A lateral 'hockey-stick' incision exposing an acute posterolateral corner injury.

Terry and Laprade (1996) are used to allow sequential evaluation of the iliotibial band, biceps femoris tendon, peroneal nerve, LCL, popliteus tendon, and popliteofibular ligament (Figure 16.7). A vertical capsular incision can be made just posterior to the LCL to allow evaluation of the popliteus tendon and the posterior joint.

The steps for repair proceed from deep to superficial using direct suture repair, soft tissue repair with suture anchors, sutures through drill holes, or fixation of avulsion injuries with screws and washers if necessary (Figures 16.8 and 16.9).

Once the exposure of the lateral knee is complete, the popliteus tendon is examined in its entirety (femoral insertion to the musculotendinous junction, including the popliteofibular ligament). Any injury to the popliteus is noted with respect to location, and the quality of remaining tissue. The popliteus is usually injured at the muscle-tendon junction. Surgical options include primary repair, advancement, augmentation, and reconstruction. Primary repair of the popliteus, when performed early, is the best option, if there is adequate tissue. If the popliteus tendon is intact but the tibial attachment or the popliteofibular ligament attachment to the fibula has been injured, tension is restored with suture fixation to the bone (Figure 16.10).

If the popliteus tendon is stretched but in continuity, its femoral insertion can be removed with a bone plug and the tendon insertion advanced by recessing the bone plug into a femoral drill hole. If the popliteus tissue is insufficient for repair, augmentation or reconstruction of the popliteus tendon can be performed using autograft hamstring tendon or allograft.

An acute avulsion injury to the LCL can be repaired with sutures, suture anchors or screws (Figures 16.8 and 16.9). If necessary, the

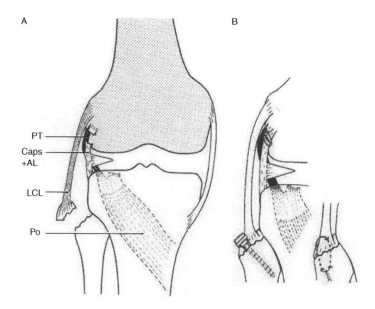

Fig. 16.8

Tears of the lateral collateral ligament (LCL) with associated lesions of
the deep capsulo-ligamentous layers and the corresponding techniques of
repair. Schematic A shows injury to the LCL and B the areas of repair,
with a cortical screw in the proximal fibula, or sutures through the proximal
fibula. PT = popliteus tendon, caps = capsule, AL = arcuate ligament,
LCL = lateral collateral ligament, Po = popliteus muscle. Reprinted,
with permission, Muller W (1982). The primary repair in special injuries.
In *The Knee: Form, function and ligament reconstruction.* pp. 195, 200.
Springer-Verlag, Heidelberg, Germany.

Fig. 16.9

Schematic C shows tears of
the LCL with associated
lesions of the capsule and
arcuate ligament. Schematic D
shows repair of the proximal
injury of the LCL and arcuate
ligament using suture
technique. Reprinted, with
permission, Muller W (1982).
The primary repair in special
injuries. In *The Knee: Form,
function and ligament
reconstruction.* pp. 195, 200.
Springer-Verlag, Heidelberg,
Germany.

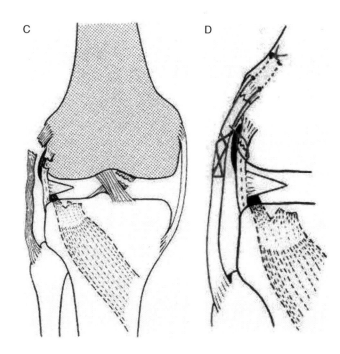

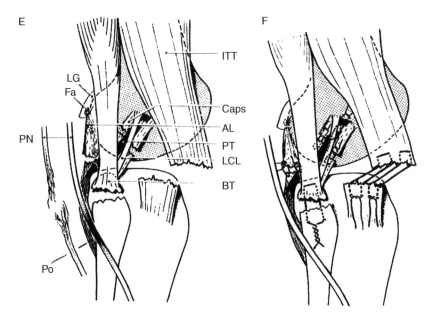

Fig. 16.10

Schematic E shows an example of a major complex lateral injury with bony avulsion of the biceps and LCL and ruptures of the popliteus tendon, posterior capsule, arcuate ligament, and both cruciate ligaments and the iliotibial tract. F shows the corresponding techniques of suture repair. LG = lateral gastrocnemius, Fa = fabella, PN = peroneus nerve, ITT = iliotibial tract, BT = biceps tendon. Reprinted, with permission, Muller W (1982). The primary repair in special injuries. In *The Knee: Form, function and ligament reconstruction*. pp. 195, 200. Springer-Verlag, Heidelberg, Germany.

LCL can be augmented with a strip of the biceps tendon. When direct repair or biceps augmentation cannot be accomplished, the LCL can be reconstructed with a patellar tendon autograft or, Achilles or patella tendon allograft.

Conclusions

- There should be a high index of suspicion of PLC injuries in patients with acute traumatic knee injuries, especially when the cruciate (ACL/PCL) ligaments are involved.
- Ecchymosis, induration and tenderness in the PLC often imply significant injury to the region. The most useful test for PLC instability is the posterior drawer test at 30° and 90° degrees of flexion and the prone external rotation test at 30° and 90° degrees of flexion and varus stress test at 0° and 30° degrees of flexion.
- Bony avulsion fractures of the fibula head and increase lateral joint space are radiographic signs of possible injury to the PLC.

- MRI is extremely useful in identifying and delineating the individual structures that are damaged and is critical to the development of a preoperative plan.
- With complete PLC injuries surgical management is usually recommended. Surgery should be performed sooner rather than later, usually within three weeks of the injury.
- The surgical approach used should allow access to all the involved structures. Identification and protection of the peroneal nerve is critical.
- Primary repair is performed only if the injured tissue is not significantly compromised. There should be a low threshold for the use of additional tissue (autogenous or allograft) in the repair of injured structures.
- The repair should be performed in layers from deep to superficial. All injured structures should be repaired.
- The postoperative rehabilitation should be individualized.

References

Albright JP (1994). Management of chronic posterolateral instability of the knee: Operative technique for the posterolateral corner sling procedure. *Iowa Orthopedics Journal*, 14, 94–100.

Baker CL, Norwood LA, and Hughston JC (1983). Acute posterolateral rotatory instability of the knee. *Journal Bone Joint Surgery*, 65A, 614–18.

Baker CL, Norwood LA, and Hughston JC (1984). Acute combined posterior cruciate and posterolateral instability of the knee. *American Journal of Sports Medicine*, 12, 204–8.

Covey DC (2001). Current concepts review: Injuries of the posterolateral corner of the knee. *Journal Bone and Joint Surgery*, 83A, 106–18.

Cooper DE, Warren RF, and Warner JJP (1991). The posterior cruciate ligament and posterolateral structures of the knee: Anatomy, function, and patterns of injury. *Instructional Course Lectures*, 40, 249–70.

DeLee JC, Riley MB, and Rockwood CA Jr (1983). Acute posterolateral rotatory instability of the knee. *American Journal Sports Medicine*, 11, 199–207.

Fleming RE Jr, Blatz DJ, and McCarroll JR (1981). Posterior problems in the knee. Posterior cruciate insufficiency and posterolateral rotatory insufficiency. *American Journal Sports Medicine*, 9, 107–13.

Grana WA, Janssen T (1987). Lateral ligament injury of the knee. *Orthopedics*, 10, 1039–44.

Greenleaf JE (1996). The anatomy and biomechanics of the lateral aspect of the knee. *Operative Techniques in Sports Medicine*, 4(3), 141–47.

Harner CD, Vogrin TM, Hoher J, Ma CB, Woo SL (2000). Biomechanical analysis of a posterior cruciate ligament reconstruction. Deficiency of the posterolateral structures as a cause of graft failure. *American Journal Sports Medicine*, 28, 32–9.

Hughston JC, Andrews JR, Cross MJ, and Moschi A (1976). Classification of knee ligament instabilities, Part II: The lateral compartment. *Journal Bone and Joint Surgery*, 58A, 173–9.

Hughston JC and Jacobson KE (1985). Chronic posterolateral instability of the knee. *Journal Bone and Joint Surgery*, 67A, 351–9.

Kannus P (1989). Nonoperative treatment of grade II and III sprains of the lateral ligament compartment of the knee. *American Journal Sports Medicine*, 17, 83–8.

Krukhaug Y, Molster A, Rodt A, and Strand T (1998). Lateral ligament injuries of the knee. *Knee Surgery, Sports Traumatology, and Arthroscopy*, 6, 21–5.

Laprade RF, Gilbert TJ, Bollom TS, Wentorf F, Chaljub G (2000). The magnetic resonance imaging appearance of individual structures of the posterolateral knee. A prospective study of normal knees and knees with surgically verified grade III injuries. *American Journal Sports Medicine*, 28(2), 191–9.

Laprade RF, Resig S, Wentorf F, and Lewis JL (1999). The effects of grade III posterolateral knee complex injuries on anterior cruciate ligament graft force. A biomechanical analysis. *American Journal Sports Medicine*, 27(4), 469–75.

Laprade RF and Terry GC (1997). Injuries to the posterolateral aspect of the knee. Association of anatomic injury patterns with clinical instability. *American Journal Sports Medicine*, 25(4), 433–8.

Maynard MJ, Deng X-H, Wickiewicz TL, and Warren RF (1996). The popliteofibular ligament. The rediscovery of a key element in posterolateral stability. *American Journal Sports Medicine*, 24, 311–6.

Muller W (1982). The primary repair in special injuries. In *The Knee: Form, function and ligament reconstruction*. pp. 195, 200. Springer-Verlag, Heidelberg, Germany.

Noyes FR and Barber-Westin SD (1996). Treatment of complex injuries of the posterior cruciate ligaments and posterolateral ligaments of the knee joint. *American Journal Knee Surgery*, 9, 200–14.

Noyes FR, Grood ES, and Torzilli PA (1989). Current concepts review. The definitions of terms for motion and position of the knee and injuries of the ligaments. *Journal Bone and Joint Surgery*, 71A, 465–72.

O'Brien SJ, Warren RF, Pavlov H, Panariello R, and Wickiewicz TL (1991). Reconstruction of the chronically insufficient anterior cruciate ligament with the central third of the patella ligament. *Journal Bone and Joint Surgery*, 73A, 278–86.

O'Donoghue DH (1950). Surgical treatment of fresh injuries to the major ligaments of the knee. *Journal Bone and Joint Surgery*, 32A, 721–38.

O'Donoghue DH (1955). An analysis of end results of surgical treatment of major injuries to the ligaments of the knee. *Journal Bone and Joint Surgery*, 37A, 1–14.

Potter HG (2000). Imaging of the multiple-ligament injured knee. *Clin Sports Med.*, 19(3), 425–41.

Seebacher JR, Inglis AE, Marshall JL, and Warren RF (1982). The structure of the posterolateral aspect of the knee. *Journal Bone and Joint Surgery*, 64A, 536–541.

Shahane SA, Ibbotson C, Strachan R, and Bickerstaff DR (1999). The popliteofibular ligament: An anatomical study of the posterolateral corner of the knee. *Journal Bone and Joint Surgery*, 81B, 636–42.

Staubli HU and Birrer S (1990). The popliteus tendon and it fascicles at the popliteal hiatus: Gross anatomy and functional arthroscopic evaluation with and without anterior cruciate ligament deficiency. *Arthroscopy*, 6(3), 209–220.

Terry GC and Laprade RF (1996). The biceps femoris muscle complex at the knee. Its anatomy and injury patterns associated with acute antero-lateral-anteromedial rotatory instability. *American Journal Sports Medicine*, 24(1), 2–8.

Terry GC and Laprade RF (1996). The posterolateral aspect of the knee. Anatomy and surgical approach. *American Journal Sports Medicine*, 24(6), 732–9.

Towne LC, Blazina ME, Marmor L, and Lawrence JF (1971). Lateral compartment syndrome of the knee. *Clinical Orthopedics*, 76, 160–8.

Veltri DM, Deng X-H, Torzilli PA, Maynard MJ, and Warren RF (1995). The role of the cruciate and posterolateral ligaments in stability of the human knee: A biomechanical study. *American Journal Sports Medicine*, 23(4), 436–43.

Veltri DM, Deng X-H, Torzilli PA, Maynard MJ, and Warren RF (1996). The role of the popliteofibular ligament in stability of the human knee: A biomechanical study. *American Journal Sports Medicine*, 24(1), 19–27.

Veltri DM and Warren RF (1994). Operative treatment of posterolateral instability of the knee. *Clinics Sports Medicine*, 13, 615–27.

17

Reconstruction methods for the lateral side of the knee: what we do

Christopher J. Wahl and Russell F. Warren

Introduction

Injuries to the lateral or posterolateral structures of the knee rarely occur in isolation. Reports by Fleming (Fleming *et al.*, 1981), Baker (Baker *et al.*, 1983, 1984), and Hughston and Jacobson (1985) have noted that posterolateral instability most commonly occurs in conjunction with multiple-ligament injuries or knee dislocations that can involve disruption to the anterior cruciate ligament (ACL), posterior cruciate ligament (PCL), or medial supporting capsular structures. Baker *et al.* (1983) found concomitant ACL ruptures in 11 of 17 patients presenting with posterolateral rotatory instability. These authors reported a second series of 13 consecutive patients with concomitant PCL and posterolateral corner injuries (Baker *et al.*, 1984). These concomitant instability patterns can make the physical examination of the posterolateral structures difficult. However, accurate and timely diagnosis of posterolateral instability is important for several reasons. First, significant potential exists for compromise of the popliteal artery, common peroneal nerve, or other neurovascular structures in the setting of knee dislocation, and if unrecognized these injures carry devastating consequences. Second, unrecognized injuries to the posterolateral capsule preclude the success of isolated repairs to other ligaments (Hughston and Jacobson, 1985). O'Brien *et al.* (1991) noted that failed ACL reconstruction was associated with unrecognized or untreated posterolateral knee instability. In another report of 23 patients who underwent surgical treatment of chronic combined posterolateral complex and cruciate injuries, Noyes and associates (Noyes and Barber-Westin, 1996a) noted that in 17 (81 per cent) the diagnosis was either missed or never addressed surgically. Fourteen ACL or PCL reconstructions failed, and 77 prior surgical procedures had been performed on the involved knees. Finally, early surgical management of acute injuries to the posterolateral structures differs dramatically from the treatment of longstanding knee joint instability. In the latter, copious scar, attenuation of tissues, and altered local anatomy add to the complexity of the procedure and can temper the expectations for optimal results (Skyhar *et al.*, 1993, Baker *et al.*, 1984, 1983).

Anatomy of the posterolateral corner

A thorough understanding of the primary supporting structures is critical to understanding both the physical diagnosis of knee ligament injuries, and the key to successful operative treatment. The three-layer system described by Seebacher *et al.* (Seebacher *et al.*, 1982) provides a simple way to conceptualize the organization of the posterolateral knee. The most superficial layer (layer I) includes the iliotibial tract and its expansion anteriorly and the superficial biceps and its expansion posteriorly (Figure 17.1). The peroneal nerve lies beneath layer I at the level of the distal femur, just posterior to the biceps tendon (Figures 17.1 and 17.2). Layer II

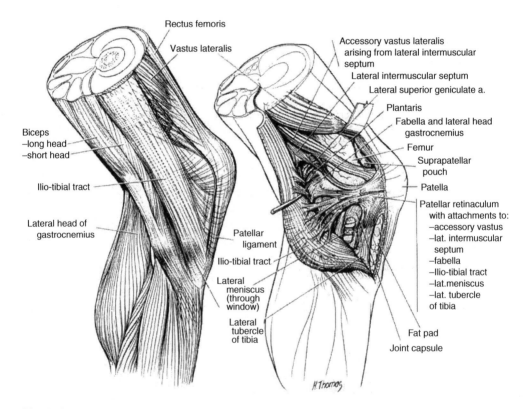

Fig. 17.1

Layers I and II of the structures of the lateral side of the knee. The drawing on the left shows the major constituents of layer I, the iliotibial tract and the superficial portion of the expansion of the biceps. On the right, layer I has been incised and peeled back from the lateral margin of the patella showing layer II. Layer II includes the vastus lateralis and its expansions as well as the patellofemoral and patellomeniscal ligaments. Reprinted with permission from Seebacher JR, Inglis AE, Marshall JL, *et al.*, The structure of the posterolateral aspect of the knee. *J Bone Joint Surg* 1982; 64A: 536–541.

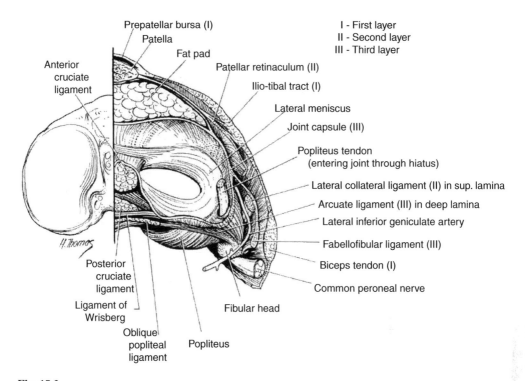

Prepatellar bursa (I)
Patella
Fat pad
Anterior cruciate ligament
Patellar retinaculum (II)
Ilio-tibal tract (I)
Lateral meniscus
Joint capsule (III)
Popliteus tendon (entering joint through hiatus)
Lateral collateral ligament (II) in sup. lamina
Arcuate ligament (III) in deep lamina
Lateral inferior geniculate artery
Fabellofibular ligament (III)
Biceps tendon (I)
Common peroneal nerve
Posterior cruciate ligament
Ligament of Wrisberg
Oblique popliteal ligament
Popliteus
Fibular head

I - First layer
II - Second layer
III - Third layer

Fig. 17.2
A view of the right knee joint from above after removal of the right femur. Note the three layers of the lateral side and the division of the posterolateral part of the capsule (layer III) into deep and superficial laminae which are separated by the lateral inferior geniculate vessels. Reprinted with permission from Seebacher JR, Inglis AE, Marshall JL, *et al.*, The structure of the posterolateral aspect of the knee. *J Bone Joint Surg* 1982; 64A: 536–541.

is formed anteriorly by the retinaculum of the quadriceps, which courses anterolaterally to its insertion at the patella. The posterior portion of layer II is incomplete, and is represented by the two lateral patellofemoral ligaments. The proximal patellofemoral ligament courses posteriorly to join the terminal fibers of the intramuscular septum, while the distal patellofemoral ligament fibers run posteriorly and distally to insert at the fabella or at the posterolateral capsule, where the lateral head of the gastrocnemius originates off the lateral femoral condyle (Figure 17.1). A patellomeniscal ligament travels obliquely postero-inferiorly from the patella toward Gerdy's tubercle beneath the iliotibial tract. It may contribute fibers to the capsule at the level of the lateral meniscus.

Layer III represents the deepest layer of the posterolateral corner, and forms the lateral and posterior joint capsule (Figure 17.2). The capsule splits into two separate laminae in the region of the posterior margin of the overlying iliotibial tract. The superficial lamina (the first encountered during a surgical dissection) envelopes the lateral collateral ligament (LCL) and continues posteriorly to insert on the fabellofibular ligament (if a fabella is present), or its structural analog, the short lateral ligament. Running in the space between the superficial and deep laminae is the lateral inferior geniculate artery, which pierces the superficial lamina where the laminae converge anteriorly and then runs between layers II and III. The deep lamina of Layer III forms the peripheral capsular attachment of the lateral meniscus (coronary ligament). The popliteus hiatus in the posterior and lateral region of the coronary ligament allows for the intraarticular passage of the popliteus tendon, as it courses superiorly and anteriorly from the posterior tibia to insert on the lateral femoral condyle. The deep lamina joins the arcuate ligament of the posterior capsule. This 'inverted Y' shaped ligament has one limb that courses inferiorly from the posterior knee capsule, over the popliteus muscle, to an insertion at the oblique popliteal ligament. The lateral limb of the arcuate ligament originates on the posterior capsule and runs inferiorly and laterally to insert at the posterior fibula.

Although not discussed by Seebacher *et al.*, several other anatomic studies have documented the presence of a static component of the popliteus tendon that attaches to the posterior fibular head (Watanabe *et al.*, 1993, Sudasna and Harnsiriwattanagit, 1990, Staubli and Rauschning, 1991, Staubli and Birrer, 1990, Lovejoy and Harden, 1970, Maynard *et al.*, 1996). This attachment has been termed the popliteofibular ligament. Thus, the popliteus is in reality another inverted Y-shaped structure with its muscular origin on the posterior tibia, a dynamic tendinous limb which courses through the popliteus hiatus in the coronary ligament of the capsule to attach at the lateral femoral condyle, and a secondary static ligamentous limb which arises at the musculotendinous junction of the popliteus and runs obliquely distally and laterally to insert on the posterior aspect of the fibular head (Figure 17.3). The relative importance of the popliteofibular ligament (PFL) is underscored by its relative strength. Maynard *et al.* (1996) reported a strength to failure of 424 N, compared to 750 N for the LCL.

It is important to consider that Seebacher and associates (Seebacher *et al.*, 1982) noted some anatomic variability in the layer system with respect to the arcuate and fabellofibular ligaments. The arcuate ligament alone reinforced the posterior capsule in 13 per cent of specimens, the fabellofibular ligament alone in 20 per cent, and both ligaments reinforced the capsule in 67 per cent. When the fabella was present, the fabellofibular ligament was stout and the arcuate diminutive. When the fabella was absent, the fabellofibular ligament was absent in favor of the short longitudinal ligament, and the arcuate ligament was stout. Watanabe and associates (1993) and Sudaasna and Harnsiriwattanagit (1990) also found some variation in the anatomy of the posterolateral capsular reinforcements, but the popliteofibular ligament was present in 98 per cent and 94 per cent of dissections, respectively.

Because the knee is not a simple hinge joint, close attention to the anatomic relationships of the origins and insertions biceps, LCL, popliteus, and popliteofibular ligament complex is warranted. Sidles and associates (Sidles *et al.*, 1988) believe the entire fibular head to be isometric to the lateral femoral epicondyle throughout the range of motion in the knee, but reported that they found slightly more isometry from the anterior aspect of the epicondyle to the posterior

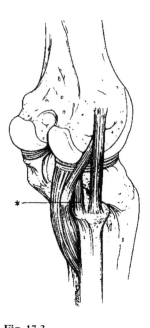

Fig. 17.3
Arising from the posterior part of the fibula, the popliteofibular ligament (*) joins the popliteus tendon just above the musculotendinous junction. (Reprinted with permission from Veltri DM and Warren RF, Posterolateral instability of the knee. *Inst Course Lect* 1995; 44: 441–453).

fibula, and from the posterior aspect of the condyle to the anterior fibula. This would seem to be consistent with the organization of the biceps insertion, LCL, popliteus and popliteofibular ligament *in vivo*. The popliteus inserts slightly anterior to the epicondyle on its sulcus in the lateral femoral condyle, and the PFL (static component of the popliteus complex) inserts posteriorly on the fibula, dorsal to the LCL and biceps insertions. The biceps serves primarily as a knee flexor and weak hip extensor and external rotator of the tibia, however; many authors feel the biceps plays an important role as a dynamic and static stabilizer of the LCL and posterolateral corner, especially as the knee flexes beyond 30° (Terry and LaPrade, 1996, Marshall *et al.*, 1978). The broad biceps insertion overlies the LCL. We believe these relationships are important considerations for accurate, isometric reconstructions of the posterolateral corner. It is the author's preference to maintain the static and dynamic functions of the biceps whenever possible.

The biomechanics of the posterolateral corner and implications for diagnosis and treatment

Basic science research and biomechanical studies have clearly defined the anatomic and functional relationships of the structures that make up the posterolateral corner: the lateral collateral ligament (LCL), the arcuate ligament, the popliteus tendon complex, the popliteofibular ligament (PFL) and the posterolateral joint capsule. Selective ligament-cutting studies in cadaveric specimens at our institution and by Noyes and other authors have defined the contributions of the cruciate ligaments and the posterolateral knee structures to overall stability. A comprehensive review of these studies is beyond the scope of this chapter, but a fundamental understanding of the contributions of the ACL, PCL, LCL, popliteus, and popliteofibular ligament aids in both diagnosis and appropriate surgical management. For simplicity, the stabilizing forces around the knee are defined as follows:

1 Primary posterior stability to applied posterior translation force
2 External rotation that is coupled to an applied posterior translation force
3 Primary varus stability to applied varus moments
4 Primary internal–external rotation stability to applied internal–external rotation moments.

Primary posterior stability to applied posterior translation force

Gollehon *et al.* (1987) studied isolated and combined sections of the lateral collateral ligament, 'deep ligament complex' (without specific isolation of the popliteofibular ligament), and posterior cruciate ligament. They found that the PCL was the primary restraint to posterior translation at all angles of knee flexion, and its contribution to stability became pronounced at higher flexion angles. Isolated section of the LCL or the deep ligament complex had no effect on anterior-posterior stability. However, combined section of the LCL and deep ligaments increased posterior translation at low flexion angles (3 mm at angles less than 30°). Combined section of the PCL, LCL, and deep ligament complex resulted in large increases (20–25 mm) in posterior translation at all flexion angles when compared to intact knees or knees with isolated section of the PCL. Further sectioning studies by Veltri and associates (Veltri and Warren, 1995, Veltri et al., 1995a, b) isolated and recognized the PFL as the static structure of the 'deep ligament complex' that contributes stability to posterior translation at low (less than 30°) flexion angles. This role of the PFL has been confirmed in further studies (Shahane et al., 1999).

External rotation that is coupled to applied a posterior translation force

In the intact knee, anterior translation causes a coupled internal rotation and posterior translation causes a coupled external rotation (Gollehon et al., 1987). The PCL and other posterolateral structures do not affect the coupled internal rotatory motion with anterior translation. The studies demonstrated that isolated section of the PCL eliminated the coupled external rotation with posterior translation. Combined lesions to the LCL and deep ligament complex substantially increased the coupled external rotation at all angles of knee flexion, probably by changing the axis of rotation about the proximal tibia. This coupled rotation was most pronounced at 30° of knee flexion. Moreover, sectioning of the PCL did not further increase the coupled external rotation.

Primary varus stability to applied varus moments

In the intact knee, varus and valgus rotation is minimal at full extension and increases progressively as the knee flexion angle increases. Gollehon and associates found that the PCL, LCL, and deep ligament complex had no effect on valgus rotation. The LCL provided the primary restraint to varus rotation, and isolated section of the LCL gave 1° to 4° of increased varus to a varus moment. The deep ligament complex provided secondary restraint to varus, and combined LCL and deep ligament complex sectioning increased varus instability to 5° to 9°. This effect was most pronounced at low (30°) flexion angles. The PCL provided a tertiary stabilizing effect, and complete sectioning of the PCL, LCL, and deep ligaments resulted in as much as 15° to 19° of varus instability to varus moments. This varus instability was most pronounced at mid- to high flexion angles (60°). Markolf et al. (1993) found that sectioning of the LCL increased varus rotation 103 per cent at full extension, and 30 per cent at 20° and 40° of flexion. Grood and associates (Grood *et al.*, 1981) alternatively found a relatively constant increase in varus instability as flexion progressed from 0° to 90°. Sectioning studies by Veltri and associates (1995a) identified the popliteofibular ligament and the popliteus insertion to the tibia as the structures in the deep ligament complex which contributed most to secondary varus stability to varus rotational moments.

Primary internal–external rotation stability to applied internal–external rotation moments

The amount of primary internal rotation of the tibia in response to an internal rotation moment was not affected by sectioning of the PCL, the LCL, or the deep ligament complex. Isolated section of the PCL did not affect the primary external tibial rotation in response to external rotatory moments at any angle of knee flexion. Isolated section of the deep ligament complex gave rise to significant increases ($6° \pm 3°$) external rotation at 90° of knee flexion. Isolated section of the LCL gave small increases (2° to 3°) at all angles of knee flexion. Combined section of the LCL and deep ligament complex caused large increases in primary external rotation at all knee flexion angles, but this was most pronounced at 30°. Additional sectioning of the PCL further increased the primary external rotation in response to an external rotatory moment at higher flexion angles (60° and 90°). These studies seem to indicate that the LCL and posterolateral ligament complex act in concert to provide resist external rotatory moments, while the PCL plays a secondary role. Indeed, Markolf *et al.* (1993) found that increased forces resulted on the PCL at 45° and 90° after sectioning of the posterolateral structures. Veltri *et al.* (1995a) confirmed that the LCL contributed only slightly to stability to primary external rotation, with the PFL and/or intact popliteus attachment to the tibia providing the primary restraint to rotational instability. The results of ligament-cutting studies by Shahane and associates (Shahane *et al.*, 1999) support the work done by Veltri *et al.* It should be noted that studies performed by Veltri *et al.* (1995b) indicate that combined ACL and posterolateral corner injuries result in a knee with *no* significant increase in *primary external rotation* compared to the intact state – a situation which can make the diagnosis of PLC injury difficult if ACL insufficiency exists.

The results of selective-cutting studies performed by Nielson and Helmig (1986), Grood *et al.* (1988), Markolf *et al.* (1993), and Wascher *et al.* (1993) utilize slightly different techniques and methods, but are consistent and substantiate the work done by Gollehon *et al.* (1987) and Veltri and associates (Veltri and Warren, 1994a, b, Veltri *et al.*, 1995a, b).

Mechanism of injury

The mechanism of injury that leads to posterolateral instability will frequently cause combined injury to the cruciate ligaments as well. Hughston and Jacobson (1985), in a review of 140 patients with posterolateral instability, found that the injury mechanism was almost always a direct blow to the tibia with the knee flexed or extended, or a twisting injury. In the author's experience with acute combined ACL/PLC injury the mechanism is frequently an hyperextension and varus load. Additional mechanisms include a direct blow to the medial tibia (resulting in hyperextension), hyperextension with external rotation, or massive direct blunt trauma (such as a motor vehicle accident).

Clinical implications, physical examination, and classification

With the above anatomic and biomechanical concepts in mind, the physical examination of posterolateral knee injuries can usually be made accurately, and the overall injury classified appropriately (see Table 17.1). Anterior-posterior translation is tested and recorded at both 30° and 90°. Slight increases in posterior tibial translation at 30° knee flexion, but not at 90°, indicates a posterolateral injury. Increases at both low and high flexion angles indicate injury to the PCL. The PCL is additionally evaluated using the quadriceps active, reverse pivot-shift, and posterior drawer tests.

For the diagnosis of posterolateral instability patterns, we find varus stress testing at 0° and 30° and the dial test at 30° and 90° to be most useful. Varus instability will not be present with isolated injury to the cruciates, however combined injury to the LCL and

Table 17.1 Classification system for posterolateral rotational instability

	Functional instability	Dysfunctional instability	Nonfunctional instability
VARUS	0–0.5 cm	0.5–1.0 cm	1.0 cm
(structures injured)	(LCL)	(LCL ± PFL, popliteus)	(LCL, PFL, popliteus ± ACL, PCL)
EXTERNAL ROTATION*	<10°*	10°–15°*	>15°*
(structures injured)	(PFL or popliteus)	(PFL, popliteus, ± LCL)	(PFL, popliteus, LCL, ± PCL)
CLINICAL FEATURES	pain, occasional instability	pain, frequent giving way, ± varus thrust gait	pain, frequent giving way, varus thrust gait, hyperextension
MANAGEMENT	**usually nonoperative**	**operative** *except* **in very low demand patients**	**operative in ambulatory patient**

*Rotational instability measured in degrees of rotation *in excess of contralateral limb*.

posterolateral structures will present with varus when tested at 30°. A large degree of varus instability, especially in full extension usually indicates combined injuries to the LCL, posterolateral structures, the PCL, and possibly the ACL. The diagnosis of knee dislocation should be entertained. The prone tibial external rotation test, or 'dial' test (Figure 17.4) is performed at 30° and 90° as well, and compared to the contralateral side (Veltri and Warren, 1993). Isolated injury to the posterolateral structures will be most evident at low flexion angles, while increased external rotation at both 30° and 90° suggests instability secondary to injury to the PCL and posterolateral corner. We consider a 10° difference between sides to be suggestive of instability. We palpate both tibial plateaus during the maneuver to differentiate between rotation occurring with posterior translation of the lateral tibial plateau versus anterior translation of the medial tibial plateau, which is caused by medial subluxation and not posterolateral instability. Again, the reader is cautioned that combined injury to the ACL and posterolateral corner may not manifest with increased external rotation with the dial test. In any patient with a reasonable mechanism and an increased anterior drawer, the surgeon must maintain a high suspicion of PLC injury; for an isolated ACL reconstruction is likely to fail in this setting (O'Brien *et al.*, 1991) (Figure 17.4).

Fig. 17.4

The prone tibial external rotation test is performed at both 30° and 90° of knee flexion. Side to side increase of more than 10° of external rotation at 30° of flexion, but not at 90° is indicative of an isolated posterolateral corner injury. Reprinted with permission from MacGillivray JD and Warren RF, Treatment of acute and chronic injuries to the posterolateral and lateral knee. *Operative Tech Sports Med* 1999.

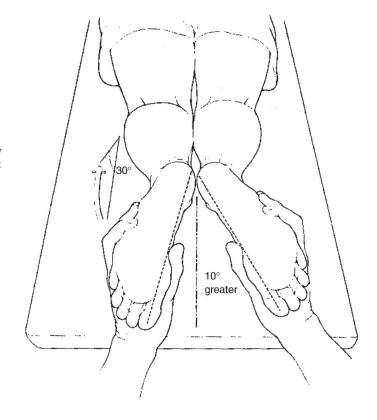

The external-rotation recurvatum test (Hughston and Norwood, 1980), posterolateral drawer test (Hughston and Norwood, 1980), and reverse pivot-shift tests are less specific, but routinely employed to confirm the suspected diagnosis of posterolateral and cruciate injury. For the external rotation recurvatum test, we grasp the great toes on the supine patient and lift them from the examining table. Relative hyperextension and external rotation with apparent tibia vara on the affected side is an indicator of posterolateral instability. During the posterolateral drawer test, the supine patient's hip is flexed 45°, the knee flexed 80°, and the foot firmly planted on the examination table in 15° of external rotation. A posterior drawer force is applied, and the test considered positive for posterolateral laxity if a significant amount of external rotation of the tibial plateau with reference to the tibia is obtained. The reverse pivot shift test is performed by bringing the 90° flexed knee into 0° of extension while a valgus stress and external rotatory moment are applied to the tibia. Because the PCL- or posterolateral corner-deficient knee will be subluxated posteriorly in flexion, the examiner will note a palpable shift or jerk as the iliotibial band shifts forward of the knee center of rotation in extension, reducing the posterior subluxation. LaPrade and Terry (1997) noted in their clinical series that the reverse pivot shift test correlated with injury to the LCL, popliteal complex, and lateral capsular ligament. Isolated PCL injury, without damage to the posterolateral structures, will not cause a reverse pivot shift on examination.

Historically, injuries to the posterolateral corner have been graded as mild (grade I), moderate (grade II) and severe (grade III); this grading was based on the physical examination. Due to the complexity of possible injury patterns to this region, this classification can not be used to accurately guide operative management or predict functional outcome. At our institution, we have implemented a descriptive anatomic and functional grading scheme. Criteria for grading include combined assessment of posterolateral rotational instability (dial test) and instability to varus rotation (Table 17.1).

Treatment

Historically, there have been several procedures described for the treatment of posterolateral instability. Baker and colleagues (1983, 1984) performed primary repair of injured structures. When poor tissue quality made primary repair impossible, they advocated advancement of the arcuate ligament, a technique also employed by Hughston and Jacobson (1985). Clancy et al. (1983) advocated rerouting the biceps to the lateral epicondyle, leaving its distal insertion intact. This technique was validated in a cadaver model by Wascher and associates (Wascher et al., 1993), who found that this tenodesis restored stability to varus and external rotation moments equal to that of the intact knee. Noyes and Barber-Westin (1995) reported a 76 per cent success rate with allograft reconstruction of the LCL and posterolateral structures in patients with insufficient or severely attenuated tissues. They describe a 'more simplified' proximal advancement procedure for patients with structurally intact ligaments that were lax (Noyes and Barber-Westin, 1996a). Although there was a 9 per cent failure rate, 91 per cent of the reconstructions were at least partially functional. Albright and Brown (1998) described the creation of a sling from the posterolateral tibia to the isometric point of the lateral femur. The procedure eliminated posterolateral rotational instability and the reverse pivot shift and reduced varus laxity and hyperextension in 87 per cent of patients.

Noyes and Barber-Westin (1996b) and Latimer and associates (Latimer *et al.*, 1998) both reported success following a complex ligament reconstruction using autograft and allograft tissues to repair the injured posterolateral knee. Based on the biomechanical and anatomic studies performed at our institution, we prefer to anatomically reestablish the essential supporting structures of the posterolateral knee (LCL, popliteus tendon, and popliteofibular ligament). In acute cases, we attempt to repair or augment damaged tissues. In chronic cases, or acute cases with severe tissue destruction, we reconstruct these structures. It should be noted that in all cases (acute and chronic), the complex reconstruction of multiple ligaments requires the best possible environment for healing. The senior author mandates that smokers avoid nicotine throughout the perioperative period.

Acute posterolateral instability

Arthroscopic and surgical evaluation, with reconstruction of the cruciates

When possible, it is preferable to address posterolateral instability in the acute setting. After a 2–3 week period, scarring, attenuation of tissues, and disrupted anatomy will make primary repair of injured structures difficult or impossible, and the surgeon must consider reconstructive options. We have developed a treatment algorithm for acute posterolateral injury (see Figure 17.5). The sequence of reconstruction progresses as follows: PCL > ACL > MCL > popliteus/ PFL > LCL > others (iliotibial band, extensor mechanism repair, etc.) We routinely begin the surgical phase of treatment with a comprehensive arthroscopy; gravity distention or a pump may be used. However, the surgeon must be aware of the possibility of an iatrogenic compartment syndrome caused by the penetration of arthroscopy fluid into the lower leg through the disrupted knee joint capsule. Concomitant chondral injury at the patellofemoral, medial or lateral tibiofemoral joints is addressed, meniscal injuries evaluated and treated, and the intraarticular portion of the popliteus evaluated. Not uncommonly, the popliteofibular ligament origin at the tendon can be identified and both the popliteus and PFL checked for subtle laxity with provocative anterior-posterior translation and rotation. The degree of varus instability is checked at 0° and 30° and quantified in millimeters using the arthroscopic probe. A comprehensive pre-repair/reconstruction evaluation can be used to intraoperatively assess the surgical result.

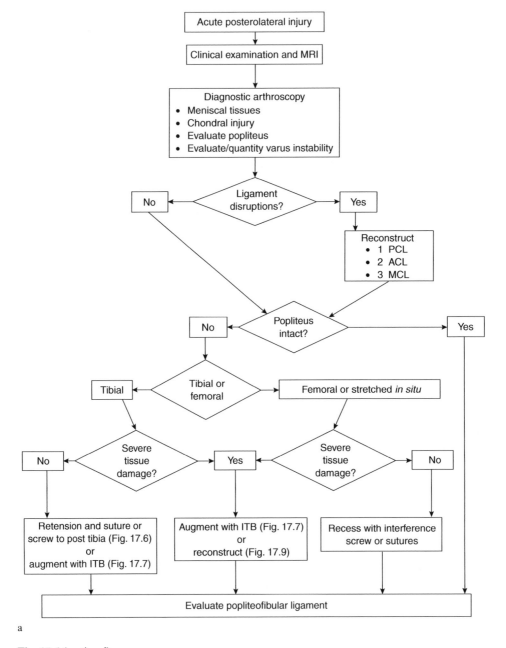

a

Fig. 17.5 (*continued*)

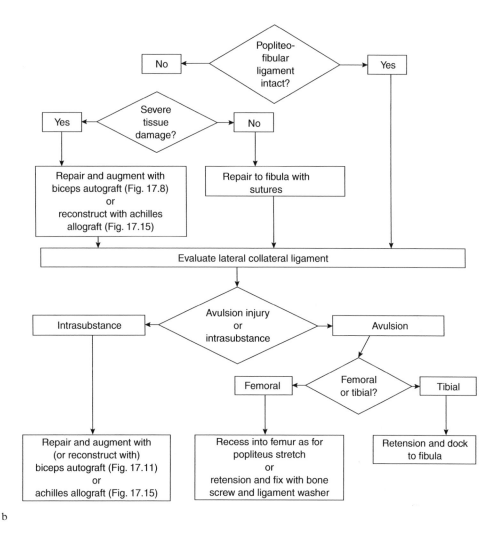

b

Fig. 17.5

Treatment algorithm for acute posterolateral knee instability.

Next, tears of the ACL and/or PCL are reconstructed using arthroscopically-assisted techniques. The ACL is reconstructed following the PCL, and then attention is turned to the posterolateral corner. The posterolateral structures are exposed through a curvilinear incision beginning midway between the tibial tubercle and the fibular head, and curves proximal and posteriorly toward the dorsal edge of the iliotibial band. As the dissection continues, we sequentially examine the ITB, biceps insertion, peroneal nerve, LCL, the popliteus, and the PFL. In severe injuries, a complete split down to the joint may be noted after skin incision, indicating injury to all of the above structures. The peroneal nerve is routinely explored proximally and distally, and if hematoma is present the epineurium is released.

The open lateral dissection begins between the internervous plane in layer I between the biceps and iliotibial band, so that the ITB can be retracted anteriorly. If necessary for exposure, the ITB

285

can be split 5 cm along the length of its fibers at the level of the lateral femoral epicondyle. This allows a 5 cm wide strip to be retracted anteriorly and posteriorly to facilitate the exposure.

As layer II is incomplete posteriorly, the dissection continues through the superficial lamina of the posterior capsule (layer III), just posterior the LCL, which is evaluated at this time. The window in the superficial lamina allows for examination of the posterolateral joint capsule and the popliteus tendon. This tendon is followed proximally to ensure that its femoral insertion is intact, and then attention is turned distally toward the musculotendinous junction (where the PFL originates) and the popliteus origin on the posterior tibia. With the entire extent of the popliteus/PFL and its injury visible, surgical options are considered.

Repair and augmentation of the popliteus tendon and popliteofibular ligament

If the popliteus tendon tissue is not severely attenuated, and its femoral insertion intact, it can be retensioned and attached statically to the posterior tibia. Sutures are placed in the tendon proximal to the injury and the tibial attachment, and either brought through

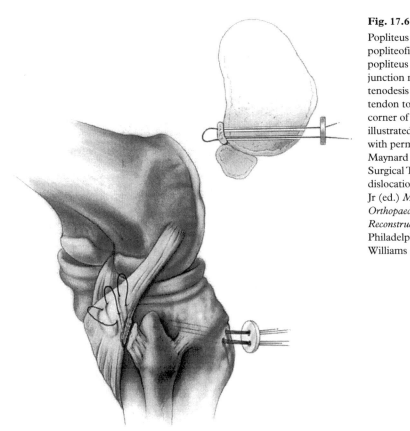

Fig. 17.6

Popliteus tendon injury at the popliteofibular ligament or popliteus muscle-tendon junction may be treated with tenodesis of the popliteus tendon to the posterior lateral corner of the tibia, as illustrated above. Reprinted with permission from Maynard MJ and Warren RF. Surgical Technique for knee dislocation. In RC Thompson Jr (ed.) *Master Techniques in Orthopaedic Surgery: Reconstructive knee surgery.* Philadelphia: Lippincott Williams & Wilkins; 1995.

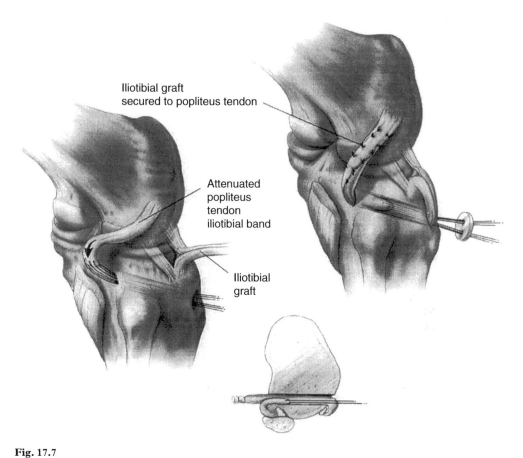

Iliotibial graft
secured to popliteus tendon

Attenuated
popliteus
tendon
iliotibial band

Iliotibial
graft

Fig. 17.7

Technique for popliteus tendon augmentation using an iliotibial band autograft. Reprinted with permission from Maynard MJ and Warren RF, Surgical technique for knee dislocation. In RC Thompson Jr (ed.) *Master Techniques in Orthopaedic Surgery: Reconstructive knee surgery*. Philadelphia: Lippincott Williams & Wilkins; 1995.

posterior to anterior drill holes in the tibia and tensioned, or tensioned and reattached using a 6.5 mm cancellous bone screw and ligament washer (Figure 17.6). The tibial site is first prepared using a burr or rongeur down to bleeding bone, and the foot internally rotated during tensioning and fixation. If the popliteofibular ligament is disrupted at its attachment site to the fibula, this can be primarily repaired using sutures securing the PFL to a posterior to anterior bone tunnel in the posterior fibula. With severe injuries and marked attenuation of the popliteus or popliteofibular ligament tissue, augmentation is mandatory (Figure 17.7). We prefer to harvest a 2 cm strip of iliotibial tract from the anterior aspect of the posterior band. This long autograft is left attached at Gerdy's tubercle distally, and a tunnel is drilled from the anterolateral aspect of the tibia to the tibial attachment site of the popliteus utilizing the ACL guide and reamers. The ITB graft is then brought from anterior to posterior through the tunnel and the sutures securing the attenuated popliteus brought reciprocally from posterior to anterior. The attenuated ligament is tensioned and secured to a ligament button at the anterior tibia, and the autograft oversewn to the native popliteus tendon from tunnel to femoral insertion. Augmentation of the PFL is

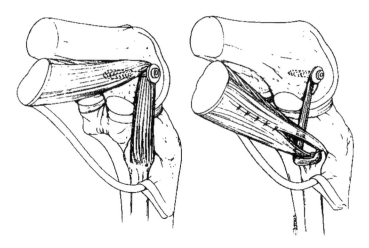

Fig. 17.8

The method of posterolateral corner reconstruction as first described by Clancy *et al.* (1983) (left). We prefer to reconstruct the popliteofibular ligament anatomically with the central slip of the biceps tendon (right). Reprinted with permission from Veltri DM, Warren RF, Operative treatment of posterolateral instability of the knee. *Clin Sports Med* 1994; 13(3): 615–627.

performed using a slip of biceps autograft (Figure 17.8). The central third of the biceps insertion is left intact on the fibula and harvested proximally for approximately 12 cm and incised. This graft is then tubularized using sutures and routed behind the remaining posterior third of biceps insertion and sutured using anchors to the posterior fibula, which is closer to the anatomic insertion site of the PFL. The autograft is then swung proximally to the anatomic insertion of the popliteus, just anterior to the lateral epicondyle in the femoral sulcus. We routinely confirm the isometry of the graft by passing the graft over a K-wire drilled at the intended insertion point (approximately 25 mm proximal to the joint line with the knee at 30° of flexion), and mark the point where the graft passes over the wire with methylene blue. The knee is then cycled from flexion to extension, and the K-wire repositioned to the point at which minimal graft excursion develops with knee motion. When an acceptable insertion point is identified, the graft is secured using a screw and ligament washer. The graft can be sutured to the native popliteus tendon as reinforcement. Care must be taken during all aspects of the augmentation to be sure the grafts to not compress the peroneal nerve.

When the popliteus complex is stretched in continuity, or the femoral attachment has been avulsed, it can be recessed under tension. It is imperative that distal injury at the level of the fibular and tibial origins does not exist, or the recession will not function. If stretched, but not avulsed, the author will harvest the femoral insertion with an attached bone plug. A reinforcing Bunnell or Krackow stitch is used to tension the proximal tendon, and is passed through a lateral to medial femoral tunnel at the insertion site. Fixation is achieved by tying the sutures over a ligament button and or using a bioabsorbable interference screw. The PFL can be reconstructed as previously described, or can be retensioned with the LCL by performing a fibular osteotomy, and advancing the fibular head distally, securing it with an intramedullary cancellous screw (Figures 17.6, 17.7, and 17.8).

If there is an injury to the ITB and biceps tendon, or if poor tissue quality is noted in the popliteus complex (i.e. PFL, popliteus muscle) these structural elements must then be reconstructed using a split Achilles tendon allograft (Figure 17.9). The posterior to anterior tunnel for the tibial insertion of the popliteus is made using an ACL guide positioned 2 cm below and parallel to the joint line, where the popliteus crosses the posterior part of the tibia. This tunnel is sized to admit the popliteus limb of the graft. A second tunnel is made transversely across the fibula just distal and posterior to the fibular styloid. Using these tunnels, the isometric point on the femur is located using a K-wire isometer. The site for the femoral tunnel is located near the sulcus, on the anterior half of the lateral femoral epicondyle, about 5 mm anterior to the femoral origin of the LCL. A 12 mm lateral to medial tunnel is created at the isometric point, and the Achilles bone block is introduced and fixed with a 7 mm interference screw. With the tibia in neutral rotation, the popliteus limb of the graft is passed through the tibial tunnel and secured using an interference screw or ligament button and sutures. The popliteofibular limb is brought through the fibular tunnel from posterior to anterior and secured to itself proximally. The popliteus and popliteofibular limbs are then tenodesed together from the level of the femoral tunnel to just above the joint line (Figure 17.9).

Fig. 17.9

Reconstruction of the popliteus and popliteofibular ligaments using a split Achilles tendon autograft. Reprinted with permission from MacGillivray JD and Warren RF, Treatment of acute and chronic injuries to the posterolateral and lateral knee. *Operative Tech Sports Med* 1999.

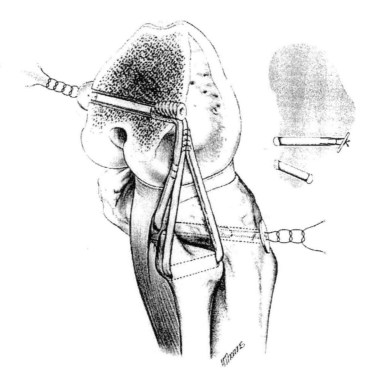

Repair and augmentation of the lateral collateral ligament

Injury to the LCL can occur within its substance or at the bony attachments. For avulsion type injuries, the torn ligament is isolated and prepared using Bunnell and Thompson sutures for retensioning. For femoral avulsions, the ligament is recessed using the technique described above for popliteus repair. Alternatively, the ligament can be retensioned and fixed isometrically using a bone screw and ligament washer. Distal avulsions are similarly prepared with sutures, and the fibular attachment achieved through a docking technique (Figure 17.10). A shallow bone tunnel is made at the fibular footprint of the LCL, and two small drill holes are continued distally to the fibular neck. The LCL is docked into the blind fibular tunnel and tensioned using the draw sutures which are tied over the bone bridge.

Intrasubstance attenuation of the LCL must be tensioned and repaired as above, or augmented. We prefer to augment the repair using the central slip of the biceps tendon (Figure 17.11). The central third of biceps tendon is harvested as described above for

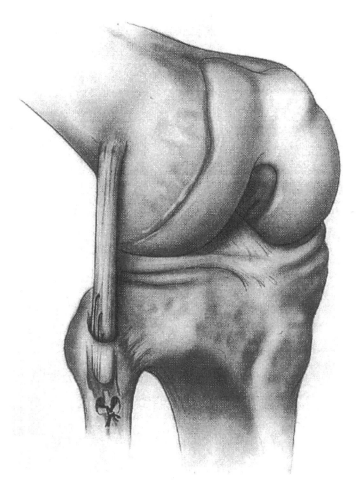

Fig. 17.10

Repair of a fibular avulsion of the LCL. Reprinted with permission from Maynard MJ and Warren RF, Surgical technique for knee dislocation. In RC Thompson Jr (ed.) *Master Techniques in Orthopaedic Surgery: Reconstructive knee surgery.* Philadelphia: Lippincott Williams & Wilkins; 1995.

Fig. 17.11

Technique for LCL reconstruction using the central slip of the biceps tendon. Note the technique of using a K-wire isometer to confirm the position of the femoral insertion prior to fixation (right). Reprinted with permission from Bowen MK, Warren RF, Cooper DE, Posterior cruciate ligament and related injuries. In J Insall (ed.) *Surgery of the Knee*, 2nd edn. New York, NY, Churchill Livingstone, 1993, pp. 505–554.

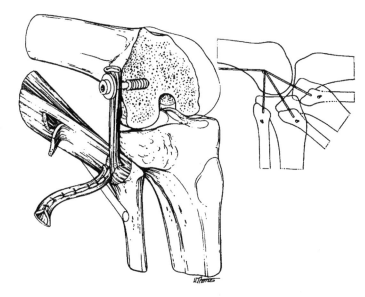

popliteofibular ligament augmentation (Figure 17.8). This slip is not rerouted, however, as the LCL and biceps insertions are relatively close on the fibula. The graft is brought proximally to the lateral femoral epicondyle, where the isometric point is established as described above and the graft fixed using a 6.5 mm cancellous bone screw and ligament washer. If the tissues are severely attenuated, or the ITB and biceps injured, the author recommends using the techniques described below for the reconstruction of chronic LCL injuries.

Chronic posterolateral instability

Reconstruction of the chronic posterolateral corner insuffiency represents a clinical challenge. We have previously mentioned poor tissue quality and altered anatomy as potential complicating factors that may make the treatment of PLC injuries more difficult. Many patients will present after having undergone one or more failed procedures for the treatment of PLC insufficiency (O'Brien *et al.*, 1991, Noyes and Barber-Westin, 1996a). As a result, autograft availability and bone stock may be compromised. Chronic disuse, functional deconditioning, abnormal hyperextension moments, varus malignment or a lateral thrust gait will result in abnormally high loads being transmitted to posterolateral complext reconstructions; these issues must be addressed in the surgical plan. Still, some patients may present suffering from the sequelae of longstanding PCL and posterolateral complex instability, with pain, osteoarthrosis, and radiographic changes in as little as four years following injury (Clancy *et al.*, 1983). In a cadaveric model, Skyhar and associates (Skyhar *et al.*, 1993) were able to demonstrate increased patellofemoral pressures and quadriceps load following PCL and posterolateral complex sectioning. Medial tibiofemoral compartment pressures increased after isolated PCL sectioning. In advanced cases, patients must be given realistic expectations for surgical outcome, and may not be surgical candidates at all.

Valgus osteotomy and posterolateral advancement

We have developed a treatment algorithm for chronic posterolateral instability (Figure 17.12). In the patient with chronic posterolateral

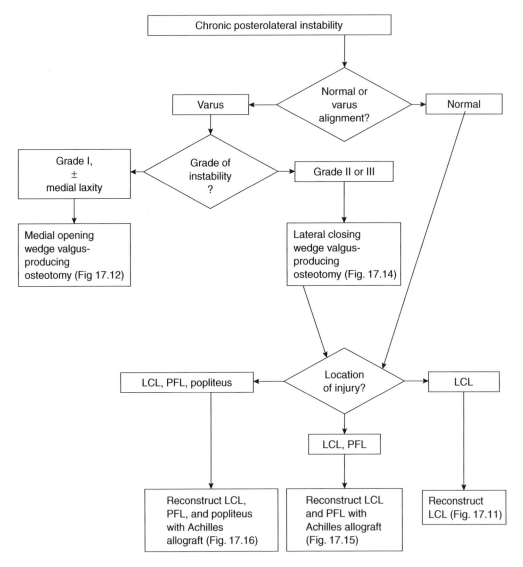

Fig. 17.12

Treatment algorithm for chronic posterolateral knee instability.

instability, varus alignment must be addressed prior to or during the surgical reconstruction of the posterolateral structures. Some patients, particularly those whose primary complaints may be related to medial tibiofemoral arthrosis, may obtain relief from osteotomy alone. It is prudent, however, to perform a diagnostic arthroscopy prior to beginning the corrective osteotomy for diagnostic purposes. The status of the ACL, PCL, popliteus tendon complex, patellofemoral and tibiofemoral compartments can be directly evaluated, and the degree of varus instability can be quantified as described above.

We have corrected angular deformities using both medial opening-wedge and lateral closing wedge valgus producing osteotomies. In persons with varus angulation with or without associated medial laxity and mild posterolateral rotational instability, we prefer an medial opening-wedge osteotomy to restore tension to the medial side of the knee (Figure 17.13). This procedure can be performed via a midline parapatellar or medial incision, using a specialized plate or external fixation system. Frequently, no posterolateral reconstruction is required, and the avoidance of a lateral closing wedge does not further destabilize the posterolateral structures.

Patients who suffer from moderate to severe varus are candidates for a laterally based, closing-wedge proximal tibial osteotomy. We favor a lateral incision through which immediate or delayed posterolateral reconstruction can be performed as well (Figure 17.14). The iliotibial band (ITB) is isolated from anterior to posterior down to its insertion at Gerdy's tubercle. A 2 cm × 2 cm bone block is prepared, drilled, and pretapped for fixation with a 6.5 mm cancellous bone screw. Next, the bone block is elevated with the attached ITB using an oscillating saw, and the proximal tibial valgus-producing osteotomy performed. The bone block/ITB complex is then secured distally on the tibia using a 6.5 mm cancellous screw after fixation of the osteotomy with a specialized plate. Care is taken not to disrupt the proximal tibiofibular joint so as not to further add to the posterolateral laxity.

If the patient and surgeon elected to perform a concurrent posterolateral procedure, attention is turned next to reconstruction of the PCL and ACL, if indicated, using patellar autograft, or more commonly allograft. When the cruciates are functional, attention is turned back to the lateral knee, which is exposed as described above for acute management, the peroneal nerve explored and protected, and the popliteus, popliteofibular ligament, and LCL explored.

Reconstruction of the popliteus tendon and popliteofibular ligament

When laxity is mild and the tissues are of good quality, it is always the author's preference to attempt recession and augmentation of the existing popliteus and popliteofibular ligament as described above. However, with chronic injuries, usually a reconstruction is

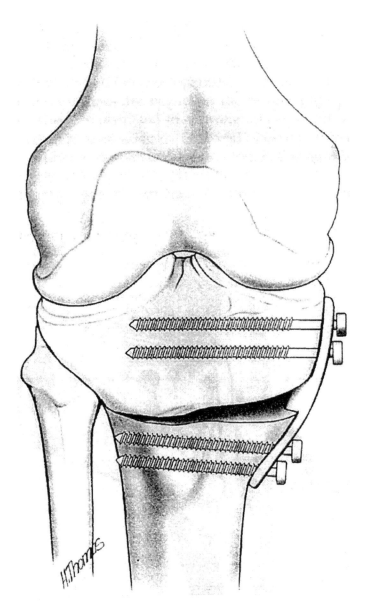

Fig. 17.13
In a varus knee with mild
posterolateral rotatory
instability and associated
medial laxity, a medial
valgus-producing proximal
tibial osteotomy restores
tension to the medial side of
the knee and corrects angular
alignment. Reprinted with
permission from MacGillivray
JD and Warren RF, Treatment
of acute and chronic injuries
to the posterolateral and
lateral knee. *Operative Tech
Sports Med* 1999.

warranted. It is possible to reconstruct using a patellar tendon
autograft, but we find that Achilles allograft provides a forgiving
alternative in terms of overall graft length and availability.

For grade II posterolateral instability, the popliteus tendon may be
left intact, with disruption of the LCL and popliteofibular ligament
(Figure 17.15). The femoral and popliteofibular insertions are created as described above for acute reconstruction of the popliteofibular ligament. Care must be exercised to protect the peroneal nerve.
When the appropriate isometric femoral attachment is identified, a
lateral to medial femoral tunnel is drilled to accommodate an achilles

Fig. 17.14

A lateral valgus-producing proximal tibial osteotomy is performed in the patient with moderate or severe posterolateral instability and varus alignment. The iliotibial band is removed with its insertion on a bone block and advanced across the ostoetomy site. Reprinted with permission from MacGillivray JD and Warren RF, Treatment of acute and chronic injuries to the posterolateral and lateral knee. *Operative Tech Sports Med* 1999.

Fig. 17.15

Reconstruction of the popliteofibular ligament and lateral collateral ligament in a patient with Grade II chronic posterolateral corner instability. The popliteus tendon is intact. Reprinted with permission from MacGillivray JD and Warren RF, Treatment of acute and chronic injuries to the posterolateral and lateral knee. *Operative Tech Sports Med* 1999.

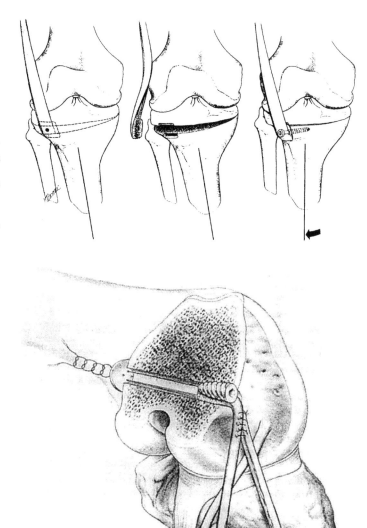

allograft bone plug. The plug is secured in the femoral tunnel using an interference screw and/or sutures and a ligament button. Next, the graft is drawn from posterior to anterior through the fibular tunnel (to recreate the popliteofibular ligament), tensioned, and then brought superiorly and sewn back upon itself (to recreate the LCL).

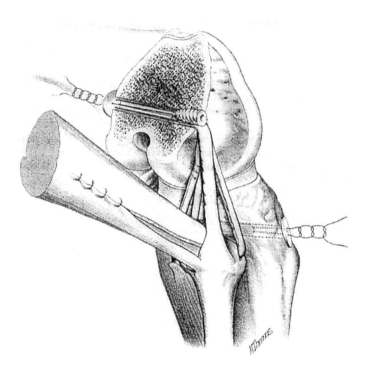

Fig. 17.16
Severe, chronic (Grade III) posterolateral corner instability. Reconstruction of the popliteus and popliteofibular ligament using a split Achilles tendon allograft with reconstruction of the LCL using the central slip of the biceps tendon. Reprinted with permission from MacGillivray JD and Warren RF, Treatment of acute and chronic injuries to the posterolateral and lateral knee. *Operative Tech Sports Med* 1999.

For severe posterolateral instability patterns (Grade III), reconstruction of the popliteus, popliteofibular ligament, and LCL is often required (Figure 17.16). For reconstruction of the popliteus and popliteofibular ligament, the Achilles or patellar graft should be split at the end opposite the larger bone plug and two separate limbs fashioned and tubularized using sutures. Achilles allograft affords the surgeon more flexibility both in the size of the bone plug and the individual limb diameter and length. An anterior to posterolateral tibial tunnel is created using an ACL guide as described above for popliteus augmentation, and the posterior to anterior fibular tunnel is created for popliteofibular reconstruction. Next, the bone plug is drawn into the femoral tunnel and secured using an interference screw and/or sutures and a ligament button. With the limb in neutral rotation, each limb is then tensioned and provisionally secured in the tibial or fibular tunnel by clamping the graft or sutures at the distal tunnel aperture. Rotatory stability of the knee is then confirmed at both 30° and 90°. The popliteus limb can then be definitively secured in the tibial tunnel using an interference screw, sutures and ligament button, or tenodesed using a cancellous bone screw and ligament washer. The popliteofibular limb is drawn through the fibular tunnel, tensioned, and sewn back upon istelf as described above.

Reconstruction of the lateral collateral ligament

The chronically attenuated LCL can usually be recessed and augmented with the biceps tendon as described above for acute injury (Figure 17.10). If the condition of the biceps tendon tissue precludes augmentation or reconstruction, patellar tendon autograft or Achilles allograft can be used to reconstruct the LCL. After exploration and protection of the peroneal nerve, a blind tunnel is fashioned atop the fibula into which the graft bone plug will be docked. This graft can be secured using sutures through two smaller tunnels exiting on the fibular neck, and tied over a bone bridge, or secured using an interference screw. The femoral attachment of the LCL reconstruction is identified using a K-wire isometer, as described above. Once an acceptable position is identified, the K-wire is over-reamed, the graft passed using sutures, and secured using an interference screw or ligament button.

Postoperative rehabilitation

In both acute and chronic posterolateral procedures, the postoperative program must first protect the repair from undue repetitive stretching and loading, but maintain motion to avoid stiffness. We place our patients on a continuous passive motion program beginning on the first postoperative day. Patients are kept non weight-bearing with crutches in a full-leg hinged knee brace locked in extension for six weeks. Care is taken to be sure the brace is well-fitted, and hyperextension and varus moments are avoided at all costs. A supervised active-assisted range of motion exercises are begun in the hospital on the second postoperative day and the patient is instructed to continue these exercises at home, and supervised in formal physical therapy as well. In the earliest postoperative weeks, return to full extension is encouraged, but bridging exercises (which create a hyperextension moment) or passive manipulation into hyperextension is avoided. The patient is advanced to partial weight-bearing from 6 to 8 weeks. After that time, as the supervised patient regains muscle control and gait normalizes, the brace is unlocked and full weight-bearing is allowed. A more normal gait is usually achieved and assistive devices no longer necessary within 12 to 16 weeks. Bracing is continued and active hamstring strengthening avoided for six months. Running is delayed for about nine months to one year, at which time athletics can be resumed if the patient desires.

Summary

Posterolateral instability usually accompanies a constellation issues for the surgeon. Concomitant injuries to neurovascular structures, the cruciate ligaments, and other supporting structures about the knee must be diagnosed and addressed. The complex anatomy and biomechanical function of the posterolateral corner, combined with associated instability patterns can make diagnosis challenging, and if posterolateral injuries are missed, they will preclude the success of other reconstructive efforts (O'Brien *et al.*, 1991, Noyes and Barber-Westin, 1996a). The treatment of these injuries in the acute period often involves primary anatomic repair with or without recession and augmentation. Biomechanical selective ligament-cutting studies have led the authors to favor the anatomic reconstitution of the posterolateral corner, concentrating on the popliteus, popliteofibular ligament, and lateral collateral ligament following cruciate reconstruction (Gollehon *et al.*, 1987, Marshall *et al.*, 1978, Shahane *et al.*, 1999, Veltri and Warren, 1993, 1994a, b, 1995, Veltri *et al.*, 1995a, b, Watanabe *et al.*, 1993). The reported results of reconstructive efforts in the acute period appear to be more favorable (Baker *et al.*, 1983, 1984).

Many patients will present with the correct diagnosis missed or ignored, having undergone previous failed procedures. The reconstruction of chronic posterolateral instability patterns is exponentially more complex. Patients may suffer from the pain, deformity, arthrosis, and other sequelae associated with longstanding instability (Clancy *et al.*, 1983, Skyhar *et al.*, 1993). Varus deformity must be addressed prior to or during reconstructive efforts. Frequently tissues are badly attenuated or absent, requiring reconstruction with allografts rather than recession or augmentation. However, the authors still favor an anatomic approach to restore stability to the posterolateral corner of the knee, and excellent results can be obtained.

Acknowledgements

The authors wish to thank Daniel M. Veltri MD and John D. Macgillivray MD for their previous work on the subject and guidance in preparing this chapter.

References

Albright JP and Brown AW (1998). Management of chronic posterolateral rotatory instability of the knee: Surgical technique for the posterolateral corner sling procedure. *Instr Course Lect*, 47, 369–378.

Baker CL, Norwood LA and Hughston JC (1983). Acute posterolateral rotatory instability of the knee. *J Bone Joint Surg*, 65-A, 614–618.

Baker CL, Norwood LA and Hughston JC (1984). Acute combined posterior cruciate and posterolateral instability of the knee. *Am J Sports Med*, 12, 204–208.

Clancy WG, Shelbourne KD, Zoellner GB, *et al.* (1983). Treatment of knee joint instability secondary to rupture of the posterior cruciate ligament. Report of a new procedure. *J Bone Joint Surg (Am)*, 65-A, 310–322.

Fleming RE, Blatz DJ and McCarroll JR (1981). Posterior problems in the knee: Posterior cruciate insufficiency and posterolateral rotatory insufficiency. *Am J Sports Med*, 9, 107–113.

Fukubayashi T, Torzilli PA, Sherman MF, *et al.* (1982). An in vitro biomechanical evaluation of anterior-posterior motion in the knee. *J Bone Joint Surg*, 64-A.

Gollehon DL, Torzilli PA and Warren RF (1987). The role of the postero-lateral and cruciate ligaments in the stability of the human knee. *J Bone Joint Surg*, 69-A, 233–242.

Grood ES, Noyes FR, Butler DL, *et al.* (1981). Ligamentous and capsular restraints preventing straight medial and lateral laxity in intact human cadaver knees. *J Bone Joint Surg (Am)*, 63-A, 1257–1269.

Grood ES, Stowers SF and Noyes FR (1988). Limits of movement in the human knee: Effect of sectioning the posterior cruciate ligament and posterolateral structures. *J Bone Joint Surg*, 69A, 233–242.

Hughston JC and Jacobson KE (1985). Chronic posterolateral rotatory instability of the knee. *J Bone Joint Surg*, 67A, 351–359.

Hughston JC and Norwood LAJ (1980). The posterolateral drawer test and external rotational recurvatum test for posterolateral rotatory instability of the knee. *Clin Orthop*, 147, 82–87.

LaPrade RF and Terry GC (1997). Injuries to the posterolateral aspect of the knee. Association of anatomic injury patterns with clinical insta-bility. *Am J Sports Med*, 25, 433–438.

Latimer HA, Tibone JE, ElAttrache NS, *et al.* (1998). Reconstruction of the lateral collateral ligament of the knee with patellar tendon allo-graft. Report of a new technique in combined ligament injuries. *Am J Sports Med*, 26, 656–662.

Lovejoy J and Harden T (1970). Popliteus muscle in man. *Anat Rec*, 169, 727–730.

MacGillivray JD and Warren RF (1999). Treatment of acute and chronic injuries to the posterolateral and lateral knee. *Operative Tech Sports Med.*

Markolf KL, Wascher DC and Finerman GA (1993). Direct in vitro mea-surement of forces in the cruciate ligaments: Part II. The effect of sec-tion of the posterolateral structures. *J Bone Joint Surg*, 70A, 88–97.

Marshall JL, Girgis FG and Zelko RR (1978). The biceps femoris tendon and its functional significance. *J Bone Joint Surg (Am)*, 66-A, 1444.

Maynard MJ, Deng X, Wickiewicz TL, *et al.* (1996). The popliteofibular ligament. Rediscovery of a key element in posterolateral instability. *Am J Sports Med*, 24, 311–316.

Maynard MJ and Warren RF (1995). Surgical technique for knee disloca-tion. *Master techniques in Orthopaedic Surgery: Reconstructive knee surgery.*

Nielsen S and Helmig P (1986). The static stabilizing function of the popliteal tendon in the knee: An experimental study. *Arch Orthop Trauma Surg*, 104, 357–362.

Noyes FR and Barber-Westin SD (1995). Surgical reconstruction of severe chronic posterolateral complex injuries of the knee using allograft tis-sues. *Am J Sports Med*, 23, 2–12.

Noyes FR and Barber-Westin SD (1996). Surgical restoration to treat chronic deficiency of the posterolateral complex and cruciate liga-ments of the knee joint. *Am J Sports Med*, 24, 415–426.

Noyes FR and Barber-Westin SD (1996). Treatment of complex injuries of the knee using allograft tissues. *Am J Sports Med*, 9, 200–214.

O'Brien SJ, Warren RF and Pavlov H (1991). Reconstruction of the chron-ically insufficient anterior cruciate ligament with the central third of the patellar tendon. *J Bone Joint Surg*, 73-A, 278–286.

Seebacher JR, Inglis AE, Marshall JL, *et al.* (1982). The structure of the posterolateral aspect of the knee. *J Bone Joint Surg*, 64-A, 537–541.

Shahane SA, Ibbotson C, Strachan R, *et al.* (1999). The popliteofubular ligament. *J Bone Joint Surg*, 81-B, 636–642.

Sidles JA, Larson RV, Garbini JL, *et al.* (1988). Ligament length relation-ships in the moving knee. *J Orthop Res*, 6, 593–610.

Skyhar MJ, Warren RF, Oritz GJ, *et al.* (1993). The effects of sectioning of the posterior cruciate ligament and the posterolateral complex on the articular contact pressures within the knee. *J Bone Joint Surg*, 75-A, 694–699.

Staubli HU and Birrer S (1990). The popliteus tendon and its fasicles at the popliteal hiatus: Gross anatomy and functional arthroscopic evaluation with and without anterior cruciate ligament deficiency. *Arthroscopy*, 6, 209–220.

Staubli HU and Rauschning W (1991). Popliteus tendon and lateral meniscus. *Am J Knee Surg*, 4, 110–121.

Sudasna S and Harnsiriwattanagit K (1990). The ligamentous structures of the posterolateral aspect of the knee. *Bull Hosp Joint Dis*, 50, 35–40.

Terry GC and LaPrade RF (1996). The biceps femoris muscle complex at the knee: Its anatomy and injury patterns associated with acute anterolateral-anteromedial rotatory subluxation. *Am J Sports Med*, 24, 2.

Veltri DM, Deng X, Torzilli PA, *et al.* (1995). The role of the popliteofibular ligament in stability of the human knee. A biomechanical study. *Am J Sports Med*, 24, 19–27.

Veltri DM, Deng X, Torzilli PA, *et al.* (1995). The role of the cruciate and posterolateral ligaments in stability of the knee. A biomechanical study. *Am J Sports Med*, 23, 336–443.

Veltri DM and Warren RF (1993). Isolated and combined posterior cruciate ligament injuries. *J Am Acad Orthop Surg*, 1, 67–75.

Veltri DM and Warren RF (1994). Anatomy, biomechanics, and physical findings in posterolateral knee instability. *Clin Sports Med*, 13, 599–614.

Veltri DM and Warren RF (1994). Operative treatment of posterolateral instability of the knee. *Clin Sports Med*, 13, 615–627.

Veltri DM and Warren RF (1995). Posterolateral instability of the knee. *Instr Course Lect.*, 44, 441–453.

Wascher DC, Grauer JD and Markolf KL (1993). Biceps tendon tenodesis for posterolateral instability of the knee: An in vitro study. *Am J Sports Med*, 21, 400–406.

Watanabe Y, Moriya H, Takahashi K, *et al.* (1993). Functional anatomy of the posterolateral structures of the knee. *Arthroscopy*, 9, 57–62.

Part 5. Arthritic ACL Deficient Knees

18

Arthritis in the ACL deficient knee: what is the best approach?

Riley J. Williams and David P. Johnson

Introduction

In the USA over 250,000 patients are diagnosed with new anterior cruciate ligament (ACL) tears each year (Johnson and Warner, 1993). Arthroscopic techniques for reconstruction of the ACL have proven very reliable and successful. Early surgical reconstruction is generally advised for the young athletically active individual and for chronic instability in the ACL-deficient knee. Early and accelerated rehabilitation protocols have been successful in achieving an early return to function, work and sport. It has also been associated with a reduction in the incidence of knee stiffness and arthrofibrosis. This has resulted in the surgical option being more appealing to the young active ACL-deficient patient. It is reasonable to conclude that surgical stabilization of the knee would result in less instability, a lower incidence of subsequent meniscal and articular cartilage damage and therefore minimize the incidence of subsequent degenerative change. However, patients presenting with knee joint arthrosis and ACL deficiency remain a common problem and are difficult patients to treat (Miller and Fu, 1993; Noyes et al., 1993).

It has been suggested that the instability associated with the ACL-deficient knee results in an increased risk of meniscal injury (Thompson and Fu, 1993). This might be expected because of the abnormal movement, mechanics and forces experienced by the unstable knee. Although meniscal injury and total meniscectomy are believed to increase the incidence of knee joint arthrosis, the association between anterior cruciate ligament insufficiency and the development of arthritis remains controversial (Fairbank, 1948; Miller and Fu, 1993; O'Brien et al., 1991). None the less it is generally accepted and regarded as best practice that in association with ACL injury, the menisci should be preserved whenever possible to preserve one of the restraints to instability, and to avoid premature degeneration.

The etiology of osteoarthritis of the knee is generally regarded as a result of the abnormal mechanical environment (Phillips and Krackow, 1998). Predisposing pathologic conditions include malalignment, articular cartilage defects, meniscal injury, meniscectomy, avascular necrosis, and ligamentous insufficiency (Allen *et al.*, 1984). In a often quoted study Daniel reported an increased incidence of arthrosis with ACL reconstruction rather than in those patients not undergoing surgery (Daniel *et al.*, 1994). However the technique for ACL reconstruction was that of a ligament augmentation device (LAD) augmentation device which appeared to result in over constraint of the knees and subsequent arthrosis. The study was also an uncontrolled historical study, which does not reflect the experience of most surgeons today. As it is known that meniscal or articular cartilage damage and knee instability is related to premature degeneration, it is reasonable to expect surgical stabilization to reduce the incidence or progression of any such degenerative changes. This is one factor used by the authors in the multifactorial decision to undertake surgical stabilization of a knee.

It has been suggested by various authors that the success of ACL reconstruction is reduced in the presence of a constitutional various deformity or a lateral thrust of the knee on weight-bearing. It has been suggested that the lateral thrust weakens and stretches the ACL graft resulting in late failure. Noyes described these factors as secondary and tertiary varus deformities and reported combined ACL reconstruction and high tibial osteotomy (HTO) in these combined complex cases. He suggested that the deforming forces of a lateral thrust or constitutional varus deformity increased the chance of a failure of the reconstructed ACL and suggested that consideration should be given to correcting the constitutional varus deformity prior to or at the time of ACL reconstruction.

Johnson *et al.* reported a combined technique of extraarticular ACL reconstruction and HTO for patients with ACL instability and medial unicompartmental arthritis. In this study an extraarticular lateral tenodesis ACL reconstruction was used (Johnson, 1996). Although long-term follow-up demonstrated that the knees generally had ACL laxity, most patients had no symptomatic instability and had returned to sporting activities with a successful functional outcome (Johnson, 1996). It was concluded that in the presence of varus deformity and medial degeneration HTO alone resulted in an improvement in the patients symptoms of pain and instability, and that if ACL reconstruction was necessary then an intraarticular hamstring or patellar-tendon technique should be utilized.

Holden *et al.* also described a sub-group of patients less than fifty years old who were treated with high tibial osteotomy for unicompartmental osteoarthritis (OA) (Holden *et al.*, 1988), with coexisting ACL laxity. The primary problem of this group of patients was antecedent knee instability and meniscal injury with subsequent medial compartment deterioration.

High tibial osteotomy (HTO) or proximal tibial osteotomy was described by Jackson in 1958 as a means of treating medial unicompartmental arthrosis of the knee joint. Since that time, numerous authors have demonstrated that osteotomies about the knee are an effective means of addressing isolated medial or lateral compartment osteoarthritis (Coventry, 1985; Coventry et al., 1993; Holden et al., 1988; Insall et al., 1984; Matthews et al., 1988; Odenbring et al., 1989; Yasuda et al., 1992). Success rates of 80–90 per cent at five years and 60–70 per cent at 10 years have been reported (Coventry et al., 1993; Ivarsson et al., 1990; Rudan and Simurda, 1991). However many of these studies are historical. Today patient expectations, patient's physical demands and activity levels make tibial osteotomy, with its invasive and extensive nature, subsequent immobilization and prolonged rehabilitation less appealing. This is to some extent reduced by recent modifications of the surgical technique. High tibial osteotomy is used for the treatment of symptomatic medial compartment OA, but it is generally reserved for patients up to 60 years of age who have early degenerative changes and wish to maintain a high-demand lifestyle (Hutchison et al., 1999).

The traditional surgical technique for HTO was that described by Coventry. This included a lateral approach to the tibial plateau and superior tibio-fibular joint. A closing full width wedge excision osteotomy was performed with non-rigid fixation by staples. The problem of disruption and subluxation of the tibio-fibular joint was addressed by others and fibular osteotomy, excision of the tibio-fibular joint, fibular osteotomy or excision of the fibular head was variously used. Puddu and Mohtardi have recently described a new technique using a medial approach, an opening osteotomy and a fixation plate for semi-rigid fixation of the osteotomy (Puddu et al., 1994). This allows a much simpler medial procedure, semi-rigid plate fixation, early mobilization and range of motion exercises.

Patients in which ACL laxity, medial degeneration and HTO generally present in the following common ways:

1   At or soon after the time of injury where ACL laxity is associated with:
    meniscal damage,
    primary varus,
    a lateral thrust,
    articular damage.
2   Late presentation where ACL laxity is associated with:
    further meniscal damage,
    progressive degenerative changes,
    medial pain,
    primary varus deformity,
    a lateral thrust,
    lax secondary lateral restraints.

This review focuses upon the management of symptomatic uni-compartmental degeneration associated with chronic symptomatic anterior cruciate ligament insufficiency.

Pathophysiology

Osteoarthritis is a slowly progressive disorder, which is character-ized, in its early stages, by increased water content and decreased cartilage matrix synthesis. These changes lead to macroscopic lesions (fissuring and focal cartilage loss) (Mankin et al., 1994). Experimental evidence supports the theory that knee malalignment contributes to the development of knee joint arthritis by placing abnormally high stresses upon the articular cartilage of the affected compartment (Phillips and Krackow, 1998; Reimann, 1973; Tetsworth and Paley, 1994; Wu et al., 1990). Thus, clinicians have historically recommended knee osteotomy as means of correcting knee malalignment, reduction in stress through the medial com-partment, slowing the degenerative process, and relieving symptoms associated with unicompartmental OA.

The biomechanical effects of ACL injury may also predispose the knee to degenerative arthritis. Magnetic resonance imaging of acute, ACL injured knees generally reveals a typical bone bruise pattern in the lateral femoral condyle and the lateral tibial plateau (Dimond et al., 1998). In a study by Rangger et al. (1998) the authors demonstrated that bone bruise lesions of the knee were characterized by microfrac-ture of cancellous bone and fragmentation of the overlying hyaline cartilage. The imaging of articular cartilage damage itself, rather than the underlying osseous changes is not clearly defined within the resolution of normal MRI scan sequences. The recurrent femoral-tibial translation ('giving way') episodes, which are charac-teristic of chronic ACL-deficient knees, can also cause this described bone bruise pattern, and may also place unusually high loads upon the articular surfaces of the knee leading to degeneration (Kaplan et al., 1999; Zeiss et al., 1995). The pattern of loading may also be different in ACL laxity with more AP movement, sliding or sheer forces on the articular surface. Articular cartilage is well suited to resist compressive loads, but sheer loads may be more destructive and this may account for the chondral fragmentation often seen in association with chronic ACL laxity.

In addition to causing functional knee instability, acute ACL rup-ture also results in the development of a joint effusion and a local inflammatory response. A number of studies have provided some insight into the biochemical changes which occur following acute knee injury (Dahlberg et al., 1994; Lohmander et al., 1993a, 1993b). Lohmander et al. and Dahlberg et al. analyzed the levels of inflam-matory cytokines, matrix metalloproteases, and cartilage matrix components in the synovium of patients who suffered ACL rupture or meniscal injury (Dahlberg *et al.*, 1994; Lohmander *et al.*, 1993a, b). These authors demonstrated that significant increases in stromelysin (a cartilage degrading metalloprotease), tissue inhibitor of metalloprotease (TIMP), and proteoglycan fragments occur following knee trauma compared to normal, uninjured knees (Dahlberg *et al.*, 1994; Lohmander *et al.*, 1993a, b). The observed increases in protease activity far exceeded those increases noted in TIMP, a natural inhibitor of metalloprotease in the joint space. In another study by Cameron *et al.*, the authors showed that elevated levels of certain inflammatory cytokines (Interleukin 1, Interleukin 6, tumor necrosis factor alpha) and keratan sulfate are present in the synovial fluid from ACL injured knees compared to uninjured knees. These facts suggest that at the time of ACL injury, a biochemical imbalance favoring cartilage catabolism exists within the knee joint. The effect of this has not been defined but may be a significant factor in the degeneration seen in the longer term.

Thus, it appears that those individuals with malaligned, ACL-deficient knees are particularly at risk for developing degenerative arthritis. As such, the clinician should attempt to eliminate both knee instability and to correct the mechanical malalignment to protect the knee from arthritic degeneration. Consideration to preservation of the meniscus and reconstruction of the articular cartilage is addressed by other authors in this volume.

Diagnosis

The initial evaluation of the patient with ACL deficiency and unicompartmental arthritis is dedicated to differentiating between symptoms of instability and symptoms of joint degeneration. However it is also necessary to determine the state of the leg alignment, menisci and secondary restraints.

History

The mechanisms of ACL injury are well described (Johnson and Warner, 1993). The most common symptoms associated with ACL-deficiency include recurrent swelling and repeated episodes of instability ('giving way'), which are typically noted with daily activities or sports. Patients may also complain of vague knee pain (Noyes *et al.*, 1983). True 'giving way' associated with the ACL-deficient knee is due to anterior subluxation of the tibia relative to the femur, and is noted during pivoting, jumping or twisting activities.

A history of previous meniscal injury is common in patients with unicompartmental arthritis and chronic ACL-deficiency. Several authors have shown that a history of medial meniscectomy was present in a majority of patients (60–100 per cent) who were treated for arthritic ACL-deficient knees (Lattermann and Jakob, 1996; O'Neill and James, 1992; Williams *et al.*, 2003; Noyes *et al.*, 1983). These patients tend to present with medial joint line pain and tenderness, varus malalignment, and radiographic evidence of medial compartment degeneration (Miller and Fu, 1993). Isolated lateral compartment arthritis combined with ACL deficiency has also been reported, but occurs less frequently (Phillips and Krackow, 1998; Edgerton *et al.*, 1993). These patients present with lateral joint line tenderness, genu valgum and radiographic changes consistent with lateral compartment osteoarthritis. Patients with early OA complain of pain with high demand activities. These patients usually report significant symptomatic relief from non-steroidal anti-inflammatory drugs, acetaminophen (Bradley *et al.*, 1991) or physical therapy. In contrast, patients who complain of chronic pain, or symptoms with lesser activities (i.e. walking) are likely to suffer from a meniscal tear, moderate to severe cartilage damage and exposed subchondral bone (DeLee and Drez, 1994). It is important to delineate the nature, location and duration of pain symptoms, and the level of activity which precipitates the symptoms.

Functional scoring may be used to evaluate the ACL-deficient patient with arthritis, longitudinally. Functional scores including the International Knee Documentation Committee (IKDC) rating scale, the Hospital for Special Surgery Knee Ligament Form, and the Lysholm and Gillquist Knee Score are typically used to evaluate younger patients who have undergone ligament reconstruction or meniscal surgery (Lysholm and Gillquist, 1982). In contrast, the WOMAC knee rating scale, the Hospital for Special Surgery Knee Score, and the Knee Society clinical rating system were developed to evaluate an older group of patients undergoing osteotomy or total knee replacement for pain associated with joint degeneration (Hefti *et al.*, 1993; Insall *et al.*, 1976, 1989; Roos *et al.*, 1999). One rating scale from each of the aforementioned groups should be used in following this group of patients.

Physical examination

The physical examination is focused, thorough, and should consist of the following assessments: stance, gait, range of motion, ligamentous stability, localization of tenderness, lower extremity alignment and neurological evaluation. Unicompartmental OA is manifest by crepitation, localized joint line tenderness, and joint space narrowing. Ligamentous stability in the coronal plane is assessed in both full extension and thirty degrees of knee flexion. Pseudo-laxity of the medial or lateral collateral ligaments may be noted at physical examination with the application of a valgus or varus force to the knee. The observed joint space opening is due to isolated joint space collapse, and does not normally indicate incompetence of the collateral ligaments. The presence of a firm endpoint confirms that the collateral ligament is functional. This is an important determination in these patients, as a valgus osteotomy in the presence of true medial collateral laxity beyond neutral will lead to symptoms of medial instability. However such pseudo-laxity must be distinguished from the increased and progressive laxity of the lateral structures. Popliteus and posterio-lateral corner which can complicate chronic ACL instability and is a common feature in the presence of a primary varus or a lateral thrust on weight-bearing.

Findings consistent with ACL deficiency are also noted. Patients may demonstrate persistent hyperextension of the knee with ambulation due to ACL deficiency (quadriceps avoidance gait) (Berchuck *et al.*, 1990), the anterior drawer, Lachman test, and pivot shift phenomena. These tests are graded according to established parameters (DeLee and Drez, 1994). These tests are generally reliable, and easily demonstrated in the chronic situation (DeLee and Drez, 1994). In the acute setting, the nature and history of the injury, the Lachman and anterior draw signs, and the presence of a haemarthrosis are important features. It is important to note that in some patients with ACL deficiency and advanced OA, osteophyte formation may result in a decreased or absent pivot shift phenomena.

Imaging studies

Full length (hip-knee-ankle) double stance weight-bearing radiographs are obtained in all ACL-deficient patients in whom osteoarthritis is suspected. Accurate determination of the mechanical and anatomic axes of the normal and affected lower extremities is important for both surgical indication and planning (Coventry, 1985; Fujisawa *et al.*, 1979; Insall *et al.*, 1984). Weight-bearing postero-anterior (40 degrees flexion), weight-bearing antero-posterior, lateral and Merchant's view radiographs of the affected knee are also taken (Merchant *et al.*, 1974; Rosenberg *et al.*, 1988). An assessment of overall alignment is made by determining the radiographic axes of both lower extremities. Radiographic changes consistent with the development of osteoarthritis are noted (osteophytosis, spurring of the tibial spine, joint space narrowing, joint space collapse, loose bodies, and subchondral cyst formation). In the osteoarthritic knee, joint line tenderness should correlate to radiographic joint space degeneration (Buss *et al.*, 1993).

MRI scanning is an important imaging modality. In these knees determination of the integrity of the ACL, PCL and menisci is reliably accurate. Thus the MRI scan is important in determining whether or not an initial arthroscopy is indicated. The imaging of the integrity of the articular surface is more difficult. Proton density, fast spin echo (FSE) and STIR MRI sequences can be helpful. The proton density and FSE sequences are able to some degree to delineate the articular cartilage. However resolution of localized defects remains difficult and inexact. STIR or Fat Saturation Gradient Echo sequences are useful to delineate subchondral increase in signal strength beneath articular cartilage defects and osteoarthritic areas of the knee (Bredella *et al.*, 1999).

Scintigraphy or bone scanning detects an alteration in the equilibrium or homeostatis in the subchondral bone architecture. Thus it is an analysis of the metabolism of the bone not a pictorial depiction of the structure. In this way it may detect early OA in the medial or lateral compartment prior to changes visualized radiographically, on MRI or at arthroscopy (Coventry, 1985; Dieppe *et al.*, 1993). Both scintigraphy and MRI provide helpful information that may aid the clinician in deciding whether to proceed with an osteotomy.

Clinical approach

Based upon their primary symptom, patients with an arthritic, anterior cruciate ligament-deficient knee fall into one of three groups. One group consists of patients for whom the primary symptom is knee instability. These persons tend to report a relatively short history of ACL injury, are active and often wish to continue athletic activities. The second group of patients consists of individuals who complain primarily of knee pain. These patients complain of long-standing progressive pain with activities of daily living in addition to knee instability secondary to chronic ACL deficiency. The third group of patients complain of both pain and instability. These finding have been reported consistently by a several authors (Lattermann and Jakob, 1996; Noyes *et al.*, 1993; Williams *et al.*, 2003).

Upon initial presentation, the authors recommend the utilization of a systematic approach, which includes the use of non-operative treatment methods. Current treatment options include the use of nonsteroidal anti-inflammatory medicine. With the availability of the cyclooxygenase-2 inhibitors (refocoxib and celecoxib), patients may be treated with a daily maintenance dose of oral nonsteroidal anti-inflammatory drug therapy. This decreases the risk of gastrointestinal side effects (Merck and Company, 1999; Searle and Company, 1999). Other metabolic supplements including glucosamine and chondroitin sulfate may prove useful in relieving symptoms in some patients with pain due to osteoarthritis (da Camara and Dowless, 1998; Kelly, 1998). Other non-operative interventions include activity modification and physical therapy. Physical therapy protocols are dedicated to quadriceps rehabilitation and joint flexibility in the affected extremity. The use of knee braces is also recommended and may result in a significant functional improvement. For patients with symptomatic knee instability due to ACL injury, a functional ACL brace may prevent giving way of the affected knee. Patients with symptomatic unicompartmental OA may be treated with an unloading type brace. In a study by Kirkley *et al.*, the authors demonstrated a potential benefit of the use of such braces in decreasing pain and increasing function in patients who presented with unicompartmental osteoarthritis (Kirkley *et al.*, 1999). We employ the use of these braces for therapeutic purposes, and as a predictor of the potential effectiveness of osteotomy in relieving the symptoms of arthritis in any particular patient.

Patients presenting with significant or persistent instability or progressive symptomatic degeneration may be considered by the patient and treating physician to be too significant for such non-operative measure to be effective in the medium to long term. Therefore in the first instance it is sometimes appropriate to consider surgical intervention.

The initial consideration for surgery should include the possibility of an initial arthroscopy, this may not be necessary for individuals who will require ACL reconstruction. Some patients' symptoms can be relieved by an initial arthroscopy menisectomy and debridement. If this results in alleviation of pain, swelling and a return to an acceptable functional level of activity then subsequent ACL reconstruction or osteotomy may be avoided. However such patients should be cautioned about the long term prospects and progression of degenerative changes. The initial arthroscopy may also delineate the extent of the degenerative changes much more accurately than clinical examination, radiographs or MRI scanning. This may be helpful in determination as to whether arthroscopic debridement, chondroplasty, articular cartilage reconstruction, osteotomy or arthroplasty may be applicable.

Patients with chronic ACL insufficiency and OA may develop osteophytes in the femoral notch, on the tibial eminence and peripherally around the joint. These arthritic changes can result in a loss of terminal extension due to notch impingement. Arthroscopic removal of these osteophytes combined with a limited notchplasty is performed in all patients at the time of the initial arthroscopy to improve knee extension, whether or not subsequent ACL reconstruction or HTO is planned. Excision of the peripheral osteophytes is important to restore the correct length orientation and function of the collateral ligaments and popliteus tendon.

Once the extent of the articular degeneration is known, surgery is considered in those individuals who fail conservative management. In our approach to all patients with ACL deficiency we consider the following parameters: pain, instability and alignment. We recommend the following algorithms for treatment of the arthritic ACL deficient patient (Tables 18.1 and 18.2). The clinician must determine the primary functional derangement of the affected knee: arthritis versus instability.

Surgical considerations for the patient who presents primarily with symptoms of instability are delineated in the following – Algorithm 1. These patients require ligament reconstruction to stabilize the unstable knee during activities. Patients with primary symptomatic instability and normal knee alignment are indicated

Table 18.1

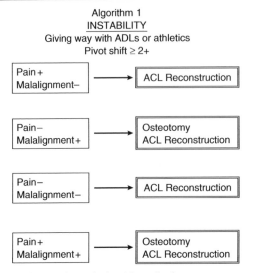

Algorithm 1
INSTABILITY
Giving way with ADLs or athletics
Pivot shift ≥ 2+

Pain + Malalignment–	→	ACL Reconstruction
Pain– Malalignment+	→	Osteotomy ACL Reconstruction
Pain– Malalignment–	→	ACL Reconstruction
Pain+ Malalignment+	→	Osteotomy ACL Reconstruction

All procedures to include exam under anesthesia and diagnostic arthroscopy
Combined osteotomy/ACL reconstruction can be staged or performed simultaneously. Osteotomy
precedes ACL reconstruction.
Key: + : positive, –: negative, ADLs: activities of daily living

Table 18.2

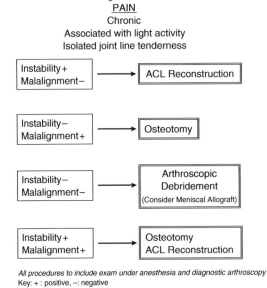

Algorithm 2
PAIN
Chronic
Associated with light activity
Isolated joint line tenderness

Instability + Malalignment–	→	ACL Reconstruction
Instability– Malalignment+	→	Osteotomy
Instability– Malalignment–	→	Arthroscopic Debridement (Consider Meniscal Allograft)
Instability + Malalignment+	→	Osteotomy ACL Reconstruction

All procedures to include exam under anesthesia and diagnostic arthroscopy
Key: + : positive, –: negative

for ACL reconstruction alone. Pain complaints in these individuals are usually secondary to instability and should be relieved with ACL reconstruction. Combined ACL reconstruction and osteotomy is performed for symptomatic instability, varus malalignment and knee pain. This surgical approach eliminates clinical instability, returns the knee to a more normal alignment, and gives the patient a more functional knee.

In contrast, the patient for whom the primary complaint is pain requires a different approach – Algorithm 2. As symptoms of instability are less problematic in these patients, surgery is performed to provide pain relief with total knee arthroplasty representing the eventual definitive treatment. The surgical plan is based upon the presence or absence of symptomatic instability and malalignment in addition to pain symptoms. Patients with pain, instability and normal knee alignment are treated with ACL reconstruction alone. The use of meniscal allografts in young patients may also be considered. Documented pain, instability and malalignment requires a combined approach with ACL reconstruction and osteotomy. In patients with pain and malalignment alone without symptomatic instability we recommend arthroscopic debridement combined with osteotomy as these procedures work well in obtaining pain relief, despite the persistence of anterior knee instability (Holden *et al.*, 1988; Noyes *et al.*, 1993). If any residual symptomatic instability is experienced then a secondary ACL reconstruction can be performed. Finally, in the third group of individuals, in which the only symptom experienced is pain without instability or knee malalignment, then should non-operative intervention fail, arthroscopic debridement is preferred.

The majority of patients with combined unicompartmental arthritis and ACL deficiency present with varus malalignment and medial degenerative joint disease. The surgical technique utilized in the treatment of these patients is described.

Preoperative evaluation

Multiple methods of preoperative planning for high tibial osteotomy have been described (Coventry, 1985; Dugdale, 1991; Insall *et al.*, 1984; Matthews *et al.*, 1988). It is our preference to use the full length standing radiographs as described. Measurements of the tibio-femoral angle (normal: 5–7° valgus) or mechanical axis (normal: 0°) are made on both extremities. Coventry recommended achieving approximately 10° of anatomic valgus, while Kettlecamp *et al.* prefer to overcorrect an additional 3–4° of valgus versus the mechanical axis of the normal knee (Coventry, 1985; Kettlecamp and Chao, 1972). Preoperative planning for HTO as described by Fujisawa *et al.* and Dugdale *et al.*, attempts to move the WBL to the medial third of the lateral compartment (Dugdale *et al.*, 1991; Fujisawa *et al.*, 1979). Whichever method is employed, the clinician should avoid under-correction, which remains one of the most common modes of failure following HTO. Overcorrection produces an ugly cosmetic deformity and is disliked by patients. The authors have used a lateral proximal tibial closing wedge or medial opening wedge osteotomy which results in an anatomic tibio-femoral axis in the range of 8–10° of valgus (Figure 18.1). More recently the technique described by Puddu and Mohtardi of an opening medial wedge osteotomy with medial plate fixation and bone grafting is preferred. The technique allows an easier surgical approach, a greater degree of control during the procedure in adjusting the alignment and secure semi-rigid fixation (Fowler *et al.*, 1991; Stevens *et al.*, 1996).

MCL insufficiency is uncommon in these patients. Use of a closing lateral wedge osteotomy in the presence of MCL insufficiency can lead to increased anteromedial instability and progressive genu valgum. This is another advantage of using the technique of a medial opening wedge osteotomy (Fowler *et al.*, 1991; Stevens *et al.*, 1996).

Technique

The usefulness of arthroscopic debridement of the arthritic knee has been documented by several authors (O'Rourke and Ike, 1994; Rand, 1991; Arnold, 1992). Thus, prior to HTO, we routinely perform a knee arthroscopy. The menisci are assessed along with the intraarticular ligaments. All cartilaginous surfaces are evaluated and graded according to Outerbridge (Outerbridge and Dunlop, 1975). While relatively normal (Grade I-II) cartilage is preferable in the post-osteotomy weight-bearing compartment, the presence of Grade III-IV chondromalacia in either joint space does not preclude good results following HTO (Keene and Dyreby, 1983). Exposed subchondral bone usually precludes a long term improvement. None the less in these patients a short to medium term improvement can often be obtained with the subsequent added benefit of a correctly aligned and stable knee at the time of joint arthroplasty. The extent and degree of the articular cartilage lesions

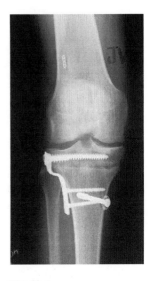

Fig. 18.1

Weight-bearing radiograph of a patient following surgery. Eight degrees of anatomic valgus was achieved. A quadrupled hamstring autograft was used for ACL reconstruction.

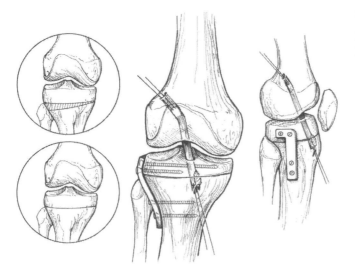

Fig. 18.2

Surgical technique for combined HTO/ACL reconstruction. High tibial osteotomy is performed initially followed by ACL reconstruction as depicted.

Fig. 18.3

MRI (axial section) of the proximal tibia from a patient status post combined HTO/ACL reconstruction. Please note that the screws are placed divergently, and that the anterior screw is sufficiently short to allow for proper placement of the tibial tunnel used for the ACL reconstruction.

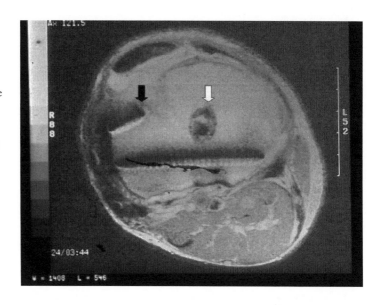

detected at arthroscopy do not necessarily correlate with clinical symptoms (Keene and Dyreby, 1983). Thus, varus malaligned patients, who report no lateral-sided pain, may undergo HTO with expected good results, even if minor isolated lateral compartment lesions are noted at arthroscopy. Arthroscopy also allows the treatment of meniscal damage and degeneration which may contribute to the symptoms of joint line pain. Osteotomy should be avoided if clinical, radiographic and arthroscopic parameters suggest the presence of degeneration or symptoms in both the medial and lateral compartments.

In the fixation of the HTO, in order to allow placement of a tibial tunnel for ACL reconstruction, any proximal anterior screw should be short and both proximal screws should be placed divergently into the proximal tibia to allow for proper tibial tunnel placement (Figures 18.2 and 18.3). A medial opening wedge osteotomy is performed using an external fixator or a wedge-plate (Figure 18.4) (Fowler *et al.*, 1991; Stevens *et al.*, 1996).

Anterior cruciate ligament reconstruction

Whether done simultaneously or in stages, ACL reconstruction should follow HTO. We recommend the use of a central third bone-patellar tendon-bone (BTB) allograft for this procedure (O'Brien *et al.*, 1991; O'Neill and James, 1992). The use of an ipsilateral BTB autograft may result in increased morbidity when ACL reconstruction is combined with HTO (Lattermann and Jakob, 1996). Use of allograft tissue reduces the overall morbidity at the operative knee, decreases postoperative pain, and may decrease the incidence of postoperative

(a)

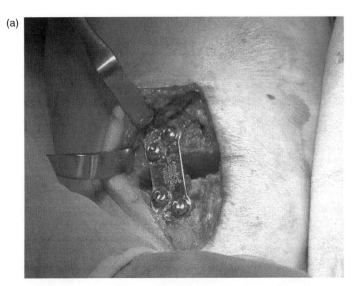

Fig. 18.4

A medical opening wedge osteotomy can be performed using a wedge-plate as depicted (Arthrex, Naples, Florida). The plate is inserted above the distal insertion of the medial collateral ligament.

(b)

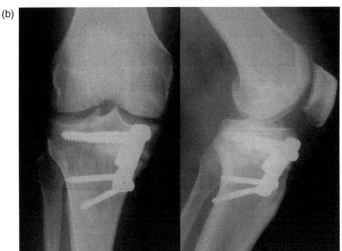

patella baja (Miller and Fu, 1993). We have also utilized the four-stranded hamstring construct for this procedure (Brown *et al.*, 1993). Although the inherent risk of disease transmission associated with the use of allograft tissue is very low, patients may object to the use allograft tissue. However the use of allograft is associated with a higher rate of failure (Noyes and Barber-Westin, 1996). The use of allograft also relies upon the availability of suitable tissue and the consideration of the additional cost. The quadruple hamstring graft is efficacious for ACL reconstruction, and its use eliminates the potential risks associated with allografts. In such cases, the semi-tendinosus and gracilis tendons are harvested through a longitudinal 2 cm incision over the pes anserinus; this same incision is used for the tibial tunnel. It has been suggested that the failure rate for hamstring

ACL reconstruction is higher than for PT (Viola *et al.*, 1999). However in these older, degenerative patients who usually have lower sporting demands, the easier rehabilitation associated with hamstring ACL reconstruction and avoidance of the donor site complications of PT reconstruction may be advantageous.

Following graft preparation, knee arthroscopy is continued. The tibial and femoral tunnels are made using commercially available guides and cannulated reamers. Proper sizing of the tunnels is determined at the time of graft preparation. Intraarticular margins of the tunnels are smoothed to prevent graft damage. The femoral tunnel should be made with the knee in at least 80° of flexion and, a posterior rim of cortex (1–2 mm) should remain. Subsequently, the ACL graft is passed, tensioned and fixed proximally and distally (Figure 18.2). In the presence of a simultaneous HTO particular attention must be paid to providing adequate fixation within the tibial tunnel. This may be difficult in the presence of an opening tibial osteotomy. Secondary supplementary cortical fixation external to the tunnels may be necessary in additional to screw fixation within the tibial tunnel.

Postoperative management

Immediately after surgery, HTO and HTO/ACL reconstruction patients are placed into a full length hinged knee brace. Radiographs are obtained following surgery to assess and document the alignment achieved, the adequacy of the fixation and the site of the ACL tunnels. Continuous passive motion is started immediately. Patients are restricted to limited toe-touch weight-bearing for at least three weeks following surgery. Weight-bearing is increased to partial (50 per cent) weight-bearing at approximately three to six weeks. Patients participate in a physical therapy protocol consisting of active flexion, passive extension, straight leg quadriceps strengthening, and gait training. The brace is continued for approximately six to eight weeks or until clinical healing of the osteotomy site occurs. In those patients undergoing concomitant ACL reconstruction an accelerated ACL rehabilitation program is then implemented.

For patients undergoing staged procedures, ACL reconstruction may be performed from six weeks after the osteotomy. However if adequate time is allowed for 6 to 12 months the tibial hardware may be removed at the time of ACL reconstruction. This obviates the need for a possible third operative procedure.

Patients are counseled before and after surgery as to the expected outcomes following surgery and the risks of progressive knee degeneration. Realistic goals should be set according to the patient's preoperative functional status, state of the knee and functional aspirations. It should be noted that a return to the preinjury level of function is not to be expected. Patients with severe pain should expect an improvement in symptoms but will not likely become pain free.

Patients are advised to avoid high-level impact or pivoting sporting activities because of the risk of further symptoms, injury or progressive degeneration.

Clinical results

To date, little has been published on the results of surgical treatment in this group of patients. Both Holden *et al.* and Odenbring *et al.*, in examining the results of HTO in patients under 50 years of age, found that most patients did experience decreased pain (Holden *et al.*, 1988; Odenbring *et al.*, 1989). However, only 32–60 per cent of patients were able to return to recreational activities. Most patients were either unable to return to jumping/pivoting athletics or experienced pain with such activities which limited their participation. Based upon these results, several authors attempted to address the observed inability to return to vigorous sports by performing ACL reconstruction in these patients.

One of the first studies addressing the problem of symptomatic genu varum and ACL deficiency reported on the use of a valgus HTO combined with ACL reconstruction (O'Neill and James, 1992). O'Neill *et al.* reviewed the results of ten patients (mean age 32 years) at three years follow-up (O'Neill and James, 1992). All patients had failed trials of physical therapy and bracing in attempts to relieve the symptoms associated with chronic anterior knee instability and symptomatic genu varum. While both objective International Knee Documentation Committee (IKDC) score and subjective functional ratings were improved following surgery, only 30 per cent of these patients were able to return to sports. These results lead the authors to conclude that the combined HTO/ACL reconstruction should be regarded as a salvage procedure for young active patients.

Johnson described follow-up of a small number of patients who had undergone simultaneous HTO by a closing lateral wedge osteotomy and a Losee type lateral ilio-tibial band tenodesis. The results demonstrated that all patients had an improvement in their pain, their function improved and all returned to recreational sporting activities. Only one patient complained of symptomatic knee instability. However more than 80 per cent of the knee were unstable to objective clinical examination. The conclusion was that HTO alone may improve the symptoms of pain and instability, and that if ACL reconstruction is undertaken then a more substantial intraarticular technique should be used.

Neuschwander *et al.* (1993) performed concomitant ACL reconstruction and HTO in five patients whose average age was 27 years. Indications for surgery included pain with ambulation, instability occurring during activities of daily living (ADLs), varus alignment, positive pivot shift, medial joint line tenderness and radiographic evidence of medial compartment arthrosis. At a mean follow-up of 2.5 years, patients were evaluated using the Lysholm scale, the Hospital for Special Surgery Knee Ligament Rating Form and the Tegner Activity Scale. Four patients had good to excellent results by the stated parameters. The fifth patient had a fair result, which was thought to be secondary to undercorrection at the osteotomy site. Additionally, all episodes of instability were eliminated, joint line tenderness was reduced, and all patients were able to return to sport to some degree. The authors stated that the combined HTO-ACL reconstruction is performed to give functional stability for activities of daily living and possibly delay the progression of degenerative arthritis. However, they reiterated that higher levels of activity should not be expected in this patient group (Neuschwander et al., 1993).

In one of the larger series, Dejour et al. retrospectively reviewed 44 combined HTO/ACL reconstructions in 43 individuals with symptomatic ACL deficiency and varus malalignment (Dejour et al., 1994). All patients were treated with concomitant intraarticular central one-third BTB grafts, and 28 patients also had extraarticular iliotibial band augmentation. At a mean follow-up of approximately three and a half years, 91 per cent of these patients were either very satisfied or satisfied with their result. A significant increase in clinical stability and symptomatic improvement was noted following surgery. Moreover, radiological assessment of these patients failed to demonstrate progression of osteoarthrosis. However, combined ACL reconstruction and valgus HTO did not return these patients to preinjury functional levels. Only 65 per cent of patients returned to sports, and only one patient was able to return to competitive contact sporting activities. Thus, the authors conclude that this combined procedure is indicated for young symptomatic patients who wish to return to leisure sports.

Noyes et al. performed a retrospective review of their experience with combined valgus HTO with and without ACL reconstruction over a two to seven year period (Noyes et al., 1993). Forty-one patients presenting with ACL deficient knees with varus angulation were treated one of three ways: HTO alone (11), combined HTO and extraarticular ACL reconstruction (14) and combined HTO and intraarticular ACL reconstruction (16). Preoperatively, 73 per cent of patients complained of pain with ADLs and only 27 per cent could perform light sports. Patients who underwent HTO with the extraarticular procedure (iliotibial band tenodesis) had significantly increased anterior tibial translation versus those patients undergoing HTO with the intraarticular ACL reconstruction. Although improvements in the knee rating scores improved in all groups following surgery, no significant differences in functional outcomes or symptoms were found between the three treatment groups. Overall patient satisfaction was high (88 per cent), and 78 per cent could perform light sports without pain. The authors were careful to note that most patients had modified their athletic activities following injury, and even after surgery no patients returned to high level athletics (jumping, pivoting). These findings suggest that HTO alone improves symptoms in the ACL deficient knee with medial gonarthrosis. Even in a subset of patients with exposed bone noted at arthroscopy, HTO improved pain and giving way in approximately two-thirds of these patients (Noyes *et al.*, 1993).

Latterman *et al.* reviewed their experience with ACL deficient patients who also presented with unicompartmental osteoarthrosis (Lattermann and Jakob, 1996). The authors divided these patients into three treatment groups. High tibial osteotomy alone was indicated in those patients in whom pain was the predominant symptom (mean age 48 years). Staged HTO/ACL reconstruction was indicated for patients presenting with both pain and instability (mean age 35 years). Simultaneous HTO/ACL reconstruction was indicated for young athletic patients in whom stability was the primary complaint (mean age 32 years). At follow-up, the IKDC scores had increased or remained unchanged in 25 of 27 patients. No significant differences in pain, stability or IKDC scores were noted in the different treatment groups. However, a significant morbidity rate was noted in this study. Consequently, the authors conclude that HTO alone was adequate in the treatment of older patients in whom pain was problematic; they suggest that younger patients should be treated with HTO initially, followed by ACL reconstruction after an interval of at least 6 weeks should there be symptoms of instability (Lattermann and Jakob, 1996).

Williams *et al.* reported the clinical results of 25 patients treated for symptomatic medial arthritis and ACL deficiency was reviewed (Williams *et al.*, 2003). All patients had clinical evidence of medial joint osteoarthritis and varus malalignment. Patients were treated with high tibial osteotomy alone (12), or combined HTO/ACL reconstruction (13). At surgery, the mean age was 38 years in the HTO group, and 33 years in the HTO/ACL group. Medial meniscectomy had been performed in 96 per cent of patients. At a mean follow-up of 43 months, significant increases in the Hospital for Special Surgery Knee Score, Tegner Activity Scale and Lysholm and Gillquist Knee Score were noted in both groups at follow-up examination. A review of the Lysholm pain and instability scores demonstrated that these symptoms were significantly decreased in patients in both treatment groups. Those patients who were treated with HTO-alone reported decreased symptomatic instability despite the persistence of objective clinical signs (pivot shift). Objective examination of preoperative and follow-up radiographs failed to demonstrate significant osteoarthritic progression in either group. Clinical outcomes did not correlate with the degree of angular correction or cartilage grading noted at arthroscopy. Overall patient satisfaction was high (92 per cent), and 23 of 25 patients were able to participate in recreational sports. The good functional results observed in this study suggest that HTO, alone and in combination with ACL reconstruction, is effective in returning arthritic ACL-deficient patients to recreational athletic activity (Williams *et al.*, 2003).

The long-term results of patients undergoing either HTO or combined HTO/ACL reconstruction are not available as yet. The results of the current studies focusing upon the management of medial compartment arthritis in the face of chronic ACL deficiency contain few patients and report on a myriad of treatment regimens. The consensus of the published reports suggests that the primary goal should be to correct the varus malalignment, which should probably be undertaken as a single procedure. This should be expected to improve the symptoms of both pain and instability. In older patients this may be adequate for good function and recreational sports. However in younger or patients with higher physical demands or a desire to minimize the possibility of progressive degeneration then a second stage intraarticular ACL reconstruction is indicated.

From an analysis of the published series (Table 18.3) the observed complication rate for HTO/ACL reconstruction was highly variable. While two studies noted no complications, Noyes *et al.* (1993), Dejour *et al.* and Latterman *et al.* reported major complication rates of 7 per cent, 5 per cent, and 37 per cent respectively. The most common complication was technical error at the osteotomy site which often required repeat osteotomy. Latterman *et al.* noted a disturbingly high rate of complication in those patients who underwent combine HTO/ACL reconstruction simultaneously (Lattermann and Jakob, 1996). Five of eight (63 per cent) patient in this group suffered a major complication which required treatment. There does appear to be a possible correlation between combined HTO and simultaneous intraarticular ACL reconstruction and the development of complications. Given the potential risk of complication, and the observed clinical improvement in those patients treated with osteotomy alone, the staged approach (HTO followed by ACL reconstruction) may represent the optimal surgical approach.

Table 18.3 Complications of Combined HTO and ACL reconstruction

Major complications
Over or under correction
Loss of correction
Intraarticular fracture
Delayed union
Arterial injury
Peroneal nerve injury
Arthrofibrosis
Deep venous thrombosis
ACL graft rupture
Instability at osteotomy site

Minor complications
Postoperative hematoma
Painful hardware
Superficial wound infection

The role of isolated ACL reconstruction in the presence of degenerative changes was analyzed by Shelbourne *et al.* who described a group of thirty-three patients (average age 29) who had documented grade 3 or 4 changes noted in at least one compartment (Shelbourne and Wilckens, 1993). While osteoarthritic changes were graded on radiographs, unfortunately the lower limb alignment was not assessed. Thirty of the thirty-three patients had a history of previous medial meniscectomy. At a mean follow-up of approximately 45 months, all patients reported subjective improvements in pain and activity level. KT-1000 arthrometer measurements also improved significantly following surgery, and all but one patient rated their knee as functionally stable. It should be noted from this study that stabilizing the knee in such patients, results in a significant improvement in the pain experienced. This is particularly appropriate for those patients without significant varus malalignment.

Meniscal allografts

In the discussion of the arthritic ACL-deficient knee, the use of meniscal allografts should be mentioned. According to Veltri *et al.*, the indications for meniscal transplant include previous meniscectomy, pain, early arthrosis, and neutral alignment (Veltri *et al.*, 1994). Thus, meniscal allograft may be considered in cases where young patients who are at a significant risk of developing premature arthritis present with significant unicompartmental pain in the absence of a meniscus. It is important to ensure that the knee is stable and correctly aligned and if not then this must be addressed to avoid early failure. In older patients the long term benefits are less well defined. An increased incidence of failure has been reported in the presence of significant osteoarthritis (Garrett *et al.*, 1991). Early to intermediate results of meniscal transplantation combined with ACL reconstruction have been encouraging (Cameron and Saha, 1997; van Arkel and de Boer, 1995; Veltri *et al.*, 1994). Some authors have combined meniscal allograft procedures with osteotomy to correct malalignment.

Summary

The ACL-deficient knee in the presence of unicompartmental arthritis is a difficult clinical problem. The incidence is increasing as ACL rupture is increasingly recognized and surgical reconstruction is established as a safe and reliable surgical technique. Symptomatic ACL instability is not a benign condition. There is a recognized incidence of increasing laxity, meniscal tears and articular degeneration. In the presence of a varus deformity or a lateral thrust on weight-bearing there may be a higher incidence of failure of any reconstruction, and premature arthritis. Careful consideration should be given to the history, examination and in determination of the patients' goals, reasonable aspirations and levels of activity. Investigations must include leg alignment radiographs and MRI scanning. Particular MRI scanning sequences may be necessary to determine the state of the particular cartilage and any subchondral changes.

In the treatment of this group of patients an initial arthroscopy to assess the extent of articular cartilage damage may be helpful. This also allows menisectomy, notchplasty and the excision of inter-condylar osteophytes and debridement of the knee. In some cases in which the activity level may be restricted, in older patients, or where surgery is to be avoided this arthroscopic technique may suffice.

Consideration of reconstruction of any damaged secondary restraints should be undertaken – this would include collateral ligament or posterior lateral ligament laxity. As in any case of ACL laxity, meniscal preservation is important. Mensical repair rather than menisectomy should be practiced wherever possible. In the presence of unicompartmental pain in the absence of a meniscus in a correctly aligned and stable knee meniscal transplantation may be indicated.

One factor which may be significant in the progression of degen-erative changes in these patients is damage to the articular surface which may result from the initial injury, for subsequent giving way episodes, or to the chronic laxity. These lesions are increasingly recognized at the time of the injury, on MRI scanning or at the time of arthroscopy. Surgical reconstruction may be indicated because of pain or to avoid the presumed progressive degeneration. Reliable reconstruction of the articular cartilage damage may be possible by arthroscopic chondroplasty techniques, osteo-chondral transplan-tation from a local site or osteocyte cell transplantation. These techniques are considered elsewhere.

High tibial osteotomy, whether by a lateral closing wedge or medial opening wedge osteotomy, is necessary if there is significant varus malalignment which is the most common deformity encoun-tered in these patients. This may reliably be expected to improve both the symptomatic pain and instability. Osteotomy is particularly indicated in the presence of a lateral thrust, lateral or posterio-lateral instability. The combination of HTO with a simultaneous intra-articular ACL reconstruction is associated with a significant inci-dence of complications and the procedures should probably be staged. The ACL reconstruction requires particular attention to fix-ation in the tibial tunnel and double fixation may be required. In low-demand, arthritic or older patients there may be some benefit in utilizing a hamstring graft rather than a PT graft.

Conclusion

Active patients complaining of instability and pain secondary to ACL deficiency and unicompartmental gonarthrosis present the clinician with a therapeutic dilemma. Knee osteotomy is an effective means of treating patients with isolated medial or lateral compartment arthritis, even in the setting of anterior knee instability. However, a thorough assessment of pain, stability and lower extremity alignment is important in the development of a treatment plan. Typically, active patients with chronic symptoms associated with unicompartmental OA and ACL deficiency can be treated with arthroscopic debridement, knee osteotomy, ACL reconstruction or a combination of these procedures. Most patients can expect symptomatic improvement and a return to recreational activities. However, a return to high level sports is not expected. The establishment of reasonable long term goals and activity modification are crucial to the success of this approach and to ensure patient satisfaction.

References

Allen PR, Denham RA and Swan AV. Late degenerative changes after meniscectomy. Factors affecting the knee after operation. *J Bone Joint Surg [Br]*. 1984; 66(5):666–71.

Arnold WJ. Arthroscopy in the diagnosis and therapy of arthritis. *Hosp Pract (Off Ed)*. 1992; 27(3A):43–6, 49, 52–3.

Berchuck M, Andriacchi T, Bach B and Reider B. Gait adaptations in patients who have a deficient anterior cruciate ligament. *J Bone Joint Surg*. 1990; 72A:871–7.

Bradley J, Brandt K, Katz B, Kalasinski L and Ryan S. Comparison of an antiinflammatory dose of ibuprofen, an analgesic dose of ibuprofen and acetaminophen in the treatment of patients with osteoarthritis of the knee. *New Engl J Med*. 1991; 325(2):87–91.

Bredella M, Tirman P, Peterfy C, Zarlingo M, Feller J, Bost F, Belzer J, Wischer T and Genant H. Accuracy of T2-weighted fast spin-echo MR imaging with fat saturation in detecting cartilage defects in the knee: Comparison with arthroscopy in 130 patients. *AJR Am J Roentgenol*. 1999; 172(4):1073–80.

Brown C, Steiner M and Carson E. The use of hamstring tendons for anterior cruciate ligament reconstruction. *Clin Sports Med*. 1993; 12(4):723–56.

Buss D, Warren R, Wickiewicz T, Galinat B and Panariello R. Arthroscopically assisted reconstruction of the anterior cruciate ligament with use of autogenous patellar-ligament grafts. *J Bone Joint Surg*. 1993; 75-A(9):1346–59.

Cameron J and Saha S. Meniscal allograft transplantation for unicompartmental arthritis of the knee. *Clin Orthop*. 1997; 337:164–71.

Coventry M. Current concepts review: Upper tibial osteotomy for osteoarthritis. *J Bone Joint Surg*. 1985; 67A:1136–40.

Coventry M, IIstrup D and Wallrichs S. Proximal Tibial Osteotomy. *J Bone Joint Surg*. 1993; 75A:196–201.

da Camara CC and Dowless GV. Glucosamine sulfate for osteoarthritis [see comments]. *Ann Pharmacother*. 1998; 32(5):580–7.

Dahlberg L, Friden T, Roos H, Lark MW and Lohmander LS. A longitudinal study of cartilage matrix metabolism in patients with cruciate ligament rupture – synovial fluid concentrations of aggrecan fragments, stromelysin-1 and tissue inhibitor of metalloproteinase-1. *Br J Rheumatol*. 1994; 33(12):1107–11.

Daniel D, Stone M, Dobson B, Fithian D, Rossman D and Kaufman K. Fate of the ACL-injured patient: A prospective outcome study. *Am J Sports Med*. 1994; 22:632–44.

Dejour H, Neyret P, Boileau P and Donell S. Anterior cruciate reconstruction combined with valgus tibial osteotomy. *Clin Orthop.* 1994;
299:220–8.

DeLee J and Drez D, eds. *Anterior Cruciate Ligament Injuries.* Orthopedic
Sports Medicine. W.B. Saunders Co.: Philadelphia, PA. 1994;
1313–1501.

Dieppe P, Cushnagan J, Young P and Kirwan J. Prediction of the progression of joint space narrowing in osteoarthritis of the knee by bone
scintigraphy. *Ann Rheum Dis.* 1993; 52:557–63.

Dimond PM, Fadale PD, Hulstyn MJ, Tung GA and Greisberg J. A comparison of MRI findings in patients with acute and chronic ACL tears.
Am J Knee Surg. 1998; 11(3):153–9.

Dugdale T, Noyes F and Styer D. Preoperative planning for high tibial
osteotomy. *Clin Orthop.* 1991; 271:105–21.

Edgerton B, Mariani E and Morrey B. Distal femoral varus osteotomy for
painful genu valgum. *Clin Orthop.* 1993; 288:263–9.

Fairbank T. Knee joint changes after meniscectomy. *J Bone Joint Surg.*
1948; 30-B:664–70.

Fowler J, Gie G and Maceachern A. Upper tibial valgus osteotomy
using a dynamic external fixator. *J Bone Joint Surg [Br].* 1991; 73(4):
690–1.

Fujisawa Y, Masuhara K and Shiomi S. The effect of high tibial osteotomy
on osteoarthritis of the knee. *Orthop Clin North Am.* 1979; 10:
585–608.

Garrett J, Steensen R and Stevensen R. Meniscal transplantation in the
human knee: A preliminary report. *Arthroscopy.* 1991; 7(1):57–62.

Hefti F, Müller W, Jakob R and Stäubli H-U. Evaluation of knee ligament
injuries with the IKDC form. *Knee Surg Sports Traumatol Arthrosc.*
1993; 1:226–34.

Holden D, James S and Larsen R. Proximal tibial osteotomy in patients
who are fifty years old or less: A long term follow-up study. *J Bone
Joint Surg.* 1988; 70A:977–82.

Insall J, Joseph D and Msika C. High tibial osteotomy for varus gonarthrosis. A long term follow-up study. *J Bone Joint Surg.* 1984; 66A:
1040–8.

Insall J, Ranawat C, Aglietti P and Shine J. A comparison of four models of total knee-replacement prostheses. *J Bone Joint Surg.* 1976;
58-A:754–65.

Insall JN, Dorr LD, Scott RD and Scott WN. Rationale of the knee society clinical rating system. *Clin Orthop.* 1989; (248):13–14.

Ivarsson I, Myrnerts R and Gillquist J. High tibial osteotomy for medial
osteoarthritis of the knee: A 5 to 7 and an 11 to 13 year follow-up. *J
Bone Joint Surg.* 1990; 72B:238–44.

Johnson D and Warner J. Diagnosis for anterior cruciate ligament surgery.
Clin Sports Med. 1993; 12(4):671–84.

Kaplan PA, Gehl RH, Dussault RG, Anderson MW and Diduch DR.
Bone contusions of the posterior lip of the medial tibial plateau (con-
trecoup injury) and associated internal derangements of the knee at
MR imaging. *Radiology.* 1999; 211(3):747–53.

Keene J and Dyreby J. High tibial osteotomy in the treatment of
osteoarthritis of the knee. *J Bone Joint Surg.* 1983; 65-A(1):36–42.

Kelly GS. The role of glucosamine sulfate and chondroitin sulfates in the
treatment of degenerative joint disease. *Altern Med Rev.* 1998;
3(1):27–39.

Kettlecamp D and Chao E. A method for quantitative analysis of medial
and lateral compressive forces at the knee during standing. *Clin
Orthop.* 1972; 83:202–13.

Kirkley A, Webster-Bogaert S, Litchfield R, Amendola A, MacDonald S, McCalden R and Fowler P. The effect of bracing on varus gonarthrosis. *J Bone Joint Surg Am.* 1999; 81(4):539–48.

Lattermann C and Jakob R. High tibial osteotomy alone or combined with ligament reconstruction in anterior cruciate ligament-deficient knees. *Knee Surg Sports Traumatol Arthrosc.* 1996; 4:32–8.

Lohmander L, Hoerrner L, Dahlberg L, Roos H, Bjornsson S and Lark M. Stromelysin, tissue inhibitor of metalloproteinases, and proteoglycan fragments in human knee joint fluid after injury. *J Rheum.* 1993; 20(8):1362–8.

Lohmander LS, Hoerrner LA and Lark MW. Metalloproteinases, tissue inhibitor, and proteoglycan fragments in knee synovial fluid in human osteoarthritis. *Arthritis Rheum.* 1993; 36(2):181–9.

Lysholm J and Gillquist J. Evaluation of knee ligament surgery results with special emphasis on use of a scoring scale. *Am J Sports Med.* 1982; 10:150–4.

Matthews L, Goldstein S, Malvitz T, Katz B and Kaufer H. Proximal tibial osteotomy: Factors that influence the duration of satisfactory function. *Clin Orthop.* 1988; 229:193–209.

Merchant A, Mercer R, Jacobsen R and Cool C. Roentgenographic analysis of patellofemoral congruence. *J Bone Joint Surg.* 1974; 56A: 1391–6.

Merck and Company, *Rofecoxib: Prescribing Information.* 1999: Whitehouse Station, NJ.

Miller M and Fu F. The role of osteotomy in the anterior cruciate ligament deficient knee. *Clin Sports Med.* 1993; 12(4):697–708.

Neuschwander D, Drez D and Paine R. Simultaneous high tibial osteotomy and ACL reconstruction for combined genu varum and symptomatic ACL tear. *Orthopedics.* 1993; 16(6):679–84.

Noyes F, Barber S and Simon R. High tibial osteotomy and ligament reconstruction in varus angulated, anterior cruciate ligament-deficient knees. *Am J Sports Med.* 1993; 21(1):2–12.

Noyes F and Barber-Westin S. Reconstruction of the anterior cruciate ligament with human allograft. Comparison of early and later results. *J Bone Joint Surg Am.* 1996; 78(4):524–37.

Noyes F, Mooar P, Matthews D and Butler D. The symptomatic anterior cruciate deficient knee. *J Bone Joint Surg.* 1983; 65A:154.

O'Brien S, Warren R, Pavlov H, Panariello R and Wickiewicz T. Reconstruction of the chronically insufficient anterior cruciate ligament with the central third of the patellar ligament. *J Bone Joint Surg.* 1991; 73-A(2):278–86.

Odenbring S, Tjornstrand B and Egund N. Function after tibial osteotomy for medial gonarthrosis below age 50 years. *Acta Orthop Scand.* 1989; 60:527–31.

O'Neill D and James S. Valgus osteotomy with anterior cruciate ligament laxity. *Clin Orthop.* 1992; 278:153–9.

O'Rourke KS and Ike RW. Diagnostic arthroscopy in the arthritis patient. *Rheum Dis Clin North Am.* 1994; 20(2):321–42.

Outerbridge R and Dunlop J. The problem of chondromalacia patellae. *Clin Orthop.* 1975; 110:177–96.

Phillips MJ and Krackow KA. High tibial osteotomy and distal femoral osteotomy for valgus or varus deformity around the knee. *Instr Course Lect.* 1998; 47:429–36.

Puddu G, Cipolla M, Cerullo G and Scala A. Arthroscopic treatment of the flexed arthritic knee in active middle-aged patients. *Knee Surg Sports Traumatol Arthrosc.* 1994; 2(2):73–5.

Rand JA. Role of arthroscopy in osteoarthritis of the knee. *Arthroscopy.* 1991; 7(4):358–63.

Rangger C, Kathrein A, Freund MC, Klestil T and Kreczy A. Bone bruise of the knee: Histology and cryosections in 5 cases. *Acta Orthop Scand.* 1998; 69(3):291–4.

Reimann I. Experimental osteoarthritis of the knee in rabbits induced by alteration of the load-bearing. *Acta Orthop Scand.* 1973; 44(4): 496–504.

Roos EM, Roos HP and Lohmander LS. WOMAC Osteoarthritis Index – additional dimensions for use in subjects with post-traumatic osteoarthritis of the knee. Western Ontario and MacMaster Universities. *Osteoarthritis Cartilage.* 1999; 7(2):216–21.

Rosenberg T, Paulos L, Parker R, Coward D and Scott S. The forty-five-degree posteroanterior flexion weight-bearing radiograph of the knee. *J Bone Joint Surg.* 1988; 70A:1479–83.

Rudan J and Simurda M. Valgus high tibial osteotomy: A long term follow-up study. *Clin Orthop.* 1991; 268:157–60.

Searle and Company, *Celecoxib: Prescribing Information*, P. Incorporated, Editor. 1999: Chicago, Illinois.

Shelbourne K and Wilckens J. Intraarticular anterior cruciate ligament reconstruction in the symptomatic arthritic knee. *Am J Sports Med.* 1993; 121(5):685–9.

Stevens P, Edelson R, Keeve J, Chamberlain S and Brewster R. Opening wedge high tibial osteotomy: Rationale and technique. *J Orthop Tech.* 1996; 4:16–22.

Tetsworth K and Paley D. Malalignment and degenerative arthropathy. *Orthop Clin North Am.* 1994; 25(3):367–77.

Thompson WO and Fu FH. The meniscus in the cruciate-deficient knee. *Clin Sports Med.* 1993; 12(4):771–96.

van Arkel E and de Boer H. Human meniscal transplantation. *J Bone Joint Surg.* 1995; 77-B:589–95.

Veltri D, Warren R, Wickiewicz T and O'Brien S. Current status of allograft meniscal transplantation. *Clin Orthop.* 1994; 303:44–55.

Viola R, Steadman J, Mair S, Briggs K and Sterett W. Anterior cruciate ligament injury incidence among male and female professional alpine skiers. *Am J Sports Med.* 1999; 27:792–5.

Williams Rr, Kelly B, Wickiewicz T, Altchek D and Warren R. The short-term outcome of surgical treatment for painful varus arthritis in association with chronic ACL deficiency. *J Knee Surg.* 2003; 16(1):9–16.

Wu DD, Burr DB, Boyd RD and Radin EL. Bone and cartilage changes following experimental varus or valgus tibial angulation. *J Orthop Res.* 1990; 8(4):572–85.

Yasuda K, Majima T, Tsuchida T and Kaneda K. A ten to 15-year followup observation of high tibial osteotomy in medial compartment osteoarthrosis. *Clin Orthop.* 1992; 282:186–95.

Zeiss J, Paley K, Murray K and Saddemi SR. Comparison of bone contusion seen by MRI in partial and complete tears of the anterior cruciate ligament. *J Comput Assist Tomogr.* 1995; 19(5):773–6.

19

Arthritic ACL-deficient knees – is there increased patient morbidity following combined high tibial osteotomy/ACL reconstruction?

Christoph B. Marti and Roland P. Jakob

Introduction

The use of high tibial osteotomy as a surgical procedure for the treatment of osteoarthritis of the knee was first reported by Jackson in 1958. High tibial osteotomy (HTO) is widely accepted as a treatment option in patients with a unicompartmental osteoarthritis and varus angulated knees. When adequate correction was obtained, Fujisawa observed arthroscopically that repair of the ulcerated region was initiated by both surviving cartilage in the affected area and by cartilage bordering the affected area (Fujisawa et al. 1979). Two years after osteotomy, he observed that the ulcerated region was thoroughly covered with fibrous and membranous tissue (Fujisawa et al. 1979). High tibial osteotomy is performed if there are early but definite osteoarthritic changes in the medial compartment, if the limb shows evident deformity like a varus morphotype or there is lateral collateral ligament instability, and if the lateral compartment shows no degenerative changes on the valgus stress radiograph.

For high tibial osteotomy we perform a medial opening wedge osteotomy if it is also necessary to tighten the medial collateral ligament and if the osteotomy was to be combined with an ACL reconstruction. We use three tri-cortical bone grafts, retrieved from the ipsilateral iliac crest, to fill the medial gap. The osteotomy is fixed with an AO-cervical spine plate and four 4.0 mm cancellous screws. By establishing normal or overcorrected axial alignment while indirectly restoring ligamentous tension, the opening wedge osteotomy permits immediate postoperative mobilization of the operated limb. This is even more desirable when the osteotomy is combined with anterior cruciate ligament reconstruction. To stimulate the formation of a

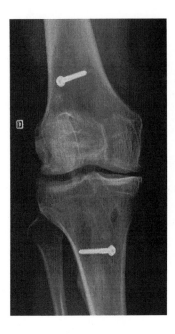
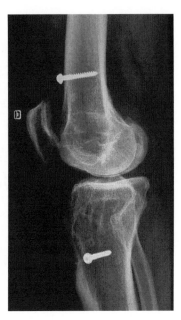

Fig. 19.1
A patient of 40 years with a prior medial meniscectomy and a failed ACL reconstruction. He developed a chronic anterior instability and a medial osteoarthritis.

fibro-cartilagineous coverage we routinely perform microfracturing on the bare bone surfaces of the dieased compartment (Steadman *et al.* 2000, Sledge 2001). If microfractures are performed, immediate continuous passive mobilization is desirable to induce a better fibrocartilage regeneration (Steadman *et al.* 2000, Sledge 2001). If needed, the medial collateral ligament is detached subperiostally with a sliver of bone to avoid excessive loading of the medial compartment after correction.

There is no data available in the literature that answers the question if the intraarticular pressure changes after open wedge high tibial osteotomy. Chronic instability of the ACL and failure of a competent reconstruction commonly leads to overload of the medial compartment, medial meniscal tears, cartilage wear and osteoarthritis (Figure 19.1). The presence of even minimal joint-space narrowing (Figure 19.2), squaring of the femoral condyles, and osteophytosis of the condylar notch and posterior medial tibial plateau are warning signs that an ACL reconstruction alone might greatly accelerate the degenerative process, especially in patients over 30 years of age (Jakob 1990). A cruciate ligament reconstruction is generally subject to increased loads in the osteoarthritic knee. Presumably this is due largely to the alteration of joint kinematics by the osteoarthritic changes but may also relate to the synovitis and bathing of the graft in a enzyme-rich synovial fluid, which can attack the autologous graft and disrupt the remodeling of its fibers (Jakob 1990). For that reason, the articular forces must be reduced by combining the ligament reconstruction with a high tibial osteotomy in patients who have loss of lateral

Fig. 19.2

The valgus/varus stress view shows the narrowing of the medial compartment.

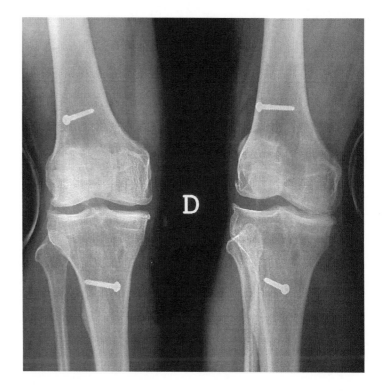

coaptation accompanied by significant constitutional varus deviation (Jakob 1990).

Simultaneous ACL reconstruction using a closing wedge osteotomy has been shown to have a higher complication rate than staged procedures. On the other hand an opening wedge osteotomy can be combined with an ACL reconstruction when there is a varus morphotype with mild osteoarthritis, when motion is not restricted and when symptoms relating to anterior instability are subjectively and objectively disabling (Jakob 1990, Noyes *et al.* 1993). Medial opening wedge osteotomy with interposition of a tricortical graft and plate fixation has become popular due to the absence of peroneal nerve problems, its simplicity, shorter surgery time and faster healing. Because this osteotomy is less invasive and is associated with less morbidity, it is relatively simple to combine with a cruciate ligament reconstruction in the same sitting (Jakob 1990). A combined high tibial osteotomy and anterior cruciate ligament reconstruction has been proposed by several authors (Boss *et al.* 1995, Dejour *et al.* 1994, O'Neill and James 1992, Holden *et al.* 1988, Noyes *et al.* 1993). Successful valgus tibial osteotomy combined with an intraarticular ACL reconstruction stabilizes the knee, reduces pain and stops early progression of osteoarthritis in symptomatic patients who have chronic rupture of the ACL and acquired varus malalignment (Dejour *et al.* 1994). There is no agreed treatment rationale available at the present time.

HTO in young patients

The current literature includes several studies discussing the short- and long-term results after high tibial osteotomy. Most of them deal with patients over 50 years of age (Marti *et al.* 2000, Aglietti *et al.* 1983, Bauer *et al.* 1969, Herningou *et al.* 1987, Ivarsson *et al.* 1990), while only a few studies address the young adult patient with osteoarthritis (Dejour *et al.* 1994, O'Neill and James 1992, Insall *et al.* 1984, Noyes *et al.* 1993). In recent years we have increasingly treated young adults aged between 20 and 40 who present with a varus aligned knee and unicompartmental medial osteoarthritis combined with a marked anterior instability due to anterior cruciate ligament insufficiency. These patients usually are very active and pose high demands on their knee joint. High tibial osteotomy in young adults has been reported to be effective for the treatment of medial osteoarthritis (Noyes *et al.* 1993, Holden *et al.* 1988). However, treatment options for patients with unicompartmental osteoarthritis and combined anterior cruciate ligament insufficiency are not clearly defined. It is unclear whether the osteoarthritis or instability has to be treated first.

Combined HTO/ACL-reconstruction

In 1996, Latermann and Jakob reported in a retrospective study of closing wedge osteotomy alone or combined with ACL reconstruction, 27 patients with a mean age of 37 years treated for a medial unicompartimental osteoarthritis and chronic anterior instability of the knee. Patients were divided into three different groups according to treatment. In the first group, only HTO was performed. In the second group, HTO and simultaneous anterior cruciate ligament reconstruction (Figures 19.3 and 19.4) and in the third group high tibial osteotomy and 6–12 months later an anterior cruciate ligament reconstruction was performed.

The authors conclude that high tibial osteotomy is a good treatment option for younger patients with medial osteoarthritis and chronic anterior instability of the knee. The presenting symptoms of these patients have to be carefully assessed in terms of instability and pain so that treatment can be fashioned to the individual's symptoms. In patients aged 40 and older high tibial osteotomy alone is an excellent treatment option with reproducibly good results. In younger patients the authors advise a high tibial osteotomy first. If instability persists, they recommend that the anterior cruciate ligament reconstruction can be done 6–12 months later. They warn that a simultaneous combined procedure has a significantly higher complication rate. The two-staged procedure is equally effective in the long run and in addition, there is the advantage that a patient can adjust to the changed weight-bearing axis. This leads to a significant reduction of instability in some patients and thus renders anterior

Fig. 19.3

Six weeks after combined open wedge HTO and ACL reconstruction. The osteotomy site was filled with three tricortical bone grafts and the osteotomy was fixed with an AO-cervical spine plate and four 4.0 mm cancellous screws.

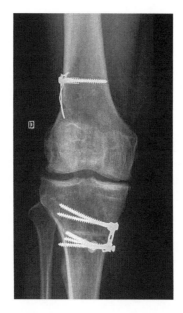
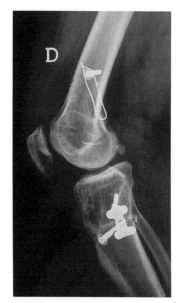

Fig. 19.4

Three months after combined HTO/ACL-reconstruction, the osteotomy has united and the patient is full weight-bearing.

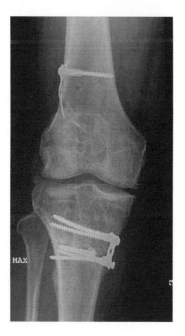
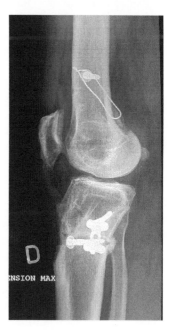

cruciate ligament replacement unnecessary. Because it is not known whether ACL replacement in a knee which lacks a medial meniscus can prevent an early progression of osteoarthritis, the identification of patients not requiring additional ACL reconstruction should be done carefully.

In their series most of the patients did not return to their preinjury sports level and the authors conclude that the aim of operative treatment should be a pain-free knee joint during light or moderate activities of daily living (Lattermann and Jakob 1996).

Discussion

The authors conclude that the simultaneous procedure carries several risks, and a high degree of surgical skill and experience is necessary (Lattermann and Jakob 1996). These findings have to be assessed with reference to the fact that the osteotomy technique practiced in the mid-eighties and early nineties as reported in this series was almost exclusively a closing wedge type osteotomy undertaken from the lateral aspect.

Complications of combined HTO/ACL reconstruction

In the light of this publication by Lattermann and Jakob (Lattermann and Jakob 1996), let us look at the various complications of the combined technique.

The development of acute compartment syndrome after arthroscopic knee surgery has been described by several authors. Peek and Haynes (1984) and Fruensgard and Holm (1988) reported two cases of compartment syndrome of the leg after arthroscopic knee surgery. In both cases, a four compartment fasciotomy was performed. A posterior capsular tear was thought to have caused the irrigation fluid extravasation. Matsen *et al.* (1980) noted that elevated compartmental tissue pressures without clinical symptoms are not an absolute indication for fasciotomies. They identified 13 patients with tissue pressures in excess of 30 mmHg who had no clinical symptoms. These patients were observed and did not develop sequelae of compartment syndrome. These findings support those of Kaper *et al.* (1997), who reported two cases with elevation of intracompartmental pressures of all four compartments of the leg without clinical symptoms. The size of the calf and the measured intracompartmental pressures decreased by simply elevating and icing the affected leg. We had one case with combined high tibial osteotomy and anterior cruciate ligament reconstruction with an undetermined amount of fluid extravasation into the calf. We suppose that the main cause for the fluid extravasation was the repeated drilling of the tibial guide wire for tunnel placement which produced several small tunnels into the proximal tibia; this allowed the fluid to cross the osteotomy gap and invade the dorsal compartment of the leg. After drilling the tibial tunnel with the 10 mm reamer, fluid extravasation into the calf increased. We were unable to document other reasons for extravasation such as a tear in the capsule or excessively high intraarticular pressure. Although the calf was tense on palpation and the compartment pressure elevated, no clinical symptoms of compartment syndrome were found.

Ekman and Poehling (1996) showed in an experimental study with pigs that even in the presence of significant fluid extravasation and elevated compartment pressures, the risk of developing compartment syndrome and subsequent neuromuscular damage is minimal. They supposed that the extravasated fluid accumulates within the extracompartmental rather than the intracompartmental tissue. Because of this, the extravasated fluid is resorbed quickly. We recommend careful observation of the patient without immediate fasciotomy. We performed a small incision and subcutaneous release of the flexor compartment of the leg, which we regarded as a reliable measure to prevent a compartment syndrome. The patient did not develop any sequelae. We conclude that high tibial osteotomy combined with simultaneous arthroscopic ACL-reconstruction has to be performed carefully, and potential complications must be detected immediately to prevent a compartment syndrome (Marti and Jakob 1999).

Tibial slope

Special attention is given to the tibial slope (Dejour *et al.* 1990). We define the tibial slope as the angle between the slope of the medial plateau and the long axis of the tibia (minus 90°). The average value is 6°. We performed a study (Marti *et al.* 2001) where we evaluated whether a frontal plane correction influences the sagittal slope of the proximal tibia in unstable knees. Twenty-four patients with the mean age of 35 years had anteroposterior knee instability and were available for a follow-up evaluation at a minimum interval of eight months. Eighteen patients had an anterior knee instability, six patients a posterior instability. In both groups, the mean postoperative tibial slope increased. In the posterior instability group, the mean tibial slope increased 1.3° more than in the anterior instability group. We conclude that a medial opening wedge osteotomy not only alters frontal plane axis but affects the posterior slope of the tibial plateau in the sagittal plane as well. We have observed that the posterior slope increases after performing an opening wedge proximal tibial osteotomy. This confirms the result of Dejour *et al.* (1990). The increase of tibial slope undesirably increases anterior translation of the tibia due to the anterior force vector induced by load transfer from the femur to the tibial plateau in a standing and walking position. Such force stretches an ACL transplant performed either simultaneously or in a staged fashion. This effect may be beneficial with a posterior instability which would unload a PCL reconstruction (Dejour *et al.* 1990). For every 10° increase in the backward inclination of the tibial plateau, anterior tibial translation is increased by 6 mm.

The theoretical load on the ACL with anterior tibial translation is three times greater when the posterior slope of the tibia exceeds 10° (Dejour *et al.* 1990). One should aim at a tibial slope of not more than 6°. In ACL-associated osteoarthritis, a preoperative tibial slope of 10° or more should be reduced provided that there is no hyperextension of the knee, because this is poorly tolerated where residual ACL instability exists. This mandates a closing wedge technique (Dejour *et al.* 1994). The closing wedge osteotomy is, however, inherently more unstable, dependent on more stable internal fixation and may be more difficult to combine with an ACL reconstruction because heavier implants may be in the way of the tibial tunnel to drill. However, with a medial opening wedge osteotomy, it is far more difficult to decrease the posterior tibial slope. If we decide to go for an opening wedge technique it is important to free the soft tissues posteriorly, to make the osteotomy by completing the cut laterally, thus allowing the sagital correction, and to shape tricortical grafts correspondingly. With ACL pathology, we recommend careful assessment of the preoperative anteroposterior stability and the posterior tibial slope and careful planning of the frontal and sagittal axis when performing a high tibial osteotomy.

Patella baja

The patellar height is, in principle, affected differently by the various osteotomy techniques. An osteotomy below the tibial tuberosity should not modify the proximal distal position of the tubercle, whereas an opening wedge should render it more distal and a closing wedge more proximal. The length of the patellar tendon can also be altered after high tibial osteotomy, as a consequence of scarring or immobilization. This is a strong argument for using rigid internal fixation and early mobilisation. It also suggests that a closing wedge osteotomy should be preferred to an opening wedge osteotomy in case of preoperative patella baja or patellofemoral arthritis. If opening wedge osteotomy is undertaken and no alteration in patellar height is desired the osteotomy may be performed below the tibial tuberosity.

Discussion

In the literature, it was thought that with the combined procedure, the greater amount of surgery could hinder early rehabilitation and therefore be harmful to the ACL graft. Many studies, however, clearly show that results after this procedure are satisfactory, and that the patients cope well (Dejour *et al.* 1994, O'Neill and James 1992, Lerat *et al.* 1993). Dejour *et al.* (1987) recommend HTO in a knee with medial osteoarthrosis because of anterior instability and in the case of symptomatic subjective and objective instability also ACL reconstruction. Noyes *et al.* (1993) do not propose HTO in all varus knees with anterior instability, especially not in asymptomatic patients, even when there is arthroscopic evidence of medial femorotibial arthritis because of the lack of long-term results and the complication rate of HTO. They perform a two-staged procedure where in most cases the osteotomy is first performed, allowing the patient time to fully recover from the procedure. This staged approach allows the surgeon to treat any complication from the osteotomy, before proceeding with the ligament stabilization procedure. This also allows assessment of giving way symptoms after the osteotomy. In selected knees, a combined procedure is performed, but the authors are mindful that the added surgery, operative time, and general complexity of both procedures performed together may increase the complication rate. Lerat *et al.* (1993) recommend a simultaneous procedure because of a lack of studies proving that HTO alone can prevent instability, because there is no progression of arthritis using a correct technique, and because there is no higher rate of complications or technical problems in a combined operation. Boss *et al.* (1995) support this opinion, since they did not have an elevated rate of complications or technical problems with a combined procedure. Rehabilitation was not prolonged or complicated, and there was only one rehabilitation period and inability to work.

Dejour *et al.* (1994) showed in here study that a combined procedure is a safe operation with a low morbidity. The rate of osteoarthrosis did not show progression at three-and-a-half-years after the operation. They recommend a combined operation for those symptomatic sportsmen with chronic rupture of the ACL who have developed varus malalignment of their knee either from medial tibiofemoral compartment joint narrowing, especially after a medial meniscectomy, or those who have lateral tibiofemoral compartment joint opening secondary to a posterolateral lesion that occurred at the time of the original injury, and where reconstruction has failed. The lateral compartment can also open up as a late sequelae of marked medial compartment narrowing. Dejour *et al.* (1994) recommends a valgus tibial osteotomy in all cases where there is lateral compartment opening, whatever is decided for the ruptured anterior cruciate ligament.

We believe that the treatment options strongly depend on the patient's specific symptoms and expectations as well as on the surgeon's operative skills. In particular, patients aged 40 years and older and not primarily presenting with a high degree of instability can be optimally treated with high tibial osteotomy alone. An additional ACL replacement is not always necessary and in many situations does not improve the functional outcome.

If a simultaneous procedure has been taken into account, we prefer a medial opening wedge osteotomy because it is relatively simple, less invasive and is associated with less morbidity. The duration of the surgical procedure is shorter, there are no peroneal nerve problems and the healing is faster than with a closing wedge osteotomy. The stability of the opening wedge osteotomy with interposition of three tricortical bone grafts and fixation with a plate is better than with the closing wedge technique, because the osteotomy is performed at a supra-ligamentous level and the musculotendinous structures are tensioned and not weakened as with the closing wedge technique. However it is not known if the opening wedge osteotomy at a supra-ligamentous level increases the pressure in the medial compartment. In a case of an advanced medial arthrosis and a tight medial collateral ligament, medial opening wedge osteotomy could be contraindicated. If there is significant articular cartilage damage then we consider an additional mosaicplasty. However, because of the prolonged nature of the procedure, which is restricted by the tourniquet time, we recommend a two-stage procedure. We first perform an opening wedge high tibial osteotomy, combined with an arthroscopic debridement, notchplasty and an open mosaicplasty. As a second step the ACL reconstruction is undertaken with removal of the metalwork.

Summary

We believe that simultaneous osteotomy and ACL replacement can be a valuable procedure if patient selection is done thoroughly. A high degree of surgical skill and experience as well as patient cooperation and motivation for the rehabilitation program is necessary. However, there is a higher risk of postoperative complications, which has to be taken into account.

References

Aglietti P, Rinonapoli E, Strisnga G, Taviani A (1983). Tibial osteotomy for the varus osteoarthritic knee. *Clin Orthop* 176: 239–251.

Bauer GC, Insall J, Koshino T (1969). Tibial osteotomy in gonarthrosis (osteoarthritis of the knee). *J Bone Joint Surg (Am)* 51: 1545–1563.

Boss A, Stutz G, Oursin C, Gächter A (1995). Anterior cruciate ligament reconstruction combined with valgus tibial osteotomy (combined procedure). *Knee Surg, Sports Traumatol, Arthroscopy* 3: 187–191.

Dejour H, Neyret P, Boileau P, Donell S (1994). Anterior cruciate reconstruction combined with valgus tibial osteotomy. *Clin Orthop* 299: 220–8.

Dejour H, Neyret P, Bonnin M (1990). Monopodal weight-bearing radiography of the chronical unstable knee. In R.P. Jakob and H.U. Stäubli, eds. *The knee and cruciate ligaments*, pp. 568–576. Springer, Berlin.

Dejour H, Walch G, Deschamps G, Chambat P (1987). Arthrose du genou sur laxité chronique antérieure. *Rev Chir Orthop* 73: 157–170.

Ekman EF, Poehling GG (1996). An experimental assessment of the risk of compartment syndrome during knee arthroscopy. *Arthroscopy* 12, 2: 193–9.

Fruensgaard S, Holm A (1988). Compartment syndrome complicating arthroscopic surgery: Brief report. *J Bone Joint Surg (Br)* 70: 146–147.

Fujisawa Y, Masuhara K, Shiomi S (1979). The effect of high tibial osteotomy on osteoarthritis of the knee. *Orthop Clin North Am* 10: 585–608.

Herningou P, Medeviell D, Debeyre J, Goutallier D (1987). Proximal tibial osteotomy for osteoarthritis with varus deformity. A ten- to thirteen-year follow-up study. *J Bone Joint Surg (Am)* 69: 332–354.

Holden DL, James SL, Larson RL, Solcum DB (1988). Proximal tibial osteotomy in patients who are fifty years old or less. *J Bone Joint Surg (Am)* 70: 977–982.

Insall JN, Joseph DM, Msika C (1984). High tibial osteotomy for varus gonarthrosis. A long-term follow-up study. *J Bone Joint Surg (Am)* 66: 1040–1048.

Ivarsson I, Myrnerts R, Gillquist J (1990). High tibial osteotomy for medial arthritis of the knee. A 5 to 7 and a 11- to 13-year follow-up. *J Bone Joint Surg (Br)* 72: 238–244.

Jackson JP (1958). Osteotomy for osteoarthritis of the knee. *J Bone Joint Surg (Br)* 40: 826.

Jakob RP (1990). Instability-related osteoarthritis: special indications for osteotomies in the treatment of the unstable knee. In R.P. Jakob and H.U. Stäubli, eds. *The knee and cruciate ligaments*, pp. 543–567. Springer, Berlin.

Kaper BP, Carr CF, Shirreffs TG (1997). Compartment syndrome after arthroscopic surgery of knee. A report of two cases managed non-operatively. *Am J Sports Med* 25: 123–125.

Lattermann C, Jakob RP (1996). High tibial osteotomy alone or combined with ligament reconstruction in anterior cruciate ligament-deficient knees. *Knee Surg Sports Traumatol Arthrosc* 4(1): 32–8.

Lerat JL, Moyen B, Garin C, Mandrino A, Besse JL, Brunet-Guedj E (1993). Laxité antérieure at arthrose interne du genou. Résultat de la réconstruction du ligament croisé antérieure associée à une ostéotomie tibiale. *Rev Chir Orthop* 79: 365–374.

Marti CB, Jakob RP (1999). Accumulation of irrigation fluid in the calf as a complication during high tibial osteotomy combined with simultaneous arthroscopic anterior cruciate ligament reconstruction. *Arthroscopy* 15(8): 864–866.

Marti CB, Rodriguez M, Zanetti M, Romero J (2000). Spontaneous osteonecrosis of the medial compartment of the knee: a MRI follow-up after conservative and operative treatment, preliminary results. *Knee Surg Sports Traumatol Arthrosc* 8(2): 83–88.

Marti CB, Wachtl SW, Jakob RP (2001) Is the sagittal slope of the tibial plateau influenced by open wedge high tibial osteotomy in the unstable knee? Presented at the ISAKOS Congress, Montreux, Switzerland, May 2001.

Matsen FA, Winquist RA, Krugmire RB (1980). Diagnosis and management of compartmental syndromes. *J Bone Joint Surg* 62A: 286–291.

Noyes FR, Barber SD, Simon R (1993). High tibial osteotomy and ligament reconstruction in varus angulated, anterior cruciate lligament deficient knees, a two- to seven-year follow-up study. *Am J Sports Med* 21: 2–12.

O'Neill DF, James SL (1992). Valgus osteotomy with anterior cruciate laxity. *Clin Orthop* 278: 153–159.

Peek RD, Haynes DW (1984). Compartment syndrome as a complication of arthroscopy. A case report and a study of interstitial pressure. *Am J Sports Med* 12: 464–468.

Sledge SL (2001). Microfracture techniques in the treatment of osteochondral injuries. *Clin Sports Med* 4; 20(2): 365–377.

Steadman JR, Rodkey WG, Rodrigo JJ (2000). Microfracture: surgical technique and rehabilitation to treat chondral defects. *Clin Orthop* 10(391 Suppl): 362–369.

Part 6. Posterior Cruciate Ligament (PCL)

20

Natural history of PCL injuries

K. Donald Shelbourne and Cary Guse

Introduction

Posterior cruciate ligament (PCL) injuries have been recognized since the early 1900s. The reported incidence of PCL injury is between 1 and 44 per cent (Fanelli *et al.* 1994, Hughston and Degenardt 1982, Johnson and Bach 1990, Parolie and Bergfeld 1986). As interest in the PCL increased, so has the debate over appropriate management of PCL injuries. The lack of prospective studies elucidating the natural history of isolated intrasubstance PCL injuries has led to significant controversy in the management of these injuries. The literature abounds with retrospective studies that show good clinical results with non-operative treatment, but there is just as much literature supporting operative treatment for the very same injuries. These studies have traditionally been small, reporting on mixed populations, and retrospective in nature. Without prospective natural history studies, the science behind the management of these injuries has been lacking and the identification of those factors leading to dysfunctional outcomes had yet to be clearly identified.

Only two prospective natural history studies have been completed on PCL injury. Fowler and Messieh (1987) prospectively examined 13 patients with isolated PCL injuries and evaluated them at 2.6 years after injury. The investigators found 100 per cent with good or excellent subjective results, but only three patients with good objective results. More recently, Shelbourne *et al.* (1999a) reported on 133 patients with average follow-up of 5.4 years and found that non-operative treatment allowed 67 patients to return to their sport at the same level, 42 to return at a lower level, and only 22 were forced to change sports. These recent studies have shed new light on PCL injuries and the complexities associated with the anatomy, examination, treatment and rehabilitation of the posterior cruciate ligament.

Mechanism of injury

The history and physical examination are crucial in the accurate diagnosis of patients with PCL injuries. The usual mechanisms include a posteriorly directed force on a flexed knee (Clancy *et al.* 1983). Shelbourne and Rubinstein (1993) recently described an unusual mechanism PCL injury wherein a force is applied to the lower extremity that is in mild knee flexion and external rotation on a planted, but unloaded foot (Figure 20.1). The PCL is most often injured in conjunction with other major knee ligament disruptions and dislocations of the knee, and is the result of major trauma. Trickey (1968), in a series of 17 patients with PCL injuries, found that motorcycle or motor vehicle accidents accounted for 94 per cent of the injuries. Most PCL injuries in athletes are the result of lower energy mechanisms rather than mechanisms involved with a motor vehicle accident and, therefore, more isolated in nature. The percentage of PCL injuries caused from athletic injury is reported to be from 40–76 per cent (Cross and Powell 1984, Hughston *et al.* 1980, Kennedy *et al.* 1979). The PCL is normally torn in midsubstance or at its tibial insertion. Because the posterior capsule is usually relaxed, it only rarely sustains damage. It has been shown in cadaver studies that it takes 75–100 inch/pounds to rupture the posterior cruciate ligament (Bautigan and Johnson 2000).

Posterior cruciate ligament injuries typically occur in association with other ligamentous injuries following exposure of the affected limb to high energy trauma. Both the posterior capsule and the PCL are usually involved in such cases. Cross and Powell (1984) found 25 per cent of combined injuries occurred occur after a severe knee twist with an applied concomitant varus or valgus force. Shelbourne *et al.* (1990) identified a combined PCL-medial collateral injury in patients who had sustained a valgus external rotation force to a flexed knee with a planted but nonweightbearing foot (Figure 20.2).

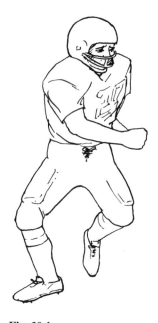

Fig. 20.1
An unusual mechanism of isolated PCL injury is anterior translation and external rotation of the femur over the weight-bearing leg when the knee is near full extension. Reprinted by permission from Reider, B., *Sports Medicine: The school age athlete*, 2nd edn, W.B. Saunders & Co. 1996.

History

Most isolated PCL injuries acutely present with posterior knee pain, swelling. The patient reports the sensation of 'something not feeling right' in the knee. Some chronic PCL-deficient knees remain asymptomatic and stay that way for an undetermined amount of time (Parolie and Bergfeld 1986). Consequently, the true incidence of PCL injuries is unclear, as many affected patients may not be symptomatic. For patients who sought treatment, pain was the main presenting symptom in 52–70 per cent of patients, and instability symptoms were usually secondary and present in 20–45 per cent of chronic PCL-deficient knees (Dandy and Pusey 1982, Parolie and Bergfeld 1986). Shelbourne *et al.* (1996) noted that many patients were asymptomatic at a jog or slow run but

Fig. 20.2

Rotation combined with additional valgus stress or an anterior pretibial blow to the flexed knee has been associated with complex injuries including the PCL. Reprinted by permission from Reider, B., *Sports Medicine: The school age athlete*, 2nd edn, W.B. Saunders & Co. 1996.

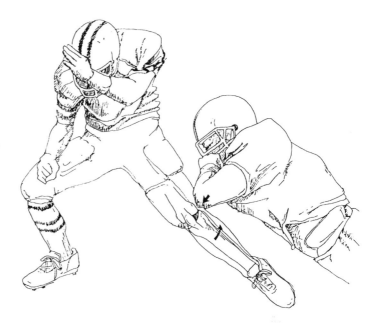

experienced severe pain when running at full speed. The authors theorized that the increased stride length caused a more complete extension and produced more posterior forces with the hamstrings pulling the tibia posteriorly. The authors theorized a similar mechanism with quick deceleration.

Physical examination

Patients with an acute isolated PCL usually have a mild effusion, and tenderness at the posterior knee; they may also experience difficulty squatting, but can bear weight. Often, knee range of motion is mildly restricted, and the patient will ambulate with a slightly flexed knee to avoid terminal extension and the feeling of instability associated with this leg position. When the injury is preceded by trauma, an abrasion or bruise on the anterior aspect of the proximal tibia may be noted (Fowler and Messieh 1987). The patient's gait pattern and overall limb alignment should be observed thoroughly as an abnormally increased thigh foot angle may also be present (Gollehon *et al.* 1987).

In a study that evaluated the ability of trained sports medicine orthopedists to detect PCL laxity by physical examination alone, Rubinstein *et al.* (1994) found that the accuracy was 96 per cent, sensitivity was 90 per cent, and specificity was 99 per cent. These authors also found the posterior drawer test to be the most sensitive and specific of physical examination maneuvers in detecting PCL injury. However, in the acute setting, knee swelling and the patient's inability to comfortably flex the knee to 90 degrees, may make physical examination less accurate in detecting these injuries. False negative findings can be minimized by carefully noting the starting position of the tibia relative to the femur. The examination in an acute injury will reveal a positive posterior drawer test with a soft endpoint and posterior tibial translation. In some circumstances, the end ranges of anterior-posterior tibial translation may be very painful during the examination. Interestingly, in many of our patients examined acutely after the injury and then 2–3 weeks later, we later find the posterior drawer endpoint to already be firm and the drawer test itself to be totally painless. Examination of the uninjured knee and the clincian's ability to detect side-to-side differences may be the only remaining clues to the injury.

Examination of the other knee ligaments should be performed as well. Normally the tibia lies 1 cm anterior to the tibial condyles in the 90° flexed knee. Grading is based on this normal anterior step off and referenced in relation to the normal contralateral knee. Most knee surgeons describe the PCL-deficient knee laxity finding using three grades. This grading was recently modified by Shelbourne and Rubinstein (1994) to include categories for those patients between grades 1–2 (grade 1.5) and grades 2–3 (grade 2.5):

Grade 1:   3–5 mm posterior displacement
Grade 1.5: 6–8 mm displacement
Grade 2:   9–10 mm posterior displacement (Tibial condyles are flush)
Grade 2.5: 11–13 mm (Tibial condyle posterior to femur)
Grade 3:   >13 mm posterior displacement.

Other less sensitive tests include the posterior sag sign, reverse Lachman, and reverse pivot shift test. The posterior sag sign may be the most characteristic diagnostic finding in the PCL-ruptured knee (Figure 20.3). The sag results from a gravity-assisted posterior displacement of the tibia in relation to the femur. It manifests as the

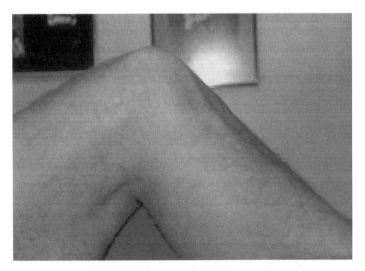

Fig. 20.3
The knee in the foreground illustrates the posterior sag usually seen in a PCL-deficient knee. Reprinted by permission from Reider, B., *Sports Medicine: The school age athlete*, 2nd edn, W.B. Saunders & Co. 1996.

(a)

(b)

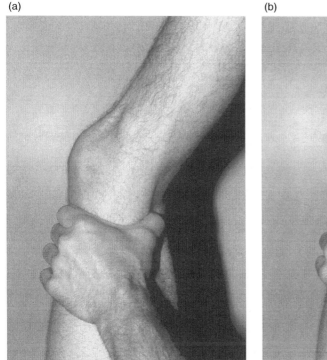
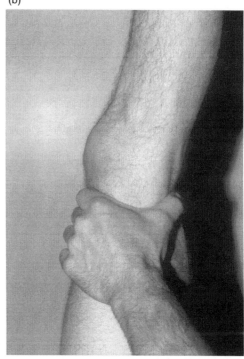

Fig. 20.4

(a) The tibia is subluxated posteriorly by pull of tightened hamstring tendons. (b) The tibia dynamically reduced as the knee nears full extension. Reprinted by permission from Shelbourne *et al.*, (1989) Dynamic posterior shift test. An adjuvant in evaluation of posterior tibial subluxation. *American Journal of Sports Medicine*, vol 17: 276.

apparent disappearance of the tibial tubercle from the lateral view of the 90° flexed knee. The quadriceps active test described by Daniels *et al.* is another adjunctive test. In their study, 41 of 42 PCL deficient knees were accurately diagnosed with this simple maneuver (Daniel *et al.* 1988).

Shelbourne *et al.* (1989) described a dynamic posterior shift test (Figure 20.4). The patient's hip and knee is flexed to 90°. The examiner places one hand on the anterior thigh just above the knee and the other hand supports the distal calf while extending the leg slowly. The test is positive when a posteriorly subluxed tibia reduces with a visible and palpable jerk when the knee is in near full extension. They found this test to be much more reliable than the reverse pivot shift test (Shelbourne *et al.* 1989). The basic theory behind all of these tests is to demonstrate posterior tibial displacement relative to the femur at 90° of flexion.

A helpful adjunct to the physical examination is the use of a knee ligament arthrometer. Rubinstein *et al.* (1994) found the KT-1000 arthrometer to have an 89 per cent overall accuracy, 76 per cent sensitivity, and 93 per cent specificity. It was much more sensitive for high-grade tears relative to lower grade tears in their study. The arthrometer has become a regular and vital part of the examination in the preoperative, peri-operative and postoperative program of many experienced clinicians.

347

Radiographic studies

In the evaluation of the acutely injured knee plain radiographs remain the gold standard. Posteroanterior (weight-bearing 45° flexed), lateral, and Merchant views should be obtained to rule out major fractures and dislocations. In the PCL-deficient knee, posterior translation or an avulsion off the tibia are the most common findings. Fibular head and Gerdy tubercle avulsions may suggest severe lateral or posteriolateral involvement. These findings should be distinguished from Segond's lateral capsule sign, which is more closely associated with anterior cruciate ligament injury.

Historically, the use of anterior and rotational stress views was commonplace. However, the development of magnetic resonance imaging (MRI) and, more importantly, improved physical examination methodology has made these radiographic views less necessary.

MRI is the gold standard for imaging of the ligaments in the knee. Excellent visualization can usually be obtained. Normally, the PCL appears as a signal void on the T1 imaging scans. The PCL commonly appears swollen and will demonstrate foci of increased signal in the injured ligament. Gross *et al.* (1992) found MRI to be 100 per cent sensitive and specific in the diagnosis of PCL injuries. The accuracy of MRI with chronic PCL injuries has recently been challenged. Tewes *et al.* (1997) looked at 13 patients with high-grade PCL injuries and found that ten had regained continuity. In this study, there was no correlation between functional status and posterior knee laxity, as 7 of the 10 patients still had positive posterior drawer tests on physical examination.

Shelbourne *et al.* (1999b) also looked at acute and follow-up MRI on 40 posterior cruciate ligament injuries. The authors found that all partial PCL tears and most complete PCL tears appeared in continuity on the follow-up MRI scan. This phenomenon was not affected by tear location, the presence of associated ligament injuries or injury severity. Moreover, altered ligament morphology was observed in 25 of 37 'continuous' posterior cruciate ligaments; this may indicate that these injured PCLs do not return to their preinjury status. Based on these studies and our clinical experience that typically has observed that the PCL injured knee regains a firm endpoint within weeks of injury, we believe that MRI should be used as an *adjunct* to a thorough history and clinical examination.

Natural history

The purpose of any natural history study is to aid the clinician in determining prognosis for an injury if left untreated. A natural history study provides invaluable information to the clinician on when and how to intervene. Much of the difficulty in treating PCL injuries begins with the poor understanding of the natural history of the PCL-deficient knee. This problem is further compounded by the lack of uniform standard in diagnosing and treating these injuries. The natural history of PCL injuries has only recently been elucidated. In fact, to date there have been only two *true* natural history studies performed on isolated PCL injuries to date (Fowler and Messieh 1987, Shelbourne *et al.* 1999a). There are many retrospective studies that describe various surgical treatments for the PCL-deficient knee. On the whole, the literature is scant on this topic, and oftentimes would suggest both conservative and operative management for PCL-injured knees with similar physical findings. There is also an inherent bias in the operative studies, as the majority of these reports include only those patients that were symptomatic and returned for treatment due to continued to pain or instability.

In the literature, most authors agree that a PCL injured, when combined with other knee ligament injuries, has a worse prognosis and tends to develop degenerative changes earlier compared to the knee with an isolated PCL injury. Satku *et al.* (1984) found that the best prognostic sign in the PCL-deficient knee was the presence or absence of associated ligamentous injuries. Fowler and Messieh (1987) presented the first truly prospective natural history study on isolated posterior cruciate ligament injuries. They found that 100 per cent of the non-operatively treated patients achieved good subjective results. However, they also found that only 3 of the 13 patients in their study achieved good objective results at a mean follow-up only 2.6 years after injury.

The most recent and largest prospective natural history study on isolated PCL injuries was reported by Shelbourne *et al.* in 1999a. His study reported on 133 patients at a mean follow-up 5.4 years. No change in knee laxity was demonstrated between those findings of the initial examination and the follow-up examination. Pain scores did not correlate with the amount of posterior knee laxity or increasing time from injury. Patients with greater laxity did not have significantly worse subjective modified Noyes knee scores, Lysholm scores, or mean Tegner activity scores. Radiographic evaluation showed that 39 of 65 patients demonstrated no radiographic changes and only 10 patients had degenerative changes in the involved knee only. Fifteen patients had degenerative changes in both knees. Although there was a trend toward medial joint arthrosis, this finding was not statistically significant; this finding did not correlate with the degree of PCL laxity. Symptomatic meniscus tears were rare, and those patients with grade 2 laxity did not develop more symptomatic meniscus tears compared to knees with grade 1 laxity. Fifty per cent of all patients were able to return to sport at the same level, 33 per cent returned to sport but at a lower level, and 17 per cent were not able to return to the same sport (Shelbourne *et al.* 1999a).

These two studies represent the only true prospective natural history studies in the literature. Other PCL injury studies have been published, but are typically retrospective in nature, and biased toward treating symptomatic patients who were seeking relief; other studies have examined the treatment of both isolated and combined PCL injuries (Cross and Powell 1984, Dandy and Pusey 1982, Keller *et al.* 1993, Kennedy *et al.* 1979, Parolie and Bergfeld 1986, Torg *et al.* 1989). On the basis of these true natural history studies, clinicians can begin to think more objectively about their treatment options. While neither study solves the debate regarding operative versus non-operative treatment modalities, they do provide the basis upon which to compare operative treatment methods.

Treatment

Treatment of isolated posterior cruciate ligament injuries remains a controversial issue. There are proponents of both operative and non-operative treatment for these injuries, and the literature is replete with studies supporting both approaches. Loss of the posterior cruciate ligament indisputably results in abnormal knee biomechanics. There is increased posterior tibial translation, and increased shear force across the articular surfaces of the knee as demonstrated in biomechanical studies. What is not known is whether these forces ultimately result in compromised knee function or whether operative treatment restores normal knee kinematics.

In developing a treatment plan for PCL-deficient patients, the clinician must consider patient symptoms, current and desired activity level, patient goals and expectations, and the overall nature of the injured knee. The ultimate goal of treatment is to restore normal knee stability and kinematics, reduce the likelihood of degenerative changes and allow a return to activity at the preinjury level. While this may be the goal of treatment the reality may be that our current surgical techniques are not able to attain such a result. If this is the case then our goal must be to offer the treatment that can best approximate the preinjury level with the minimal amount of risk.

Operative treatment

A variety of surgical techniques and a myriad of graft types have been advocated for PCL reconstruction. Arthroscopic techniques, tibial inlay reconstruction and traditional open approaches are described techniques. Autologous tissues including patellar tendon, hamstring tendon, Achilles tendon, biceps femoris tenodesis, and gastrocnemius augmentation have all been well described.

This authors' preference for PCL repair is reconstruction using an autogenous bone-patellar tendon-bone graft. The harvest site follows the same course as that observed for ACL reconstruction. Shelbourne and Rubinstein (1994) reported on 23 patients with a bone-patellar-bone repair with an average follow-up of 3.6 years. They found laxity decreased from an average grade of 2.5 to an average of grade 1. The postoperative subjective score was an average of 76 points.

Their primary indications for operative treatment are those cases involving severe combined instability or dislocation. Noyes and Westin (1994) reported that PCL reconstruction using an allograft improved stability at low flexion angles but not at high angles. They did not find ligament augmentation improved their results. The authors, however, continued to recommend reconstruction with autograft.

Clancy *et al.* (1983) reported on 23 bone-patella-bone reconstructions with 21 having good or excellent results at two years follow-up. They found that, at four years after the injury, 90 per cent of patients had developed moderate to severe articular changes in the medial compartment at the time of surgery. They demonstrated a decrease in posterior laxity to 1+ in most of the cases. Keller *et al.* (1993) found that even with isolated PCL injuries, patients had a significant decrease in functional status and an increase in subjective complaints as time passed after the injury. The authors also recommended operative treatment on the basis of these findings and felt that a decrease from grade 2 to grade 1 laxity was helpful in decreasing subjective complaints in their series. However, the study did not evaluate patients from initial time of injury, they were not followed at regular intervals and were potentially biased by patients specifically presenting for treatment of their pain.

Fanellli *et al.* (1994) reported on 30 patients who underwent PCL reconstructions utilizing either Achilles allograft or autogenous patellar tendons. They reported a decrease in KT-1000 arthrometer measurements from 4.64 mm to 1.95 mm postoperatively and increase in Lysholm scores from an average of 48.2 to a post-operative score of 93.0.

Certainly, the published results of PCL reconstruction have yet to equal the results produced by ACL-reconstructive procedures. In addition, no one has been able to biomechanically reconstruct the posterior ligament in a manner approaching an anatomic reconstruction. All studies have shown results of residual posterior laxities of 1+. Significant work on single isometric graft placement continues and split and dual graft reconstructions are being developed, but because of the complexities of PCL biomechanics, an ideal solution has yet to be developed.

Non-operative treatment

Historically, the general recommendation for treatment of mild, isolated PCL insufficiency has been non-operative treatment, the belief being that these patients will achieve acceptable results. Parolie *et al.* (1986) reported their six year follow-up on 25 athletes with acute PCL injuries and found 80 per cent were satisfied with their knees and 68 per cent returned to their same level of performance. Their study, however, included both isolated and combined injuries.

Torg *et al.* (1989) reported on 43 patients divided into two groups. Group 1 consisted of 14 isolated PCL injuries, and group 2 consisted of 29 patients with multidirectional instability. With an average follow-up of 6.3 years, group 1 patients had significantly better subjective results than did group 2 patients. Good or excellent results were obtained in 86 per cent of group 1 patients as opposed to 48 per cent in group 2 patients. Poor results were reported in as many as 28 per cent of group 2 patients, but only 7 per cent of group 1 patients. They also did not find any correlation between arthrometer testing and functional results. They recommended non-operative treatment for isolated injuries and advocated surgical repair for combined injuries. Many in the literature have taken a similar approach.

Fowler and Messieh (1987) looked at 13 patients with isolated PCL injuries and found that acceptable functional stability did not require absolute static stability. They believed that non-operative treatment was a viable alternative to operative management and recommended treatment on a case-by-case basis.

Controversy still exists about appropriate treatment for interstitial tears. Unlike a ruptured anterior cruciate ligament and more similar to a medial collateral ligament, the posterior cruciate ligament can heal on its own. As was discussed previously, patients with acute injuries without a solid endpoint can re-present a few weeks later with a firm endpoint. MRI imaging has demonstrated the ligament's ability to heal, albeit with abnormal morphology (Shelbourne *et al.* 1999b). Currently, we are not able to exactly predict the timeframe for regeneration, but it has been observed clinically as early as two weeks.

The goal of any rehabilitation program should be to restore function as quickly and efficiently as possible, at the same time minimizing any long-term sequelae. Traditionally, knee rehabilitation has involved strengthening the musculature surrounding the knee and minimizing the forces crossing the knee.

The initial non-operative management of PCL injuries must address the issues of pain, effusion, and decreased range of motion. This can usually be accomplished using combinations of anti-inflammatories, immobilization, and cold therapy. The authors prefer the use of the Cyro/Cuff (Aircast, Inc., Summit, NJ) to provide both cold and compression simultaneously. As pain and effusion subside, range of motion and quadriceps muscle therapy is initiated. We prefer the use of closed chain kinetic exercises as activity progresses. Once adequate strength and range of motion have been acquired, a functional progression to running and eventually a return to competitive sport are allowed. We have found that three-quarters speed running is usually well tolerated, but full speed sprinting is often painful and not well tolerated. Although this is seen in the early rehabilitation phase (3–8 weeks), the pain seems to subside with time. We have not seen any worsening of posterior laxity with this early return to activity.

Cross and Powell (1984), in a study of 116 patients, found that patients with good quadriceps muscle strength were less symptomatic than patients with poor quadriceps muscle strength. They did concede, however, that eventual degenerative change and arthrosis was inevitable. Conversely, Keller *et al.* (1993) found no correlation between functional outcome and the maintenance of good quadriceps strength. In the natural history study by Shelbourne *et al.* (1999a) the quadriceps muscle strength of the injured quadriceps was found to be 94 per cent of the non-injured knee. In those patients in whom quadriceps strength was diminished, the investigators were not able to distinguish if the injury was the cause of any pain or the result of existing pain.

Bracing the PCL-deficient knee is occasionally performed. However, there are few studies that have actually looked at the efficacy of bracing. There are several investigators who question the use of a brace on the basis of the fact that instability is rarely a significant problem in the isolated posterior cruciate deficient knee. Many investigators have found no correlation between KT-1000 arthrometer testing and functional complaints. Furthermore, there is a significant question as to whether any brace is truly capable of preventing posterior translation during daily or sporting activities. Bracing may be of some benefit, especially during the initial rehabilitation phase.

Because of the results reported in the most recent natural history study, we are now able to give patients a better idea of what to expect after an isolated PCL injury. Athletes with acute isolated PCL injuries can be counseled that the amount of posterior laxity will slightly improve over time. Unfortunately, this improvement in laxity has not correlated with subjective improvement. We cannot attribute low subjective scores to quadriceps muscle weakness as the natural history has shown >90 per cent strength relative to the uninjured side. We agree that patients with chronic isolated PCL laxity who are symptomatic and show significant quadriceps weakness may benefit from quadriceps muscle strengthening, but there is little supportive evidence that patients with normal strength will benefit from continued strengthening exercises.

There have been multiple studies indicating that the PCL-deficient knee is more susceptible to the development of degenerative changes (Boynton and Tietjens 1996, Clancy *et al.* 1983, Dejour *et al.* 1988). Macdonald *et al.* (1996) showed in cadaver studies that PCL-deficient knees have increased medial compartment pressure. This finding might bias the surgeon towards choosing surgical management of the PCL-injured knee, because, in theory, reducing the amount of knee laxity would prevent the development of arthritic changes. In the study by Shelbourne *et al.* (1999a), only 10 of 67 patients developed degenerative changes and no episodes of patellofemoral arthritis were noted. The authors found no correlation between degree of laxity and degenerative changes. However, longer follow-up would be required to determine the true likelihood of one developing arthritis following PCL injury.

As previously discussed, the indications for operative interventions are quite varied in the literature. In most cases, the patient assessment is based on subjective interpretation of symptoms and physical findings by the treating clinician. How accurately can a clinician distinguish between 9 and 12 mm of posterior tibial translation? How long should one wait for reconstruction of the ligament? How does the clinician decide which arthritic changes are severe enough that surgery would be contraindicated? Perhaps the most important question to be answered is, 'Does surgical intervention improve the natural history of the injury?' To date, no operative procedure has been shown to restore normal biomechanics to the knee or alter the course of degenerative changes. The amount of posterior laxity has not been shown to correlate to function or degenerative changes in any way. Therefore, operative reconstructions that decrease the grade of laxity from 2 + to 1 + may not have any effect on the long-term function of patients with PCL-deficient knees. In contrast, it has been shown that ACL reconstruction can prevent instability episodes and protect the menisci when tibiofemoral translation is less than 3 mm (Shelbourne *et al.* 1999a). Posterior cruciate ligament-deficient patients with residual grade 1 posterior laxity (3–5 mm) still have functional complaints similar to patients who have much greater posterior laxity. This suggests that decreasing but not normalizing PCL laxity may not be of significant help to these patients. Therefore, in order to significantly alter the natural history of the PCL-deficient knee, a surgical technique that restores normal knee biomechanics needs to be developed.

Shelbourne *et al.* (1999a) also identified an interesting trend. Patients who had subjective modified Noyes scores that were greater than 90 at one year had a 90 per cent chance of maintaining high levels of knee function over time. Those patients with scores less than 75 points at one year had only a 30 per cent chance of improved knee function over time. Unfortunately, the investigators could not find any identifiable characteristics or objective findings that could reliably predict which patients would show improvement or deterioration of knee function in the future. They were able to show that 50 per cent of patients were able to return to their sport at the same level, 31 per cent of patients returned to their sport but at a lesser level, and 18 per cent could not return to their sport whatsoever. Once again, no reliable prognostic indicators were found that might aid clinicians in predicting into which category a patient might fall.

We are not suggesting that non-operative management is the only solution for all acute isolated PCL injuries. It is well known that there is a subset of patients that do not fare well with PCL-deficient knees from the outset. There is also a subset of patients that remain totally asymptomatic despite significant laxity. At the annual National Football League evaluation of prospective players, nearly 2 per cent of the participants typically present with posterior laxity; these patients, based on their participation in the NFL event, remain asymptomatic and able to participate in elite level athletics (unpublished data). We believe that most patients will eventually develop some difficulty. Conversely, operative management has not been shown to alter the natural history of isolated PCL injuries, either subjectively or objectively. This is likely due to the fact that the cause of the difficulties is still not truly known. It is likely that pressure changes occur even with the smallest amount of PCL laxity. These pressure changes can cause an alteration in the load sharing effects of the meniscus and lead to variable amounts of pain or disability. We suspect that there is a critical amount of laxity that occurs and results in medial joint pressure changes. The exact amount of laxity remains unknown. We hypothesize that this laxity renders the meniscus non-functional. We are not advocating any specific treatment methods (non-operative, operative, or physical therapy). The ideal operative procedure would restore posterior laxity to preinjury status, as merely reducing posterior laxity is clearly not enough. However to be considered successful, an intervention must give better results than the natural course of the injury. Currently, we cannot prove that any operative intervention can definitely improve on the natural course of the PCL-deficient knee.

Conclusion

For the assessment of any knee ligament injury, the first step is to establish the diagnosis accurately. Recent improvements and advancements in physical examination, as well as biomechanics and imaging, have allowed clinicians to accurately identify and diagnose the PCL-deficient knee. The diagnosis must be determined in the context of both chronicity and the number of ligaments involved. Treatment decisions should take into consideration the symptoms, timing, expectations, and activity level of the patient and need to be tailored to the individual. Although non-operative treatment will not give these patients a normal knee, it may give the most predictable results. Surgical treatment may play a significant role in the future, but normal PCL stability must be established before improvement in results can be found compared with the natural history of the injury.

References

Brautigan B, Johnson DL (2000). The epidemiology of knee dislocations. *Clin Sports Med*, 19, 387–397.

Boynton MD, Tietjens BR (1996). Long-term follow-up of the untreated isolated posterior cruciate ligament-deficient knee. *Am J Sports Med*, 24, 306–310.

Clancy WG, Shelbourne KD, Zoellner GB, Keene JS, Reider B, Rosenberg TD (1983). Treatment of knee joint instability secondary to rupture of the posterior cruciate ligament. *J Bone Joint Surg*, 65-A, 310–322.

Cross MJ, Powell JF (1984). Long-term follow-up of posterior cruciate ligament rupture: A study of 116 cases. *Am J Sports Med*, 12, 292–297.

Dandy DJ, Pusey RJ (1982). The long-term results of unrepaired tears of the posterior cruciate ligament. *J Bone Joint Surg*, 64-B, 92–94.

Daniel DM, Stone ML, Barnett P, Sachs R (1988). Use of the quadriceps active test to diagnose posterior cruciate-ligament disruption and measure posterior laxity of the knee. *J Bone Joint Surg*, 70-A, 386–391.

Dejour H, Walch G, Peyrol J, Eberhard P (1988). The natural history of rupture of the posterior cruciate ligament. *French J Orthop Surg*, 2, 112–120.

Fanelli GC, Giannotti BF, Edson CJ (1994). Current concepts review. The posterior cruciate ligament. Arthroscopic evaluation and treatment. *Arthroscopy*, 10, 673–688.

Fowler PJ, Messieh SS (1987). Isolated posterior cruciate ligament injuries in athletes. *Am J Sports Med*, 15, 553–557.

Gollehon DL, Torzilli PA, Warren RF (1987). The role of posterolateral and cruciate ligaments in the stability of the human knee. *J Bone Joint Surg*, 69-A, 233–242.

Gross ML, Grover JS, Bassett LW, Seeger LL, Finerman GA (1992). Magnetic resonance imaging of the posterior cruciate ligament. Clinical use to improve diagnostic accuracy. *Am J Sports Med*, 20, 732–737.

Hughston JC, Bowden JA, Andrews JR, Norwood LA (1980). Acute tears of the posterior cruciate ligament. *J Bone Joint Surg*, 62-A, 438–450.

Hughston JC, Degenhardt TC (1982). Reconstruction of the posterior cruciate ligament. *Clin Orthop*, 164, 59–77.

Johnson JC, Bach BR (1990). Current concepts review. Posterior cruciate ligament. *Am J Knee Surg*, 3, 143–153.

Keller PM, Shelbourne KD, McCarroll JR, Rettig AC (1993). Nonoperatively treated isolated posterior cruciate ligament injuries. *Am J Sports Med*, 21, 132–136.

Kennedy JC, Roth JH, Walker DM (1979). Posterior cruciate ligament injuries. *Orthop Digest*, 7, 19–31.

MacDonald P, Miniaci A, Fowler P, Marks P, Finlay B (1996). A biomechanical analysis of joint contact forces in the posterior cruciate deficient knee. *Knee Surg Sports Traumatol Arthroscopy*, 3, 252–255.

Noyes FR, Barber-Westin SD (1994). Posterior cruciate ligament allografts reconstruction with and without a ligament augmentation device. *Arthroscopy*, 10, 371–382.

Parolie JM, Bergfeld JA (1986). Long-term results of nonoperative treatment of isolated posterior cruciate ligament injuries in the athlete. *Am J Sports Med*, 14, 35–38.

Rubinstein RA Jr, Shelbourne KD, McCarroll JR, VanMeter CD, Rettig AC (1994). The accuracy of clinical examination in the setting of posterior cruciate ligament injury. *Am J Sports Med*, 22, 550–557.

Satku K, Chew CN, Seow H (1984). Posterior cruciate ligament injuries. *Acta Orthop Scand*, 55, 26–29.

Shelbourne KD, Benedict F, McCarroll JR, Rettig AC (1989). Dynamic posterior shift test. An adjuvant in evaluation of posterior tibial subluxation. *Am J Sports Med*, 17, 275–277.

Shelbourne KD, Davis TJ, Patel DV (1999a). The natural history of acute isolated non-operatively treated posterior cruciate ligament injuries. A prospective study. *Am J Sports Med*, 27, 276–283.

Shelbourne KD, Foulk DA, Nitz P (1996). Posterior cruciate ligament injuries. In B Reider, ed. *Sports Medicine. The school-age athlete*, pp. 349–362. WB Saunders, Philadelphia.

Shelbourne KD, Mesko JW, McCarroll JR, Rettig AC (1990). Combined medial collateral ligament–posterior cruciate rupture. Mechanism of injury. *Am J Knee Surg*, 3, 41–44.

Shelbourne KD, Jennings RW, Vahey TN (1999b). Magnetic resonance imaging of posterior cruciate ligament injuries: assessment of healing. *Am J Knee Surg*, 12, 209–213.

Shelbourne KD, Rubinstein RA Jr (1993). Isolated posterior cruciate ligament rupture: an unusual mechanism of injury. A report of three cases. *Am J Knee Surg*, 6, 84–86.

Shelbourne KD, Rubinstein RA Jr (1994). Methodist Sports Medicine Center's experience with acute and chronic isolated posterior cruciate ligament injuries. *Clinics in Sports Med*, 13, 531–543.

Tewes DP, Fritts HM, Fields RD, Quick DC, Buss DD (1997). Chronically injured posterior cruciate ligament. Magnetic resonance imaging. *Clin Orthop*, 335, 224–232.

Torg JS, Barton TM, Pavlov H, Stine RS (1989). Natural history of posterior cruciate ligament-deficient knee. *Clin Orthop*, 246, 208–216.

Trickey EL (1968). Rupture of the posterior cruciate ligament of the knee. *J Bone Joint Surg*, 50-B, 334–341.

21

PCL reconstruction: is it necessary following PCL rupture?

Todd M. Herrenbruck and John A. Bergfeld

Introduction

Injuries to the posterior cruciate ligament (PCL) may lead to significant disability. The incidence of PCL injuries has been reported to be as high as 20 per cent in severe knee ligament injuries (Bianchi, 1983). The primary challenge to the clinician lies in predicting the effect of these injuries on our patient's day to day activities. As progressive disability from untreated PCL injuries has become more evident, and as successful reconstruction of the anterior cruciate ligament (ACL) has become commonplace, interest in surgical treatment of PCL injuries has experienced a crescendo over the past ten years. Most literature to date has emphasized diagnosis and treatment, while information regarding long-term results of either operative or non-operative treatment has lagged behind. As a result, controversy continues regarding the appropriate treatment for injuries to the PCL. Only in the last few years have laboratory and clinical studies become available to help guide the clinician in the decision-making process. In this chapter, we will present a decision-making algorithm that clarifies the recommendations for operative treatment of a PCL injury. We will first discuss the important anatomic and biomechanical properties of the injured PCL as well as the history and physical findings that predict the need for operative treatment. An important distinction is made to classify these injuries as either isolated unidirectional injuries or combined multidirectional injuries, and to label them as acute or chronic. We emphasize the importance of the distinctions as we find them critical in predicting the necessity for operative intervention. Injuries isolated to the PCL spare the menisci, capsule, and ligaments about the knee. Successful non-operative treatment is predictable (Shelbourne *et al.*, 1999a). When PCL injuries are associated with concomitant damage to one or more of the surrounding capsuloligamentous restraints however, operative treatment is frequently required. The combined, multidirectional injuries often include a PCL tear in addition to an injury to the posterolateral structures of the knee. Other injury combinations include concomitant ACL and PCL tears, and PCL tears associated with medial collateral ligament complex injuries. The incidence of these combined injuries may be as high as 60 per cent acutely (Clancy et al., 1983) and the laxity may worsen over time as a chronically PCL-deficient knee stretches the surrounding secondary restraints. Defining these injury patterns, and clearly understanding the scope of abnormal knee laxity, is critical in deciding to proceed with operative reconstruction of the PCL.

Functional anatomy

The PCL is an intraarticular, extrasynovial ligament that arises from the posterior aspect of the tibia and attaches on the medial femoral condyle. The total length of the ligament averages between 32–38 mm (Girgis et al., 1975) and has been divided into various components by different authors. Traditionally, the PCL has been described as containing inseparable but functionally distinct posterolateral and anteromedial bundles with variably present meniscofemoral ligaments (Harner et al., 1995). These two bundles have recently been found to equally contribute to the overall mid-substance diameter of the PCL. Others have proposed the PCL contains a large anterior component representing 95 per cent of the ligament and a small posterior oblique component emanating from the postero-superior aspect of the femoral attachment and attaching obliquely onto the posterolateral aspect of the tibia (O'Brien and coworkers unpublished, 1989). Still others have classified the PCL as having four distinct fiber regions divided into the anterior, central, posterior longitudinal and posterior oblique (Covey et al., 1996). Regardless of the classification, it is generally accepted that the anterior bulk of the ligament tightens in flexion and the posterior aspect of the ligament tightens in extension. It has been shown that the PCL insertion area on the medial femoral condyle is half moon shaped and located where the intercondylar notch joins the wall, approximately 1 cm posterior to the articular cartilage (Harner et al., 1999). This area is of critical importance when considering the femoral tunnel placement for reconstruction and the best position for graft placement is still debated. The tibial attachment of the PCL is centered in a mediolateral direction and is generally 1 cm distal to the joint line (Girgis et al., 1975). The attachment lies on the posterior cortex of the tibia, a critical point that influences our choice of the inlay graft for PCL reconstruction.

One or both of the meniscofemoral ligaments are present in over 90 per cent of normal knees. The anterior meniscofemoral ligament of Humphrey originates distal and posterior to the PCL attachment on the femur and attaches at the most anterior aspect of the posterior horn of the lateral meniscus. The posterior meniscofemoral ligament of Wrisberg originates from the femur proximal and posterior to the PCL footprint and attaches on the posterior horn of the lateral meniscus. It is evident from the literature that the size and contribution of these ligaments to the overall function of the PCL is variable and poorly understood. In our laboratory, we have found the meniscofemoral ligaments to provide considerable contribution to the overall resistance and bulk of the PCL complex. It is important to keep these ligaments in mind when assessing isolated PCL tears as they may provide essential stability and should be left intact if found during PCL reconstruction.

Functional biomechanics

Understanding the role of the PCL in maintaining global knee stability is important when considering operative treatment for PCL injuries. The PCL complex (PCL and meniscofemoral ligaments) has been shown to contribute 95 per cent of the overall restraint to posterior tibial translation with the knee at 90 degrees of flexion (Butler *et al.*, 1980). Our experience has been that this number may be closer to 85 per cent with a 10 per cent contribution from the meniscofemoral ligaments. The ultimate load capacity of the PCL is only slightly higher than that of the ACL, but significant differences have been found with respect to the anterior lateral bundle and posterior medial bundle. The anterior lateral bundle fails on average at 1120 N, while the posterior medial bundle and meniscofemoral ligaments fail at 419 N and 297 N respectively (Harner *et al.*, 1995). The PCL appears to provide its greatest restraint to posterior translation at higher knee flexion angles. At angles closer to full extension, the secondary stabilizers about the knee provide increasing amounts of resistance to posterior translation. The lateral collateral ligament and the posterolateral capsuloligamentous complex provide primary resistance to varus and external rotation moments at all flexion angles and act as secondary stabilizers to posterior translation of the tibia (Gollehon *et al.*, 1987). Other secondary restraints include the posterior knee capsule, the meniscofemoral ligaments, and the medial capsuloligamentous structures. At terminal extension, all of these structures may play a role in decreasing posterior laxity in an isolated tear of the PCL. Additionally, the senior author has recently demonstrated that sectioning of the PCL and meniscofemoral ligaments results in a significant increase in posterior knee laxity at 30, 60, and 90° that is significantly decreased at 60 and 90° with the tibia held in internal rotation. Intact or sectioned meniscofemoral ligaments did not affect this decrease in posterior laxity (Bergfeld *et al.*, 2001). Our biomechanical studies show that this decrease in posterior translation with internal rotation of the tibia represents a tightening of the intact medial capsuloligamentous structures (Ritchie *et al.*, 1998). These structures and possibly other posterolateral structures represent additional important secondary stabilizers to posterior translation. A clear understanding of these secondary stabilizers is critical in determining the need for operative reconstruction of the PCL, and is addressed further in the discussion on the clinical exam.

Mechanisms of injury

When considering operative intervention for PCL injuries, the mechanism of injury should be elucidated. The most common mechanism, the so-called dashboard injury, involves a posterior directed force on a flexed knee. This mechanism most often results in a mid-substance tear of the PCL and often injures other secondary restraints. A similar mechanism in the athlete is a fall on a fully flexed knee with the foot in plantar flexion. This causes elongation and often loss of continuity of the anterior component of the PCL. This injury pattern often spares the posterior capsule and other secondary restraints. A less common mechanism is an anteriorly directed force against an extended knee resulting in varus and hyperextension. The PCL and posterolateral structures are injured in this scenario and result in a combined ligamentous laxity. When considering the treatment options for a PCL-deficient knee, the mechanism of injury can provide essential information in the treatment algorithm.

Clinical evaluation (history)

When evaluating patients with knee injuries, it is critical to uncover the patient's chief complaint. In the acute setting, this is primarily revealed in a detailed history of the injury mechanism. As described above, there a variety of mechanisms which can result in a tear of the PCL. The history, eyewitness accounts, and occasionally videotape may be available to clarify the injury mechanism. This important piece of the puzzle will provide insight into the integrity of the secondary stabilizers. In addition, a thorough history of any prior knee problems should be completed. It is not uncommon to uncover previous injuries and disabilities that will influence the treatment algorithm. Specifically, previous injuries to the medial and lateral secondary stabilizers should be questioned.

For the patients with chronic knee problems and abnormal posterior laxity, functional symptoms may predominate. Intermittent episodes of instability, pain while going up and down stairs, down ramps, squatting, or taking long walks have been noted to be the most common complaints (Dandy and Pusey, 1982). Often walking on uneven ground or a sudden change in direction may result in pain or instability. Over time, these symptoms may worsen as the secondary stabilizers lengthen and the articular surfaces are required

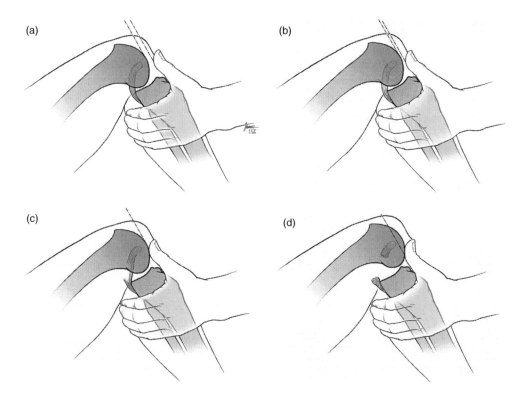

Fig. 21.1

Posterior drawer examination of the knee. (a) The examiner's thumbs are placed just anterior to the femoral condyles and in the normal knee, will rest approximately 10 mm anterior to the condyles. (b) The grade I injury with posterior drawer testing demonstrates approximately 5 mm of increased posterior translation. (c) The examination of the grade II injury will allow the thumbs to become flush with the condyles. (d) A grade III PCL injury will allow the tibial plateau to translate posterior to the anterior edge of the femoral condyles.

to support increasingly abnormal forces. A common scenario involves an initially asymptomatic patellofemoral joint that later develops retro-patellar pain and intermittent effusions (Cross and Powell, 1984).

Clinical evaluation (physical examination)

The exam of the knee with an acute PCL injury critically influences the decision as to whether surgical reconstruction will be required. This exam varies according to the time of presentation and the nature of the injury. Patients with injuries to the PCL may present following significant trauma, as may be seen in vehicular accidents, or they may present in the office with vague symptoms and no known mechanism of injury. The spectrum of associated ligamentous injuries often parallels the force of the injury and must be considered in the examination. In the severely traumatized knee, acute swelling and pain may limit the examination. The physician must then either obtain ancillary studies at that time to aid in the diagnosis or immo-bilize the knee in the acute period for later examination. If the knee is too painful to be taken through a range of motion, information regarding the integrity of the secondary stabilizers may be obtained by examining for ecchymosis, local tenderness and gross instability.

The most sensitive test for a PCL injury is the posterior drawer (Figure 21.1, a–d). Our current technique involves testing posterior laxity at 90 degrees of flexion in neutral, internal, and external tibial rotation. The medial tibial plateau, as compared to the medial femoral condyle, is graded as normal if the plateau is 10 mm anterior to the medial femoral condyle with posterior drawer testing. From this position of normal, grades of abnormal laxity are assigned based on the amount of posterior excursion from this point. Grade I laxity is 0–5 mm of posterior laxity with the plateau still anterior to the condyle. Grade II laxity is 5–10 mm of posterior translation while the tibial plateau remains anterior or flush with the medial femoral condyle. Grade III laxity is more than 10 mm of posterior translation as the plateau continues posterior to the medial femoral condyle. We find that placing the IP joints of the examiner's thumbs on the tibial plateau with the thumbs anterior to the condyles allows a 95 per cent reliable clinical reproduction of this classification (Rubinstein *et al.*, 1994). If when performing the exam the thumbs hit the condyles and yet the tibia continues to subluxate past this point, a grade III injury exists. Additionally, we repeat this maneuver with the tibia held in maximal internal rotation. We have found that decreased posterior laxity with internal rotation represents intact, functional capsuloligamentous structures, especially the superficial medial collateral ligament. An isolated grade III PCL injury will demonstrate 2–4 mm decreased posterior translation when held and tested in internal rotation. This decrease to a grade II on internal rotation indicates proper functioning medial capsuloligmentous structures and portends a better prognosis with nonsurgical treatment. If the posterior tibial displacement remains unchanged or increases with internal rotation, operative treatment may be necessary. This has been our observation in the clinical setting and has been demonstrated through work in our laboratory (Ritchie *et al.*, 1998). Two clinical series of non-operatively treated PCL injuries have demonstrated this important sign (Warren personal communication; Rubinstein *et al.*, 1994). A decrease in posterior laxity with tibial external rotation may also be seen but is less specific for these structures. A more reliable examination for the posterolateral corner (PLC) structures is external rotation asymmetry (Veltri and Warren, 1994). This examination may be completed in the prone or seated position with the knees at 30° of flexion. It is important however, to ensure that the tibia is reduced under the femur in an anatomic position. If the tibia remains subluxated posteriorly, PLC laxity may be diminished on exam and go undiagnosed. When external rotation is increased 15° as compared to the contralateral side, a significant PLC disruption is present. If this is seen at 30° and at 90° of knee flexion, the PCL and PLC have been injured. This combined ligamentous injury will require operative treatment. Other tests such as the external recurvatum test, the posterolateral drawer test, and the reverse pivot shift add important information about the integrity of the capsuloligamentous structures and impact the decision-making process. Additional testing of the collateral ligaments to varus and valgus stress at 0 and 30° should be completed. Side to side differences in the examination of these ligaments will indicate the degree of injury to these important secondary restraints. Gait analysis and standing alignment should also be evaluated. Varus alignment with or without a varus thrust indicates a shift of the weight-bearing axis to the medial joint line. If varus alignment exits without a thrust, a high tibial osteotomy may be needed to redirect the weight-bearing axis through the lateral compartment. A thrust indicates deficient lateral and posterolateral secondary restraints and if not addressed at the time of PCL reconstruction, will place abnormal forces on the PCL graft.

Imaging studies

Imaging studies contribute significantly in the decision as to whether surgery is indicated for PCL injuries. All patients should have plain radiographs. If pain allows, standing anterior-posterior, 45° flexion anterior-posterior, lateral, and Merchant patellar views are evaluated for the presence of associated fractures, avulsion injuries, and concomitant arthritis. Reduction of the tibia under the femur should first be evaluated to rule out persistent subluxation or dislocation. Avulsion fractures seen at the PCL insertion sites are a strong indication for surgical repair. Results are favorable for these surgeries, although they encompass only a small part of the entire spectrum of PCL injuries. Capsuloligamentous avulsion injuries from the tibial plateau represent a more serious combined injury and should be noted. Bone avulsions from the fibular head indicate additional damage to the posterolateral corner structures. Primary repair of the capsuloligamentous injuries, especially in the posterolateral aspect of the knee, is indicated and produces more reliable results than delayed reconstruction techniques.

Some authors, primarily in the European literature, have advocated stress radiographs (Puddu et al., 2000). The goal of any of the described methods is to evaluate the posterior tibial subluxation in comparison to the contralateral side. Different measurements and sensitivity have been reported and these techniques appear to be user-dependent. Currently, we use stress radiographs to supplement our clinical exam and have found them to be particularly helpful when the exam is equivocal.

Magnetic residence imaging (MRI) contributes significantly to the ligamentous evaluation about the knee. The sensitivity and specificity of detecting an acute, complete tear of the PCL with MRI has been reported to be as high as 100 per cent in one study (Gross et al., 1992). It is important to note, however, that signal changes within the PCL may indicate partial disruption of the ligament that does not clinically result in abnormal PCL laxity (Shelbourne et al., 1999b). The normal MRI appearance is curvilinear as the PCL passes over the ACL and the anterolateral component loosens in extension.

Careful examination of the signal changes on MRI may indicate the location and extent of the tear. If a soft tissue avulsion from either insertion site, particularly the femoral side, is seen, a primary repair may be performed with predictably good healing. Additionally, the MRI provides critical information about the integrity of the surrounding capsuloligamentous structures, menisci, and articular surfaces. All of this information should be carefully correlated with the physical exam, as the decisions regarding surgical necessity and timing are contemplated. In the chronic PCL injury, the MRI may not clearly indicate lose of PCL integrity. Occasionally, a PCL avulsion may heal back to the bone attachment sties, or in the case of midsubstance tears, to the adjacent ACL. In this setting, we again refer back to the critical nature of a detailed history and physical exam. An apparently intact ligament may lack important biomechanical properties with resultant functional instability and abnormal laxity.

A bone scan may be utilized in a chronic PCL injury for patients with primary complaints of pain. Increased uptake in the medial and patellofemoral compartments may indicate early stress reaction and articular cartilage damage secondary to abnormal mechanical stresses. In these patients, and especially in the younger athletes, reconstruction of the PCL may reduce abnormal laxity, change the mechanical stresses in these compartments, and decrease symptomatic complaints.

Natural history

Our goal is to present to the patient the associated risks and benefits of non-operative versus operative treatment for a PCL injury. The natural history of PCL injuries is not known, although some data exists to help educate the patient. Studies by various authors have indicated that 80–85 per cent of all PCL injuries may have satisfactory knee function at short term follow-up and the results may be correlated with better quadriceps strength (Cross and Powell, 1984, Parolie and Bergfeld, 1986). Others have shown that with longer follow-up, the risk of progressive arthritis approaches over 50 per cent and the risk of meniscal tears reaches approximately 30 per cent (Boynton and Tietjens, 1996, Dejour et al., 1988, Geissler and Whipple, 1993, Torg et al., 1989). Shelbourne recently reported that 50 per cent of patients with isolated PCL tears returned to the same sport at the same or higher level, 33 per cent returned to the same sport at a lower level, and the subjective and objective knee function did not correlated with the grade of laxity (Shelbourne et al., 1999a). Keller showed that at six year follow-up, 90 per cent of patients with isolated PCL tears had persistent pain and 65 per cent had limited activity as a result (Keller et al., 1993). Unfortunately, all studies except those reported by Parolie et al. and Shelbourne et al. did not define exactly the isolated PCL injury and may include patients outside the definition an isolated PCL injury.

The studies above provide some valuable information regarding the natural history of PCL injuries. At minimum, it is apparent that athletes with PCL-deficient knees will have unsatisfactory outcomes 15–20 per cent of the time. These numbers may rise significantly if symptoms of knee pain and arthritis are attributed to the altered mechanics of a PCL deficient knee. Functional instability is also difficult to correlate with objective findings. Moreover, few nonoperative studies clearly delineate the problems encountered with severe combined multiligamentous injuries and subtle secondary capsuloligamentous laxities. Finally, there may be some correlation with improved quadriceps strength and better subjective outcomes, but this benefit may deteriorate over time. Obviously a void exists in grasping the entire spectrum of the PCL deficient knee's natural history. For this reason it is imperative the clinician weigh the available outcomes data, basic science information, and patient specific goals when determining which athletes may benefit from a PCL reconstruction.

Operative treatment results

In light of the poor outcome that undoubtedly will occur in some patients with a PCL-deficient knee, surgical reconstruction is offered to those who meet specific criteria. Ideally, recommendations for operative treatment should be based on prospective randomized studies that indicate a benefit of operative over nonoperative treatment. Such studies do not exist. There is, however, literature available that suggests operative treatment may offer improved results in certain cases.

Initial reports of operative treatment for isolated PCL tears generally depicted mixed results. The results of Bianchi and Loos were generally rated as good or fair (Loos *et al.*, 1981, Bianchi, 1983). The patients in these studies had little functional instability but the procedures often did not completely reduce the abnormal laxity. Richter reported 53 patients with acute isolated and combined PCL instabilities with 8-year follow-up (Richter *et al.*, 1996). In this study, 46 patients improved to 1+ or better on the posterior drawer test. However, no patient in this series had normal International Knee Documentation Committee scoring and only 13 per cent were graded as nearly normal. Clancy reported excellent subjective and objective results in 15 patients treated operatively for acute PCL insufficiency (Clancy *et al.*, 1983). The technique used included a ligament repair that was supplemented with a central third patellar tendon autograft passed through bony tunnels. The two-year follow-up of eight patients with isolated PCL injuries showed seven excellent and one good result. They also found improvement in objective laxity was seen with seven patients demonstrating trace posterior drawer findings and one patient with improvement to a 1+ exam.

Acute PCL injuries with combined instabilities are treated operatively by most surgeons because this combination results in a large degree of instability that is not tolerated well. Reviewing the literature regarding these injuries becomes even more complex as either numerous injury patterns are combined into one series, the series are too small with short follow-up, or a wide arrange of treatment modalities have been utilized. In our review of the literature we have found no studies that utilize a modern PCL reconstruction technique with adequate description of the combined injury treatment. The studies quoted in the literature generally involve either a substantial subset of mid-substance PCL tears repaired with suture, reconstruction techniques believed to be inadequate today, or insufficient follow-up data.

Operative indications

Our treatment of PCL injuries derives from a collective understanding of the broad scope of information presented above. This incorporates our current understanding of the pathophysiology, clinical and imaging diagnostics, purported natural history, and modern operative techniques to reconstruct the biomechanical function of the PCL. Undoubtedly, some of the influences on our decision-making are a result of clinical gestalt. We feel, however, that this gestalt is guided by science. Our goal for the athlete with a PCL-deficient knee is to optimize the acute function and preserve the long term stability of the reconstructed knee.

Acute isolated PCL injuries

Our recommendation for acute isolated PCL injuries is nonoperative treatment. This recommendation is based on a clinical exam that demonstrates less than 10 mm of posterior tibial translation, a decrease in posterior translation with internal rotation on exam, a side to side rotary laxity of less than 5°, no significant valgus or varus testing laxity, and negative x-ray findings for bone avulsions (Figure 21.2). If these criteria are met, the treatment involves early brace immobilization that blocks full extension and encourages early weight-bearing. Ice, anti-inflammatory medication, and early rehabilitation exercises concentrate on improving quadriceps control and strength. Generally, return to sports can occur from 4 to 10 weeks after the injury providing a near full range of motion occurs. In the athlete, we like to lock the knee brace from extending past 15° of flexion. In sports competition, we believe this will result in near full extension with loading.

An important distinction in isolated PCL injuries is the presence of subtle increased laxity secondary to mild capsuloligamentous insufficiency. This is a distinct entity from the traditional combined ligamentous injuries with obvious disruption of either the lateral collateral ligament, medial collateral ligament, or anterior cruciate

Fig. 21.2

Algorithm for the diagnosis
and treatment of isolated
PCL tears.

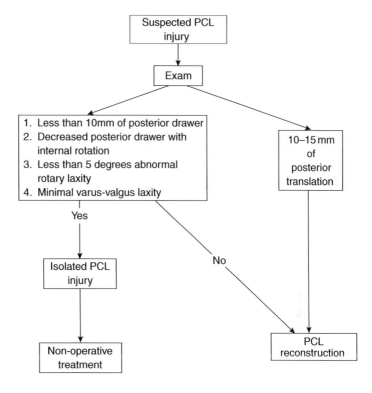

ligament. In this scenario, the physical exam will reveal 10 mm or greater of abnormal posterior laxity without demonstrating a firm endpoint or tightening with internal rotation of the tibia. Here, the secondary restraints, specifically the superficial medial collateral ligament and medial capsule, are in continuity but have lost critical stabilizing properties. If the exam of the acutely injured knee reveals a soft posterior endpoint, or a 10 mm or greater posterior drawer that does not decrease on internal rotation, an initial trial of nonoperative treatment is warranted. If these findings persist four weeks after the injury, however, the need for surgical reconstruction becomes increasingly likely. It is important to note that not all cases will require surgical reconstruction and continued quadriceps strengthening should be encouraged. These patients should be followed regularly, though, to evaluate for early signs of arthritis or increased functional instability.

Isolated PCL injuries that involve avulsions from the insertion sites warrant early surgical repair. These early repairs heal well and more closely reproduce normal restraint patterns than current reconstruction techniques. Occasionally, acute MRI findings may not reveal a bony avulsion but rather a pealing away of the Sharpey's fibers at the bone insertion site. These Sharpey's fibers have the same healing potential as bone avulsions and should be repaired acutely.

Acute PCL with combined ligamentous injury

With higher energy injuries, PCL disruptions are often found in combination with injuries to the posterolateral corner, anterior cruciate ligament, or medial collateral ligament (MCL) complex. Accurate diagnosis of these injuries in the acute setting becomes critical, as we prefer to treat this combination early with surgical repair and reconstruction as warranted. We have found that if left untreated, the combined injury pattern leads to excessive laxity and functional instability that is often quite debilitating. MRI is a valuable adjunct in this instance and can guide the preoperative planning of the associated injuries.

Acute injuries to the posterolateral structures and PCL are best treated operatively within the first three weeks after injury. This allows for a primary repair of the injured posterolateral corner structures. A preoperative MRI will often help clarify the extent of the posterolateral injury and adds critical information to the physical exam. Our preference is to reconstruct the PCL and then directly repair the posterolateral structures through a lateral approach. This acute repair offers the best opportunity to reproduce the normal anatomy and is critical in the rehab of the reconstructed PCL.

Posterior cruciate ligament injury combined with acute MCL disruption is less common but does occur. As described previously, a PCL injury with a grade II or III MCL sprain may result in sufficient patholaxity to require reconstruction of the PCL. A grade II or III MCL sprain may be diagnosed on physical exam with increased laxity to valgus stress at 30° of flexion that dissipates with the leg held in extension. The PCL tear in this instance will have 10 mm or greater posterior drawer exam. An MRI scan will also help define the extent of the medial sided injury. The initial treatment involves brace protection, early range of motion, and quadriceps exercises with hamstring avoidance. As the knee progresses in therapy, careful attention is paid to the posterior drawer test in neutral and internal rotation of the tibia. If over the next 4–6 weeks a tightening of the valgus laxity or a decrease in posterior drawer with internal rotation does not occur, we will discuss reconstruction of the PCL with the athlete. In this instance, we feel substantial injury has occurred to the capsuloligamentous structures on the medial side of the knee and problems will ensue. A reconstruction of the PCL will provide the necessary stability to posterior translation and the medial side will be addressed indirectly with this reconstruction.

A PCL tear with an MCL injury that demonstrates increased laxity to valgus stress at full extension represents a grade III MCL injury plus disruption of the posterior medial capsular structures. This injury has little chance of recovering sufficient restraints on the medial side to allow nonoperative treatment of the PCL tear. An MRI scan in this instance may demonstrate femoral, tibial, or mid-substance disruption of the MCL and posterior capsular structures.

Operative treatment can then be directed toward the site of injury. Initial brace immobilization followed by range of motion exercises are begun in the preoperative period as operative treatment is planned. Early operative intervention includes reconstruction of the PCL followed by primary repair of the medial structures in an isometric fashion.

Injuries to the ACL and PCL represent significant injuries and are often unrecognized knee dislocations. As such, vascular integrity to the lower extremity should be evaluated prior to initiating any treatment modalities. Our preference for this injury pattern once the knee is reduced, is to begin early weight-bearing in a brace locked in extension. This is followed by early range of motion as pain and swelling permit. When the range of motion is at least 110° of flexion and the patient has good control of the injured leg and musculature, we will proceed with reconstruction of the ACL and PCL. Our ACL reconstruction utilizes and a 2 incision arthroscopically assisted technique which is then followed by a PCL reconstruction. In these instances, it is critical to obtain accurate reduction of the tibia under the femur prior to final tensioning of the two ligament reconstructions. Our grafts for this technique will be allograft bone-patellar-tendon bone for the ACL and Achilles tendon allograft for the PCL reconstruction. If the PCL attachment is avulsed from the femoral attachment site, or less commonly the tibial attachment site, a primary repair with sutures through bone tunnels will have excellent results.

Chronic PCL insufficiency

. Complaints of knee pain by patients with chronic isolated PCL laxity are a not uncommon and are seen at least 15 per cent of isolated injuries. The mechanism of initial injury is often lower impact and the patient may describe a variable interval of good function. Problems in the knee are associated with either increased or persistent functional instability or disabling pain with daily activities. A posterior drawer exam of 10 mm or greater with a soft endpoint is often seen and this may have increased over time as the secondary restraints slowly stretched under added load. If the exam indicates an isolated PCL-deficiency with tightening of the posterior drawer on internal rotation, no external rotation asymmetry, and a firm end point, a trial of physical therapy emphasizing quadriceps strengthening is warranted. The new onset of symptoms may be a result of a gradual loss of quadriceps strength and control. Additionally, radiographic examination should be completed to evaluate for early signs of articular cartilage changes. A gradual progression of knee arthrosis may present as functional instability, mechanical symptoms, or pain in the PCL-deficient knee. If radiographs appear normal, a positive bone scan may indicate localized bone turnover and early arthritis.

If rehabilitation efforts do not alleviate the symptoms, surgical reconstruction should be considered. A search must be made for additional abnormal capsuloligamentous laxity that will require treatment at the time of the PCL reconstruction. Insufficient secondary restraints will often lead to increased symptoms and be can be diagnosed on careful physical exam. In addition to the soft tissue restraints, evidence for a varus thrust and poor alignment should be evaluated during gait. Reconstruction of the PCL and the soft tissue restraints alone in the setting of faulty alignment will portend a poor result. Our preference is to proceed with a high tibial osteotomy that realigns the weight-bearing axis over the medial half of the lateral compartment. This procedure is initially done alone and may alleviate the symptoms by itself. If symptoms of instability and pain persist, we will then proceed with a PCL reconstruction and address the secondary soft tissue restraints as warranted.

Operative technique

A complete review of our operative technique and rationale is beyond the scope of this chapter. A brief mention of our preferences is warranted however (Figure 21.3). Our current technique utilizes an arthroscopically assisted single bundle posterior tibial inlay technique that has evolved and been modified from the original techniques described by Benedetto, Jakob, Gaechter, and Berg (Thomann and Gaechter, 1994, Berg, 1995). Studies in our laboratory (Bergfeld et al., 2001) have shown that the tibial inlay technique is

(a) (b)

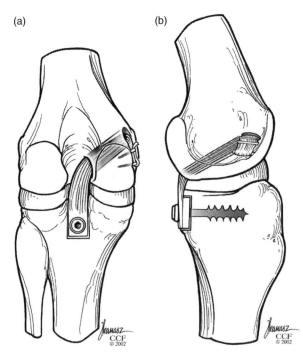

Fig. 21.3
These represent our current technique for PCL reconstruction. (a) Anterior view showing the staple soft tissue fixation of the Achilles tendon allograft after it passes through the single femoral tunnel. (b) Lateral view showing the tibial inlay graft fixed with a 6.5 mm cancellous screw.

more stable than the tibial tunnel technique to posterior translation at all flexion angles, and especially at higher angles of flexion. Markolf and colleagues' laboratory data indicates that while the initial stability of the tibial tunnel technique is similar, increased laxity ensues following the tunnel technique if the knee is put through cyclic loading forces (Markolf KL, Zemonavic JR, McAllister DR, presented at AAOS 2002). This information corroborates our laboratory data that suggests long-term stability of the graft is improved with the inlay technique. Laboratory cyclic loading of the knee has demonstrated thinning, damage, and rarely rupture of the graft just above the bone tendon junction at the 'killer curve' as the graft exits around the back of the tibia. We feel the posterior inlay technique more reliably provides improved stability in the acute setting and avoids the long-term complications of graft wear and stretching at the 'killer curve'. Currently we use an Achilles tendon allograft for a single bundle PCL reconstruction with a posterior inlay technique. The 11 mm by 20 mm bone block is fixed to the tibial side with a 6.5 cancellous screw through a posterior approach to the knee. The femoral tunnel is 10 mm in diameter and placed at the anatomic footprint of the PCL with the Achilles tendon passed through it. The femoral side is fixed upon the medial femoral condyle with two bone staples. Our rehab protocol involves early weight-bearing with brace immobilization at full extension until good quadriceps control is obtained. Early active and active assisted range of motion is begun at one week, and as strength and range of motion improve, light strengthening is added to the regimen. At approximately 4–6 weeks, the patient is fitted with a functional PCL brace and the rehab is progressed on an individual basis. As the patient progresses through full range of motion, full weight-bearing, and full strength gains, the program is advanced to include functional activity rehabilitation tailored to the athletes' needs.

Summary

The treatment of PCL injuries continues to be an issue of considerable debate. Undoubtedly, a subset of patients who have suffered isolated PCL injuries will go on to have significant disability. This may occur despite good participation in a well developed nonoperative treatment program. As a result, determining which patients can benefit from operative intervention is a constant challenge. We have found that those patients who demonstrate any of the following have a high potential for dissatisfaction with their knee as a result of pain or functional instability: greater than 10 mm of posterior drawer laxity, no decrease in posterior drawer laxity with internal tibial rotation, greater than 5° of abnormal rotary laxity, or appreciable increased varus or valgus laxity. Additionally, those patients with injury patterns of combined major ligament disruption predictably will have progressive problems of pain and instability. We recommend operative reconstruction of the PCL for those patients with the above findings who wish to remain active. Our experience has led us to believe that these patients' symptoms and activity levels are improved by our attempts at establishing more normal knee kinematics and we feel our current technique of PCL reconstruction accomplishes that goal.

References

Berg, E. E. (1995) *Arthroscopy*, 11, 69–76.

Bergfeld, J. A., McAllister, D. R., Parker, R. D., Valdevit, A. D. and Kambic, H. (2001) *J Bone Joint Surg Am*, 83-A, 1339–43.

Bianchi, M. (1983) *Am J Sports Med*, 11, 308–14.

Boynton, M. D. and Tietjens, B. R. (1996) *Am J Sports Med*, 24, 306–10.

Butler, D. L., Noyes, F. R. and Grood, E. S. (1980) *J Bone Joint Surg Am*, 62, 259–70.

Clancy, W. G., Jr., Shelbourne, K. D., Zoellner, G. B., Keene, J. S., Reider, B. and Rosenberg, T. D. (1983) *J Bone Joint Surg Am*, 65, 310–22.

Covey, D. C., Sapega, A. A. and Sherman, G. M. (1996) *Am J Sports Med*, 24, 740–6.

Cross, M. J. and Powell, J. F. (1984) *Am J Sports Med*, 12, 292–7.

Dandy, D. J. and Pusey, R. J. (1982) *J Bone Joint Surg Br*, 64, 92–4.

Dejour, H., Walch, G., Peyrot, J. and Eberhard, P. (1988) *Rev Chir Orthop Reparatrice Appar Mot*, 74, 35–43.

Geissler, W. B. and Whipple, T. L. (1993) *Am J Sports Med*, 21, 846–9.

Girgis, F. G., Marshall, J. L. and Monajem, A. (1975) *Clin Orthop*, 106, 216–31.

Gollehon, D. L., Torzilli, P. A. and Warren, R. F. (1987) *J Bone Joint Surg Am*, 69, 233–42.

Gross, M. L., Grover, J. S., Bassett, L. W., Seeger, L. L. and Finerman, G. A. (1992) *Am J Sports Med*, 20, 732–7.

Harner, C. D., Baek, G. H., Vogrin, T. M., Carlin, G. J., Kashiwaguchi, S. and Woo, S. L. (1999) *Arthroscopy*, 15, 741–9.

Harner, C. D., Xerogeanes, J. W., Livesay, G. A., Carlin, G. J., Smith, B. A., Kusayama, T., Kashiwaguchi, S. and Woo, S. L. (1995) *Am J Sports Med*, 23, 736–45.

Keller, P. M., Shelbourne, K. D., McCarroll, J. R. and Rettig, A. C. (1993) *Am J Sports Med*, 21, 132–6.

Loos, W. C., Fox, J. M., Blazina, M. E., Del Pizzo, W. and Friedman, M. J. (1981) *Am J Sports Med*, 9, 86–92.

Parolie, J. M. and Bergfeld, J. A. (1986) *Am J Sports Med*, 14, 35–8.

Puddu, G., Gianni, E., Chambat, P. and De Paulis, F. (2000) *Arthroscopy*, 16, 217–20.

Richter, M., Kiefer, H., Hehl, G. and Kinzl, L. (1996) *Am J Sports Med*, 24, 298–305.

Ritchie, J. R., Bergfeld, J. A., Kambic, H. and Manning, T. (1998) *Am J Sports Med*, 26, 389–94.

Rubinstein, R. A., Jr., Shelbourne, K. D., McCarroll, J. R., VanMeter, C. D. and Rettig, A. C. (1994) *Am J Sports Med*, 22, 550–7.

Shelbourne, K. D., Davis, T. J. and Patel, D. V. (1999a) *Am J Sports Med*, 27, 276–83.

Shelbourne, K. D., Jennings, R. W. and Vahey, T. N. (1999b) *Am J Knee Surg*, 12, 209–13.

Thomann, Y. R. and Gaechter, A. (1994) *Arch Orthop Trauma Surg*, 113, 142–8.

Torg, J. S., Barton, T. M., Pavlov, H. and Stine, R. (1989) *Clin Orthop*, 246, 208–16.

Veltri, D. M. and Warren, R. F. (1994) *Clin Sports Med*, 13, 599–614.

22

PCL reconstruction: the double-bundle method is most effective for restoring posterior tibiofemoral laxity

Andrew A. Amis

Introduction

The function of the posterior cruciate ligament (PCL), and PCL reconstruction form a subject area that remains relatively unexplored, when compared to the many studies of the anterior cruciate ligament (ACL) and its reconstruction. There is much that is unexplained, even at the most fundamental level. Why, for example, do many people with a ruptured PCL not appear to need a PCL reconstruction, when we know that it is the largest and strongest ligament crossing the knee?

The biomechanical case for PCL reconstruction rests on the PCL being the primary restraint to posterior tibial translation (Butler *et al.*, 1980; Race and Amis, 1996), and so its absence can allow the tibia to sublux posteriorly, under the influence of the hamstrings. When this occurs, the patellar tendon slants further posteriorly as it passes to the tibia, and this raises the compressive force on the patellofemoral joint. This may tilt the patella, altering the congruence of the joint, the combined effect causing patellofemoral joint pain. The posterior subluxation leads to greater anteromedial impact at the moment of heelstrike during gait, a situation linked to the onset of unicompartmental arthritis. Chronic cases may have a fixed posterior subluxation, that must be overcome if the PCL reconstruction is to restore a normal tibiofemoral articulation (Strobel *et al.*, 2002). This may contribute to the well-known problem of partial recurrence of posterior tibial subluxation following PCL reconstruction, that relates to the influences of hamstrings tension and gravity while the patient is recumbent. One reason for moving to a double-bundle graft is to place more tissue across the joint, to resist this stretching-out.

PCL reconstruction is most commonly considered when there has been damage to both the PCL and other structures, usually posterolaterally. While the PCL is the primary restraint to tibial posterior translation in the mid-range of knee flexion, it is less important in extension (Race and Amis, 1996). This makes the reconstruction of these other structures vital, if knee stability is to be re-established in extension. The corollary is that an isolated PCL rupture may not cause functional problems if the posterolateral corner remains intact, since it is those other structures that are important for knee stability in walking.

The title of this chapter was chosen by the editors to be controversial, in order to provoke debate, and the author must provide the evidence that will allow the reader to decide if it is justified. Given that PCL reconstruction is a clinical problem, the ideal treatment of this subject would be to quote comparative, prospectively randomized, blinded studies, with enough cases to ensure statistical power, and more than adequate length of follow-up, that have compared double-bundle PCL and single-bundle reconstructions, and to no reconstruction, for series of 'isolated' and combined ligament injuries. Of course, this is fantasy: if studies such as this had been done, then this subject would no longer be controversial – we would know what to do. In the absence of clinical data, the case for double-bundle PCL reconstruction must rely on anatomical and biomechanical studies.

Functional anatomy of the PCL

The concept of double-bundle reconstruction is supported principally by two anatomical observations: that the fibres of the PCL diverge widely as they pass from the tibia to the femur, and so must pull in different directions, and secondly that the fibres in different parts of the PCL are clearly not isometric, and are tight at different positions in the arc of knee flexion. From an anatomical and biomechanical viewpoint, an ideal reconstruction would reproduce all the important functional aspects of the natural PCL. This would include having the correct orientation, tightness and stiffness for the fibres, so that the tension in the reconstruction loads the knee normally, and the resistance to elongation builds up normally, in response to tibiofemoral relative motion. This requires reproduction of the many collagen fascicles of the natural structure, with correct mapping of their bone attachments. Man-made structures might approximate this in the future, via tissue engineering, but for now we are limited to autogenous tissue grafts. These are discrete bundles of fibres, approximately parallel-fibred, that may not have the same tensile stiffness as the ligament being replaced. Clearly the simplest method is to use a single graft, and the use of more grafts must be justified by significant improvements, because the surgery will become more complex and time-consuming.

When the PCL is viewed in a lateral-medial direction, the divergent paths of the fibres are apparent. The anterolateral fibres

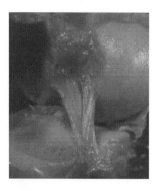

Fig. 22.1

View of left knee from posterolateral aspect after removal of lateral femoral condyle. The PCL has been separated into an anterolateral (aPC) bundle, attaching to the roof of the intercondylar notch, and a posteromedial (pPC) bundle, attaching to the medial femoral condyle. Reproduced with permission from Race and Amis (1994). The mechanical properties of the two bundles of the human posterior cruciate ligament. *J Biomechs* 27: 13–24.

(aPC) pass to the antero-distal region of the roof of the femoral intercondylar notch; the posteromedial fibres (pPC) pass to the lateral aspect of the medial femoral condyle, adjacent to the postero-distal margin of the condylar articular cartilage (Figure 22.1). This article uses standard anatomical nomenclature for positions and directions; surgeons usually view the flexed knee, when distal femoral attachments are shallow, proximal are deep, anterior are high, and posterior are low in the field of view (Amis *et al.*, 1994).

The anterolateral (aPC) fibres take a curved path when the knee is extended. This appearance is seen commonly in MRI, and shows that these fibres are slack. The posteromedial fibres (pPC) of the PCL are tensed in full knee extension, but Figure 22.1 shows that they are then oriented in a proximal-distal direction. This means that they are not set up to resist posterior tibial translation, the function for which the PCL is the primary restraint. The pPC slackens as knee flexion commences and tightens in full knee extension, and so appears to restrain hyperextension along with the posterior knee joint capsule and gastrocnemius, that wrap over the prominent posterior femoral condyles. These observations, that the aPC is slack and the pPC pulling in the wrong direction, explain why the PCL is not the primary restraint to posterior tibial translation when the knee is at or close to full extension.

The aPC tightens as the knee flexes, and is then well-aligned to resist tibial posterior translation. At 6 mm translation, the aPC becomes the primary restraint (i.e., it contributes 50 per cent or more of the resistance to movement) by 30° knee flexion. With increasing knee flexion, the aPC swings upwards, away from the tibial plateau, and this means that it becomes less well-oriented to resist posterior tibial draw. Because of its large stiffness (Race and Amis, 1994), the aPC is the primary restraint until 120° knee flexion (Race and Amis, 1996). The aPC wraps against the roof of the femoral intercondylar notch by 120° knee flexion (Figure 22.2), and there is then a small gap between the posterior outlet of the notch and the edge of the tibial plateau. The PCL is vulnerable to injury during a fall onto the tibial tubercle of the flexed knee because it is sheared between the two bones.

While the knee is flexing, and the aPC is tight, the posteromedial fibres of the PCL (the pPC) crumple and pass through the narrow gap between the aPC and the medial wall of the intercondylar notch. In deep knee flexion, the pPC retightens, as its femoral attachment moves anteriorly and superiorly. The pPC is well-aligned to resist tibial posterior draw in deep knee flexion (Figure 22.2), and it is the primary restraint beyond 120 degrees.

The reciprocal pattern of fibre bundles tightening and slackening as the knee flexes supports the double-bundle concept for PCL reconstruction. Although the idea of two bundles is entirely artificial, the natural PCL being a continuous array of fibres, there is a clear demarcation between the aPC and pPC, when the PCL is examined in a cadaveric knee that is flexed and extended cyclically, approximately between fibres that attach to the roof of the intercondylar notch, and those that attach to the side wall (Figure 22.1). This examination does not lend support to the idea of going to three or even more bundles; the bulk of the PCL fits well with the two-bundle description.

The PCL is not an isometric structure. The isometric zone is at the proximal edge of the femoral attachment, where the split between the fibre bundles is shown in Figure 22.1 (Sidles *et al.*, 1988; Friederich and O'Brien, 1992; Grood *et al.*, 1989). Overall, attachments in the central bulk of the PCL distal to this point tighten across the arc of knee flexion, while the pPC swings distally and anteriorly around it, thus initially slackening and then retightening in deep flexion.

The natural PCL and posterior draw resistance

The PCL was shown to be the primary restraint against tibial posterior translation by Butler and Grood (1980), whose work led to the concept of primary and secondary restraints (Noyes *et al.*, 1980). They used selective cutting of the structures during cyclic AP draw tests. The contribution of the PCL was found by measuring how much the posterior draw force fell when the tibia was pushed a fixed distance posteriorly, from the intact to PCL cut states.

Race and Amis (1996) used a similar method, cycling the tibia with the PCL intact, after cutting the aPC, then after cutting the pPC. Figure 22.3 shows the average percentage contributions of the aPC, pPC and other structures that had been the secondary restraints while the PCL was intact, to resisting 6 mm posterior tibial translation from 0–130° knee flexion.

At full knee extension, structures other than the PCL provided 65 per cent of the resistance to posterior draw. The majority of the restraint was provided by the aPC from 30–120° knee flexion. The role of the pPC rose as knee flexion increased, and it was the major contributor (57 per cent mean) at 130° flexion.

These results suggest at first glance that the aPC alone should be reconstructed, except for those patients who require a stable knee in deep flexion, when the pPC has a role. However, the pPC contributes from 30–50 per cent of the posterior draw resistance across the mid range of knee flexion, and so not reconstructing it would undoubtedly increase the forces acting on any single-bundle graft. This would increase the risk of creep elongation during graft remodelling, leading to a return of posterior laxity. The graph also shows why an isolated PCL reconstruction, whether single or double-bundle, will not stabilize the knee in extension, if the posterolateral structures have been damaged and not repaired or reconstructed.

A PCL reconstruction should aim to return posterior tibiofemoral laxity to normal across the arc of knee flexion. In the laboratory,

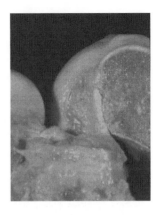

Fig. 22.2

In deep knee flexion the aPC wraps against the roof of the intercondylar notch. The pPC is now tight and well-aligned to resist tibial posterior translation. Note the small posterior outlet, which puts the PCL at risk of shearing between the bones in hyperflexion. Reproduced with permission from Amis AA (1999). Anatomy and biomechanics of the posterior cruciate ligament. *Sports Med Arthroscopy Rev* 7: 225–234.

Fig. 22.3

The percentage contributions of the aPC, pPC, and other structures to resisting 6 mm posterior tibial translation, across the range of knee flexion. Reproduced with permission from Race and Amis (1996). Loading of the two bundles of the posterior cruciate ligament: an analysis of bundle function in A-P drawer. *J Biomechs* 29: 873–879.

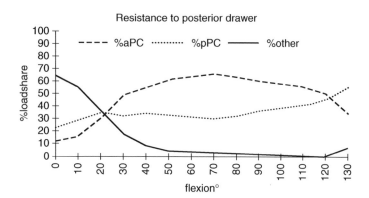

posterior draw was measured at a displacement force of 100 N. The PCL was ruptured in isolation by applying a rapid, posterior tibial displacement at 90° flexion, with failure occurring at a displacement of 14.6 + 2.8 mm, at a force of 1.94 + 0.74 kN (Race and Amis, 1998). The PCL rupture caused only 1.4 mm extra posterior laxity at full extension, which increased to 13 mm at 90° flexion. This shows why PCL integrity is tested at 90° knee flexion. A similar trend was found by Galloway *et al.* (1996) and Harner *et al.* (2000) (see Figure 22.6).

Biomechanical comparison of single versus double-bundle reconstructions

Three biomechanical studies have compared single versus double-bundle reconstructions of the PCL. They all measured the success of the reconstructions at restoring posterior tibial translation to normal across the range of knee flexion *in vitro*. All three found that the double-bundle methods were better able to restore posterior laxity than single-bundle methods, although the ways in which the reconstructions were performed differed in important details such as graft tunnel placement and graft tensioning.

The first of these studies (Race and Amis, 1998) compared three reconstructions: an isometric graft, a single-bundle aPC graft, and a double-bundle reconstruction, that had a pPC graft added to the aPC graft. The reconstructions used two patellar tendon grafts, 10 mm wide for the aPC, 8 mm for the pPC (Figure 22.4). The femoral attachments used screw-mounted tensiometers, that could adjust the graft tension/tightness, and measure graft tension. The isometric graft was first placed in a 10 mm femoral tunnel at the isometric point that had been identified using an isometer when the knee was intact. This was located approximately at the roof-wall transition at the proximal edge of the natural PCL attachment. It was decided not to apply a fixed level of graft tension, because knees have a wide range of AP laxity (Amis, 1989). Instead, to simulate clinical practice, the knees were subjected to cyclic AP loading and

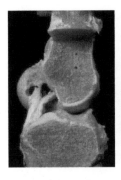
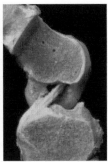
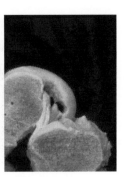

Fig. 22.4

Double-bundle PCL reconstruction, with patterns of graft tightening and slackening that mimic the natural structure: in extension the aPC is slack and the pPC is tight; in mid flexion the aPC is tight and the pPC is slack; in deep flexion the pPC is tight and well-aligned.

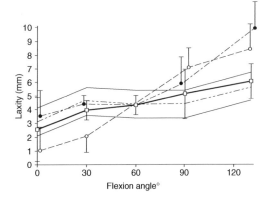

Fig. 22.5

Variation of posterior laxity across the range of knee flexion for isometric (iso) (○), aPC (●), and double-bundle (aPC + pPC) PCL (□) reconstructions. The thin lines show the zone of intact knee laxity ±1 mm.

the tensiometer adjusted until the normal AP laxity had been restored, at 60° knee flexion for the isometric and aPC grafts, and at 130° for the pPC. These tensioning angles were chosen because they are when the grafts act to stabilise the knee. The knee was then tested under the same load cycles at other angles of flexion, and the graft tension monitored throughout. The isometric graft had a high tension when the knee was extended, that overconstrained AP laxity (Figure 22.5). Conversely, in deep flexion the knee was significantly laxer than when intact. The aPC graft alone restored normal laxity within 1 mm up to 60° knee flexion, but then allowed excess laxity. Posterior draw in greater flexion was controlled by adding the pPC graft (Figure 22.5). Thus, this experiment showed a clear advantage for the double-bundle reconstruction when compared to the isometric and aPC reconstructions.

Harner *et al.* (2000) used a 10 mm Achilles tendon and a doubled semitendinosus tendon 8 mm diameter for their aPC and pPc grafts. The graft tunnels were drilled through the PCL bundle femoral attachment sites. Fixed tensions were used: 88 N was applied to the aPC at 90° knee flexion, while the tibia was pulled anteriorly by 134 N. The pPC was tensed to 67 N and fixed in full knee extension. The aPC graft alone allowed significantly more laxity than for the intact knee at all angles of flexion, and a tendency

Fig. 22.6

Variation of posterior laxity for intact, PCL-deficient, aPC reconstruction (PCL-1), and double-bundle (aPC + pPC) (PCL-2) reconstructions. From Harner *et al.*, 2000, with permission.

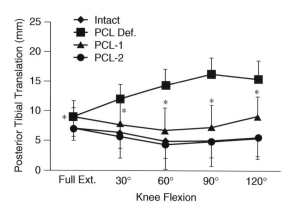

for this deficit to increase in deep flexion. In contrast, the double-bundle reconstruction did not differ significantly from normal at all angles of knee flexion (Figure 22.6).

Mannor *et al.* (2000) used a 10 mm patellar tendon graft, split to form a Y with two 5 mm bundles proximally. The aPC graft was tensioned at 90° knee flexion to restore normal AP knee laxity, then caused overconstraint in extension. Mannor *et al.* did not try pPC grafts, but looked at the effects of distal (shallow) or proximal (deep) grafts at the middle of the PCL femoral attachment. The distal graft alone could restore AP laxity within 2 mm across the range of knee flexion, but with high graft tension in flexion. The proximal graft alone allowed excessive laxity in flexion. When used alone, the proximal graft allowed excessive laxity in flexion. When the shallow and deep grafts were used in double-bundle reconstructions with the aPC graft, they showed reciprocal patterns of tension as the knee flexed: the distal graft caused overconstraint in flexion, the proximal graft caused overconstraint in extension. These results fitted with earlier work on PCL isometry (Grood *et al.*, 1989) and show how important it is to place the graft at the correct distance from the distal articular cartilage margin.

Conclusions

The double-bundle PCL reconstruction evolved from earlier work on the ACL (Radford and Amis, 1990). The PCL has a much more divergent fibre structure, and so is more clearly appropriate for this treatment. Despite this, and the clear biomechanical data supporting the concept, it was with some trepidation that the author suggested to surgeons that they should move to a more complex technique. However, the logic of the approach is attractive, once the natural PCL behaviour is seen clearly, and so the method is now in widespread clinical use (e.g. Stahelin *et al.*, 2001). There were reports at the ISAKOS conference in Montreux in 2001 that double-bundle reconstruction did not offer a significant advantage, but the author's observation was that the two bundles had not been spaced apart far enough to reproduce the extensive natural PCL femoral attachment, and so could not act in a manner significantly different to a single-bundle reconstruction.

A key attraction of the double-bundle method is that it provides more collagen fibres across the joint, and thus is likely to be better able to withstand the common tendency for PCL reconstruction to be spoilt by chronic stretching-out. However, for the patient who is not demanding stability in deep knee flexion, the aPC reconstruction, in combination with restoration of the posterolateral structures, may be sufficient to ensure functional stability. Overall, the biomechanical studies all support the double-bundle reconstruction method, so now the clinical studies must be performed, to either confirm or refute these claims.

Acknowledgements

The work on the PCL in the author's laboratory was done largely by Dr Amos Race, whose project, and the Instron machine, were funded by the Arthritis Research Campaign, a charity based in Chesterfield, England.

References

Amis AA (1989) Anterior cruciate ligament replacement – knee stability and the effects of implants. *J Bone and Jt. Surg* 71B: 819–824.

Amis AA (1999) The kinematics of knee stability. In: Jakob RP, Fulford P, Horan F (eds) European instructional course lectures vol 4. *J Bone Jt Surg, London*, 96–104.

Amis AA, Beynnon B, Blankevoort L, Chambat P, Christel P, Durselen L, Friederich N, Grood E, Hertel P, Jakob R, Muller W, O'Brien M, O'Connor J (1994) Proceedings of the ESSKA scientific workshop on reconstruction of the anterior and posterior cruciate ligaments. *Knee Surg, Sports Trauma, Arthroscopy* 2: 124–132.

Butler DL, Noyes FR, Grood ES (1980) Ligamentous restraints to anterior-posterior drawer in the human knee: a biomechanical study. *J Bone Jt Surg (Am)* 62: 259–270.

Friederich NF, O'Brien WR (1992) Functional anatomy of the cruciate ligaments. In: Jakob RP, Staubli HU (eds) *The Knee and the Cruciate Ligaments*, pp. 78–91. Springer-Verlag, Berlin.

Galloway MT, Grood ES, Mehalik JN *et al.* (1996) Posterior cruciate ligament reconstruction. An *in vitro* study of femoral and tibial graft placement. *Am J Sports Med* 24: 437–445.

Grood ES, Hefzy MS, Lindenfield TN (1989) Factors affecting the region of most isometric femoral attachments. Part 1: The posterior cruciate ligament. *Am J Sports Med* 17: 197–207.

Harner CD, Janaushek MA, Kanamori A, Yagi M, Vogrin TM, Woo SLY (2000) Biomechanical analysis of a double-bundle posterior cruciate ligament reconstruction. *Am J Sports Med* 28: 144–151.

Mannor DA, Shearn JT, Grood ES, Noyes FR, Levy MS (2000) Two-bundle posterior cruciate ligament reconstruction. An *in vitro* analysis of graft placement and tension. *Am J Sports Med* 28: 833–845.

Noyes FR, Grood ES, Butler DL, Paulos LE (1980) Clinical biomechanics of the knee: ligament restraints and functional stability. In *AAOS Symposium on the Athlete's Knee*, pp. 1–35. CV Mosby, St Louis.

Race A, Amis AA (1994) The mechanical properties of the two bundles of the human posterior cruciate ligament. *J Biomechs* 27: 13–24.

Race A, Amis AA (1996) Loading of the two bundles of the posterior cruciate ligament: an analysis of bundle function in A-P drawer. *J Biomechs* 29: 873–879.

Race A, Amis AA (1998) PCL reconstruction: *in vitro* biomechanical comparison of 'isometric' versus single and double-bundled 'anatomic' grafts. *J Bone Jt Surg* 80B: 173–179.

Radford WJP, Amis AA (1990) Biomechanics of a double prosthetic ligament in the anterior cruciate ligament deficient knee. *J Bone Jt Surg* 72B: 1038–1043.

Sidles JA, Larson RV, Garbini JL, Downey DJ, Matsen FA (1988) Ligament length relationships in the moving knee. *J Orthop Res* 6: 593–610.

Stahelin AC, Sudkamp NP, Weiler A (2001) Anatomic double-bundle posterior cruciate ligament reconstruction using hamstrings tendons. *Arthroscopy* 17: 88–97.

Strobel MJ, Weiler A, Schulz MS, Russe K, Eichhorn HJ (2002) Fixed posterior subluxation in posterior cruciate ligament-deficient knees. Diagnosis and treatment of a new clinical sign. *Am J Sports Med* 30: 32–38.

Part 7. Meniscus and Cartilage Injury

23

Meniscus and cartilage injury: Does meniscal allograft transplantation prevent articular cartilage degeneration?

Scott A. Rodeo

Introduction

Meniscal allografts present a useful reconstructive option for patients following the loss of the meniscal tissue following prior meniscectomy. The menisci serve several important functions, including load transmission and shock absorption across the knee, knee stability, and joint lubrication. Numerous clinical and experimental studies demonstrate the progressive degenerative changes that occur following meniscectomy. This chapter will review the functions of the meniscus, which will serve as a background for a discussion of the rationale and indications for meniscus transplantation. Clinical results of meniscus transplantation will then be reviewed, in order to allow resolution of the question: does meniscal allograft transplantation prevent articular cartilage degeneration?

Function of the meniscus

The principal function of the meniscus is to transmit load across the tibio-femoral joint. The menisci improve the congruency of the articulating surfaces and increase the surface area of joint contact. The medial meniscus transmits 50 per cent of joint load in the medial compartment and the lateral meniscus transmits 70 per cent of joint load in the lateral compartment (Seedhom and Hargreaves 1979). The menisci transmit 50 per cent of the joint load when the knee is in extension and 85–90 per cent of the joint load when the knee is in flexion (walker and Erkman 1975). With joint loading the meniscus experiences radially extrusive force, which results in tensile stress ('hoop stress') in the circumferential collagen fibers. The meniscus also experiences high compressive forces, which are resisted by the swelling pressure provided by proteoglycans and water. Experimental studies demonstrate that total or partial meniscectomy increases the peak stress across the articular surfaces from 40 per cent to 700 per cent (Seedhom and Hargreaves 1979). The excessively high articular contact stresses that occur following meniscectomy predictably result in hyaline cartilage degeneration with time. The meniscus may also aid in articular cartilage nutrition by helping to maintain a synovial fluid film over the articular surface and by compressing synovial fluid into articular cartilage.

The menisci also play a role in joint stability. The medial meniscus serves as a significant restraint to anterior tibial translation in the ACL-deficient knee (Levy et al. 1982). Load sharing occurs between an ACL graft and the medial meniscus, and there are increased forces in an ACL graft in the setting of medial meniscus deficiency (Allen et al. 2000). The menisci also play a role in varus-valgus stability. There is increased varus-valgus rotation in the ACL-deficient and medial meniscus deficient knee (Markolf et al. 1984). Furthermore, it may be difficult to stabilize a knee with collateral ligament instability if both medial and lateral menisci are absent; consideration should be made for transplantation in this rare circumstance. The meniscus may also contribute to joint proprioception, given the presence of nerve endings and mechanoreceptors near the horn insertions and capsular attachments.

The rationale behind meniscal allograft transplantation is to replace these important functions of the meniscus and thus potentially prevent or forestall progressive degenerative changes. Laboratory studies have provided the impetus for the clinical use of meniscal allografts, and subsequent clinical and basic science investigations have further refined its application.

Biomechanical studies of meniscus transplantation

Several in vitro studies have examined the ability of a meniscus transplant to normalize load transmission in the meniscus-deficient knee. Paletta et al. demonstrated that a lateral meniscus transplant could partially normalize articular contact pressures and contact area in the lateral compartment (Paletta et al. 1997). In that study, peak local contact pressures were elevated 235–335 per cent following total lateral meniscectomy. Lateral meniscus replacement reduced these joint contact pressures by 55–65 per cent. These authors also found that contact pressures were only improved if the anterior and posterior horns of the transplant were secured. Alhalki et al. carried out similar experiments for a medial meniscus transplant, and reported that a medial meniscus transplant could partially restore contact mechanics compared to absence of the meniscus (Alhalki et al. 1999). These studies provide support for the ability of a meniscus transplant to prevent articular cartilage degeneration.

Sequelae of meniscectomy

Clinical studies of post-meniscectomy knees support the experimental models of meniscus deficiency. In general, degenerative changes gradually progress following meniscectomy. There is generally more rapid progression of degenerative changes following lateral meniscectomy than for medial meniscectomy. There are large series in the literature that report long-term follow-up of meniscectomized knees; however, it must be noted that patients underwent open meniscectomy in these historical studies. Furthermore, the degree and nature of concomitant knee joint pathology (such as anterior cruciate ligament (ACL) pathology) was not always documented. Nonetheless, these studies clearly demonstrate the adverse sequelae of meniscectomy. Fairbank was one of the first to describe the radiographic changes that ensue following meniscectomy; so-called 'Fairbank's changes' include formation of a ridge on the margin of the condyle, flattening of the condyle, and joint space narrowing (Fairbank 1948). The major factors that affect outcome following meniscectomy include the degree of concomitant articular cartilage degeneration, the amount of meniscus removed, medial versus lateral meniscectomy, the status of the ACL, and the type of meniscus tear (inferior results with degenerative tears).

Tapper and Hoover reported 10–30 year follow-up on 113 patients out of 1005 that had undergone total meniscectomy at the Mayo Clinic from 1936–1956 (Tapper and Hoover 1969). They found that 45 per cent of males were asymptomatic at that time, while only 10 per cent of females were asymptomatic. Johnson et al. reported on 99 out of 440 patients who had undergone meniscectomy at the University of Iowa between 1927 and 1964. At an average 17 year follow-up, degenerative joint disease was diagnosed in the operative knee in 40 per cent of patients compared to 6 per cent in the contralateral knee (Johnson et al. 1974). They also reported better results following medial meniscectomy compared to lateral meniscectomy. Further evidence of the morbid sequelae of lateral meniscectomy is reported by Yocum et al. who reported on the results following isolated lateral meniscectomy in 26 patients at early follow-up (35 months). They found satisfactory results in only 54 per cent of patients (Yocum et al. 1979).

The results of partial meniscectomy reported in the literature are generally better than those following total meniscectomy. For example, Northmore-Ball and Dandy reported on 99 patients at three year follow-up and found 90 per cent satisfactory results in normal knees compared to 67 per cent satisfactory results in knees with ACL-insufficiency and/or degenerative changes (Northmore-Ball and Dandy 1982). Jaureguito et al. reported the early and late results (8 years) of 26 isolated partial lateral meniscectomies and found satisfactory results at early follow-up in 92 per cent of patients, with deterioration to 62 per cent satisfactory results at early follow-up

(Jaureguito *et al.* 1995). They also found that although 85 per cent of patients had returned to full activity at early follow-up, only 48 per cent were still active at later follow-up. Further evidence of the different outcomes following partial versus complete meniscectomy is provided by direct comparisons. McGinty *et al.* compared the outcome of 39 partial meniscectomies to 89 total meniscectomies at 5.5 year follow-up. The subjective results following partial meniscectomy were better than total meniscectomy, and there were radiographic changes in 60 per cent of the total meniscectomy group compared to 30 per cent in the partial meniscectomy group (McGinty *et al.* 1977).

The influence of concomitant pathology on outcome following meniscectomy is also demonstrated in outcome studies. McBride *et al.* reported 96 per cent satisfactory results following partial meniscectomy for non-degenerative tears, compared to only 65 per cent satisfactory results for degenerative tears. The best results were found in patients who underwent meniscectomy for mechanical symptoms (McBride *et al.* 1984). Similarly, Schimmer *et al.* reported 95 per cent satisfactory results 12 years following partial meniscectomy in patients with no degenerative joint disease, compared to 62 per cent satisfactory results for patients with concomitant degenerative changes (Schimmer *et al.* 1998). Burks *et al.* found 88 per cent satisfactory results 15 years following partial meniscectomy in ACL-intact knees compared to only 48 per cent satisfactory results in ACL-insufficient knees (Burks *et al.* 1997).

Rationale and indications for meniscus transplantation

The indications and rationale for meniscus transplantation are logically derived from consideration of the functions of the meniscus (for example, as a contributor to joint stability) and clinical outcomes. The indications for meniscus transplantation continue to evolve as clinical studies report outcomes of this procedure. Meniscus transplantation was initially undertaken in patients with degenerative knees who had undergone previous total meniscectomy in an effort to prevent the progressive joint degeneration that predictably follows meniscectomy. It is now clear that there is a high failure rate in patients with advanced arthrosis; however, early clinical results are encouraging for patients with only early degenerative changes. I will discuss specific clinical situations in which meniscus transplantation may be considered.

Articular cartilage damage

The most common indication for meniscus transplantation is for the patient with symptoms referable to a meniscus-deficient tibio-femoral compartment. The most common symptoms are pain and swelling. Mechanical symptoms such as catching and locking are less frequently reported. Most authors currently recommend limiting transplantation to those patients with only partial-thickness cartilage loss, as the results of meniscus transplantation are much less predictable in knees with advanced degenerative changes (Carter 1999; Garrett 1993; Noyes and Barber-Westin 1995; Rodeo *et al.* 1998; Van Arkel and de Boer 1995). The presence of a large area of subchondral bone exposure (grade IV lesions) with radiographic joint space narrowing and malalignment is generally a contraindication to this procedure. The mechanical axis of the limb should not go through the involved compartment (for example, isolated lateral meniscus transplantation should not be performed in a valgus knee).

It is likely that the size and location of a hyaline cartilage lesion plays an important role in the fate of a meniscus transplant. For example, a small, focal lesion may permit load-bearing around its periphery and thus not present a deleterious mechanical environment. There are usually varying degrees of cartilage damage on different parts of the articular surfaces, making it difficult to accurately grade such surfaces and difficult to interpret published reports. Many patients with meniscus deficiency demonstrate focal erosive lesions on the flexion weight-bearing (posterior) zone of the femur and tibia (Fairbank 1948; Noyes and Barber-Westin 1995). Such lesions may result in early joint space narrowing on flexion weight-bearing radiographs. Since the posterior aspect of the meniscus is loaded in flexion (Walker and Erkman 1975), the presence of focal erosive lesions on the flexion weight-bearing zone of the femur and the posterior tibia should be carefully evaluated. Although meniscus transplantation may be particularly advantageous in an individual with articular cartilage degeneration in the meniscal weight-bearing zone of the femoral condyle or tibial plateau, loss of cartilage in these areas may also predispose the meniscus transplant to failure. Further studies are required to define how the size, location, and depth of articular cartilage lesions affect the biologic incorporation and mechanical function of a meniscus transplant.

Protection of cartilage resurfacing procedure

Since these patients often have some hyaline cartilage damage, meniscus transplantation could be performed in conjunction with a cartilage-resurfacing procedure, such as osteochondral autograft/ allograft transplantation or autologous chondrocyte implantation. Concomitant meniscus transplantation may help to protect the healing cartilage surface by aiding in stress transmission across the involved compartment. It is likely that the results of cartilage resurfacing procedures will be superior if the ipsilateral meniscus is present, and similarly, it is established that healing and biologic incorporation of a meniscus transplant is better with an intact hyaline cartilage surface. Given these considerations, it is possible that the best results will come with concomitant meniscus transplantation and cartilage resurfacing. However, there is currently very little clinical evidence available to support these complicated procedures. Further studies are required to determine the amount of meniscal loss that would necessitate meniscus transplantation to maximize the outcome of a cartilage resurfacing procedure. Likewise, further studies are required to define the critical size and location of a hyaline cartilage lesion that would mandate concomitant resurfacing in order for concomitant meniscus transplantation to be successful. Until further information is available to help refine the indications for such combined procedures, their use is not routinely recommended.

Meniscus transplantation with osteotomy

Meniscectomy may result in progressive varus or valgus deformity. Osteotomy is often indicated in this setting in order to shift the mechanical axis to the more normal compartment. Recurrence of symptoms following osteotomy is often due to gradual progression of arthrosis in the compartment that was unloaded (Holden *et al.* 1988). It is possible that replacement of the meniscus in the involved compartment would forestall recurrence of symptoms; thus, consideration may be made for concomitant or staged meniscus transplantation if it could be demonstrated that meniscus transplantation could delay such recurrence. Such a procedure would be considered in very few select candidates, such as a young patient with largely intact articular cartilage. Meniscus transplantation at the same time as the osteotomy may be technically challenging since drill holes in the proximal tibia are required if the meniscus is transplanted with bone plugs attached to the anterior and posterior horns. Careful placement of any internal fixation devices for the osteotomy is necessary to avoid the bone tunnels. Alternatively, meniscus transplantation can be performed as a staged procedure after the osteotomy has healed. There is currently very little data to support concomitant osteotomy and meniscus transplantation.

Ligament instability

Many knees undergoing ACL reconstruction have early arthrosis due to previous meniscectomy. The majority of the meniscal transplantations reported to date have been done with concomitant anterior cruciate ligament (ACL) reconstruction. Ligament stabilization is recommended if meniscus transplantation is being undertaken in an unstable knee. Biomechanical studies have demonstrated that the medial meniscus is a secondary restraint to anterior tibial translation in the ACL-deficient knee (Allen *et al.* 2000; Levy *et al.* 1989). Thus, medial meniscus transplantation at the time of anterior cruciate ligament reconstruction may help to protect the anterior cruciate ligament graft. A recent cadaveric study reported significant increases in the *in situ* forces in an ACL graft in medial meniscus-deficient knees compared to meniscus-intact knees (Papageorgiou *et al.* 2001). Clinical evidence for the role of the medial meniscus in knee stability is provided in a recent report by Shelbourne and Gray who demonstrated greater laxity as measured with KT-1000 arthrometry following ACL reconstruction in patients that had undergone previous medial meniscectomy compared to knees with intact menisci (Shelbourne and Gray 2000). Also, Garrett has reported significantly improved KT-1000 arthrometer results for ACL reconstructions performed with concomitant medial meniscus transplantation compared to a group of patients who underwent isolated ACL reconstruction with persistent medial meniscus deficiency (Garrett 1992). Thus, a medial meniscus transplant may protect an ACL graft by diminishing the forces on the graft. In contrast, the lateral meniscus has not been demonstrated to act as a secondary restraint to anterior tibial translation in the ACL-deficient knee in cadaveric studies (Levy *et al.* 1989), and clinical follow-up has demonstrated no difference in KT-1000 arthrometer results following ACL reconstruction in lateral meniscus-deficient knees compared to knees with intact menisci (Shelbourne and Gray 2000). Further studies are required to determine if concomitant meniscus transplantation can improve the results of ACL reconstruction.

The absence of both the medial and lateral menisci may result in slightly increased varus/valgus rotation, and meniscus transplantation may be considered in this setting if collateral ligament repair or reconstruction is performed. It has been noted in such patients that replacing both the medial and lateral meniscus may help improve varus and valgus laxity. Further support for this strategy comes from Markolf *et al.* who demonstrated greater varus-valgus laxity in the ACL-deficient and medial meniscus-deficient knee compared to the ACL-deficient knee with an intact medial meniscus (Markolf *et al.* 1984). It can be difficult to restore posterolateral knee stability (with repair or reconstruction of the lateral ligaments) if the lateral meniscus is absent, due to the convex tibial and femoral condylar surfaces in the lateral compartment. Lateral meniscus transplantation may be considered in that setting.

Early meniscus transplantation

Eventual joint degeneration is well-documented sequelae of meniscectomy, with more rapid degeneration in the lateral compartment than in the medial compartment (Fairbank 1948). It is possible that the best time to perform meniscus transplantation is at the time of meniscectomy, prior to development of significant hyaline cartilage degeneration. The goal of meniscus replacement in this situation would be to prevent or delay degenerative joint changes. It is possible that such prophylactic meniscus transplantation may especially play a role in the lateral compartment, where there is a more rapid progression of degenerative changes following meniscectomy. This may be considered following resection of an irreparable bucket-handle tear that involves the majority of the lateral meniscus, resection of a symptomatic discoid lateral meniscus, or with a radial split tear, in which the loss of hoop stress transmission is functionally equivalent to a total lateral meniscectomy. However, routine prophylactic meniscus transplantation cannot currently be recommended until further long-term results are available.

A current dilemma is how early to perform prophylactic meniscus transplantation. Although it is becoming evident that meniscus transplantation should probably be performed earlier than it has been in most reported series, patients typically have no symptoms in the early years following meniscectomy in the otherwise normal knee. Most authors do not recommend meniscus transplantation for the asymptomatic patient. An objective indicator is needed for the detection of early compartment degeneration, to allow for detection of pathologic changes prior to the development of significant cartilage injury. High-resolution MRI is currently the most sensitive method to detect early degenerative changes (Potter *et al.* 1996). In the near future it is likely that metabolic markers, such as synovial fluid analyses of collagen or proteoglycan breakdown products, matrix metalloproteinase activity, and/or cytokines will provide information that will assist in the identification of the appropriate time to consider meniscus replacement in a patient with known meniscus deficiency.

Contraindications

Most authors currently recommend limiting transplantation to patients with only early articular cartilage degeneration and relatively normal axial alignment (Carter 1999; Garrett 1993; Noyes and Barber-Westin 1995; Rodeo *et al.* 1998). The presence of diffuse subchondral bone exposure is a contraindication to this procedure. The location of chondral lesions is probably as important as the size and depth. Since most failures of meniscus transplantation occur due to progressive degeneration of the posterior part of the transplanted meniscus, the presence of full-thickness articular cartilage lesions on the posterior part of the femoral condyle or tibia that are greater than 10–15 mm in width or length are currently considered a contraindication to meniscus transplantation (Noyes and Barber-Westin 1995; Rodeo *et al.* 1998). Changes in bone morphology should also be considered. Several reports have demonstrated poorer results when there is remodeling and flattening of the femoral condyle (Noyes and Barber-Westin 1995; Rodeo *et al.* 1998). Uncorrected knee instability or axial malalignment are also contraindications to meniscus transplantation.

Graft sizing and surgical technique

Appropriate size matching of the meniscus transplant to the recipient knee is likely to be critical for optimal mechanical function. Studies have demonstrated a consistent relationship between meniscus size and radiographic landmarks (Pollard *et al.* 1995). Radiographic methods that may be used to size the transplant include plain radiographs, MRI, and CT scans, and there is currently no agreement in the literature as to the most accurate imaging modality (Garrett 1992; Johnson *et al.* 1994; Kuhn and Wopjtys 1996; Shaffer *et al.* 2000). It is important to note that the tolerance of the tibio-femoral compartment to meniscus size mismatch is not known. The author currently recommends use of plain radiographs (taken with a size marker to aid in correcting for magnification) and MRI to determine tibial plateau dimensions. A matching tibial plateau (or hemi-plateau) graft with attached meniscus is then obtained from the tissue bank. However, if only the meniscus is supplied by the tissue bank (such as if using a fresh or cryopreserved graft) it will be necessary to use some formula to derive meniscus dimensions from the bone measurements. It is recommended that the clinician familiarize him or herself with the technique used at the tissue bank supplying their grafts.

Meniscal grafts may be transplanted using either open or arthroscopically assisted techniques, and comparable results have been reported with both techniques (Noyes and Barber-Westin 1995; Pollard *et al.* 1995; Rodeo *et al.* 1998; Yoldas *et al.* 1998). Perhaps more important than the particular surgical technique used is the selection of appropriate sites for anchoring the anterior and posterior horns. The clinician needs to be familiar with normal meniscus anatomy and the relationship of the insertion sites to other intraarticular structures, including the tibial spines and cruciate ligaments.

Implantation with attached bone appears to result in more secure anchorage of the horn attachment sites. Cadaver models have demonstrated superior load transmission with meniscal horn bone plug fixation compared to no bone plugs (Alhalki *et al.* 1999; Chen *et al.* 1996; Paletta *et al.* 1997). The graft may be inserted either as a free graft, with separate bone plugs attached to the horns, or using the keyhole technique (or a variation thereof), in which the graft contains a common bone bridge attached to both anterior and posterior horns. This bone bridge is then inserted into a similarly-shaped slot in the recipient tibia. The usual diameter of the bone plugs is 9 mm.

The author currently recommends use of bone plugs for medial meniscus transplants. The graft is brought into the knee through an enlarged anterior portal. The graft is sutured to the capsule using standard meniscal repair techniques. The author uses an inside-out technique to suture the posterior aspect and an outside-in approach for the anterior part of the transplant. Consideration may be made for use of absorbable meniscal fixation devices, but studies have demonstrated that the holding strength of these devices is inferior to

(a)

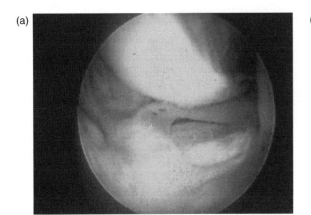

(b)

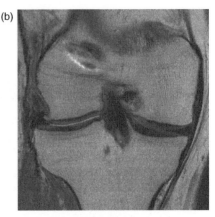

Fig. 23.1

(a) Operative photograph of a
lateral meniscal allograft
placed in the knee of a
36-year-old male four months
following implantation. This
procedure was performed
concomitantly with ACL
reconstruction. (b) MRI of the
same patient made 62 months
following transplantation.

vertical mattress sutures (Albrecht-Olsen *et al.* 1997; Dervin *et al.* 1997). The sutures attached to the horns are then tied together over a bone bridge over the anterior tibia. Lateral meniscus transplants are inserted with a common bone slot connecting both horns. The recipient slot in the tibia is made with an arthroscopic burr and small osteotomes, under direct arthroscopic visualization. The graft is then inserted through a small arthrotomy. Sutures placed through the bone slot are then retrieved through a drill hole made into the base of the recipient trough from the outside. Standard arthroscopic meniscal suturing is then performed as described above for medial meniscus transplants (Figure 23.1).

If concomitant ACL reconstruction is performed with medial meniscal transplantation, the starting point for the ACL tibial tunnel on the outside of the tibia is moved slightly more medially to allow central placement of the two smaller tunnels for the anterior and posterior horn meniscus bone plugs. Attempts should be made to avoid having the ACL tibial tunnel and the anterior horn tunnel break into each other. For combined lateral meniscus transplantation and ACL reconstruction, the ACL tibial tunnel may partially violate the meniscus bone slot, but the overall integrity of the slot usually remains intact. The other option is to consider staged ACL reconstruction and lateral meniscus transplantation. If both medial and lateral transplants are being performed, an arthrotomy is used and the grafts are implanted with one common bone bridge containing the attachments of both menisci.

Results of meniscus transplantation

There are reports in the literature of the early clinical results following meniscus transplantation, but there is very little objective information available on the results of this procedure. Most of the reported series are small with limited follow-up, and it is difficult to interpret and compare the reports that are available due to variability in graft processing techniques (cryopreserved vs. fresh-frozen, irradiated vs. non-irradiated), surgical technique (whether implanted with attached bone or not), degree of arthrosis, and method of evaluation. One of the principal limitations in the existing literature is the fact that the majority of the patients reported underwent other concomitant procedures (most commonly ACL reconstruction), making it difficult to evaluate the contribution of the meniscus transplant to the overall result. Accordingly, the most definitive information about the status of the meniscal allograft has been gained from studies that have directly evaluated the meniscus using either arthroscopy or MRI. Overall, the current clinical literature demonstrates improvements in symptoms of pain and swelling following meniscus transplantation. This is presumably due to improvement of load transmission across the tibio-femoral joint. The question of whether meniscus transplantation can prevent articular cartilage degeneration can only be answered with long-term follow-up. The definitive way to answer this question would be a prospective, randomized study, which does not currently exist.

Objective evaluations of meniscus transplants have demonstrated that the meniscus heals well to the joint capsule and the bone plugs heal reliably to the recipient tibia in the majority of patients (Noyes and Barber-Westin 1995; Rodeo *et al.* 1998). Arthroscopic inspection reveals that the meniscus has a normal appearance, consistency, and position in the joint in knees with minimal articular cartilage degeneration. Degenerative changes are common in the posterior horn. There is frequently abnormal intrameniscal signal in the posterior horn on MRI (Figures 23.1 and 23.2) (Noyes and Barber-Westin

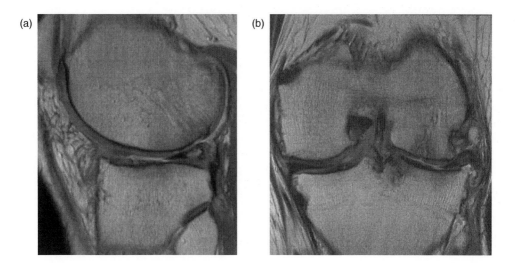

(a)   (b)

Fig. 23.2

(a) Forty-one-year-old male, 35 months following lateral meniscus transplantation using a bone slot. Note the increased signal in the transplant. (b) Coronal MRI image of same patient. The image demonstrates thinning of articular cartilage over the lateral femoral condyle. The apparent extrusion of the graft relative to the femur is due to the presence of a tibial plateau osteophyte.

1995; Rodeo *et al.* 1998). In knees with more advanced degenerative changes and with flattening of the femoral condyle, some degree of extrusion into the medial or lateral gutter is sometimes observed. Extrusion is usually associated with breakdown of the meniscus adjacent to the posterior horn attachment. Potter *et al.* demonstrated that allograft degeneration is associated with articular cartilage degeneration, and reported frank extrusion of the transplant in patients with full-thickness chondral degeneration, condylar flattening, and posterior horn meniscal degeneration (Potter *et al.* 1996).

Meniscus transplantation was initially used as a salvage procedure in young, active patients with relatively advanced joint degeneration. This is a difficult group of patients for whom there are no highly predictable reconstructive options, and the results in these patients have been variable. The majority (60–100 per cent) of the patients in these series reported improvements in pain, swelling, and function, with significant improvements reported on standardized knee scales. The overall results are related to the degree of arthrosis at the time of transplantation, with poorer results in patients with more advanced degeneration in the involved compartment (Garrett 1993; Noyes and Barber-Westin 1995; Rodeo *et al.* 1998). Only long-term follow-up will determine whether a meniscus transplant can delay or prevent the progression of degenerative changes.

The outcome of meniscal transplantation may be best evaluated by analysis of isolated meniscal transplants, but there are very few follow-up reports on such patients. The largest series of isolated transplants appears to be reported by van Arkel and de Boer (1995). These authors reported clinical follow-up at a minimum of two years for 23 patients with cryopreserved transplants and performed arthroscopic evaluation in 12 of the transplants. Partial detachment was found in five menisci, and three of these were eventually removed. There were signs of degeneration in five transplants but there was no change in the articular surfaces. Cameron and Saha reported good to excellent results in 19 out of 21 knees (90 per cent) that underwent isolated meniscus transplantation, but the majority of these transplants were not evaluated objectively (Cameron and Saha 1997).

Important information can be gained by review of several of the larger series on the results of this procedure. The largest and most carefully studied group of patients was reported by Noyes and Barber-Westin (1995). These authors reported on 96 fresh-frozen, irradiated transplants in 82 patients. All patients had objective evaluation of the transplant with either MRI or arthroscopy. Of the total 96 transplants, 56 (58 per cent) failed, 30 (31 per cent) were partially healed, 9 (9 per cent) healed, and one (2 per cent) was unknown. The high failure rate appears to be due to the presence of advanced arthrosis at the time of transplantation, as well as possible irradiation-induced weakening of the meniscus. Failure was found to be related to joint degeneration as graded by MRI.

The longest follow-up report comes from Wirth *et al.* who reported 14-year follow-up of 23 transplants (17 freeze-dried, six fresh frozen) (Wirth *et al.* 2002). Patients with deep-frozen transplants had better results than patients with lyophilized transplants. Shrinkage was noted in the freeze-dried transplants. MRI demonstrated good preservation of the deep-frozen transplants even after 14 years. The authors concluded that the long-term results were affected by the initial condition of the cartilage. Several other studies have demonstrated higher failure rates in knees with more advanced degenerative changes. Garrett evaluated 28 transplants with arthroscopy and found eight (29 per cent) failures (Garrett 1993). Failures were related to the degree of arthrosis: in the overall group of 43 patients, there were only two failures out of 32 transplants in patients with grade III chondral changes, while six out of 11 transplants failed in patients with grade IV changes.

We have reported our results of 33 fresh-frozen, non-irradiated meniscus transplants performed at The Hospital for Special Surgery at a minimum two-year follow-up (Rodeo *et al.* 2000). Each meniscus transplant was evaluated objectively with MRI and/or arthroscopic inspection. MRI and arthroscopic inspections of the meniscus transplants demonstrated consistent healing of the meniscus transplant to the capsule and at the bone plug attachment sites. MRI frequently demonstrated some degree of extrusion of the transplant from the tibio-femoral compartment, with the most extrusion in knees with more advanced articular degeneration. MRI also demonstrated variable amounts of increased intra-meniscal signal within the substance of the meniscus (most frequently observed in the posterior horn), indicating ongoing remodeling of the transplant and/or degeneration.

The overall outcome was graded based on the objective evaluation of the transplant. Of the 33 total meniscal transplants, there were eight good, 14 moderate, four poor, and seven failures. There was no significant change in joint degeneration at this follow-up interval. There were significant improvements ($P < 0.05$) in the final IKDC and Lysholm ratings, visual analog scale scores for both pain and function, and the Lysholm scores for locking, pain, swelling, and instability. The results were significantly better for menisci that were transplanted with attached bone plugs as compared to those implanted without bone plugs. Fourteen out of 16 (88 per cent) of the menisci implanted with bone plugs were rated as good or moderate, while eight out of 17 (47 per cent) of the menisci implanted without bone plugs were rated as good or moderate ($P = 0.03$).

Fresh meniscal transplants have the theoretical advantage of providing viable cells at the time of transplantation. Verdonk transplanted 40 fresh menisci in 36 patients and found intact grafts using MRI in all patients and arthroscopic inspection in 12 patients (Verdonk 1997; Verdonk *et al.* 1994). Analysis of DNA from cells cultured from a small biopsy of the transplanted meniscus demonstrated donor DNA in some (indicating survival of donor cells) and host DNA in others (indicative of cellular repopulation from the host). However, it must be noted that animal studies have not definitively established that viable donor cells survive following transplantation. Jackson *et al.* used DNA probe analysis in a goat model to demonstrate that donor cells in a fresh meniscus transplant were rapidly replaced by host cells (Jackson *et al.* 1993). Garrett transplanted 16 fresh menisci and 27 cryopreserved menisci and found no significant difference between the two types of transplants (Garrett 1993). Zukor *et al.* transplanted 28 fresh menisci as part of a tibial plateau osteochondral allograft (Zukor *et al.* 1988). Objective evaluation with arthroscopy or arthrotomy was carried out for 14 transplants. The transplants were found to be structurally intact and well-attached. No significant immune rejection has been noted in these series, although there are isolated patients with persistent effusions and synovitis following transplantation reported in these and other series.

The ability of a meniscus transplant to 'protect' a cartilage resurfacing procedure is supported by a few studies in the literature. Zukor *et al.* and Garrett have reported favorable results following meniscal transplantation in conjunction with osteochondral allograft resurfacing of major chondral defects (Garrett 1993; Zukor *et al.* 1988). Further studies with careful objective evaluation of the status of the articular surface are required to determine the ability of a transplanted meniscus to prevent articular cartilage degeneration and/or improve the outcome of a cartilage resurfacing procedure.

Graft processing is likely to affect clinical outcome; however, at this time there is limited information available in the literature to allow accurate comparisons of different graft types. Essentially comparable results have been reported for fresh, fresh-frozen, and cryopreserved transplants. The overall results reported for freeze-dried grafts appear to be inferior to other graft types. Graft shrinkage has been reported with freeze-dried grafts. Similarly, the effect of irradiation is unclear. Noyes reported a high failure rate using fresh-frozen grafts that had received 2.5 mrads of irradiation (Noyes and Barber-Westin 1995). The poor results with irradiated menisci may be secondary to weakening of the tissue by the irradiation (Yahia and Zukor 1994). Another important factor related to graft processing is whether the graft is transplanted with attached bone. Our group found improved healing rates in menisci transplanted with attached bone plugs, suggesting that healing of bone plugs in a bone tunnel is more secure than healing of the meniscus to bone (Rodeo *et al.* 1998). This finding supports cadaver models that have demonstrated superior load transmission with meniscal horn bone plug fixation compared to no bone plugs (Chen *et al.* 1996; Paletta *et al.* 1997). There is very little information available on the healing of meniscus to bone, and no studies have compared healing of bone plugs to healing of meniscal tissue in a bone tunnel. It is likely that secure fixation of the allograft is critical for initial healing, remodeling of the allograft, and long-term function.

Mechanisms of failure of meniscus transplants

A careful analysis of the mechanisms of failure of meniscus transplants aids in identifying factors that are critical to the success of this procedure. Lessons learned from such failures will help to define new methods to improve the results of this procedure and improve our ability to offer meniscus transplantation as a viable option to prevent articular cartilage degeneration. It is likely that both biomechanical and biological factors combine to result in failure of meniscal transplants. The principal factor involved in failure appears to be advanced articular cartilage degeneration. The presence of bony remodeling of the tibio-femoral compartment, with flattening of the femoral condyle, is associated with degeneration of the meniscus (Noyes and Barber-Westin 1995). Degeneration and tears most commonly occur adjacent to the posterior horn attachment, where the contact stresses on the meniscus are highest (Figure 23.2).

Surgical technique and graft sizing play important roles in outcome. Proper placement of the anterior and posterior horn fixation sites will affect the ability of the meniscus to transmit hoop stresses and to ultimately function in load transmission across the knee. Cadaveric studies demonstrate that secure, anatomic fixation of bone plugs attached to the anterior and posterior horns is required to best restore normal contact mechanics for both medial (Alhalki et al.) and lateral transplants (Chen et al. 1996). A recent biomechanical study demonstrated that non-anatomic placement of the posterior horn attachment site of a medial meniscus transplant by only 5 mm resulted in abnormal contact area and contact stress (Sekaran et al. 2002). The use of bone plugs is likely to provide more secure fixation of the horn attachments.

Similarly, proper graft sizing is critical for restoration of normal contact mechanics. An undersized graft would likely be exposed to excessive loads due to poor congruity with the femoral condyle, while an oversized graft is likely to extrude from the compartment and thus fail to transmit compressive loads across the knee. There is currently no data available as to the tolerance of the tibio-femoral compartment for graft size mismatch.

Biologic factors are also likely to play a role in failure of meniscal transplants. Histologic studies demonstrate significant structural remodeling of the matrix associated with the process of graft revascularization and cellular repopulation. This remodeling may weaken the tissue and predispose to tears and graft failure. Since it appears that the presence of viable cells is critical for the long-term maintenance and repair of the tissue, it is possible that results may be improved by transplantation of meniscus with viable cells. However, it has not been definitively established that viable donor cells in the meniscus at the time of transplantation (using either fresh or cryopreserved tissue) survive following transplantation (De Boer and Koudstaal 1994; Jackson *et al.* 1993). An immune response may also occur against transplanted tissue. Although frank immune rejection does not appear to occur, there is microscopic evidence of an immune response against the transplant. It is possible that such a subclinical immune response may contribute to the graft shrinkage and persistent effusions that have been reported, and may modulate allograft revascularization and cellular repopulation.

Summary

Meniscus transplantation has emerged as a useful treatment option for selected patients with meniscus deficiency. Biomechanical studies support the possibility that meniscus transplantation can prevent articular cartilage degeneration. Predictable improvements in pain, swelling, and knee function have been demonstrated in early reports. Results are poor in patients with advanced articular cartilage degeneration, and this procedure should not be performed in patients with subchondral bone exposure and/or flattening of the femoral condyle. Results are likely to be improved by earlier transplantation. The use of biomarkers such as serum, synovial fluid, or urinary metabolites of articular cartilage may allow earlier identification of early cartilage breakdown and aid in identifying appropriate timing for meniscus transplantation. Further information about the basic biology of the transplanted meniscus will also refine the use of this technique. In particular, improved understanding of the process of cell migration into the meniscus during cellular repopulation and the effect of an immune response on graft remodeling will aid in identifying methods to improve graft healing and graft survival. Finally, the experience gained from meniscal transplantation will be useful in the future as other meniscal replacement options become available, such as synthetic devices and tissue-engineered menisci.

References

Albrecht-Olsen P, Lind T, Kristensen G, Falkenberg B. (1997) Failure strength of a new meniscus arrow repair technique: Biomechanical comparisons with horizontal suture. *Arthroscopy* 13: 183–187.

Alhalki MM, Howell SM, Hull, ML. (1999) How three methods for fixing a medial meniscal auto graft affect tibial contact mechanics. *American Journal of Sports Medicine* 27: 320–328.

Allen CR, Wong EK, Livesay GA, Sakane M, Fu FH, Woo SL. (2000) Importance of the medial meniscus in the anterior cruciate ligament-deficient knee. *Journal of Orthopaedic Research* 18: 109–15.

Burks RT, Metcalf MH, Metcalf RW. (1997) Fifteen-year follow-up of arthroscopic partial meniscectomy. *Arthroscopy* 13: 673–679.

Cameron JC, Saha S. (1997) Meniscal allograft transplantation for unicompartmental arthritis of the knee. *Clinical Orthopaedics and Related Research* 337: 164–171.

Carter TR. (1999) Meniscal allograft transplantation. *Sports Medicine and Arthroscopy Review* 7: 51–62.

Chen MI, Branch TP, Hutton WC. (1996) Is it important to secure the horns during lateral meniscal transplantation? A cadaveric study. *Arthroscopy: The Journal of Arthroscopic and Related Surgery* 12: 174–181.

De Boer HH, Koudstaal J. (1994) Failed meniscus transplantation. A report of three cases. *Clinical Orthopaedics and Related Research* 306: 155–162.

Dervin GF, Downing KJW, Keene GCR, McBride DG. (1997) Failure strengths of suture versus biodegradable arrow for meniscal repair: An *in-vitro* study. *Arthroscopy* 13: 296–300.

Fairbank TJ. (1948) Knee joint changes after meniscectomy. *Journal of Bone and Joint Surgery* 30B: 664–670.

Garrett JC. (1993) Meniscal transplantation: a review of 43 cases with 2- to 7-year follow-up. *Sports Medicine and Arthroscopy Review* 1: 164–167.

Garrett JC. (1992) Meniscal transplantation. In Aichroth PM and Cannon WD (editors): *Knee Surgery: Current practice*. Martin Dunitz Ltd, London, pp. 95–103.

Holden DL, James SL, Larson RL, Slocum DB. (1988) Proximal tibial osteotomy in patients who are fifty years old or less. A long-term follow-up study. *Journal of Bone and Joint Surgery* 70: 977–982.

Jackson DW, Whelan J, Simon TM. (1993) Cell survival after transplantation of fresh meniscal allografts. DNA probe analysis in a goat model. *American Journal of Sports Medicine* 21: 540–550.

Jaureguito JW, Elliot JS, Lietner T, Dixon LB, Reider B. (1995) The effects of arthroscopic partial lateral meniscectomy in an otherwise normal knee: a retrospective review of functional, clinical, and radiographic results. *Arthroscopy* 11: 29–36.

Johnson RJ, Kettelkamp DB, Clark W, Leaverton P. (1974) Factors effecting late results after meniscectomy. *Journal of Bone and Joint Surgery* 56A: 719–29.

Johnson DL, Swenson TM, Harner CD. (1994) Meniscal reconstruction using allograft tissue: An arthroscopic technique. *Operative Techniques in Sports Medicine* 2: 223–231.

Kuhn JE, Wojtys EM. (1996) Allograft meniscus transplantation. *Clinics in Sports Medicine* 15: 537–556.

Levy IM, Torzilli PA, Gould JD, Warren RF. (1989) The effect of lateral meniscectomy on motion of the knee. *Journal of Bone and Joint Surgery* 71A: 401–406.

Levy IM, Torzilli PA, Warren RF. (1982) The effect of medial meniscectomy on anterior-posterior motion of the knee. *Journal of Bone and Joint Surgery* 64A: 883–888.

Markolf KL, Kochan A, Amstutz HC. (1984) Measurement of knee stiffness and laxity in patients with documented absence of the anterior cruciate ligament. *Journal of Bone and Joint Surgery* 66A: 242–253.

McBride GG, Constine RM, Hofmann AA, Carson RW. (1984) Arthroscopic partial medial meniscectomy in the older patient. *Journal of Bone and Joint Surgery* 66A: 547–551.

McGinty JB, Geuss LF, Marvin RA. (1977) Partial or total meniscectomy: a comparative analysis. *Journal of Bone and Joint Surgery* 59A: 763–766.

Northmore-Ball MD, Dandy DJ. (1982) Long-term results of arthroscopic partial meniscectomy. *Clinical Orthopaedics* 167: 34–42.

Noyes FR, Barber-Westin SD. (1995) Irradiated meniscus allografts in the human knee: A two to five year follow-up study. Presented at the American Orthopaedic Society for Sports Medicine Specialty Day Meeting, Orlando, February 1995.

Paletta GA, Manning T, Snell E, Parker R, Bergfeld J. (1997) The effect of allograft meniscal replacement on intraarticular contact area and pressures in the human knee: A biomechanical study. *American Journal of Sports Medicine* 25: 692–698.

Papageorgiou CD, Gil JE, Kanamori A, Fenwick JA, Woo SL, Fu FH. (2001) The biomechanical interdependence between the anterior cruciate ligament replacement graft and the medial meniscus. *American Journal of Sports Medicine* 29: 226–231.

Pollard ME, Kang Q, Berg EE. (1995) Radiographic sizing for meniscal transplantation. *Arthroscopy* 11: 684–687.

Potter HG, Rodeo SA, Wickiewicz TL, Warren RF. (1996) MR imaging of meniscal allografts: Correlation with clinical and arthroscopic outcomes. *Radiology* 198: 509–514.

Rodeo SA, Potter HG, Berkowitz M, Wickiewicz TL, Cohen S, Warren RF. (1998) A clinical and objective evaluation of meniscal allograft transplantation: Minimum two-year follow-up. Presented at Annual Meeting of the American Academy of Orthopaedic Surgeons, New Orleans, March 1998.

Rodeo S, Seneviratne A, Suzuki K, Felker K, Wickiewicz T, Warren R. (2000) Histological analysis of human meniscal allografts: a preliminary report. *Journal of Bone and Joint Surgery* 82: 1071–1082.

Schimmer RC, Brulhart KB, Duff C, Glinz W. (1998) Arthroscopic partial meniscectomy: a 12-year follow-up and two-step evaluation of the long-term course. *Arthroscopy* 14: 136–142.

Seedhom B, Hargreaves D. (1979) Transmission of the load in the knee joint with special reference to the role of the menisci: II. Exprimental results, discussion, and conclusions. *Engineering in Medicine* 8: 220.

Sekaran SV, Hull ML, Howell SM. (2002) Nonanatomic location of the posterior horn of a medial meniscal autograft implanted in a cadaveric knee adversely affects the pressure distribution on the tibial plateau. *American Journal of Sports Medicine* 30: 74–82.

Shaffer B, Kennedy S, Klimkiewicz J, Yao L. (2000) Preoperative sizing of meniscal allografts in meniscus transplantation. *American Journal of Sports Medicine* 28: 524–533.

Shelbourne KD, Gray T. (2000) Results of anterior cruciate ligament reconstruction based on meniscus and articular cartilage status at the time of surgery. Five-to fifteen-year evaluations. *American Journal of Sports Medicine* 28: 446–452.

Tapper EM, Hoover NW. (1969) Late results after meniscectomy. JBJS 51A: 517–526.

Van Arkel ERA, de Boer HH. (1995) Human meniscal transplantation. Preliminary results at two to five-year follow-up. *Journal of Bone and Joint Surgery* 77B: 589–595.

Verdonk R. (1997) Alternative treatments for meniscal injuries. *Journal of Bone and Joint Surgery* 79B: 866–873.

Verdonk R, Van Daele P, Claus B, Vandenabeele K, Desmet P, Verbruggen G, Veys EM, Claessens H. (1994) Viable meniscus transplantation. *Orthopade* 23: 153–159.

Walker PS, Erkman MJ. (1975) The role of the menisci in force transmission across the knee. *Clinical Orthopaedics and Related Research* 109: 184.

Wirth CJ, Peters G, Milachowski KA, Weismeier KG, Kohn D. (2002) Long-term results of meniscal allograft transplantation. *American Journal of Sports Medicine* 30: 174–181.

Yahia L, Zukor D. (1994) Irradiated meniscal allotransplants of rabbits: study of the mechanical properties at six months post-operation. *Acta Orthop Belg* 60: 210–215.

Yocum LA, Kerlan RK, Jobe FW, Carter VS, Shields CL Jr, Lombardo SJ, Collins HR. (1979) Isolated lateral meniscectomy. A study of twenty-six patients with isolated tears. *Journal of Bone and Joint Surgery* 61A: 338–342.

Yoldas EA, Irrgang J, Fu FH, Harner CD. (1998) Arthroscopically-assisted meniscal transplantation using non-irradiated fresh-frozen menisci. Presented at Annual Meeting of the American Academy of Orthopaedic Surgeons, New Orleans, March 1998.

Zukor D, Brooks P, Gross A. (1988) Meniscal allografts-experimental and clinical study. *Ortho Review* 17: 522.

24

Indications, preservation, and implant techniques for meniscal allograft transplantation

Ewoud van Arkel

Indications

In the past it was recognized that a torn meniscus gives significant clinical symptoms and could cause secondary damage to the articular cartilage. In 1970 Smillie warned of the importance of removing the entire meniscus, because of the danger of leaving behind an unrecognized posterior horn lesion and intrameniscal defects or secondary and possible tertiary bucket handle tears. He also suggested that if total meniscectomy can only be performed by damaging the articular cartilage, the bucket handle fragment should be removed only. In his experience, a meniscus that has regenerated after total meniscectomy takes the same form and appearance as the original structure, although it may be somewhat smaller or thinner.[1]

The standard treatment at the time and for a considerable period after was total meniscectomy. However, the late results after total meniscectomy showed a high incidence of osteoarthritis of the knee. The incidence of osteoarthritis after open meniscectomy varies between 50–70 per cent after 10–20 years.[2, 3] On a radiographic review of patient's x-rays who had a total meniscectomy 10 or more years before, Tapper and Hoover identified the site of the meniscectomy correctly in 85 per cent of the cases. Like Veth, they also noted the discrepancy between the deterioration in radiological appearance and the clinical results over time following total meniscectomy.[4, 5] Their study showed that after medial meniscectomy 80 per cent had a good or excellent clinical result, whereas this was 50 per cent after medial and lateral, and 47 per cent after lateral meniscectomy alone.[4] Other studies have suggested that following menisectomy degeneration is greatest on the lateral rather than medial aspect of the joint. In a recent study, using the Ahlbäck radiological criteria as signs of osteoarthritis, the incidence of narrowing of articular cartilage was 36 per cent at 30 years of follow-up.[6]

Because of the greater role in stress protection of the lateral meniscus compared to the medial meniscus, lateral meniscectomy will show higher incidence of osteoarthritis.[3, 7, 8] After 30 years the clinical results of total medial meniscectomy were best, followed by lateral meniscectomy and worst after both medial and lateral meniscectomy of the same knee.[6]

McGinty et al. showed that partial meniscectomy gave better subjective functional results, better anatomical and radiological results, and less postoperative complications than a total meniscectomy.[9] Cox et al. resected the medial meniscus in dogs' knees and showed that the degenerative changes after meniscectomy were directly proportional to the amount of tissue removed.[10] It is now generally accepted that if meniscectomy is indicated, arthroscopic partial meniscectomy is the treatment of choice.

As a result of the interest in developments in arthroscopic surgery and the science of the meniscus, meniscal-sparing therapy such as partial meniscectomy and meniscal repair could evolve. The indications for meniscal repair are longitudinal lesions within the vascular part of the meniscus. Contraindications include stable longitudinal tears shorter than 1 cm, radial tears, partial thickness tears, degenerative tears and joint instability. Asymptomatic, stable or partial tears of less than 1 cm may heal without surgical intervention or by trephining, alone which stimulates vascular ingress and healing. If meniscal repair is possible in a knee with deficiency of the anterior cruciate ligament (ACL), the repair should be undertaken at the same time with reconstruction of the ACL.[11] Other factors that influence the results of meniscal repairs are the vascularity of the repair site, rim width, tear length and duration of symptoms.[12] Meniscus-related surgical treatment decisions between repair or partial meniscectomy are based on location, extent of the damage, size, stability of the meniscal tear and the activity level of the patient and the acceptability of a longer period of rehabilitation and inactivity associated with a repair rather than partial meniscectomy. Total meniscectomy is reserved for tears for which any other option is not suitable.[13] The subsequent osteoarthritis may prove difficult to treat if the patient is young, active, the ACL is deficient or osteotomy is inappropriate.

If the progression to degeneration and arthritis following menisectomy could be reduced or avoided by meniscus preservation or replacement then this may represent an advantage in certain circumstances. If further meniscal replacement improved the stability in unstable knees then this too would represent an advantage.

For meniscal transplantation to become a recognized and reliable part of the surgical armamentarium it must be safe, predictable, reliable and suitable tissue must be readily available. To achieve this, the meniscal allograft must not only survive without an immunilogical or chemical reaction in the host and heal into the meniscal bed but must also integrate with the knee capsule to perform the biomechanical function of the meniscus in the knee, without an immunologically provoked inflammatory response. It must also replicate the weight-bearing function of the meniscus, and reduce the symptoms experienced whether they be pain, swelling or instability. There is controversy regarding the indications for and applicability of meniscal transplantation with regards to symptoms, age and state of the articular cartilage.

The indication to transplant a meniscus is; Outerbridge grade 1 or 2 articular changes, as determined by the use of a 45° postero-anterior weight-bearing radiograph as described by Rosenberg et al.[14] Although the classification described should possibly be the grade 1 or 2 radiographic changes as described by Fairbank,[2] the study does suggest undertaking meniscal transplantation in the presence of minimal degenerative changes rather than a knee at a later stage in which degeneration has already occurred. It must be remembered that not every patient has the inevitability of pain or osteoarthritis after meniscectomy. It should also be remembered that using this indication of minimal degenerative change, no short-term results are reported in the peer-reviewed literature. Third, there is a discrepancy between the deterioration in radiological appearance and the clinical results after total meniscectomy; the patient's symptomatology must be considered and not every patient develops pain or osteoarthritis after meniscectomy.[4, 5] A fourth point is that although joint contact pressure on articular cartilage is reduced after meniscal replacement, there is no evidence to date either in animal or human studies that meniscal transplantation protects articular cartilage from degeneration.[15–19] Another aspect is that although contact pressure on articular cartilage is reduced after meniscal replacement, and a partial protective effect has been shown after meniscal transplantation, the technique should not be used as a prophylactic procedure to protect articular cartilage (Table 23.1).[15–19] Therefore transplantation, replacement or substitution of the meniscus is not indicated in every menisectomized knee.

The main indication for meniscus transplantation is disabling pain after (sub) total meniscectomy. Ligament instability is also associated with pain and degeneration and any ligament instability should be reconstructed prior to or in combination with meniscal transplantation.[20–22] Because of the predictable and good medium term results of total and uni-compartmental knee arthroplasty it is not logical or appropriate to transplant menisci in a patient over the age of 60 years and possibly over the age of 40. The average age in the series of Cameron and Saha was 41 years with only 11 patients older than twenty years of age.[23] Other studies report a mean age of 32 (range 21–40) years and 41 (range 30–55) years, respectively.[24, 25] In our own study of the preliminary results after two to five years follow-up we reduced the suggested maximum age for this procedure from 55 to 45 years. I believe that, taking the physical demands and physiological age of the patient into consideration, the current upper age limit for this procedure should be no more than 50 years of age.[22] When considering the indication for the procedure on the

Table 24.1 Articular cartilage following meniscal allograft transplantation (MAT)

Author, year	Protection	Species	Follow-up months	Evaluation
Aagaard,[38] 1999, 2002	Partial	Sheep	6	Gross/ histological
Edwards,[15] 1996	No	Sheep	Mean 21	Radiographs
Cummings,[79] 1997	Partial	Rabbit	6	Gross/histological
Szomor,[18] 2000	Partial	Sheep	4	Gross/histological
Mora,[80] 2001 (abs)	Partial	Sheep	6	Histological
Elliott,[81] 2002	No	Dog	3	Gross/histological/ biomechanical

Only experimental studies are reviewed with controlled, systematic measurements. Full protection is defined as MATs same results as controls and better then after meniscectomy. Partial protection is defined as control better results then MATs, and MATs better results then after meniscectomy. No protection is defined as MATs and meniscectomy the same results, both worse then controls. Reprinted with permission of H. Aagaard, 4de ICRS meeting, Toronto 2002.

basis of articular degeneration, one area of controversy is the presence of chondromalacia of Outerbridge grade 4. Goble *et al.* stated that it has been demonstrated in a limited fashion that transplanted menisci will provide relief of pain in properly selected joints of this grade.[26] But in general, patients with chondromalacia grade 4 are considered poor candidates for meniscal transplantation due to the extent of the pre-existing degenerative changes. The arguments are that the allograft is more susceptible to abrasion, entrapment and degeneration due to the subchondral bone exposure, flattening and irregularity of the femoral condyles.

Briefly, in my opinion the current indication for meniscal transplantation is: a patient who is under the age of 45 to 50 years with pain, disabling compartmental osteoarthritis, after (sub) total meniscectomy, in the presence of a normal knee alignment and a stable joint.

Preservation and implantation techniques

Experiments in meniscal reconstruction

Studies to substitute or reconstruct the menisci with a teflon-net, carbon fiber-polyurethane grafts, co-polymeric collagen scaffolds, tendon autografts and fat pads are described in the experimental phase.[27-31] These techniques are based on the phenomenon of creeping substitution. The scaffold forms a meshwork in which vessels and cells penetrate. From the perimeniscal capillary plexus and the vascular fringe vessels will proliferate into the scaffold with mesenchymal cells which will remodel into a new meniscus matrix. The scaffold has the function of a porous meniscal prosthesis. As a meniscal autograft the quadriceps tendon is the only meniscus substitute clinically used, but is still considered experimental.[32]

Prerequisites for the meniscal prosthesis are biocompatibility, e.g. will not give rise to a foreign body reaction, or synovitis due to particle wear. Biogradeble materials should be used. Solubility should be in balance with the growth of new meniscal tissue and it should have the same biomechanical properties as meniscal tissue. The prosthesis should gain the normal contour of a meniscus as soon as possible in order to be congruent to femoral and tibial condyles. And the prosthesis should not give rise to degeneration of the joint.[33] Clinically the effect of the prosthesis should be a decrease in pain, but the concept of a prosthetic meniscal replacement has been abandoned in the experimental phase.

Tissue engineering is a new development in orthopaedic surgery. Because of the limited resources of meniscal allografts, a tissue-engineered meniscus could solve this problem. And if it is possible to engineer a meniscus the potential risk of disease transmission is also eliminated.

Experiments with meniscal transplantations

After total meniscectomy, a meniscal allograft transplantation is an alternative to meniscal replacement. In animals menisci have been transplanted in merino sheep, dogs and goats.[34-38] In humans, meniscal transplantation had been performed with or without additional procedures[23-25, 34, 39, 40] (see Figure 24.1). The results of these meniscal transplantations showed that the transplanted menisci were firmly attached to the knee capsule by fibrovascular tissue, without

Fig. 24.1

A cryopreserved meniscal allograft is transplanted in the knee using an open technique and no bone blocks. Under direct vision all the needles, with the posterior horn first, were pulled through the capsule. Gradually pulling on the sutures puts the allograft in place. Knots are made on the outside of the capsule.

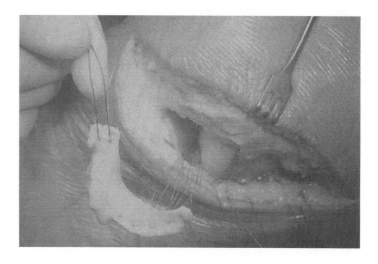

signs of an inflammatory response or rejection.[34-36] Although no cellular and humoral responses to fresh meniscal allografts in mice were found, a minimal lymphocyte invasion into the allogeneic meniscus was observed.[41] Serological HLA typing in humans after meniscal transplantation showed that 11 of 18 recipients became sensitized.[42] Histological evidence of a subtle immune response directed against the allograft was shown, but again this response does not appear to affect the clinical outcome.[43]

This subtle immune response probably evokes the phenomenon of creeping substitution in the meniscal allograft. If creeping substitution takes place than incorporation, revascularization and cellular repopulation of the allograft will take place. Evidence of this phenomenon is given because recipient DNA material has been found in biopsy material of transplanted meniscal allografts.[44, 45] But the statement of Debeer et al. that repopulation is nearly completed one year after transplantation of the allograft seems to be a little too optimistic. This conclusion can be made only after a complete analysis of the allograft and not after analysis of biopsy specimens.

Meniscal transplantation – the donor side

Transplanting allografts includes a potential risk of infectious disease transmission through the meniscal transplant. In blood transfusion it is known that many transfusion-transmissible viruses are found in paid donors at higher rates than in volunteer donors, and patients receiving blood from volunteers have fewer transfusion-transmitted infections.[46] Therefore the United States and Europe converted from paid blood donors to totally voluntary, none-remunerated donor sources for blood donation. The World Health Assembly condemned payment of blood donors as 'exploitation of the poor'. Transplantation of organs, tissue and cells has resulted in transmitting, bacterial, viral and fungal diseases from donor to recipient.[47] Simonds et al. reported a male donor who died 32 hours after a gunshot wound; he had no risk factors for HIV-1 infection and was sero-negative. Of the 48 recipients who obtained tissues and organs from the donor, all four recipients of organs and three recipients of unprocessed fresh-frozen bone were infected with HIV-1.[48] It is generally accepted that after HIV exposure, 95 per cent of the individuals will have HIV antibody at detectable levels by 6 months.[49] Because of this 'window of sero-negativity' re-testing is advised after the window-period of six months.

To prevent or at least minimize the risk of transmission of infectious disease one should only use transplants when needed. The procurement agency should carefully obtain the donor's medical and social history and exclude those suspected to be at risk for HIV, hepatitis, or other viral or bacterial infections.[47] Sterilization of certain tissues can be very effective, although some infectious agents, such as Creutzfeld Jacobs Disease are impervious to sterilization.

Nemsek *et al.* showed that routine processing and removal of bone marrow do not inhibit the ability to transmit viruses like HIV in bone allografts.[50]

The clinical effectiveness of many organs, tissues or cells requires cellular viability. Like meniscal allografts, these grafts are unable to withstand sterilization procedures. Buck *et al.* estimated that the possibility of transplanting a bone allograft from a donor infected with HIV is 1/1667600, provided there is a combination of rigorous donor selection, screening for the HIV antigen and antibody, and histopathological studies of donor tissues. If adequate precautions are not taken the risk might be as high as one in 161.[51] In conclusion, donor selection is an important factor. Donors should meet the criteria of the American Association of Tissue Banks or the standards of the European Association of Tissue Banks and the European Association of Musculo Skeletal Transplantation.

Different banking techniques have been developed. Donor menisci could be banked fresh, frozen, or cryopreserved. Prerequisites for human meniscal allografts are viability of meniscal fibrochondrocytes after preservation and transplantation, and an intact collagen matrix in the long term to maintain the meniscal biomechanical function. Fresh meniscal preservation offers a source of living chondrocytes. A disadvantage of fresh preservation techniques of allografts is that the transplantation has to be performed within 48 hours after procurement, which necessitates an expensive organization, and patients on call.

In frozen meniscal allografts, no considerations are made to preserve cell viability. Storage, preservation and thawing are relatively easy. Transplantation of deep-frozen autografts in dogs showed cellular re-population.[52] However Milachowski *et al.* noted severe shrinkage after deep-frozen meniscal allografts in humans.[34] Although in dogs repopulation of cells was noted a general statement in transplant surgery is that it does not seem to be appropriate to implant organs or tissue of which the cells are for the most part irreversibly damaged. The timespan in which the cellular population of the organ or tissue could be held before the point of no return of irreversible damage, at low temperature and optimal medium, is significant for the possibilities and limitations of a transplantation.[53]

The cryopreservation technique has the advantage of being a source of living cells, and meniscal transplantation could be performed under elective circumstances, without extra overhead costs. As cryopreservent glycerol or dimethylsulphoxide (DSMO) are used.[54, 55] Although cryopreservation and short-term storage do not appear to have an effect on the morphological appearance or the biomechanical character of the meniscus, only a reduced number of the fibrochondrocytes were metabolically active.[36] Ohlendorf *et al.* showed that cryopreservation increased the numbers of surviving cells compared to cell survival in osteochondral allograft without cryopreservation. They also provided evidence that cryopreservation of osteochondral allografts was confined to the cells in the superficial layer of the cartilage.[56]

Meniscal transplantation – technical aspects

When meniscal transplantation is indicated there are some prerequisites:

1 The donor should meet the criteria of the American Association of Tissue Banks or the standards of the European Association of Tissue Banks and the European Association of Musculo Skeletal Transplantation, and procurement should be done accordingly.

2 Sizing the appropriate meniscal allograft should be done by radiograph, MRI or CT. Although the meniscal allograft should be as anatomical as possible to the recipient, it is not clear how important sizing of the meniscal allograft actually is and by which technique sizing is done most accurately. Pollard *et al.* demonstrated a reproducible radiographic relationship between each meniscus and established bony landmarks.[57] Other tissue banks use CT or MRI for sizing the allograft and advise that the recipient should be sized by using the same technique. In a study of 12 cadaver knees which underwent sequential radiographs, MRI and arthrotomy, none of these imaging techniques were sufficiently accurate to measure individual meniscal dimensions. Using less strict criteria for accuracy, within 5 mm, radiography and MRI became more reliable.[58] The latter is certainly better than radiography in predicting the three-dimensional geometry of the meniscus.[59] The most appropriate and practical sizing technique currently is still based upon measurements on bone. In a study in which 16 patients had a meniscal transplantation matched by radiographs, and in which the clinical results were evaluated by MRI and arthroscopy, no mismatch of the size was noted.[19]

3 The mechanical axes provide the description of load transmission through the knee joint. When there is varus or valgus malalignment abnormal stress will occur on the medial or lateral tibial plateau respectively. The rationale for upper tibial osteotomy is to correct the abnormal loading stresses on the knee that are caused by the abnormal mechanical axis in the coronal plane. The excessive load on the medial compartment of the joint in varus deformity is transferred, in a more normal amount, to the lateral compartment, with pain relief as clinical result.[60] When meniscal transplantation is indicated in a knee joint with an abnormal mechanical axis, this malalignment is proposed to cause abnormal pressure on the meniscal allograft resulting in impaired revascularization that will lead to degeneration and loosening of the graft. For that reason a normal mechanical axis

of the knee joint in the coronal plane is advised in meniscal transplantations.

4 It is known that in knee joints with insufficiency of the ACL the menisci are at secondary risk of damage; in time the frequency of meniscal tears increase significantly.[61] In meniscal repair the results show that healing occurs up to 96 per cent in stable knees,[62] and in significantly lower rates in knees with deficiency of the ACL.[63] Because the menisci are secondary stabilizers in knees with a ruptured ACL, the allografts will be at risk in unstable knees. Therefore meniscal allografts should only be transplanted in stable knee joints, or in conjunction with reconstruction of the ACL. The biomechanical interdependence between the ACL and the medial meniscus was confirmed in two recent studies. Both Hollis *et al.* and Papageorgiou *et al.* showed that anterior tibial translation and medial meniscal strain were restored to normal levels after reconstruction of the ACL.[20, 21]

5 How to fix the meniscal allograft? Different techniques have been described to fix the meniscus to the tibial plateau; open or arthroscopic assisted, with or without bone blocks to secure the meniscal horns, and with transosseous sutures and a bone bridge for tying the meniscal horn sutures.[16, 25, 64–66] There is evidence that securing the meniscal horns reduces the contact pressure on the articular cartilage in contrast to meniscal horns that are not secured.[66, 67] Fukubayashi and Kurosawa have shown that there are anatomical and biomechanical differences between the medial and lateral meniscus.[68] Van Arkel and de Boer showed it is not possible to compare the results of lateral and medial meniscal allografts.[22] The best technique to secure the donor meniscus could possibly be different for the lateral and medial allograft.

A second aspect is how to fix the meniscal allograft to the knee capsule. When an open technique is used to implant the allograft absorbable sutures could be passed under direct vision through the capsule. Knots can be made on the outside of the capsule after gradually pulling the meniscal allograft into the joint.[25] Absorbable sutures can also be used if meniscal transplantation is performed arthroscopically assisted with an inside-out or outside-in technique, combined with posterior incisions. The posterior incisions have been documented to greatly reduce the risk of vascular and nerve lesions.[69] For the arthroscopic all-inside technique different absorbable devices have been developed. In a study testing the pull-out strength of vertical and horizontal loop sutures and absorbable arrows was shown that the vertical loop sutures had the highest pull-out strength, followed by the horizontal loop sutures and least for the biogradable meniscal repair devices.[70] Second the costs are in favor of sutures. The special meniscal repair devices are far more expensive than the absorbable sutures. The arthroscopic all-inside technique has device-specific complications, including subcutaneous migration, aseptic synovitis, and chondral lesions because of the biogradable device.[71-74]

6   There is no general accepted and scientifically proved postoperative rehabilitation protocol after meniscal transplantations, but most authors include a period of non-weight-bearing, combined with continuous passive motion, with restricted range of motion, with or without brace, followed by a period of progressive weight-bearing as tolerated. Cycling and swimming is promoted. From 6 to 12 months return to previous activities is recommended, but contact sports are not advised until 12 months postoperatively.[25, 75, 76]

In summary, no deterioration or improvement of articular cartilage after meniscal transplantation was shown, but ingrowth of the allograft to the knee capsule did occur.[25] Clinical results and survival were good for the lateral, intermediate for both in the same knee and poor for the medial allografts. The results in the medial meniscal transplant will improve when instability in the knee is treated at the same time.[22] Only a subtle immune response was found after meniscal transplantation. Recipients of a meniscal allograft can become sensitized, because antibodies against human leucocyte antigens were found after transplantation.[42] This subtle immune response may induce the phenomenon of creeping substitution and incorporation and revascularization of the graft.

There is no specific scoring system to evaluate the meniscus following transplantation. There are only validated scoring systems for ligament reconstruction and prosthesis in the knee joints. To enable comparability of meniscal transplantation studies in the absence of a meniscal scoring system, the clinical evaluation protocol should contain at least the Lysholm, and the International Knee Documentation Score, a visual analogue scale for pain, and a standard and full standing radiographs of the knee joint. Unless sophisticated MRI techniques are used, arthroscopy correlates best to the clinical results.[19] Since meniscectomy is not the only prognostic factor for the development of tibio-femoral osteoarthritis in the knee, it can be useful to add a description of the other factors. The other strong risk factors for tibio-femoral osteoarthritis are obesity, previous knee injury and physical activity, while Heberden's nodes and family history, genetic predisposition, are more closely associated with patello-femoral involvement.[77, 78]

The indications for meniscal transplantation remain imprecise. Although contact pressure on articular cartilage is reduced after meniscal transplantation, there is no evidence in animal and human studies that meniscal transplantation protects articular cartilage from degeneration. Therefore transplantation of a meniscal allograft is not indicated to prevent articular cartilage degeneration after (sub) total meniscectomy, it is not a prophylactic procedure to prevent osteoarthritis. Meniscal transplantation is indicated in a patient under the age of 45 years with pain, disabling compartmental osteoarthritis after (sub) total meniscectomy, normal alignment of the knee and a stable joint.

Interesting areas for further research remain. The specific purpose of further study could be:

1 To assess what causes the HLA-sensitization after meniscal transplantation. Therefore specific analysis (particularly for HLA class 2) to confirm the anti-HLA reactivity is recommended.
2 To assess which fixation technique of meniscal allografts provides the best results. Because the medial meniscus is firmly attached, and the lateral meniscus is more loosely attached to the knee capsule, it could be possible that different fixation techniques are needed for medial and lateral allograft transplantation. Biomechanical studies and dynamic studies in an open MR imaging setting should give the answers.
3 A prospective DNA fingerprinting study should provide the answer if incorporation of the meniscal allograft takes place by the phenomenon of creeping substitution.
4 To assess how important sizing of the allograft is.
5 To investigate if it is possible to culture a meniscus with the same biomechanical properties as a native meniscus with tissue engineering techniques. If this is possible the potential risk of disease transmission is eliminated, and the procurement of allografts facilitated.
6 To develop more accurate methods to assess and document the amount and location of meniscal tissue resected, after the meniscus has been repaired and after meniscal transplantation.
7 A specific scoring system to evaluate the meniscus after meniscectomy, repair and transplantation must be developed.

Current practice, technique and experience

The operative technique for meniscal transplantation has evolved and continues to be progressively modified. Before 1998 menisci were transplanted using an open technique without bone blocks. The allograft was stitched under direct vision to the knee capsule. However since 1998 an arthroscopic assisted technique is used to transplant the meniscus. The procedure starts with an arthroscopy to evaluate the articular cartilage. When there is still a small remnant of the original meniscus this is debrided. At the insertion of the anterior and posterior horn on the tibial plateau two bone tunnels are made using an arthroscopic aiming-device. At the same time on a side table the meniscal allograft is prepared from the donor tibial plateau and sutures are placed in the anterior and posterior horn and in the meniscal area posterior to the medial or lateral collateral ligament (see Figure 24.2).

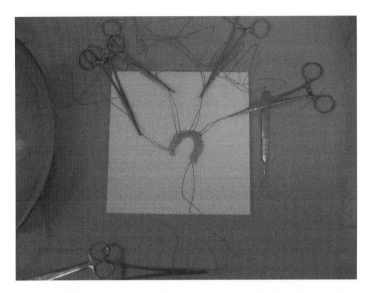

Fig. 24.2
The donor meniscus is prepared on a side table with sutures through the anterior and posterior horn and in the area posterior to the lateral or medial collateral ligament.

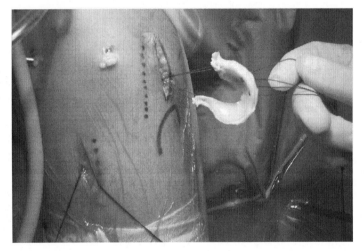

Fig. 24.3
The sutures in the anterior and posterior horn are pulled through the posterior incision and the bone tunnels. Pulling on these sutures brings the allograft into the anatomical position in the knee joint. Under direct vision and protection of the neurovascular structures posterior in the knee, the donor meniscus is stitched, inside-out, to the capsule. Finally, the two sutures of the anterior and posterior horns are knotted over the bone-bridge of the two bone tunnels, bringing the allograft under tension.

When bone tunnels and allograft are prepared a posterior lateral or medial incision is made. The sutures in the anterior and posterior horn are pulled through the posterior incision and the bone tunnels. Pulling on these sutures brings the allograft into the anatomical position in the knee joint. Under direct vision and protection of the neurovascular structures posterior in the knee, the donor meniscus is stitched, inside-out, to the capsule. Finally, the two sutures of the anterior and posterior horns are knotted over the bone bridge of the two bone tunnels, bringing the allograft under tension (see Figure 24.3).

My own experience with the arthroscopic-assisted technique is that admission to the hospital is reduced from a mean of 10 days with the open technique to 4 or 5 days with the arthroscopic technique.

Postoperative pain is less, range of motion (with in the limitation of the first six weeks between 0–90° of extension to flexion) is regained faster, and the scar is smaller.

In the evaluation of the results following meniscal transplantation it has been shown that the Knee Assessment Scoring System (KASS) was not superior to the Lysholm score[22] and in the absence of a specific scoring system form the meniscus, I now use a combination of the Lysholm score, the International Cartilage Repair Society (ICRS) evaluation pack, and a visual analogue scale (VAS) for pain and function. As a patients' outcome score I use the KOOS score. The ICRS evaluation pack includes the IKDC score and a detailed articular cartilage evaluation form. In my opinion the ICRS articular cartilage evaluation form is superior to the Outerbridge criteria, which unfortunately allows intra- and interobserver variation. The ICRS evaluation pack is available and can be downloaded from www.cartilage.org.

References

1. Smillie IS (1970). *Injuries of the Knee*. Edinburgh: Churchill Livingston.
2. Fairbank TJ (1948). Knee joint changes after meniscectomy. *J Bone Joint Surg (Br)*, 30, 664–70.
3. Johnson RJ, Kettelkamp DB, Clark W, Leaverton P (1974). Factors affecting late results after meniscectomy. *Journal of Bone and Joint Surgery (Am)*, 56, 719–29.
4. Tapper EM, Hoover NW (1996). Late results after meniscectomy. *J Bone Joint Surg (Am)*, 51, 517–26.
5. Veth RP (1985). Clinical significance of knee joint changes after meniscectomy. *Clin Orthop*, 198, 56–60.
6. McNicholas MJ, Rowley DI, McGurty D, *et al.* (2000). Total meniscectomy in adolescence, a thirty-year follow-up. *J Bone Joint Surg (Br)*, 82, 217–21.
7. Allen PR, Denham RA, Swan AV (1984). Late degenerative changes after meniscectomy. Factors affecting the knee after operation. *J Bone Joint Surg (Br)*, 66, 666–71.
8. Jorgensen U, Sonne HS, Lauridsen F, Rosenklint A (1987). Long-term follow-up of meniscectomy in athletes. A prospective longitudinal study. *J Bone Joint Surg (Br)*, 69, 80–3.
9. McGinty J, Geuss L, Marvin R (1977). Partial or total meniscectomy. *J Bone Joint Surg (Am)*, 59, 763–6.
10. Cox JS, Nye CE, Scheaffer WW, Woodstein IJ (1975). The degenerative effects of partial and total resection of the medial meniscus in dog's knees. *Clin Orthop*, 109, 178–83.
11. van Trommel MF (1999). Meniscal repair, Thesis University of Leiden; Leiden.
12. DeHaven KE (1999). Meniscus repair. *Am J Sports Med*, 27, 242–50.
13. DeHaven KE (1990). Decision-making factors in the treatment of meniscus lesions. *Clin Orthop*, 252, 49–54.
14. Johnson DL, Neef RL (2000). Meniscal allograft reconstruction: an arthroscopically assisted technique. In Harner CD, Vince KG, Fu FH. *Techniques in Knee Surgery*, pp. 10–22, Philadelphia: Lippincott Williams & Wilkins.
15. Edwards DJ, Whittle SL, Nissen MJ, Cohen B, Oakeshott RD, Keene GCR (1996). Radiographic changes in the knee after meniscal transplantation. *Am J Sports Med*, 24, 222–6.

16. Paletta GA, Manning T, Snell E, Parker R, Bergfeld J (1997). The effect of allograft meniscal replacement on intraarticular contact area and pressure in the human knee, a biomechanical study. *Am J Sports Med*, 25, 692–98.
17. Alhalki MM, Hull ML, Howell SM (2000). Contact mechanics of the medial tibial plateau after implantation of a medial meniscal allograft, a human cadaveric study. *Am J Sports Med*, 28, 370–76.
18. Szomor ZL, Martin TE, Bonar F, Murrell GAC (2000). The protective effect of meniscal transplantation on cartilage. *J Bone Joint Surg (Am)*, 82, 80–8.
19. van Arkel ERA, Goei R, de Ploeg I, de Boer HH (2000). Meniscal allografts: evaluation with magnetic resonance imaging and correlation with arthroscopy. *Arthroscopy*, 16, 517–21.
20. Hollis JM, Pearsall AW, Niciforos PG (2000). Change in meniscal strain with anterior cruciate ligament injury and after reconstruction. *Am J Sports Med*, 28, 700–4.
21. Papageorgiou CD, Gil JE, Kanamori A, Fenwick JA, Woo SLY, Fu FH (2000). The biomechanical interdependence between the anterior cruciate ligament replacement graft and the medial meniscus. *Am J Sports Med*, 29, 226–31.
22. van Arkel ERA, de Boer HH (2002). Survival analysis of human meniscal transplantations. *J Bone Joint Surg (Br)*, 84, 227–31.
23. Cameron J, Saha S (1997). Meniscal allograft transplantation for unicompartmental arthritis of the knee. *Clin. Orthop*, 337, 164–71.
24. Garrett JC, Steensen RN, Stevensen RctSR (1991). Meniscal transplantation in the human knee: a preliminary report [published erratum appears in *Arthroscopy*, 1991;7(2):256]. *Arthroscopy*, 7, 57–62.
25. van Arkel ERA, de Boer HH (1995). Human meniscal transplantation. Preliminary results at 2 to 5-year follow-up. *J Bone Joint Surg (Br)*, 77, 589–95.
26. Goble EM, Kane SM, Wilcox TR, Doucette SA (1996). Meniscal allografts. In: McGinty JB, Caspari RB, Jackson RW, Poehling CG (eds) *Operative Arthroscopy*, pp. 317–31. Lippincott-Raven, Philadelphia.
27. Toyonaga T, Uezaki N, Chikama H (1983). Substitute meniscus of Teflon-net for the knee joint of dogs. *Clin Orthop*, 179, 291–97.
28. Veth RHP, Jansen HWB, Leenslag JW, Pennings AJ, Nielsen HKL (1986). Experimental meniscal lesions reconstructed with a carbon fiber-polyurethane-poly(L-lactide) graft. *Clin Orthop*, 202, 286–93.
29. Stone K, Rodkey W, Webber R, McKinney L, Steadman J (1992). Meniscal regeneration with co-polymeric collagen scaffolds. *In vitro* and *in vivo* studies evaluated clinically, histologically and biochemicaly. *Am J Sports Med*, 20, 104–11.
30. Klompmaker J, Jansen HW, Veth RP, *et al.* (1992) Meniscal repair by fibrocartilage? An experimental study in the dog. *J Orthop Res*, 10, 359–70.
31. Kohn D, Wirth CJ, Reiss G, *et al.* (1992) Medial meniscus replacement by a tendon autograft. Experiments in sheep. *J Bone Joint Surg (Br)*, 74:910–7.
32. Goble EMK, Verdonk R, Kane SM (1999). Meniscal substitutes, human experience. *Scand J Med Sci Sports*, 9, 146–57.
33. Klompmaker J (1992). Porous polymers for repair and replacement of the knee joint meniscus and articular cartilage. Thesis University of Groningen, the Netherlands.
34. Milachowski KA, Weismeier K, Wirth CJ (1989). Homologous meniscus transplantation. Experimental and clinical results. *Int Orthop*, 13, 1–11.

35. Canham W, Stanish W (1986). A study of the biological behavior of the meniscus as a transplant in the medial compartment of a dog's knee. *Am J Sports Med*, 14, 376–9.

36. Arnoczky SP, Warren RF, McDevitt CA (1990). Meniscal replacement using a cryopreserved allograft. An experimental study in the dog. *Clin Orthop*, 252, 121–27.

37. Keating EM, Malinin TI, Belchic G (1988). Meniscal transplantations in goats. In: Orthopaedic Research Society 34th annual meeting, 1–4 February; Atalanta, Georgia.

38. Aagaard H (1998). Meniscal allograft transplantation in sheep. Thesis University of Copenhagen.

39. Zukor DJ, Cameron JC, Brooks PJ, *et al.* (1990). The fate of human meniscal allografts. In Ewing W, (ed.) *Articular Cartilage and Knee Joint Function*, pp. 147–52. Raven Press, New York.

40. Milachowski KA, Weismeier K, Wirth CJ, Kohn D (1990). [Meniscus transplantation and anterior cruciate ligament replacement–results 2–4 years postoperative]. *Sportverletz Sportschaden*, 4, 73–8.

41. Ochi M, Ishida O, Daisaku H, Ikuta Y, Akiyama M (1995). Immune response to fresh meniscal allografts in mice. *J Surg Res*, 58, 478–84.

42. van Arkel ERA, van den Berg-Loonen EM, van Wersch JWJ, de Boer HH (1997). Human leukocyte antigen sensitization after cryopreserved human meniscal transplantations. *Transplantation*, 64, 531–33.

43. Rodeo SA, Seneviratne A, Suzuki K, Felker K, Wickiewicz TL, Warren RF (2000). Histological analysis of human meniscal allografts. *J Bone Joint Surg (Am)*, 82, 1071–82.

44. Jackson DW, Whelan J, Simon TM (1993). Cell survival after transplantation of fresh meniscal allografts. DNA probe analysis in a goat model. *Am J Sports Med*, 21, 540–50.

45. deBeer P, Decoste R, Delvaux S, Bellemans J (2000). DNA analysis of a transplanted cryopreserved meniscal allograft. *Arthroscopy*, 16, 71–5.

46. Eastlund T (1998). The histo-blood group ABO system and tissue transplantation. *Transfusion*, 38, 975–88.

47. Eastlund T (1995). Infectious disease transmission through cell, tissue, and organ transplantation: reducing the risk through donor selection. *Cell Transplantation*, 4, 455–77.

48. Simonds RJ, Holmberg SD, Hurwitz RL, Coleman TR (1992). Transmission of human immunodeficiency virus type 1 from a seronegative organ and tissue donor. *N Engl J Med*, 326, 726–32.

49. Horsburgh CR, Jason J, Longini Jr IM, *et al.* (1989). duration of human immunodeficiency virus infection before detection of antibody. *Lancet*, 1, 637–40.

50. Nemsek JA, Arnoczky SP, Swenson CL (1996). Retroviral transmission in bone allografts, effects of tissue processing. *Clin Orthop*, 324, 275–82.

51. Buck B, Malinin T, Brown M (1989). Bone transplantation and human immunodeficiency virus, an estimate of risk of acquired immunodeficiency syndrome. *Clin Orthop*, 240, 129–36.

52. Arnoczky SP, DiCarlo EF, O'Brien SJ, Warren RF (1992). Cellular repopulation of deep-frozen meniscal autografts: an experimental study in the dog. *Arthroscopy*, 8, 428–36.

53. James J (1988). (The cell within the organism; on life and death). *Ned Tijdschr Geneeskd*, 132, 2348–51.

54. Malinin TI, Martinez OV, Brown MD (1985). Banking of massive osteoarticular and intercalary bone allografts – 12 years' experience. *Clin Orthop*, 187, 44–57.

55. Arnoczky SP, Warren RF, Spivak JM (1988). Meniscal repair using an exogenous fibrin clot. An experimental study in dogs. *J Bone Joint Surg (Am)*, 70, 1209–17.

56. Ohlendorf C, Tomford WW, Mankin HJ (1996). Chondrocyte survival in cryopreserved osteochondral articular cartilage. *J Orthop Res*, 14, 413–16.

57. Pollard ME, Kang Q, Berg EE (1995). Radiographic sizing for meniscal transplantation. *Arthroscopy*, 11, 684–7.

58. Shaffer B, Kennedy S, Klimkiewicz J, Yao L (2000). Preoperative sizing of meniscal allografts in meniscus transplantation. *Am J Sports Med*, 28, 524–33.

59. Haut TL, Hull ML, Howell SM (2000). Use of roentgenography and magnetic resonance imaging to predict meniscal geometry determined with a three-dimensional coordinate digitizing system. *J Orthop Res*, 18, 228–37.

60. Coventry MB (1985). Current concepts review; upper tibial osteotomy for osteoarthritis. *J Bone Joint Surg (Am)*, 67, 1136–40.

61. Keene GC, Bickerstaff D, Rae PJ, Paterson RS (1993). The natural history of meniscal tears in anterior cruciate ligament insufficiency. *Am J Sports Med*, 21, 672–9.

62. Rosenberg T, Scott S, Coward D (1986). Arthroscopic meniscal repair evaluated with repeat arthroscopy. *Arthroscopy*, 2, 14–20.

63. Warren RF (1990). Meniscectomy and repair in the anterior cruciate ligament-deficient patient. *Clin Orthop*, 252, 55–63.

64. Stone KR, Rosenberg T (1993). Surgical technique of meniscal replacement. *Arthroscopy*, 9, 234–7.

65. Shelton WR, Dukes AD (1994). Meniscus replacement with bone anchors: a surgical technique. *Arthroscopy*, 10, 324–7.

66. Chen MI, Branch TP, Hutton WC (1996). Is it important to secure the horns during lateral meniscal transplantation? A cadaveric study. *Arthroscopy*, 12, 174–81.

67. Alhalki MM, Howell SM, Hull ML (1999). How three methods for fixing a medial meniscal autograft affect tibial contact mechanics. *Am J Sports Med*, 27, 320–28.

68. Fukubayashi T, Kurosawa H (1980). The contact area and pressure distribution pattern of the knee. *Acta Orthop. Scan*, 51, 871–79.

69. Dehaven KE (1999). Meniscus repair. *Am J Sports Med*, 27, 242–50,

70. Boenisch UW, Faber KJ, Ciarelli M, Steadman JR, Arnoczky SP (1999). Pull-out strength and stiffness of meniscal repair using absorbable arrows or ti-cron vertical and horizontal loop sutures. *Am J Sports Med*, 27, 626–31.

71. Seil R, Rupp S, Dienst M, Mueller B, Bonkhoff H, Kohn D (2000). Chondral lesions after arthroscopic meniscus repair using meniscal arrows. *Arthroscopy*, 16, 7.

72. Ross G, Gabrill J, McDevitt E (2000). Chondral injury after meniscal repair with biogradable arrows. *Arthroscopy*, 16, 754–56,

73. Ganko A, Engebertsen L (2000). Subcutaneous migration of meniscal arrows after failed meniscus repair; a report of two cases. *Am J Sports Med*, 28, 252–53,

74. Song EK, Lee KB, Yoon TR (2001). Aseptic synovitis after meniscal repair using the biogradable meniscus arrow. *Arthroscopy*, 17, 77–80,

75. Kohn D, Aagaard H, Verdonk R, Dienst M, Seil R (1999). Postoperative follow-up and rehabilitation after meniscus replacement. *Scand J Med Sci Sports*, 9, 177–80.

76. Peters G. Postoperative rehabilitation after meniscal replacement. Personal communications.

77. Cooper C, McAlindon T, Snow S, *et al.* (1994). Mechanical and constitutional risk factors for symptomatic knee osteoarthritis: differences between medial tibialfemoral and patellofemoral disease. *J Rheumatol*, 21, 307–13.

78. Cooper C, Snow S, McAlindon T, *et al.* (2000). Risk factors for the incidence and progression of radiographic knee osteoarthritis. *Arthritis Rheum*, 43, 995–1000.

79. Cummings JF, Mansour JN, Howe Z, Allan DG (1997). Meniscal transplantation and degenerative articular change: an experimental study in the rabbit. *Arthroscopy*, 13, 485–91.

80. Mora G, Alvarez E, Ripalda P, *et al.* (2003). Articular cartilage degeneration after frozen meniscus and achilles tendon allograft transplantation: experimental study in sheep. *Arthroscopy*, 19, 833–41.

81. Elliott DM, Setton LA, Scully SP, *et al.* (2002). Joint degeneration following meniscal allograft transplantation in a canine model: mechanical properties and semiquantitative histology of articular cartilage. *Knee Surgery Sports Traumatol Arthroscopy*, 10, 109–18.

Editor's question:

What is the effect of irradiation of the graft for sterilisation against HIV and other transmittable diseases and is this a viable alternative without a detrimental effect on the mechanical properties of the graft.

Authors answer.

Sterilization procedures can be very effective to minimise the risk of transmission of disease, although some infectious agents, like Creuzfeldt Jacobs Disease, are impervious to sterilizants. Meniscal transplantation requires an intact collagen structure and viable cells of the allograft. Irradiation of the allograft will alter the collagen structure and decrease cell viability. In 1995, Noyes presented at the AAOS meeting in Atlanta his 2 to 5 year results with irradiated meniscal allografts in the human knee. The results showed 44 per cent failure of the transplants, although he used bone plugs and reconstructed the anterior cruciate ligament. Cryopreserved and fresh meniscal allografts show better results. Clearly, irradiation has a detrimental effect on the mechanical proportions of the meniscal allograft.

To prevent or minimize the risk of HIV, donor selection should be done rigorously, combined with screening for HIV antigen and antibody, and histopathological studies of donor tissue. The possibility of transmitting a bone (not a meniscal allograft, which contains less to no bone marrow derived cells) allograft from a donor infected with HIV is 1/1667600. If adequate precautions are not taken the risk might be as high as one in 161.

25

Microfracture arthroplasty is an effective means to treat full thickness cartilage lesions of the knee

J. Richard Steadman, William G. Rodkey, and
Karen K. Briggs

Introduction

Full thickness articular cartilage defects rarely heal without surgical intervention (Blevins *et al.* 1998; Brittberg *et al.* 1994; Buckwalter 1998; Cohen *et al.* 1998; Rodrigo *et al.* 1994; Singleton *et al.* 1995; Steadman *et al.* 2001a, 1997, 2001b; Urrea and Silliman 1995; Walker 1998). Thus, attempts at cartilage repair must focus on either enhancing an individual's own capacity for healing or upon whole tissue reconstruction of the articular cartilage surface. Although some patients with full thickness chondral defects may not be symptomatic, most affected individuals will eventually develop degenerative changes that are often irrevocably debilitating (Buckwalter 1998; Cohen *et al.* 1998; Walker 1998). Various cartilage repair techniques have been described, and include abrasion, drilling, osteochondral autograft transplantation, osteochondral allograft transplantation, and autologous cell transplantation (Blevins *et al.* 1998; Brittberg *et al.* 1994; Buckwalter 1998; Frisbie *et al.* 1999; Johnson 1990). The senior author (JRS) developed 'microfracture arthroplasty' to enhance chondral resurfacing by providing a suitable environment for the formation of reparative cartilage tissue by stimulating the body's own healing potential (Blevins *et al.* 1998; Frisbie *et al.* 1999; Rodrigo *et al.* 1994; Steadman *et al.* 2001a, 1997, 1999, 2001b). Essentially, the microfracture technique facilitates the recruitment of marrow-based mesenchymal stem cells to the area of cartilage loss. The pluripotential characteristics of theses cells is believed to enhance the likelihood of successful cartilage repair compared to those circumstances where the subchondral plate is not violated during cartilage injury. The senior author's clinical experience now includes more than 2500 patients in whom microfracture has been done. It is our contention that in the majority of patients with symptomatic, full thickness, articular cartilage lesions of the knee, microfracture arthroplasty is a safe and effective method of treating these difficult lesions.

Indications for microfracture arthroplasty

In the acute setting, active patients with symptomatic chondral lesions are usually offered surgical treatment if there are no specific contraindications as described. Typically, for at least 12 weeks after a suspected chronic or degenerative chondral lesion is diagnosed clinically, patients are treated nonoperatively. Conservative treatment includes activity modification, physical therapy, the use of nonsteroidal anti-inflammatory drugs, braces, joint injections, and perhaps dietary supplements (i.e. glucosamine sulfate, chondroitin sulfate). It is during this period of patient observation that we ascertain a given individual's suitability for operative cartilage repair. When nonoperative treatment does not yield a successful outcome, surgical treatment is offered as an alternative (Blevins *et al.* 1998; Rodrigo *et al.* 1994; Steadman *et al.* 2001a, 1997, 1999, 2001b).

Microfracture arthroplasty was conceived initially for patients with posttraumatic articular cartilage lesions of the knee that had progressed to symptomatic full thickness chondral defects. Microfracture arthroplasty is most commonly indicated for full thickness loss of articular cartilage in either the weight-bearing areas of the tibial or femoral condyles, patella, and trochlear surfaces (Blevins *et al.* 1998; Rodrigo *et al.* 1994; Steadman *et al.* 2001a, 1997, 1999, 2001b). Microfracture may also be indicated in circumstances where unstable cartilage flaps overlie the subchondral bone. In addition, microfracture arthroplasty can also be applied to those patients with degenerative joint disease in a knee that has normal axial alignment. All of these lesions involve loss of articular cartilage at the bone-cartilage interface. We believe that it is the creation of a stable cartilage rim, around the chondral lesion, that has a direct impact upon the success of the microfracture technique. Thus, even in cases of chronic knee articular cartilage degeneration, the clinician can surgically manipulate a given lesion site (i.e. create a stable cartilage rim) and enhance the likelihood of success following application of the microfracture method. For acute lesions, we place no restrictions on lesion size because we have observed excellent results in the treatment of very large lesions (i.e. greater than 400 mm^2). However we stress that surgeons must consider the quality of the cartilage surrounding a given lesion, the presence of global knee arthritis, and axial knee alignment in indicating patients for microfracture repair. For instance, symptomatic chondral lesions of the medial femoral condyle will not likely improve clinically following any type of cartilage repair procedure, in an excessively varus knee. Thus, the surgeon must consider lesion etiology and knee alignment to ensure long-term clinical success following microfracture, and other types of cartilage repair.

General considerations for use of microfracture arthroplasty include patient age, knee alignment, patient activity level, and patient expectation (Steadman *et al.* 2001a, 2001b). We will typically consider the use of microfracture arthroplasty in active patients within the first six decades of life. As the postoperative regimen is crucial to clinical success, patients must understand and submit to the rehabilitation protocol.

Microfracture arthroplasty general contraindications

Contraindications for microfracture arthroplasty include the following:

1　Tri-compartmental knee arthritis
2　Abnormal axial malalignment of the knee
3　Patients unwilling or unable to follow the required rehabilitation protocol
4　Partial thickness cartilage defects
5　An inability to use the opposite leg for weight-bearing
6　Systemic immune-mediated disease
7　Systemic arthritis (i.e. rheumatoid arthritis)
8　Age older than 65 years (relative contraindication)
9　Lesions with excessive bone loss.

The age contraindication might be reconsidered if the patient meets all the other criteria. However, we urge caution in these circumstances as the authors have observed that some older patients experience difficulty with crutch walking and the overall rehabilitation protocol (Steadman *et al.* 2001a). In addition, it is possible that the healing response, in the older patients, may be compromised; this fact may adversely affect the clinical outcome following microfracture arthroplasty. We would not consider a patient for microfracture arthroplasty in the presence of global degenerative osteoarthrosis or if the cartilage surrounding the lesion is too thin to establish the perpendicular cartilage rim that is necessary to hold the post-microfracture clot within the lesion. Such a scenario is common in patients with symptomatic cartilage lesions in the affected compartment of a malaligned knee.

We routinely use two methods for radiographic measurement of the knee alignment: the tibio-femoral angle on a standing anterorposterior (AP) view, and the weight-bearing mechanical axis drawn from the center of the femoral head to the center of the tibiotarsal joint on long standing (~51′/130 cm) radiographs. If the tibio-femoral angle is greater than 5° of varus or valgus compared to the normal knee, we consider this to represent axial knee malalignment. Preferably the weight-bearing line should be in the central quarter of the tibial plateau of either the medial or lateral compartment. If the mechanical axis weight-bearing line falls outside the most central quarter of the plateau, either medially or laterally, we consider this to be a contraindication if left uncorrected. In cases of knee malalignment, a realignment procedure (i.e. high tibial osteotomy) should be combined with the microfracture cartilage repair procedure.

Preoperative planning

Patients who present with knee joint pain undergo a thorough physical and orthopaedic examination. The physical diagnosis often can be difficult and elusive, especially in cases of isolated chondral defects. Point tenderness over a femoral condyle or tibial plateau may be indicative of such a lesion, but cannot be considered diagnostic. We believe that imaging modalities are critical for these cases. As mentioned, we recommend the use long standing radiographs to observe angular deformity and to assess joint space narrowing. We also obtain standard AP and lateral radiographs of both knees as well weight-bearing views with the knees flexed to 30° to 45°. Patellar views are useful to evaluate the patellofemoral joint. However, the most important imaging modality in the treatment of symptomatic cartilage lesion is MRI. Magnetic resonance imaging, using cartilage-specific sequencing, has become our primary method of definitive diagnosis of patients with suspected chondral lesions. These images give an accurate assessment of lesion location, size, and depth, and greatly enhance our ability to develop a preoperative plan.

Surgical technique

Three portals are routinely made about the knee for the microfracture technique; a tourniquet is typically not necessary. Following the intraarticular diagnostic examination, we perform all other intraarticular procedures prior to microfracture arthroplasty. This routine helps prevent loss of visualization that is associated with penetration of the subchondral bone (e.g. fat droplets and blood enter the knee from the microfracture holes). We also pay particular attention to soft tissues such as medial plicae and the lateral retinaculum as the presence of tight or abnormal structure in these areas may adversely affect knee cartilage by producing increased compression between cartilage surfaces (Steadman et al. 2001a, 1997, 1999, 2001b).

After carefully assessing the full thickness articular cartilage lesion, the exposed bone is debrided of all unstable cartilage. We use a handheld curved curette and a full radius resector to create a stable cartilage rim. Our experience indicates that it is critical to debride all loose or marginally attached cartilage from the surrounding rim of the lesion. The calcified cartilage layer that is often present just superficial to the subchondral bone must be removed; a curette is used for this portion of the procedure (Figure 25.1). Complete removal of this calcified cartilage layer is extremely important based on animal studies that we have completed (Frisbie et al. 1999). Care

Fig. 25.1

The calcified cartilage layer of a full thickness chondral defect is being removed with a hand-held curette.

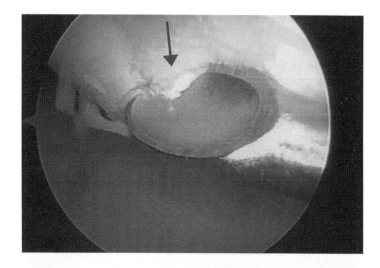

Fig. 25.2

A full thickness chondral defect on the condyle of a femur has undergone debridement prior to microfracture arthroplasty. A stable perpendicular edge of healthy cartilage (larger arrow) has been formed after removal of the damaged cartilage. The smaller arrow points to a small area of petechial hemorrhage which indicates that the curettage has completely removed the calcified cartilage layer.

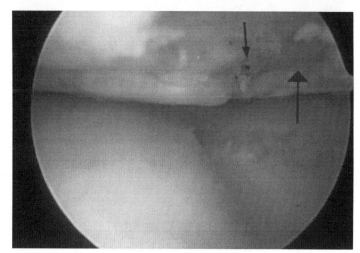

should be taken to maintain the integrity of the subchondral plate by not penetrating too deeply with the curette. Following lesion preparation, a stable perpendicular edge of healthy cartilage should surround the defect such that a firm crater has been formed that will hold the marrow clot, 'super clot' as we have termed it, as it forms (Figure 25.2).

When the lesion has been adequately prepared, we then use an arthroscopic awl to make multiple holes, or 'microfractures,' in the exposed subchondral bone plate. We use an awl with an angle that permits the tip to be perpendicular to the bone as it is advanced, typically 30° or 45°. There also is a 90° awl that should be used only on the patella or other soft bone. The 90° awl should be advanced manually, we do not use a mallet with this particular awl. The holes are made as close together as possible, but not so close that one breaks into another. This technique usually results in microfracture holes that are approximately 3 to 4 mm apart. When fat droplets can be seen coming from the marrow cavity, the appropriate depth of penetration (~2 to 4 mm) has been reached. Unlike drilling, the awls produce no thermal necrosis of the bone; we believe this is a critical characteristic of the microfracture method that makes it a more desirable option than earlier described drilling techniques. We make microfracture holes around the periphery of the defect first, immediately adjacent to the healthy stable cartilage rim (Figure 25.3). The process is completed by making the microfracture holes toward the center of the lesion (Figure 25.4). The microfracture arthroplasty is assessed to assure that a sufficient number of holes have been made. When the arthroscopic pump pressure is reduced we

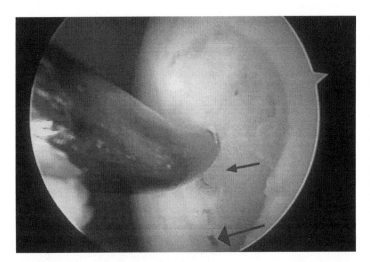

Fig. 25.3
After careful preparation and thorough debridement, a chondral defect is undergoing microfracture arthroplasty. The microfracture holes are started at the periphery of the defect adjacent to the stable cartilage (larger arrow). The smaller arrow points to a fat droplet as it is released from the marrow cavity, thus indicating adequate depth of penetration by the microfracture awl.

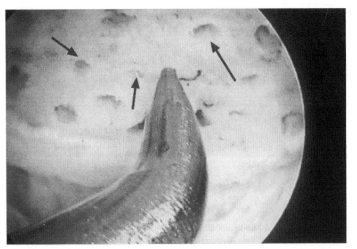

Fig. 25.4
From the periphery, the microfracture arthroplasty is continued into the central portion of the lesion (arrows). The microfracture awl is penetrating the subchondral bone approximately 2 to 4 mm in depth.

Fig. 25.5

Blood and fat droplets
(arrows) from the marrow
cavity can be seen coming
from essentially all of the
microfracture arthroplasty
holes after the arthroscopic
irrigation fluid pressure
has been reduced.

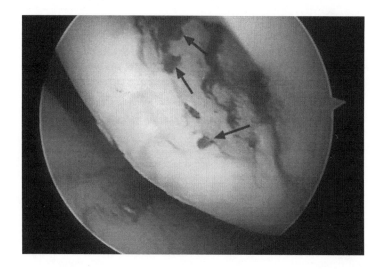

observe the release of marrow fat droplets and blood from the
microfracture holes under direct visualization. We assume that the
quantity of marrow contents flowing into the joint is adequate if we
observe blood and fat droplets emanating from all microfracture
holes (Figure 25.5). We then remove all instruments from the knee
and evacuate the joint of fluid. Intraarticular drains should not be
used because the goal is for the surgically induced marrow clot rich
in marrow elements to form and to stabilize while covering the
lesion.

Chronic degenerative chondral lesions commonly have extensive
sclerotic bone with thickening of the subchondral plate (Johnson
1990). The presence of these bony changes makes it difficult to do
an adequate microfracture procedure. In these instances, we first
make a few microfracture holes with the awls in various locations of
the lesion to assess the thickness of the subchondral plate. It may be
necessary to use a motorized burr to remove the sclerotic bone until
punctate bleeding is seen. After the bleeding appears uniformly over
the surface of the lesion, microfracture arthroplasty can be performed as previously described. In our hands, use of this technique,
in patients with chronic chondral lesions, has yielded good results.
However, if the surrounding cartilage is too thin to establish a perpendicular cartilage rim we would not recommend a microfracture
procedure.

The microfracture awl produces a roughened surface in the
subchondral bone to which the marrow clot can adhere more easily,
yet the integrity of the subchondral plate is maintained which preserves the joint surface shape. We believe that this procedure is vastly
superior to drilling. The microfracture arthroplasty method virtually
eliminates the possibility of local thermal necrosis that is associated
with drilling. Furthermore, the different angles of arthroscopic awls
available provide easy access to difficult-to-reach areas of the knee.

The awls provide not only perpendicular holes but also improved control of depth penetration compared to drilling. We believe that the key to the entire procedure is to establish the marrow clot to provide the optimal environment for the body's own pluripotential marrow cells to differentiate into stable tissue within the lesion. Moreover, the microfracture technique preserves the arthroscopic approach while allowing access to essentially the entire intraarticular space.

Postoperative management

We have designed the postoperative program to promote the ideal physical environment in which newly recruited marrow-based mesenchymal stem cells can differentiate into the appropriate artic- ular cartilage-like cell lines (Hagerman *et al.* 1995). These differen- tiation and maturation processes must be allowed to occur slowly but consistently (Hagerman *et al.* 1995; Irrgang and Pezzullo 1998). Animal studies have confirmed that both cellular and molecular changes are an essential part of the development of a durable repair tissue (Frisbie *et al.* 1999). The postoperative rehabilitation protocol is based upon facilitating the cartilage repair process. Our patients are counseled carefully so they understand that they likely will not start to experience improvement in their knees for at least six months after microfracture. Our experience and clinical research data indicate that improvement can be expected to occur slowly and steadily for at least two years (Blevins *et al.* 1998; Rodrigo *et al.* 1994; Steadman *et al.* 2001a). During this protracted period, the repair tis- sue matures, pain and swelling resolve, and the patients regain con- fidence and comfort in their knees during increased levels of activity.

Rehabilitation

The rehabilitation program after microfracture for treatment of chon- dral defects in the knee is crucial to optimize the results of the surgery (Hagerman *et al.* 1995; Irrgang and Pezzullo 1998). The rehabilitation promotes the optimal physical environment for the mesenchymal stem cells to differentiate and produce new extracellular matrix that eventually matures into a durable repair tissue. The postoperative rehabilitation program after microfracture arthroplasty requires consideration of several factors (Hagerman *et al.* 1995). The specific protocol recommended depends on both the anatomic location and defect size. Two different rehabilitation protocols are applied.

Protocol for lesions on the femoral condyle or tibial plateau

After microfracture of lesions on the weight-bearing surfaces of the femoral condyles or tibial plateaus, continuous passive motion (CPM) is started immediately in the recovery room. The initial range of motion (ROM) typically is 30°–70°, and then it is increased as tolerated by 10°–20° until full passive ROM is achieved. The rate of the machine is usually one cycle per minute, but the rate can be varied based on patient preference and comfort. Many patients tolerate use of the machine at night. For those who do not, we have observed empirically that intermittent use is sufficient. Regardless of when the CPM machine is used, the goal is to have the patient in the CPM machine for 6 to 8 hours every 24 hours. If the patient is unable to use the CPM machine, then instructions are given for passive flexion and extension of the knee with 500 repetitions three times per day. We encourage patients to gain full passive ROM of the injured knee as soon as possible after surgery. We also prescribe cold therapy for all patients postoperatively. We have observed that the cold helps control pain and inflammation, and most patients state that the cold provides overall postoperative discomfort relief. Cold therapy usually is used for 1–7 days postoperatively (Ohkoshi et al. 1999).

We prescribe crutch-assisted touchdown weight-bearing ambulation for 6 to 8 weeks, depending on the size of the lesion. However, for patients with small lesions (<1 cm diameter), weight-bearing may be advanced between 4–6 weeks. Patients with lesions on the femoral condyles or tibial plateaus rarely use a brace during the initial postoperative period. However, we now prescribe a unicompartmental unloader knee brace when the patient becomes more active in the postoperative period.

We instruct patients to begin limited strength training immediately after surgery. Patients do double leg one-third knee bends the day after surgery (Hagerman et al. 1995). Because they are touchdown weight-bearing, patients place most (75–80 per cent) of their body weight on their uninjured leg during this exercise. Patients may begin stationary biking without resistance and a deep water exercise program at 1–2 weeks postoperatively. The deep water exercises include use of a kick board and a flotation vest for water-based running. Patients progress to full weight-bearing after eight weeks, and begin a more vigorous program of active motion of the knee. Elastic resistance cord exercises are started at approximately eight weeks after microfracture arthroplasty. Our observations indicate that the ability to achieve predetermined maximum levels for sets and repetitions of elastic resistance cord exercises is an excellent indicator for progressing to weight training. We permit free or machine weights when the patient has achieved the early goals of the rehabilitation program, but not before 16 weeks after microfracture arthroplasty. We strongly emphasize the importance of proper technique when beginning a weight program. Depending on the clinical examination, we usually recommend that patients do not return to sports that involve pivoting, cutting, and jumping until at least 4–6 months after microfracture arthroplasty.

Rehabilitation protocol for patients with patellofemoral lesions

We emphasize that all patients treated by microfracture arthroplasty for patellofemoral lesions must use a long leg brace set at 0°–20° for at least eight weeks. The brace limits compression of the regenerating surfaces of the trochlea or patella, or both. We allow passive motion with the brace removed, but otherwise the brace must be worn at all times. Patients with patellofemoral lesions are placed into a CPM machine immediately postoperatively. We also use cold therapy as described above. With this regimen patients typically obtain a pain free and full passive ROM soon after surgery. For patients with patellofemoral joint lesions, we carefully observe joint angles at the time of arthroscopy to determine where the defect comes into contact with the patellar facet or the trochlear groove. We make certain to avoid these areas during strength training for approximately four months. This avoidance allows for training in the 0°–20° range immediately postoperatively because there is minimal compression of these chondral surfaces with such limited motion.

Patients with lesions of the patellofemoral joint treated by microfracture arthroplasty are allowed weight-bearing as tolerated at knee flexion where the treated lesion is not compressed. We routinely lock the brace between 0°–20° ROM to prevent flexion past the point where the median ridge of the patella engages the trochlear groove. After eight weeks, we open the knee brace gradually before it is discontinued. When the brace is discontinued, patients are allowed to advance their strength training progressively.

Potential complications from microfracture arthroplasty

Most patients progress through the postoperative period with little or no difficulty (Steadman *et al.* 2001a, 2001b). However, some patients present with mild transient pain, most frequently after microfracture arthroplasty in the patellofemoral joint. Small changes in the articular surface of the patellofemoral joint may be detected by a grating or 'gritty' sensation of the joint, especially when a patient discontinues use of the knee brace and begins normal weight-bearing through a full ROM. Patients rarely complain of pain at this time, and this grating sensation usually resolves spontaneously in a few days or weeks. Similarly, if a steep perpendicular rim was made in the trochlear groove, patients may notice 'catching' or 'locking' as the apex of the patella rides over this lesion during joint motion. Some patients may even perceive these symptoms while in the CPM machine. These symptoms usually dissipate within three months. If this perceived locking is painful, then the patient is advised to limit weight-bearing and avoid the symptomatic joint angle for an additional period. Swelling and joint effusion typically resolve within eight weeks after microfracture arthroplasty. Occasionally, a recurrent effusion develops between six and eight weeks after microfracture, usually when a patient begins to bear weight on the injured leg after microfracture arthroplasty of a defect on the femoral condyle. While this effusion may mimic the preoperative or immediate postoperative effusion, usually it is painless. We treat this type of painless effusion conservatively. It usually resolves within several weeks after onset. Rarely has a second arthroscopy been required for recurring effusions.

Microfracture arthroplasty outcomes results

We recently reported the outcomes results for 233 patients who underwent microfracture arthroplasty for full thickness chondral defects (Steadman *et al.* 2001b). These patients had a minimum two year follow-up after microfracture arthroplasty (range of 2–12 years). The time from injury to microfracture ranged from one day to ten years. Chronic patients had failed nonoperative (conservative) therapy for greater than 12 weeks. Acute patients were treated surgically within 12 weeks of chondral injury. All patients completed a detailed questionnaire preoperatively then annually following microfracture arthroplasty; most patients returned for at least one annual objective clinical examination. There were no complications directly related to microfracture arthroplasty. There was statistically significant ($P < 0.05$) improvement in all outcomes variables at each postoperative year compared to the preoperative knee condition. For example, at three years following microfracture, pain had improved for 75 per cent of patients, remained unchanged for 19 per cent, and worsened for 6 per cent. Improvements were also noted in strenuous work tolerance (66 per cent), strenuous sports participation (59 per cent), and during the execution of daily living activities (68 per cent). Virtually identical improvement rates continued through eight years with no indication of deterioration (Steadman *et al.* 2001b).

A Kaplan-Meier survivorship analysis revealed 95 per cent survival (no additional operative treatment for the same lesion) at four years and 92 per cent at seven years (Figure 25.6). Twelve of the 233 patients experienced failure following microfracture arthroplasty. These twelve patients required further operative interventions (total knee replacement [4], knee osteotomy [3], and repeat microfracture arthroplasty [5]). Further analysis of these failures revealed that negative indicators for success included preoperative joint space narrowing, age greater than 30 years, the presence of chronic cartilage lesions, and poor compliance with the use postoperative continuous passive motion therapy (Steadman *et al.* 2001b).

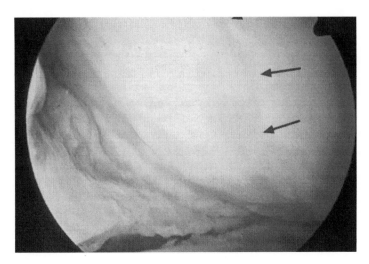

Fig. 25.6
The arrows identify the interface between microfracture repair tissue and normal articular cartilage on the femoral condyle of a large lesion that had undergone microfracture arthroplasty more than five years prior to the time of this photograph.

Conclusions

We conclude that arthroscopic microfracture arthroplasty of sub-chondral bone is safe and effective to treat full thickness chondral defects of the knee in clinical patients, both acute and chronic. Microfracture arthroplasty significantly improves functional outcomes and decreases pain in the majority of patients treated. This repair tissue appears tough and durable, yet it is smooth enough to function similar to normal articular cartilage in clinical patients. We believe that microfracture arthroplasty should be considered the initial treatment of choice for full thickness articular cartilage defects rather than more extensive procedures.

References

Blevins FT, Steadman JR, Rodrigo JJ, Silliman J (1998). Treatment of articular cartilage defects in athletes: An analysis of functional outcome and lesion appearance. *Orthopedics*, 21, 761–768.

Brittberg M, Lindahl A, Nilsson A, Ohlson C, Isakson O, Peterson L (1994). Treatment of deep cartilage defects in the knee with autologous chondrocyte transplantation. *New England Journal of Medicine*, 331, 889–895.

Buckwalter JA (1998). Articular cartilage: Injuries and potential for healing. *Journal of Orthopaedic and Sports Physical Therapy*, 28, 192–202.

Cohen NP, Foster RJ, Mow VC (1998). Composition and dynamics of articular cartilage: Structure, function, and maintaining healthy state. *Journal of Orthopaedic and Sports Physical Therapy*, 28, 203–215.

Frisbie DD, Trotter GW, Powers BE, *et al.* (1999). Arthroscopic subchondral bone plate microfracture technique augments healing of large osteochondral defects in the radial carpal bone and medial femoral condyle of horses. *Journal of Veterinary Surgery*, 28, 242–255.

Hagerman GR, Atkins JA, Dillman C (1995). Rehabilitation of chondral injuries and chronic degenerative arthritis of the knee in the athlete. *Operative Techniques in Sports Medicine*, 3, 127–135.

Irrgang JJ, Pezzullo D (1998). Rehabilitation following surgical procedures to address articular cartilage lesions of the knee. *Journal of Orthopaedic and Sports Physical Therapy*, 28, 232–240.

Johnson LL (1990). The sclerotic lesion: Pathology and the clinical response to arthroscopic abrasion arthroplasty. In JW Ewing (ed.) *Articular Cartilage and Knee Joint Function: Basic science and arthroscopy*, pp. 319–333. Raven Press, New York.

Ohkoshi Y, Ohkoshi M, Nagasaki S, Ono A, Hashimoto T, Yamane S (1999). The effect of cryotherapy on intraarticular temperature and postoperative care after anterior cruciate ligament reconstruction. *American Journal of Sports Medicine*, 27, 357–362.

Rodrigo JJ, Steadman JR, Silliman JF, Fulstone AH (1994). Improvement of full-thickness chondral defect healing in the human knee after debridement and microfracture using continuous passive motion. *American Journal of Knee Surgery*, 7, 109–116.

Singleton SB, Silliman JF (1995). Acute chondral injuries of the patellofemoral joint. *Operative Techniques in Sports Medicine*, 3, 96–103.

Steadman JR, Rodkey WG, Rodrigo JJ (2001a). 'Microfracture': Surgical technique and rehabilitation to treat chondral defects. *Clinical Orthopaedics and Related Research*, 391S, S362–S369.

Steadman JR, Rodkey WG, Singleton SB, Briggs KK (1997). Microfracture technique for full-thickness chondral defects: technique and clinical results. *Operative Techniques in Orthopaedics*, 7, 300–304.

Steadman JR, Rodkey WG, Singleton SB, Briggs KK, Rodrigo JJ, McIlwraith CW (1999). Microfracture procedure for treatment of full-thickness chondral defects: Technique, clinical results and current basic science status. In: CD Harner, KG Vince, FH Fu (eds) *Techniques in Knee Surgery*, pp. 23–31. Williams & Wilkins, Media, PA.

Steadman JR, Rodrigo JJ, Briggs KK, Rodkey WG, Silliman J, Sink E (2001b). Debridement and microfracture ('Pick Technique') for full-thickness articular cartilage defects. In JN Insall, WN Scott (eds) *Surgery of the Knee*, 3rd edn, pp. 361–373. Churchill Livingstone, New York.

Urrea LH, Silliman JF (1995). Acute chondral injuries to the femoral condyles. *Operative Techniques in Sports Medicine*, 3, 104–111.

Walker JM (1998). Pathomechanics and classification of cartilage lesions, facilitation of repair. *Journal of Orthopaedic and Sports Physical Therapy*, 28, 216–231.

Autologous chondrocyte transplantation can effectively treat most articular cartilage lesions of the knee?

Mats Brittberg and Lars Peterson

Introduction

Articular cartilage trauma is extremely common, and, until recently, methods for treatment of the cartilaginous lesions did not produce good long-term results. A better understanding of how articular cartilage responds to injury has produced various techniques that hold promise for long-term success. Among such techniques is autologous chondrocyte transplantation, in which a patient's own cartilage cells are harvested, expanded *in vitro* and reimplanted in a full-thickness articular surface defect (Brittberg *et al.* 1994). Results are available with up to 11 years' follow-up, and more than 80 per cent of the patients have shown improvement with relatively few complications (Peterson *et al.* 2002).

The fact that the damaged articular cartilage appears to have little ability to regenerate functional tissue has led to attempts at transplanting cells of various types into chondral defects. Clinical works have included autologous rib perichondrium cells, autologous periosteum, and, more recently, autologous chondrocytes. What are the facts to support the use of chondrocytes to repair cartilage defects? Pros and cons regarding the use of chondrocytes are discussed in this chapter.

The problem

In contrast to other mesenchymal tissues which all are vascularized, articular cartilage has a very low capacity for repair. Following damage to the articular surface, the chondrocytes, unable to migrate into the injured area, will increase their mitotic activity and their production of extracellular matrix components such as collagen and proteoglycan. However, this response is transient, is not sustained and is insufficient for an adequate repair (Mankin 1982). The primary factors limiting the repair potential of articular cartilage are the lack of blood vessels in the cartilage and a low concentration of cell within the extracellular matrix.

Several research centers have attempted to improve the repair of articular cartilage defects through implantation of chondrocytes or other cells or tissues with chondrogenic potential (Goldberg and Caplan 1994, Caplan *et al.* 1997). In 1984, Peterson *et al.* introduced a method of cartilage repair based on supplementing the local cell population in cartilage defects using cultured autologous articular chondrocytes (Peterson *et al.* 1984, Grande *et al.* 1989, Brittberg *et al.* 1994). The method, autologous chondrocyte transplantation (ACT), was introduced in humans in 1987 and is the first method of orthopedic tissue repair based on cells that have been biologically manipulated *ex vivo*.

Autologous chondrocyte transplantation

The primary goal of *in vitro* cell manipulation in ACT is to increase the number of cells. Chondrocytes are isolated from a small amount of tissue harvested from a minor weight-bearing area. The extra cellular matrix is removed by enzymatic digestion and the cells are expanded in monolayer culture (Figure 26.1).

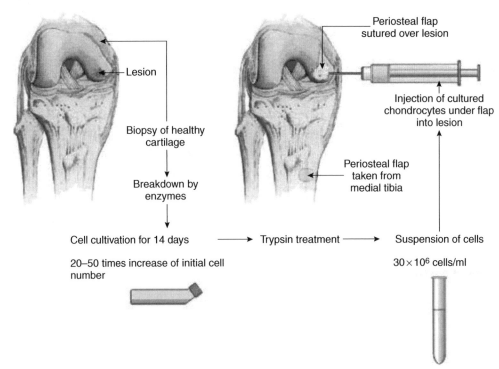

Fig. 26.1

Schematic drawing of the autologous chondrocyte transplantation techniques. Courtesy of Lars Peterson and Per Rehnström.

Once a suitable number of cells are produced, the increased numbers of chondrocytes are suspended in the culture medium and implanted into the area of cartilage defect using a periosteal patch over the defect as a method of cell containment. In order for articular surface restoration to occur, the manipulated chondrocytes must attach to the walls of the defect and revert to the normal chondrocytic phenotype.

The first patient was operated with this technology in 1987. It was the first time that a patients own cells *in vitro* expanded were used to repair a mesenchymal tissue injury. Much discussion and questions about the methodology rose during the years that have passed since that first step of biomedical surgery.

Survey of the published clinical related research

The first clinical result from patients who had been operated on with chondocyte transplantation under a flap of periosteum was presented by Brittberg *et al.* in 1994. Twenty-three patients (mean age 27) who had all local deep cartilage injuries that had been treated with conventional methods without any healing were followed for mean four years. The technique appeared to be most successful in patients who had injuries on the femoral surfaces producing a single, localized deep cartilage lesion compared with the patella patients that were less successful. This is important to note as opposed to the gradual wear and tear of advancing age. The disappointing outcome of the patella group might partly have resulted from mechanical malalignment of the patella that was not corrected at the time of transplant surgery.

A new re-examination was presented by Lars Peterson in 1998 on 219 patients with a follow-up between 2–10 years (Peterson 1998). There was a high percentage of good to excellent results in patients with single femoral condyle lesions (90 per cent of 57 patients) and in patients with osteochondritis dissecans (84 per cent of 32 patients) whereas 74 per cent of patients gained good or excellent results with femoral condyle lesions and a concomitant reconstruction of an anterior cruciate ligament injury (27 patients). Sixty nine per cent of thirty-two patients in whom patellar articular lesions were grafted improved, whilst 58 per cent of 12 patients with lesions on the femoral trochlea improved. ACT gratfing in cases where there were multiple lesions showed a 75 per cent chance of improvement (75 per cent of 53 patients). This multiple site ACT surgery is considered a salvage procedure; thus a 75 per cent change of improvement is considered satisfactory.

Of the 219 patients, second look arthroscopies were performed in 46 and twenty-six patients biopsies with 80 per cent of the biopsies showing a hyaline-like appearance (Figures 26.2, 26.3, 26.4 and 26.5). This hyaline-like cartilage more probably closely recreates the wear characteristics and durability of normal hyaline cartilage than the

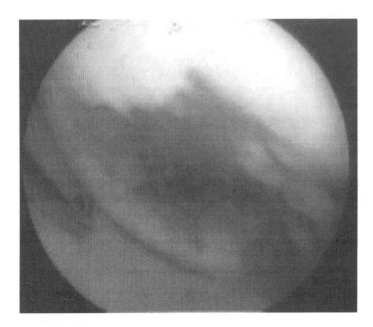

Fig. 26.2
Arthroscopic view of a
chondral lesion on the
weight-bearing central part of
the medial femoral condyle
of 17-year-old woman.

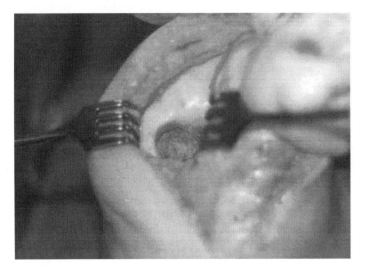

Fig. 26.3
The same lesion as in
Figure 26.2. The defect has
been debrided via a mini
arthrotomy.

fibrous or fibrocartilage repair tissue formed by pluripotential stem
cells after drilling (Gillogly 1998).

Genzyme Tissue Repair (Cambridge, Massachusetts) has initiated an international registry to assess the clinical effectiveness of
autologous chondrocyte transplantation. Thus far to date, outcome
data have been presented for 588 patients at 12 months, 220 patients
at 24 months and 40 patients at 36 month's post-implantation
(Mandelbaum *et al.* 1998). Fifty-nine per cent of these patients
had failed previous treatment. The average lesion size was 4 cm².
Clinical improvement for patients with femoral lesions, according

Fig. 26.4

The same lesion as in
Figures 26.2 and 26.3.
The defect has been
covered by a periosteal flap.

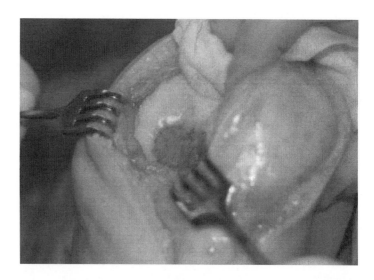

Fig. 26.5

(a–c) The same lesion as
in Figures 26.2–26.4.
Arthroscopic second look
one year post-surgery.
(d) The view of the donor
site at one year post-surgery.

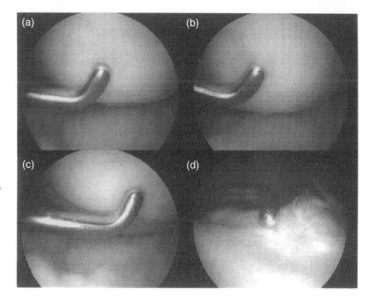

to a modified Cincinnati Knee rating system, was reported for
79 per cent of the patients at 24 months and in 85 per cent of the
patients at 36 months. Eighty-five per cent of the patients reported
an improvement at the 3 year follow-up. A 5 per cent re-operation
rate occurred (Mandelbaum *et al.* 1998).

In Germany, Lohnert in 1998 presented 52 patients that had been
treated with autologous chondrocytes since 1996 and eleven
patients were screened clinically and by MRI 18 months later. The
biopsy specimen from the transplanted area showed the formation
of hyaline cartilage.

A statistically significant improvement was found in both the
clinician and patient knee rating at one year of 25 patients treated by

ACT 12–36 months post surgery and the improvement continued between one and two years following ACT (Gillogly *et al.* 1998). When these patients were biopsied, 80 per cent of the tissue samples displayed a hyaline-like appearance.

Minas (1998) prospectively examined the efficacy of treatment and quality of life in 44 patients undergoing autologous chondrocyte transplantation (ACT) for full-thickness cartilage lesions and calculated the average cost per additional quality-adjusted life year. The 12-month results of ACT treatment showed improvement in the patient function as measured by both the Knee Society scores (114.02 to 140.67, or a 23 per cent mean improvement, $P < 0.001$) and the Western Ontario and McMaster Universities Osteoarthritis Index (35.30 to 23.82, or a 33 per cent mean improvement, $P < 0.05$). The quality of life-estimation, as measured by the Short Form-36 Physical Component Summary, was improved from 33.32 before transplantation to 41.48 ($P < 0.05$) 12 months after transplantation. Improvement on all three scales was maintained during the period from 12 to 24 months after surgery. The estimated cost per the additional quality-adjusted life year was $6791.

Bentley (2000) recently presented the early one year postoperative results from a randomized study between chondrocyte grafted patients (six patients with a periosteal membrane, 34 patients with a resorbable membrane, Chondrogide® (Geistlich Biomaterials, Wolhusen, Switzerland) and 25 multiple osteochondral graft patients. There was improvement in pain and function following both cell techniques and osteochondral grafts in 79 per cent after one year. He stated that cartilage healing can occur with the resorbable membrane Chondrogide® or with periosteum with no obvious adverse effects. The arthroscopic assessment revealed healing with hyaline-like cartilage in 9 out of 11 knees following the ACT procedure. Arthroscopic assessment revealed complete incorporation of the osteochondral graft in 6 of 14 mosaicplasties (Bentley 2000).

Mitsuo *et al.* (2000) used the transplantation of cultured chondrocytes embedded in an atelocollagen gel to treat cartilage defects in 46 patients with mean 26 years and mean cartilage defect size 3.1 cm². The cell-gel construct was covered with a periosteal flap. The authors reported the biomechanics tests demonstrated that the transplants had acquired a similar hardness to the surrounding cartilage but no biopsy specimens were taken at that time.

Knutsen and co-workers recently have operated 35 patients (36 knees) since 1996. Twelve of their first patients were more than 18 months after surgery when they performed second-look arthroscopies. Seventy-five per cent of those patients were classified as good or excellent and 85 per cent had a significant improvement in their clinical condition. Histological evaluation showed hyaline-like cartilage in 9 of the 12 patients (75 per cent). Grifka and colleges (2000) related to the prospective, multi-centre study (Euract) with 400 patients that have been treated by ACT in six centres. They presented

119 patients that had passed one year and with the longest follow-up of three years. Repeated MRI showed a complete filling of the defect sites and good integration into surrounding tissue. Hyaline-like repair with strong expression of S-100 cartilage specific antigen was found in biopsies obtained one and two years after surgery.

The histological evaluation of the repair tissue

Retrieval studies in individuals following autologous chondrocyte transplantation suggest that the process results in production of both hyaline-like tissue and fibrocartilage (Brittberg *et al.* 1994, Nehrer *et al.* 1999, Richardson *et al.* 1999, Peterson *et al.* 2000, Brittberg *et al.* 2001, Peterson *et al.* 2002). Hyaline-like tissue resembles normal articular cartilage histologically with round chondrocytes encased within an extensive extra cellular matrix. The matrix consists primarily of type II collagen and aggrecan, which are the major macromolecules of articular cartilage extracellular matrix (Figure 26.6).

A full thickness of the osteochondral biopsy is needed to get a full understanding and assessment of the repair tissue. From an ACT procedure one will normally get a biopsy specimen consisting of a superficial fibrous layer, followed by a layer with hyaline-like tissue and finally a part of the subchondral bone (Brittberg *et al.* 2001).

In a retrieval study (Nehrer *et al.* 1999) the authors evaluated the composition of reparative tissue retrieved during revision surgery from full thickness chondral defects in six patients for whom periosteal patching augmented by autologous chondrocyte implantation in cell suspension failed to provide lasting relief of symptoms. Revision after autologous chondrocyte transplantation was associated with the partial displacement of the periosteal graft from the defect site because of insufficient ongrowth or early suture failure. When the graft edge displaced, repair tissue was fibrous (55 $\pm$ 11 per cent), whereas graft tissue attached to subchondral bone displayed hyaline tissue (in 6 per cent of patients) and fibrocartilage (in 12 per cent of patients) comprising Type II collagen at three months following surgery. Evaluation of retrieved repair tissue after selected cartilage repair procedures revealed distinct histological features reflecting the mechanisms of failure.

Roberts *et al.* (2001) examined biopsy samples from the ACT grafted area using a batch of specific antibodies to investigate the cellular mechanisms involved and to determine whether remodeling of the matrix occurs. Ten full-depth core biopsy samples were obtained from patients who had undergone ACT 9–30 months previously (ages 28–53 years), in addition to 6 'control' biopsy samples. Cryosections were evaluated by standard histologic examination using polarized light and immunohistochemistry. Antibodies specific for type II collagen were used, as well as antibodies against the C-propeptide of type II collagen and its denaturation product, as indicators of anabolism or catabolism. Also, antibodies to neoepitopes of the aggrecan core protein were used to demonstrate either aggre-canase or matrix metalloproteinase activity. The authors found that all biopsy samples stained for type II collagen, even in areas of fibro-cartilaginous morphology. There was evidence of newly synthesized type II collagen besides denatured collagen. Matrix metallopro-teinase and aggrecanase activity on the proteoglycan population were evident, with aggrecanase being more active in fibrocartilagi-nous areas. The authors concluded that their results indicate that ACT is capable of not only cartilage repair but, in some cases, regeneration, achieved by the turnover and remodeling of an initial fibrocartilaginous matrix via enzymatic degradation and synthesis of newly formed type II collagen (Roberts *et al.* 2001).

There is still no purely objective evaluation of cartilage repair morphology. Perhaps in the future one will be able to better analyze the repair tissue with non-invasive methods. Magnetic resonance imaging (MRI) is a potential method to be used more in the future for such evaluations (Adil *et al.* 2000, Winalski *et al.* 2000). Ludvigsen and associate (2000) followed 24 patients that had been operated with autologous chondrocyte transplantation. They were reexamined at different intervals with MRI. At three months, MRI showed normal signals in 50 per cent, in 36 per cent at 6 months and in 57 per cent at 12 months. The clinical results at 12 months showed 81 per cent of the patients classified as excellent and good.

Different opinions

Shimizu *et al.* (1987) in their article stated that "There is no way to assess the repair of cartilage that is universally applicable, gener-ally accepted and beyond criticism". Two approaches are needed to enable the surgeon to understand the use of chondrogeneic promot-ers for cartilage repair. First we should consider the question of using either tissue-based (entailing the grafting of perichondrial, periosteal, cartilage or bone-cartilage material) or cell-based (using chondro-blasts, chondrocytes, periochondrial cells or mesenchymal stem cells) systems for chondrocyte and articular cartilage regeneration. Cell-based systems are further subdivided according to whether cells are transplanted within a matrix (biodegradable, non-biodegradable or synthetic) or free in suspension. Thus far, the application of cell sus-pensions has always been combined with the grafting of a periosteal flap. The criticisms of autologous chondrocyte implantation have been that it is not proven to what extent the chondrocytes contribute to the repair versus the effect of the overlying periosteal membrane (Lohmander 1998). The periosteum itself is known to produce carti-laginous tissue when combined with subchondral drilling. For purely scientific reasons it is important to know how near regeneration of cartilage we could come with the use of chondrogeneic cells, espe-cially as the cost of producing autologous chondrocyte cells is high.

Fig. 26.6

Histology of a femoral condylar graft biopsy three years post-surgery. The grafted area has been biomechanically examined with an indentation probe (Artscan Oy, Helsinki, Finland) with an indenter force of 3.7 N to be compared with a control area in the same knee of 3.8 N.

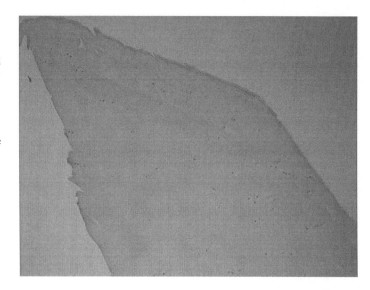

However, from the clinical view the durability of the repair as well as the ability of the neocartilage to give pain relief to the patient, is much more important than the histological morphology of the repair. Long term function also mitigates the initial cost.

Furthermore, unfortunately, the knowledge of the clinical efficacy of the other available types of articular cartilage repair is still poor, and we lack randomized studies on the various techniques available measured against each other and the indistinct natural course of articular cartilage lesions.

Other concerns regarding ACT are that there could be a leakage of grafted chondrocytes from the grafted site after mobilization and joint movement because the cells in suspension are injected beneath the periosteal flap over the cartilage defect and also in an unequal and unknown distribution of grafted chondrocytes in the three-dimensional space of the cartilage defect. There is a possibility that gravity causes all chondrocytes to go down to the base of the defect or the same portion of the defect. This results in a concern as to the uniformity and success of any individual graft site in the early stages.

Sohn *et al.* (2002), using an *ex vivo* bovine model, attempted to study if gravitational forces affect the uniformity of cell distribution within an ACT-treated defect. They reported that the orientation relative to gravity of a repaired full-thickness articular cartilage defect was found to affect the initial distribution of transplanted chondrocytes, prelabeled with 3H-thymidine. After four hours, the injected cells (3H-radioactivity) were primarily at the base of the defect in samples oriented in the up position and primarily at the dependent semi-cylindrical half of the defect in samples oriented to the side, and mostly at the periosteal top of the defect in samples oriented upside-down. Interestingly the cell distribution remained unchanged after reorientation into other positions.

The defect orientation at an early time post-seeding can be an important factor in the uniformity of cell distribution in the autologous chondrocyte transplantation procedure and may be an important determinant of the ultimate clinical outcome. Various research groups have started to test the different cell seeded scaffolds experimentally to avoid such a gravitational effect. A further effect on cell distribution is that cells in a scaffold may better retain their phenotype compared to cells that have been expanded in monolayer and that are dedifferentiated when implanted into the cartilage defect. There is a criticism that we do not know the degree of redifferentiation of implanted cells once implanted in the defect area. Furthermore, Ochi (2000) has concerns that the chondrocytes cultured by our method and then inserted may function in the grafted site as hyaline cartilage for a certain period. However the author has found that the telomeres of the grafted chondrocytes are shorter than those of the original and normal chondrocytes, indicating that the grafted chondrocytes are older than the original cells. Ochi (2000) says that this could mean that the hyaline cartilage formed by the grafted chondrocytes could display premature ageing and degenerate or breakdown at an unexpectedly early stage.

However, much of the controversy surrounding the question of whether joint lesions following ACT can heal results from a failure to assess and measure joint and function and patient satisfaction, rather than the visual cartilage appearance. The primary objective of articular cartilage reconstruction surgery should be a repair producing improved function, reduced symptoms and long term durability for the patient – rather than a short tem subjective improvement as determined by the operating surgeon.

Specific viewpoints of the author's bias and clinical practice

Regarding the evaluation of the repair tissue: the authors agree that objective rather than subjective measurement of the grafted area is important. Today the best way of studying the grafted area is an invasive study *in vivo* i.e. arthroscopy in combination with indentation measurements and biopsy. For obvious ethical reasons we have not been able to perform such invasive studies in all patients. We have evaluated the grafted area in an earlier study (Peterson *et al.* 2000), and correlated the graft histology to the clinical outcome. We found that over 90 per cent of the patients with a good or excellent clinical outcome had a hard and intact transplanted area. The strength of this study is that all consecutive patients from our start of treatment in 1987 are included and followed. The clinical outcome in this group of patients, as compared to other published results with other treatments, is convincing.

Since the first report on ACT (Brittberg *et al.* 1994) we have considered the potential durability of the repair to be an advantage over some of the other treatments. The long-term results presented in that pilot study confirm our initial belief that treatment with ACT results in a durable repair for the majority of the patients, and additionally indicates the importance of patient outcome at two years as an indicator of the future outcome after a longer term follow-up. Patients who have returned to activities of daily living and sport by two years post-ACT are able to continue these activities in the long-term. Most patients that develop a failed ACT graft do so within the first two years post-implantation. After that period the graft survival is close to 100 per cent between three and eight years later. This contrasts sharply with ACT grafts which fail and produce fibrocartilage tissue repairs which often have poor durability, even in the intermediate term.

With the increasing future clinical use of chondrocyte transplantation, other types of chondrogeneic cell research must include randomized studies to compare the different clinical repair methods available. More research is needed using different cell sources, matrices, and on the durability of grafted areas.

Implantation with autologous cultured chondrocytes allows for resurfacing of larger defect areas and the implantation appears to produce new tissue in a high percentage similar in histological and mechanical characteristics to hyaline cartilage, resulting in good clinical outcomes in more than 75 per cent of the patients. Results are best in isolated lesions of the distal femur, with good to excellent results in 90 per cent of the patients. Patellar lesions are less successfully treated by ACT and require strict attention to patellofemoral alignment. Results following treatment of femoral trochlear results are size-dependent. At the time of this writing, the consensus is that autologous cultured chondrocyte implantation could be considered as a primary treatment for lesions greater than 2 cm^2, and as a secondary treatment for all lesions, regardless of size.

Being clinical orthopaedic surgeons our main interest with any method of articular cartilage repair is to give a high percentage of the treated patients, satisfactory pain relief and an improvement in function for a significant period of time. We continue to strive to obtain this, but believe that ACT provides and with further development and understanding of the most appropriate lesion and indications may achieve the recognition as a method with rate of success and long-term durability.

As with any new technique, the right candidates for the treatment and indications must be determined over time by clinical experience. The best candidates for ACT are patients with local cartilage defects on the femoral condyles, well-contained lesions in stable knees. Several predisposing factors to cartilage injuries such as tibiofemoral malalignment, patellofemoral malalignment, and ligamentous or the bone insufficiency must be assessed so that they may be either corrected before or at the same time as the ACT surgery. Axial alignment weight-bearing and patello-femoral CT skyline views are necessary to assess tibiofemoral or patellofemoral malalignment. MRI is still not accurate enough in clinical practice in the imaging of articular cartilage lesions to determine the extent, depth, size or characteristics of a chondral injury. None the less it remains the best modality available and improved resolution which new scanning sequences has potential in this regard. Radiographs are helpful in terms of assessing advanced degeneration and malalignment; an essential part of the assessment as to whether any symptomatic patient is a candidate for ACT.

When varus or valgus malalignment is associated with a medial or lateral condyle articular cartilage injury, then a corrective osteotomy is crucial to the success of local cartilage repair with chondrocytes. Patello-femoral maltracking combined with a patello-femoral joint cartilage injury requires careful pre-operative assessment and CT or MRI analysis. The reconstruction of the extensor mechanism with the eventual deepening of a dysplastic trochlea combined with tibial tubercle realignment is the key to long-term durability of any patello-femoral ACT grafted area. The relative effect of ACT and the patello-femoral reconstruction is an unknown worthy of future study.

Cartilage repair in a knee being unstable due to the anterior cruciate ligament (ACL) insufficiency may jeopardize a chondrocyte graft, and a staged or concomitant ACL reconstruction surgery should be performed to prevent shear forces and instability episodes from damaging the ACT graft. If there is a bony deficiency greater than 1 cm in depth as commonly occurs in osteochondritis dissecans, the osteochondral lesions should be bone grafted either as a one stage procedure with concomitant ACT repair, or bone grafted as an initial part of a two-stage procedure.

Conclusion and final remarks

For successful treatment of symptomatic lesions of articular cartilage careful assessment and prior treatment of concomitant lesions must be undertaken. Additionally the facts predisposing to early failure, such as malalignment, must be corrected to ensure that any articular cartilage repair will have reasonable chance of long-term survival. All of the available cartilage repair techniques today, including ACT, can result in full articular cartilage tissue regeneration but are compromised by many preexisting or concomitant factors. The management of these other factors will be important to optimize the fate of any cell-induced repair, whatever the cell types, scaffolds and growth factors that might be used in the future.

Furthermore, for the orthopaedic surgeon the choice of the most appropriate treatment will be dependant on the reported results of the medium and long-term outcome of the various available treatment procedures. This must include documented objective measurement of the symptomatic, functional improvement, quality of life and the cost effectiveness of the treatment. Since the new technology of *in vitro* expanded autologous chondrocytes is potentially more costly and invasive than other conservative and surgical therapies, cost benefit analyses are needed. Recently, an evaluation of the effect of ACT on clinical outcome, absenteeism, disability status, and total direct economic burden in 57 patients with full-thickness chondral lesions of the knee treated between 1987 and 1996 have been presented (Lindahl *et al.* 2001). Forty-nine of the 57 patients improved clinically as a result of the ACI treatment and a dramatic cost-saving effect was demonstrated over a projected 10-year period due to reduced absenteeism and disability. Similar economical analyses are needed for all the methods of articular cartilage repair.

A comprehensive analysis of the ACT technology was presented last year (Jobanputra *et al.* 2001). The authors stated that on the basis of literature, no definite conclusions can be drawn from the clinical effectiveness of ACT, which should be regarded as an experimental procedure. However, on these grounds, almost all other techniques used for treating disabling cartilage defects, could be regarded as experimental. The cost of ACT is substantial in comparison to the other techniques, and surgeons have reported similar good results using those methods. However most of these other cartilage repair techniques have still quite short follow-ups (three years) and the authors speculate that it is possible that, by extending the time horizon and assuming that better outcomes are sustained with ACT, but not with other therapies, financial and human costs might in the long run be less with ACT. Such speculations are, say the authors, not justified until data from randomized studies becomes available. We agree with that statement but emphasize the importance of long-term follows ups in such studies with a definitions of a short-term study being two years old, mid-term for five years and a long-term study at least 10 years.

Our experience with implantation of chondrocytes in combination with periosteum is that it is a promising new treatment option for cartilage injuries and a technique with a long-term durability. Most patients in our series of follow-ups have been patients with chronic lesions of the knee and have been treated before without success; the success of ACT should be seen in terms of its application as a second line of treatment when the conventional techniques had failed. We believe that we have come into a new thrilling era of tissue engineering and repair for musculoskeletal injuries and a future cartilage repair methodology is likely to be based on cultured cells supported in engineered tissue. Different biodegradable matrices are available that could support chondrocyte growth within regenerating articular cartilage growth are under investigation. The potential for addition of growth factors and the use of different types of cell-based repair is enormous and of great clinical potential for the future.

References

Adil B, McKeon B, Scheller A, Gray M, Burstein D (2000). MR imaging of glycosaminoglycan in patients with autologous chondrocyte transplants. Hunziker E, Mainil-Varlet P (eds) *Updates in Cartilage Repair.*

A multimedia production on cartilage repair on 6 CD-ROMS. CD 6. Lippincott, Williams and Wilkins Company, Philadelphia, USA.

Bentley G (2000). Development of applied tissue engineering of articular cartilage. In *The Art of Tissue Engineering 2000*. CD-ROM, Isotis, AB Bilthoven, The Netherlands.

Brittberg M, Lindahl A, Nilsson A, Ohlsson C, Isaksson O, Peterson L (1994). Treatment of deep cartilage defects in the knee with autologous chondrocyte transplantation. *N Engl J Med* 331, 889–895.

Brittberg M, Nilsson A, Lindahl A, Ohlsson C, Peterson L (1996). Rabbit articular cartilage defects in the knee with autologous cultured chondrocytes. *Clin Orthop Rel Res* 326, 270–283.

Brittberg M, Tallheden T, Sjogren-Jansson B, Lindahl A, Peterson L (2001). Autologous chondrocytes used for articular cartilage repair: an update. *Clin Orthop* 391 (Suppl), 337–348.

Caplan AI, Elyaderani M, Mochizuki Y, Wakitani S, Goldberg VM (1997). Principles of cartilage repair and regeneration. *Clin Orthop Rel Res* 342, 254–269.

Gillogly SD (1998). Autologous chondrocyte implantation: Current state-of-the-art. In Imhoff AB, Burkart A. *Knieinstabilität-knorpelschaden*, pp. 60–66. Steinkopff Verlag, Darmstadt, Germany.

Gillogly SD, Voight M, Blackburn T (1998). Treatment of articular cartilage defects of the knee with autologous chondrocyte implantation. *J Orthop Sports Phys Ther* 28, 241–251.

Goldberg VM, Caplan AI (1994). Cellular repair of articular cartilage. In: Kuettner KE, Goldberg VM (eds) *Osteoarthritic Disorders* pp. 357–364. American Academy of Orthopedic Surgery, Monterrey, USA.

Grande DA, Pitman MI, Peterson L, Menche D, Klein M (1989). The repair of experimentally produced defects in rabbit articular cartilage by autologous chondrocyte transplantation. *J Orthop Res* 7, 208–218.

Grifka J, Löhnert J, Feldt S, Josimovic-Alasevic O, Fritsch K-G (2000). A one to three years follow-up of 119 patients treated with autologous chondrocyte transplantation using CO.DON chondrotransplant. In Hunziker E, Mainil-Varlet P (eds) *Updates in Cartilage Repair. A multimedia production on cartilage repair on 6 CD-ROMS*. CD 6, Lippincott, Williams and Wilkins Company, Philadelphia, USA.

Jobanputra P, Parry D, Fry-Smith A, Burls A (2001). Effectiveness of autologous chondrocyte transplantation for hyaline cartilage defects in knees. A rapid and systematic review. *Health Technology Assessment* 5, 1–57.

Knutsen G, Isaksen V, Johansen O (2000). Autologous chondrocyte transplantation in the knee. Histological and clinical follow-up. In Hunziker E, Mainil-Varlet P (eds) *Updates in Cartilage Repair. A multimedia production on cartilage repair on 6 CD-ROMS*. CD 6, Lippincott, Williams and Wilkins Company, Philadelphia, USA.

Lindahl A, Brittberg M, Peterson L (2001). Health economics benefits following autologous chondrocyte transplantation for patients with focal chondral lesions of the knee. *Knee Surg Sports Traumatol Arthrosc* 9, 358–363.

Lohnert J (1998). Regeneration of hyaline cartilage in the knee joint by treatment with autologous chondrocyte transplants-initial clinical results Langenbecks. *Arch Chir Suppl Kongressbd* 115, 1205–1207 (in German).

Lohmander LS (1998). Cell-based cartilage repair: do we need it, can we do it, is it good, can we prove it? *Current Opinion in Orthopedics* 9, 38–42.

Ludvigsen TC, Knopp A, Engebretsen L (2000). Autologous chondro-cyte implantation for treatment of cartilage defects in the knee. In Hunziker E, Mainil-Varlet P (eds) *Updates in Cartilage Repair. A multi-media production on cartilage repair on 6 CD-ROMS*, CD 6. Lippincott, Williams and Wilkins Company Philadelphia.

Mandelbaum BR, Browne JE, Fu F *et al.* (1998). Articular cartilage lesions of the knee. Current concepts. *Am J Sports Med* 26, 853–861.

Mankin HJ (1982). The response of articular cartilage to mechanical injury. *J Bone Joint Surg Am* 64, 460–466.

Minas T (1998). Chondrocyte implantation in the repair of chondral lesions of the knee: economics and quality of life. *Am J Orthop* 27, 739–744.

Mitsuo O, Uchio Y, Kawasaki K, Iwasa J, Kaqtsube K (2000). Treatment of osteochondral defects in the knee with transplantation of cul-tured autologous chondrocytes embedded in atelocollagen gel. In Hunziker E, Mainil-Varlet P (eds) *Updates in Cartilage Repair. A multi-media production on cartilage repair on 6 CD-ROMS*. CD 6. Lippincot, Williams and Wilkins Company, Philadelphia, USA.

Nehrer S, Spector M, Minas T (1999). Histologic analysis of tissue after failed cartilage repair procedures. *Clin Orthop* 365, 149–162.

Ochi M (2000). New and exciting information from basic science. *Isakos Newsletter* 4, 9.

Peterson L (1998). Cartilage repair/regeneration by periosteal and chon-drocyte transplantation. Symposium on articular cartilage repair, regeneration and transplantation. Presented at the sixty-fifth Annual meeting of the American Academy of Orthopaedic Surgeons, New Orleans, 214, 1998.

Peterson L, Brittberg M, Kiviranta I, Akerlund EL, Lindahl A (2002). Autologous chondrocyte transplantation. Biomechanics and long-term durability. *Am J Sports Med* 30, 2–12.

Peterson L, Menche D, Grande D, Pitman M (1984). Chondrocyte transplantation – An experimental model in the rabbit. *Trans Orthop Res Soc* 9, 218.

Peterson L, Minas T, Brittberg M, Nilsson A, Sjögren-Jansson E, Lindahl A (2000). Two- to nine-year outcome after autologous chondrocyte transplantation of the knee. *Clin Orthop* 374, 212–234.

Richardson JB, Caterson B, Evans EH, Ashton BA, Roberts S (1999). Repair of human articular cartilage after implantation of autologous chondrocytes. *J Bone Joint Surg Br* 81, 1064–1068.

Roberts S, Hollander AP, Caterson B, Menage J, Richardson JB (2001). Matrix turnover in human cartilage repair tissue in autologous chon-drocyte implantation. *Arthritis Rheum* 44, 2586–2598.

Shimizu T, Videman T, Shimazaki K, Mooney V (1987). Experimental study on the repair of full thickness articular cartilage defects. Effects of varying periods of continuous passive motion, cage activity and immobilization. *J Orthop Res* 5, 187–197.

Sohn DH, Lottman LM, Lum LY *et al.* (2002). Effect of gravity on local-ization of chondrocytes implanted in cartilage defects. *Clin Orthop Rel Res* 394, 54–62.

Winalski CS, Chiu RI, Minas T (2000). Utility of magetic resonance imag-ing for postoperative assessment of autologous chondrocyte implanta-tion: MR-arthroscopic correlation. In Hunziker E, Mainil-Varlet P (eds) *Updates in Cartilage Repair. A multimedia production on cartilage repair on 6 CD-ROMS*, CD 6. Lippincott, Williams and Wilkins Company, Philadelphia, USA.

Editor's questions:

Question 1 What is the effect of lesion size on your current practice on choice of surgical procedures for the primary treatment of articular cartilage full thickness lesions in a 25 year old patient? Say in the less than 10 mm square lesion, the less than 25 mm square lesion, and a larger lesion?

Answer The effect of the lesion size determines the management protocol in the following way: The choice of treatment depends on the size of the defect, if it is acute or chronic and if the lesion has been treated before with other repair techniques. If the lesion is acute, previously untreated and less than 2 cm², one can could choose a bone marrow stimulation technique or osteochondral autograft done arthroscopically. The patient undergoes intensive physiotherapy and if the result is not satisfactory and improved by 6 months another technique like ACT is considered.

If the defect is larger than 2 cm², acute and untreated, one can consider ACT or osteochondral autografts.

If the lesion is larger than 4 cm² the choice is between and initial ACT or osteochondral allografting.

If the lesion is chronic, or has previously been treated then ACT, osteochondral autograftsis considered or in some cases carbon fibres reconstruction.

If the lesion is of a chronic nature but untreated then bone marrow stimulation techniques should be considered or alternately osteochondral autografts. The patients require an intensive period of post-operative physiotherapy for 6 months. If the clinical result is still not satisfactory then other techniques such as ACT.

See also attached the treatment flow chart.

Question 2 What is the effect of age on your current indications for ACT grafting?

Answer The biologic age meaning that the quality of the joint and articular cartilage surrounding the lesion is more important that chronolgical age itself. A patient at the age of 65 could have a local cartilage defect with good surrounding cartilage making it suitable for ACT while a much younger patient could have a severe osteoarthritic joint not be suitable for ACT. In general, most patients chosen to undergo ACT treatment have been between 18–60 years of age. We have not had any problems in culturing chondrocytes from cartilage derived from the more elderly patients.

27

Fresh osteochondral allograft transplantation for the treatment of hyaline cartilage defects: is this a viable surgical alternative?

Beth E. Shubin Stein and Riley J. Williams III

Introduction

Injuries to the articular cartilage of the knee are frequent (Curl *et al.*, 1997). As early as 1743, physicians were aware of the inability of articular cartilage to heal itself (Hunter, 1743). Today, cartilage defects remain some of the most difficult problems that we treat. There seem to be many treatment options, none yielding reliable clinical outcomes.

Current treatment options such as lavage, drilling, abrasion, and microfracture have demonstrated variable clinical results related to long-term function. Under the best circumstances, these treatments promote a fibrocartilage scar that partially fills the articular defect. Despite early symptomatic relief, the biomechanical and histological properties of fibrocartilage are a poor substitute for normal hyaline cartilage and it has been shown to break down over time (Gerber *et al.*, 2002). Another method of cartilage repair, autologous chondrocyte implantation (ACI), has also been investigated and applied clinically (Amiel, 1985, Brittberg *et al.*, 1994, Chu *et al.*, 1995, Vacanti, 1989). Unfortunately, this technique remains technically difficult and expensive. Yet the development of the chondrocyte implantation technique over the past decade did give clinicians another useful option in the treatment of large cartilage lesions. The development of the ACI technique also refocused knee specialists on the topic of cartilage resurfacing as a result of increased patient demand. This phenomenon shed a new light on the use of allograft tissue, already popular in ligament reconstruction, as it applied to treating cartilage defects.

For over two decades surgeons at the University of Toronto and the University of California at San Diego have employed the use of fresh condylar specimens for the treatment of such lesions with good success. These fresh specimens featured live chondrocytes that could maintain the cartilage structure indefinitely in the host knee. Unfortunately, such allograft tissue was not available to the typical orthopedic surgeon or knee specialist. Now, however, stored allograft tissue is available through commercial vendors in the USA. And, unlike those grafts implanted at the aforementioned institutions, these commercial grafts are stored for intervals in excess of 30 days prior to implantation. This chapter will seeks to answer the following questions:

1   What is the role of allografts in the myriad of options available to the knee specialist in treating chondral and osteochondral defects?
2   Does stored fresh allograft (tissue) represent a reasonable option for the knee specialist wishing to treat a large chondral or osteochondral lesion of the knee?

Cartilage structure

Articular cartilage is composed of an extracellular matrix (ECM) with a few specialized chondrocytes dispersed throughout. The ECM consists of water, proteoglycans and collagen. The collagen is predominantly type II and provides cartilage with its tensile properties, in addition to stabilizing the proteoglycans within the ECM (Buckwalter, 1998, Mankin, 1994). Proteoglycans are composed of a protein core to which multiple glycosaminoglycans (GAGs) attach. The GAGs are negatively charged; this negative charge helps to push the proteoglycan units away from each other, allowing the collagen mesh to fill with water. With compression, water is driven out of the ECM, forcing the individual proteoglycans closer to one another, and increasing the tissues resistance to further compression. When the compressive force is removed, these molecules spread farther apart, and fluid is taken back into the tissue (Mankin, 1974, 1994).

Cartilage injury and repair

Curl et al. reviewed more than 31,000 knee arthroscopies and found a 3 per cent incidence of chondral lesions (Curl et al., 1997). Moreover, approximately one-third of these lesions were associated with ligament rupture (i.e. ACL tear). Though relatively uncommon, these injuries are particularly relevant to the knee specialist. The response of the cartilage to injury depends on the depth of the injury. If the damage does not penetrate the subchondral bone, no inflammatory response results, as hyaline cartilage is avascular. With no blood supply to promote the formation of a fibrin clot, the cartilage defect persists (Mankin, 1974). If the injury penetrates the subchondral bone (i.e. subchondral fracture), an inflammatory response is initiated. Initially, the defect fills with blood, and a fibrin clot forms. This fibrin clot contains pluripotential mesenchymal cells which eventually differentiate to become fibroblasts, producing a new matrix and eventually a capillary rich granulation tissue which fills the defect. At approximately 6–8 weeks, the repair tissue contains an ECM and chondrocyte-like cells (Mankin, 1971). Ultimately this newly formed ECM partially fills the defect with a fibrocartilagenous material that is functionally inferior to normal hyaline cartilage.

Mechanisms of injury

Cartilage injury can occur secondary to an impact, avulsion, or following the application of high shear forces to the knee (Matthewson, 1978). These injuries are seldom recognized initially. Matthewson *et al.* found that over 30 per cent of the osteochondral injuries in their study were not detected at the initial presentation (Matthewson, 1978). Often the mechanism of injury is complex and may involve a direct blow combined with a deceleration, rotation or valgus force to the knee (Milgram, 1978, Vellet, 1991). The forces responsible for the production of osteochondral injuries are often directed tangentially to the joint surface (Farnworth, 2000).

Diagnosis

Initial presentation of patients with chondral lesions can vary. The presence of pain or knee locking is common. There may be associated findings of joint line tenderness and/or a joint effusion. Knee radiographs are usually normal and should not be used to rule out chondral pathology; however large osteochondral defects can be detected with radiographs (Farnworth, 2000). The gold standard for the detection of chondral lesions is magnetic resonance imaging (MRI). MRI (using cartilage sensitive pulse sequencing) may be used to assess the cartilage surfaces and has been shown to be both highly sensitive and specific for chondral pathology. Potter *et al.* found little interobserver variability using this method, and concluded that MRI is an accurate, non-invasive, and reproducible method with which to diagnose chondral lesions of the knee (Potter *et al.*, 1998) (Figure 27.1).

Several authors have noted the relationship between osteochondral defects and other knee injuries. Indelicato *et al.* found chondral injuries in 23 per cent of acute anterior cruciate ligament (ACL) injuries and 54 per cent of chronic ACL injuries (Indelicato, 1985). Noyes *et al.* proposed that an increased number of subluxation episodes might account for the higher incidence of chondral pathology associated with chronic ACL insufficiency (Noyes, 1980).

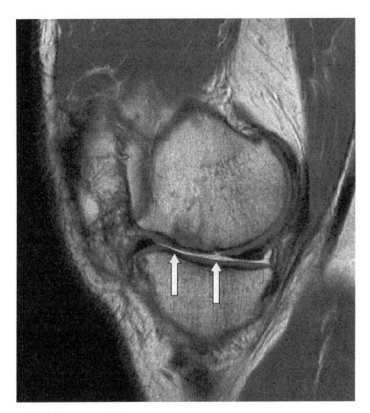

Fig. 27.1
Magnetic resonance imaging of a full-thickness chondral lesion of the femur using a cartilage sensitive fast-spin echo technique (Potter *et al.*, 1998). The articular cartilage is of intermediate signal intensity; the extent of the lesion is delineated by the arrows (white).

Many studies have shown an association between chondral injuries and meniscal lesions (Curl *et al.*, 1997, Geissler, 1993, Lewandrowski, 1997). Lewandrowski *et al.* demonstrated this combination in 76 per cent of patients with medial femoral condyle lesions and 46 per cent of patients with lateral femoral condylar lesions. The likelihood of finding a chondral injury was significantly increased with the presence of a bucket-handle tear or complex tear compared to horizontal cleavage or radial tears of the meniscus (Lewandrowski, 1997).

Surgical treatment options

As knee surgeons we are all familiar with those treatment options currently available (Table 27.1). Thinking critically about these options, clinicians should understand that the most expedient methods of treating cartilage defects are temporizing at best. Most surgeons would agree that there are first and second line treatments for cartilage lesions. However we knee specialists can seldom agree, uniformly, as the application of one method compared to another in any given clinical scenario.

Table 27.1 Options for the Treatment of Symptomatic Articular
Cartilage Lesions of the Knee

1. Non-operative
    a. Oral medications
    b. Physical Therapy
    c. Injections (Steroid, Visco-supplementation)
2. Operative
    a. Knee Arthroscopy with Lavage
    b. Chondroplasty
    c. Drilling
    d. Microfracture
    e. Abrasion Arthroplasty
    f. Mosaicplasty
    g. Autologous Chondrocyte Implantation (ACI)
    h. Osteochondral Allograft
    i. Osteotomy
    j. Arthroplasty

Enhancement of cartilage healing

The enhancement of cartilage healing depends upon the recruitment
of marrow stem cells into the cartilage defect to promote cartilage
repair. Abrasion arthroplasty, drilling, and microfracture (picking) all
fall into this category. These methods all require penetration of the
subchondral plate and bleeding into the cartilage defect. The fibrin
clot cascade promotes the formation of granulation tissue that
eventually matures into a reparative fibrocartilage (Buckwalter *et al.*,
1994, Mankin, 1982, Steadman *et al.*, 1999). This method is perhaps
the most commonly applied method of cartilage repair as it is fast,
cost-effective, and preserves the arthroscopic approach. However,
the clinical outcomes of all of these methods are highly variable. It
is known that fibrocartilage will partially fill the defect, and that
the biomechanical properties of the fibrocartilage are inferior to the
articular cartilage. Fibrocartilage has been demonstrated to degenerate as early as a year after surgery in clinical circumstances (Mankin,
1982). Surgeons must carefully monitor those patients who undergo
cartilage repair techniques that rely upon the enhancement of
cartilage healing via mesenchymal stem cell recruitment. While
smaller lesions may do well with such techniques, patients with larger
chondral lesions (>2 cm^2), should be prepared to move to a second
line of treatment in the event of recurrent symptoms.

Autologous chondrocyte transplantation

Cartilage precursor cells can also be used to treat a chondral defect
via autologous chondrocyte transplantation. Studies have proved that
the cultured chondrocytes are viable and capable of producing an

ECM that more closely resembles articular cartilage than reparative fibrocartilage (Chen, 1997). Many authors have reported good clinical results using ACI (Brittberg et al., 1994, Menche, 1998, Minas, 1999). The clinical use of autologous chondrocyte transplantation was first reported by Brittberg and Peterson; and excellent results in clinical practice are reported (Peterson et al., 2002, Brittberg et al., 1994, Peterson et al., 2000). These authors advocate the ACI method for the treatment of even large lesions (>10 cm²). Unfortunately, reports have been variable in the USA (Gillogly et al., 1998, Micheli et al., 2001, Minas, 2001, Muellner et al., 2001). Histology specimens retrieved from ACI patients reveals the presence of hyaline-like cartilage and fibrocartilage. Currently, this method requires two surgeries (cell harvest and cell implantation), and remains an expensive approach. Overall the ACI method is a good approach for large lesions, but does not effectively address the question of bony deficiency (i.e. osteonecrosis, osteochondritis dissecans) alone. The ACI method is an effective means of treating large, even irregular knee cartilage lesions; however, the clinician may require a method of cartilage resurfacing that includes the recreation of a bony deficiency.

Autogenous tissue transplantation

Another option for treating full-thickness cartilage defects is autologous whole tissue transplantation. This procedure (mosaicplasty) described by Hangody et al. (1997) uses small cylindrical osteochondral grafts or plugs harvested from the ipsilateral knee joint to fill the articular defect. Depending on the size of the defect, a single plug may suffice or multiple grafts may be used. Hangody et al. reviewed their series at five year follow-up and showed excellent results (Hangody et al., 2001, 1998). There are however, several limitations to this technique. First, there is a finite amount of donor tissue sites available, making this technique useful for relatively small lesions (<4 cm²). Second, it is very difficult to obtain a congruent surface with multiple osteochondral plugs filling a single defect. Finally, there is evidence to suggest that placing multiple grafts into a single site may weaken the normal cartilage surrounding the defect as well as possibly damaging the opposing articulating surface (Paletta and Hannafin, 1996, personal communication). Mosaicplasty results in a hyaline cartilage repair, and can be used to treat concomitant bony deficiency. The primary drawback to this technique is the lack of donor tissue, and as such, mosaicplasty is not recommended for the treatment of large cartilage lesions.

Allograft tissue transplantation

Osteochondral allografts have the advantage of providing hyaline cartilage grafts of any size and shape with no donor-site morbidity.

In contrast to ACI, which requires neochondrogenesis, osteochondral allografts techniques are a one-step process that relies on incorporation of the subchondral bone via creeping substitution. In contrast to mosaicplasty techniques, osteochondral allografting permits the use of a single orthotopic graft that completely fills the chondral defect and immediately restores joint surface congruity. Osteochondral grafts have been used to reconstruct joints for many years. (Burwell *et al.*, 1985, Convery *et al.*, 1991a, Ganel *et al.*, 1981, Highgenboten *et al.*, 1989, Locht *et al.*, 1984, Meyers *et al.*, 1983). Their use is predicated on the notion that transplantation of cartilage grafts with viable cells would enable maintenance of the ECM and would result in long-term clinical success. Although surgeons at a handful of institutions have been performing osteochondral transplantations with success, this treatment approach continues to be unavailable to a majority of knee surgeons. Several factors make the application of fresh osteochondral allograft treatment a difficult endeavor. Donor tissue availability, associated risk of disease transmission, and the maintenance of cell viability are just a few issues relevant to the implantation of harvest donor osteochondral specimens.

Graft availability has been a major barrier to the widespread use of fresh osteochondral allografts. Historically, obtaining maximal chondrocyte viability necessitated transplanting the fresh graft within 3–5 days. These time restraints tended to limit the clinical use of allograft to those institutions capable of facilitating the graft harvest, host matching and quality control. In hopes of increasing the availability of these grafts, the orthopaedic community has become interested in storage techniques that would maintain cell viability and allow for transportation of grafts to recipients farther away at a remote location from the donor. Ideally there is maximal defect congruence from these size matched grafts (Figure 27.2).

Fig. 27.2

Whole femoral hemi-condylar specimen being prepared for donor allograft transplantation.

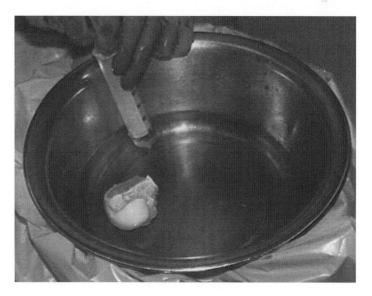

What types of donor tissue are available?

Four different types of osteochondral grafts are now available: fresh-frozen, cryopreserved, fresh, and fresh cold-stored.

Fresh-frozen

In light of the limited availability of fresh grafts, most surgeons have experience with fresh-frozen donor specimens for reconstructive purposes (i.e. bulk allografts for tumor reconstruction). Condylar specimens are typically frozen and stored at –80°C. The freezing process results in total cell death in stored specimens. Thus there is no method by which the cartilage ECM can be maintained over the long term in such grafts. Despite the absence of viable chondrocytes, fresh-frozen tissue does have one major advantage compared to fresh tissue. Fresh-frozen tissue has been shown to be less immunogenic compared to the fresh grafts; this results in a shorter interval to bony incorporation (Rodrigo, 1987). Initially, studies looking at the survival of chondrocytes extracted from their matrix after the freezing process showed promising results (Tomford, 1984). However, further investigation found that when frozen within their matrix the chondrocytes did not survive (Rodrigo, 1987). Animal studies using fresh-frozen grafts confirmed the poor chondrocyte survival and poor graft survivorship. (Schachar et al., 1999). Schahar et al. used fresh-frozen grafts to resurface cartilage defects in sheep and examined the specimens at 3, 6 and 12 months after transplantation. Their results showed poor chondrocyte survival of the fresh-frozen grafts (Schachar et al., 1999). Thus, the use of fresh-frozen osteochondral allografts, though much more available, is not recommended for the treatment of chondral or osteochondral defects.

Cryopreserved tissue

Cryopreservation has been shown to yield some chondrocyte survival (Tomford, 1984). Cryopreserved condylar specimens are frozen in a nutritive medium in an effort to promote cell survival despite freezing. Ohlendorf et al. observed chondrocyte survival in grafts that were cryopreserved; however, the viable cells were found only in the superficial layers of the articular cartilage (Ohlendorf et al., 1996). In one animal study, cell viability of cryopreserved fresh grafts was examined after immersing them in 10 per cent dimethyl sulfoxide for 30 minutes prior to freezing. This protocol resulted in 50 per cent chondrocyte viability and intermediate overall graft outcome compared with that of fresh autografts (Schachar et al., 1999). However, the cryopreservation method is not standardized, and chondrocyte viability has been shown to vary with the type and concentration of cryopreservative used (Malinin et al., 1985, Marco et al., 1992). Although Ohlendorf found viable chondrocytes limited to the superficial layer of cartilage, Muldrew et al. found that these limited number of cells maintained enough metabolic activity to produce and replenish the ECM (Muldrew, 2001). Unfortunately commercial attempts at cartilage cryopreservation have failed repeatedly, as vendors sought to make condyles with viable cells available to the knee surgeons. Thus, the use of cryopreserved osteochondral allografts may become a viable option for the treatment of full-thickness articular defects with further advances in cryopreservative methodology and a standardization of techniques. Presently, the use of these grafts, because of poor chondrocyte viability, is not recommended for cartilage resurfacing procedures.

Fresh

Fresh condylar specimens indicated for an osteochondral allografting procedure are usually implanted into a size-matched host knee within 72 hours of harvesting. This short interval to implantation ensures a high percentage of cell viability. Fresh allografts have consistently demonstrated maintained chondrocyte viability both in vitro (Rodrigo, 1987) and in retrieval studies of clinical specimens (Oakeshott, 1988). Czitrom et al. studied cell viability in biopsies taken from transplanted fresh grafts using $_{35}SO^4$ and ^3H-cytidine autoradiography. In this study, 69–99 per cent of chondrocytes were viable up to 41 months after the transplantation (Czitrom, 1990). Ten-year survival of chondrocyte viability in fresh osteochondral allografts has been demonstrated by Convery et al. (Convery et al., 1996). In this case report, Convery et al. examined the removed allograft and looked at the cell viability as well as the biochemical features of the failed allograft. They found that the graft contained a large percentage of viable cells, and that the concentrations of type-II collagen and glycosaminoglycans was essentially the same as those found in normal articular cartilage (Convery et al., 1996). They determined that the graft did not fail as a result of the metabolic activity of the cartilage, but rather as a result of resorption of the transplanted subchondral allograft bone. The authors commented that the techniques used for the initial transplant were inferior to the newer technical standards – specifically, the addition of autogenous bone graft placed beneath the allograft to fill the gap between the host bed and the allograft (Convery et al., 1996). The use of the described fresh osteochondral allografts does have a major limiting factor. In North America only two institutions (University of Toronto and UCSD) have the ability to harvest the donor graft and match the specimen to a patient, allowing the graft to be implanted in less than 72 hours. This short period between harvest and implantation significantly limits the availability of truly fresh grafts to the majority of knee surgeons. As a result, surgeons

463

have turned to commercial vendors to aid in making such allograft tissue more widely available.

Fresh cold-storage tissue

In 1998, fresh cold-stored grafts became commercially available in the United States, instantly increasing the availability of donor condyle specimens to knee surgeons. The theoretical advantage of such grafts is identical to that of fresh grafts: the presence of viable cells in these specimens allows for the potential long-term maintenance of the cartilage matrix. Unfortunately there are no reports on the use of such cold-storage tissue in humans. It is important to remember that these fresh cold-stored grafts are not the same as fresh grafts. Published studies on fresh tissue report on grafts implanted by five days; fresh cold-stored grafts are available up to 45 days post harvest. What is known is that longer storage intervals result in decreasing cartilage cell viability and compromised mechanical properties (Marco *et al.*, 1992, Rodrigo, 1987). Schachar *et al.* demonstrated that the metabolic activity of the chondrocytes persists during the cold-storage period (Schachar *et al.*, 1994). Rodrigo *et al.* looked at chondrocyte viability with cold-storage techniques. These authors found that before 24 hours, there was little effect on cell viability. However, after the first 24 hours, the number of viable cells markedly dropped (Rodrigo, 1987). These findings were supported by work done by Marco *et al.* (Marco *et al.*, 1992). Even with the rapid drop in cell viability, studies have still shown successful outcomes with osteochondral allografts stored up to 14 days in animal models (Oates *et al.*, 1995).

Just as cryopreservation with a nutritive medium enhances cell viability over its fresh-frozen counterpart, so to, has the addition of a nutritive medium enhanced cell viability with the fresh cold-storage technique. Sammarco *et al.* (1997) were able to show excellent preservation of cell viability at 48 hours. They examined human cartilage grafts taken from notchplasties and stored in cell culture medium at 4°C. Their results showed an average decrease in $_{35}$S-sulfate uptake of 0.8 per cent at 24 hours and 6.4 per cent at 48 hours, indicating a high level of chondrocyte viability after refrigeration.

Now with commercial availability of these cold-stored osteochondral allografts, a size-matched specimen is determined and the fresh cold-stored whole condylar specimens are shipped to the treating surgeons for implantation. The commercial vendors who provide these cold-stored grafts report up to 50 per cent cell viability at 45 days post harvest (Cryolife, 1998).

In an attempt at quantifying the effects of cold-storage on the material properties of the condylar specimens, we performed a series of *in vitro* experiments. In this study by Williams *et al.*, ovine condyles stored in a nutritive medium at 4°C were analyzed at 1, 8, 15, 29, 45 and 60 days post-harvest. On post-harvest day 1, 100 per cent cell viability was demonstrated. Chondrocyte viability declined from 99 per cent, 82 per cent, 83 per cent, 66 per cent and 51 per cent at subsequent intervals (Williams, 2002). Significant drops in chondrocyte viability were noted between days 8 and 15, and between days 29 and 45. In contrast to cryopreservation, viable chondrocytes were seen in all layers of the articular cartilage. Significant decreases in proteoglycan content and the dynamic modulus was also noted (Williams, 2002). This study suggests that an increasing storage interval results in a significant loss of condylar material properties, including decreasing cell viability, decreasing matrix ground substance, and decreased mechanical strength. These results bring more questions:

1   What *is* the minimum number or percentage of chondrocytes necessary for long-term graft survival? Put another way, is there a maximum storage interval for harvested condylar tissue, beyond which osteochondral allografting will fail?
2   Do the changes in matrix ground substance and mechanical properties recover after implantation? If not, does this adversely affect graft survival?
3   Finally, and perhaps most importantly, should knee surgeons use these grafts in clinical practice.

The senior author (RJW) has qualitatively analyzed the commercial allografts used clinically at the Hospital for Special Surgery since 1998. The figures demonstrate the wide variability in cell survival noted in these tissue specimens. Thus, with specific regard to question three, the authors suggest the following: the sooner the better. Clearly cold-stored tissue specimens degrade with time. Therefore, we stress the timely implantation of these grafts soon after the commercial quality control process has been completed. In light of the presented data, we seldom implant a graft that has been stored longer than 30 days. It is critical that knee specialists who wish to repair articular cartilage using the allograft technique understand that there is no published information on the material that is currently available commercially.

Immunology and osteochondral allografts

Host immune reaction to osteochondral allografts in antigen-mismatched specimens has been documented (Strong *et al.*, 1996, Stevenson *et al.*, 1989). However, the clinical significance of these findings remains unknown and this host response is typically a local phenomenon. Many researchers believe that like heart valves and corneas, articular cartilage is an 'immunologically privileged' tissue (Langer, 1974). Chondrocytes are known to be immunogenic, but only when isolated from their extracellular matrix (Langer, 1974).

When transplanted along with their extracellular matrix, chondrocytes are protected from any clinically significant host response (Oakeshott, 1988). Both humoral and cell-mediated antibodies are produced; however, the reaction is mild. This is presumably due to the fact that the antibodies are filtered by the local cartilage matrix and fail to reach the chondrocyte (Elves, 1976). According to some authors, this makes tissue typing and immunologic suppression unnecessary in cases (Langer, 1975). Transplantation of bone is, similarly, associated with an immunologic response. However, most authors believe that this reaction is not clinically significant (Garrett, 1998). The immunogenicity resulting from histocompatibility antigens is reduced by deep-freezing the allograft prior to implantation, and responses are diminished even further when tissues are freeze-dried. Collagen itself may also act as an immunogen. The magnitude and significance of these immunogens are a matter of speculation. The significance of osteochondral allograft immunogenicity, as compared with biomechanical factors in the incorporation of a bone graft, has not yet been elucidated (Friedlaender, 1983).

Technical considerations

Osteochondral allografting can be used to treat articular lesions in many locations (i.e. knee, shoulder, ankle). Although mainly used for femoral condylar defects, it has also been described for patellar defects and tibial plateau lesions. Condylar lesions ideal for osteochondral allografting are typically those between 2–3 cm in diameter. These lesions are traumatic in origin or represent an osteochondritis dessicans lesion. Bony disorders such as AVN may result in chondral damage and are also well suited for osteochondral grafting.

The surgical approach is based upon the identification of a symptomatic chondral lesion either by prior surgery or MRI. The femur is approached through a minimal parapatellar arthrotomy. Using commercially available equipment, an appropriately sized cylindrical guide is placed over the defect and a wire is placed through the guide and driven into the center of the articular defect. A powered reamer is used to sharply create a host defect followed by a reamer for penetrating and preparing the bony bed (Figure 27.3). The resulting bed is usually about 5–10 mm deep (up to 15 mm). Since the condyle is not flat, the depth will also vary within the defect. We usually measure the depth at the 12, 4, and 8 o'clock positions and mark them for reference when orienting the graft. The defect is then matched with the corresponding location on the donor condyle (thus obtaining an orthotopic graft). A core reaming device is then used to harvest the osteochondral bone plug. The result is a composite, cylindrical graft of articular cartilage and subchondral bone (Figure 27.4). The graft is then matched to the defect with respect to depth (at the 12, 4, and 8 o'clock positions).

Fig. 27.3

In clinical cases, condylar lesions were identified. These lesions were prepared for allograft transplantation by creating a cylindrical defect that is approximately 8–10 mm deep.

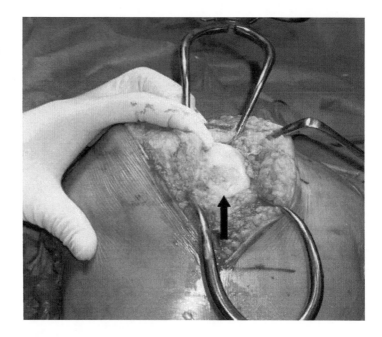

The graft height may need to be adjusted if it is too proud and this can be done with an oscillating saw to remove excess bone. If, on the other hand the graft is recessed within the defect, bone graft may be needed to build up the bed to obtain a flush graft that is flush with the defect.

Most grafts are stable with a press fit, however, some may need to be secured with headless screws. These screws also provide compression if the graft is slightly proud, without the problem of prominent screw heads on the cartilage surface. The screws are countersunk so that early motion can be started, but without making later removal of the screws too difficult. Some authors have advocated bioabsorbable pin fixation, however this option does not provide the compression that the screws offer.

For larger osteochondral defects, especially those of the far posterior condyles, customized full-width condylar osteochondral allografts have been used. However, the clinical results with these grafts are not as predictable as with the dowel allografts.

Clinical results

The largest series of osteochondral allografts have been those using fresh shell allografts. Meyers and Convery reported on their series of 59 fresh osteochondral allografts which were consecutively transplanted into the knees of 58 patients. The preoperative diagnoses consisted of chondromalacia or degenerative arthritis of the patella, osteochondritis dissecans, a traumatic defect or osteonecrosis of the

(a)

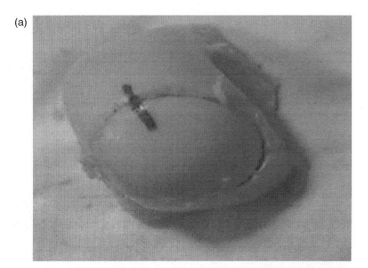

Fig. 27.4a–b
A size matched whole femoral condyle is used to obtain a cylindrical osteochondral specimen (a); this donor allograft is then press-fit into the defect to reconstruct the cartilage surface (b).

(b)

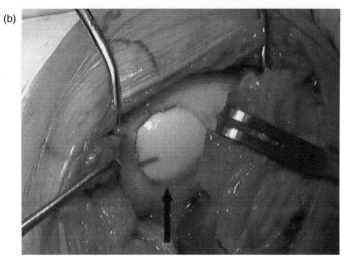

femoral condyle, a painful healed depressed fracture or traumatic defect of the tibial plateau, and unicompartmental traumatic arthritis of the knee. All of the patients had failed previous surgical attempts to treat the problem. Thirty-nine patients with 40 knees were evaluated with a minimum two year follow-up (2–10 yrs). Thirty-one out of 40 knees (77.5 per cent) had successful outcomes. For the patients in the group with traumatic unicompartmental arthritis, the results were not very good, with only 30 per cent successful outcomes. Thus, the authors concluded that fresh shell osteochondral allografting was a satisfactory treatment option for the previously named conditions, with the exception of traumatic arthritis (Meyers *et al.*, 1989). Convery later narrowed the focus of his review on the same group of patients. He looked specifically at those patients with femoral condylar lesions treated with fresh osteochondral allografting with a minimum five year follow-up. Of the 12 transplants in the group, three were lost to follow-up. Eight of the nine knees evaluated rated good or excellent. Technical insufficiencies were cited as the cause of the one poor clinical result. (Convery *et al.*, 1991b). The University of San Diego experience was reviewed by Chu *et al.* in 1999 (Chu *et al.*, 1999). The results of 55 consecutive patients with fresh osteochondral allografts were reviewed at just over six year follow-up. Patients with malalignment were excluded from the study, and the majority of patients were under 45 years of age. Overall, 76 per cent of the knees were rated as good or excellent. Unipolar transplants did significantly better (84 per cent good or excellent) compared with the bipolar group (only 50 per cent good or excellent).

Beaver *et al.* reviewed Toronto's experience with the use of fresh osteochondral allografting, reviewing 92 cases of post-traumatic chondral defects treated with the osteochondral allograft technique (Beaver *et al.*, 1992). Patients with malalignment were also treated with simultaneous osteotomies. They reported a 75 per cent success rate at 5 years, 64 per cent at 10 years and 63 per cent at 14 years. As with Chu's study, Beaver *et al.* found that unipolar transplants did significantly better than bipolar grafts. They also found poorer results in the group of patients over 60 years of age (Beaver *et al.*, 1992).

Also from Toronto, Ghazavi reported on fresh osteochondral allografting in 123 patients with 126 knees (Ghazavi *et al.*, 1997). The average age of the patients was 35 years and the mean follow-up was 7.5 years (range 2–20 yrs). Eight-five percent of the knees were rated as having successful outcomes and 15 per cent failed. Significant factors related to failure included; age greater than 50 years, bipolar transplants, varus/valgus malalignment, and workman's compensation. Based on their results, the authors recommended using fresh osteochondral allografts in patients with unipolar post-traumatic osteochondral defects of the knee in young patients.

Take-home message

There are limited options for treating full-thickness chondral lesions. Though fresh osteochondral allografts seem to be the best graft source, they are difficult to obtain and thus a represent a limited option. The problems with rapid harvest, donor matching, quality control, and graft transportation are major barriers in the way of making this a viable treatment option for most patients and surgeons. Fresh cold-stored grafts seem to be the second best choice. What are the potential pitfalls of cold storage? There is less cell viability in these grafts, and the question of 'how much is enough?' remains to be answered. For the time being the answer seems to be 'as much as possible'.

With the introduction of commercially available fresh cold-stored specimens, the option of osteochondral allografting for cartilage defects became available on a nationwide level. Though the chondrocyte survival rates are not 100 per cent (as have been reported for the fresh grafts transplanted within 24 hours), they are significantly better than the frozen or cryopreserved alternatives. Commercial package inserts quote cell survivals of 55 per cent at 45 days (Cryolife, 1998). Our experience seems to suggest that the grafts should be used within 28 days since, in our study, the cell survival percentage consistently dropped off significantly after 28 days post-harvest. Currently, no published reports are available on the clinical outcome of patients who have received stored allograft tissue for the treatment of chondral and osteochondral defects. The senior author has implanted over 20 such grafts dating from 1998. A preliminary review of the MRI appearance of over 15 patients (minimum one year follow-up) demonstrated poor bony incorporation of these grafts as late as four years following implantation. However, in most cases the articular cartilage MRI appearance remains iso-intense compared to the surrounding native cartilage. Furthermore, the MRI appearance of these grafts does not appear to correlate with validate knee outcomes measures (unpublished data). Consequently, while the authors believe that there is a role for the use of these grafts in the treatment of symptomatic knee lesions, caution and care should be employed with their use. Quite frankly, until proven otherwise with clinical outcome studies, we believe that these grafts should be considered as a salvage reconstruction option.

Osteochondral allografting is a single-stage procedure which replaces the articular defect with an orthotopic graft of hyaline cartilage containing viable chondrocytes. None of the other surgical options (microfracture, mosaicplasty, ACI) have all of these advantages. In addition, osteochondral allografts are especially useful in cases where the subchondral bone is injured, allowing bone-to-bone healing via creeping substitution from healthy underlying bone. Based on the literature reviewing fresh osteochondral allografts, our indications for using fresh cold-stored osteochondral allografts to resurface full-thickness cartilage defects (>2 cm^2) are patients with unipolar defects due to trauma, avascular necrosis or osteochondritis dessicans with grafts that have been stored no longer than ~28 days in culture.

References

Amiel D, Courts RD, Abel M: Rib perichondrial grafts for the repair of full-thickness articular cartilage defects: A morphological and biochemical assessment in rabbits. *J Bone Joint Surg Am* 67A: 911–20, 1985.

Beaver RJ, Mahomed M, Backstein D, Davis A, Zukor D, Gross A: Fresh osteochondral allografts for post-traumatic defects in the knee. A survivorship analysis. *J Bone Joint Surg Br* 74: 105–10, 1992.

Brittberg M, Lindahl A, Nilsson A, Ohlsson C, Isaksson O, Peterson L: Treatment of deep cartilage defects in the knee with autologous chondrocyte transplantation. *N Engl J Med* 331: 889–95, 1994.

Buckwalter JA, Mankin, HJ: Articular cartilage: Degeneration and osteoarthritis, repair, regeneration, and transplantation. *Instr Course Lect* 47: 487–504, 1998.

Buckwalter JA, Mow VC, Ratcliffe A: Restoration of injured or degenerated articular cartilage. *J Am Acad Orthop Surg* 2: 192–201, 1994.

Burwell RG, Friedlaender GE, Mankin HJ: Current perspectives and future directions: The 1983 Invitational Conference on osteochondral allografts. *Clin Orthop* 67: 141–57, 1985.

Chen AC NJ, Schinagl RM, Lounan LM, Sah RL: Chondrocyte transplantation to articular cartilage explants in vitro. *J Orthop Res* 15: 791–802, 1997.

Chu CR, Convery FR, Akeson WH, Meyers M, Amiel D: Articular cartilage transplantation. Clinical results in the knee. *Clin Orthop* 360: 159–68, 1999.

Chu CR, Coutts RD, Yoshioka M, Harwood F, Monosov A, Amiel D: Articular cartilage repair using allogeneic perichondrocyte-seeded biodegradable porous polylactic acid (PLA): A tissue-engineering study. *J Biomed Mater Res* 29: 1147–54, 1995.

Convery FR, Akeson WH, Amiel D, Meyers M, Monosov A: Long-term survival of chondrocytes in an osteochondral articular cartilage allograft. A case report. *J Bone Joint Surg Am* 78: 1082–8, 1996.

Convery FR, Meyers MH, Akeson WH: Fresh osteochondral allografting of the femoral condyle. *Clin Orthop* 74: 139–45, 1991.

Curl WW, Krome J, Gordon ES, *et al.*: Cartilage injuries: A review of 31,516 knee arthroscopies. *Arthroscopy* 13: 456–60, 1997.

Czitrom AA, Keating S, Gross AE: The viability of articular cartilage in fresh osteochondral allografts after clinical transplantation. *J Bone Joint Surg Am* 72: 574–81, 1990.

Elves MW: Newer knowledge of the immunology of bone and cartilage. *Clin Orthop* 120: 232–59, 1976.

Farnworth L: Osteochondral defects of the knee. *Orthopedics* 23: 146–57; quiz 158–9, 2000.

Friedlaender GE: Immune responses to osteochondral allografts. Current knowledge and future directions. *Clin Orthop* 35: 58–68, 1983.

Ganel A, Israeli A, Horoszowski H, Farine I: Osteochondral graft in the treatment of osteonecrosis of the femoral condyle. *J Am Geriatr Soc* 29: 186–8, 1981.

Garrett JC: Osteochondral allografts for reconstruction of articular defects of the knee. *Instr Course Lect* 47: 517–22, 1998.

Geissler WB WT: Intraarticular abnormalities in association with posterior cruciate ligament injuries. *Am J Sports Med* 21: 846–9, 1993.

Ghazavi MT, Pritzker KP, Davis AM, Gross A.: Fresh osteochondral allografts for post-traumatic osteochondral defects of the knee. *J Bone Joint Surg Br* 79: 1008–13, 1997.

Gillogly SD, Voight M, Blackburn T: Treatment of articular cartilage defects of the knee with autologous chondrocyte implantation. *J Orthop Sports Phys Ther* 28: 241–51, 1998.

Hangody L, Kish G, Karpati Z, Eberhart R: Osteochondral plugs: autogenous osteochondral mosaicplasty for the treatment of focal chondral and osteochondral articular defects. *Operative Tech Orthop* 7: 312–22, 1997.

Hangody L, Feczko P, Bartha L, Bodo G, Kish G: Mosaicplasty for the treatment of articular defects of the knee and ankle. *Clin Orthop* S328–36, 2001.

Hangody L, Kish G, Karpati Z, Udvarhelyi I, Szigeti I, Bely M: Mosaicplasty for the treatment of articular cartilage defects: Application in clinical practice. *Orthopedics* 21: 751–6, 1998.

Highgenboten CL, Jackson A, Aschliman M, Meske M: The estimation of femoral condyle size. An important component in osteochondral allografts. *Clin Orthop* 71: 225–33, 1989.

Hunter W: On the structure and diseases of articulating cartilage. *Philos Trans R Soc Lond B Biol Sci* 9: 267, 1743.

Indelicate P, Bittar E: A perspective of lesions associated with ACL insufficiency of the knee. *Clin Orthop* 198: 77–80, 1985.

Langer F, Czitrom A, Pritzker KP, Gross AE: The immunogenicity of fresh and frozen allogeneic bone. *J Bone Joint Surg Am* 57: 216–20, 1975.

Langer F, Gross A: Immunogenicity of allograft articular cartilage. *J Bone Joint Surg Am* 56: 297–304, 1974.

Lewandrowski K, Muller J, Schollmeier G: Concomitant meniscal and articular lesions of the tibiofemoral joint. *Am J Sports Med* 25: 486–94, 1997.

Locht RC, Gross AE, Langer F: Late osteochondral allograft resurfacing for tibial plateau fractures. *J Bone Joint Surg Am* 66: 328–35, 1984.

Malinin TI, Wagner JL, Pita JC, Lo H: Hypothermic storage and cryopreservation of cartilage. An experimental study. *Clin Orthop* 197: 15–26, 1985.

Mankin HJ, Meachim G, Roberts C: Repair of the surface from subarticular tissue in rabbit knee. *J Anat* 104: 317–27, 1971.

Mankin HJ: The reaction of articular cartilage to injury and osteoarthritis. *N Engl J Med* 291: 1285–92, 1974.

Mankin HJ: The response of articular cartilage to mechanical injury. *J Bone Joint Surg Am* 64: 460–6, 1982.

Mankin HJ, Mow VC, Buckwalter JA, Iannotti J, Ratcliffe A: Form and function of articular cartilage. *AAOS Orthopaedic Basic Science, Rosemont, Ill* 3–41, 1994.

Marco F, Leon C, Lopez-Oliva F, Perez A, Sanchez-Barba A, Lopez-Duran Stern L: Intact articular cartilage cryopreservation. In vivo evaluation. *Clin Orthop* 197: 11–20, 1992.

Matthewson MH, Dandy D: Osteochondral fractures of the lateral femoral condyle: A result of indirect violence on the knee. *J Bone Joint Surg Br* 60: 199–202, 1978.

Menche DS, Vangsness C, Pitman M, Gross AK, Peterson L: The treatment of isolated articular cartilage lesions in the young individual. *Instr Course Lect* 47: 505–15, 1998.

Meyers MH, Akeson W, Convery FR: Resurfacing of the knee with fresh osteochondral allograft. *J Bone Joint Surg Am* 71: 704–13, 1989.

Meyers MH, Jones RE, Bucholz RW, Wegner D: Fresh autogenous grafts and osteochondral allografts for the treatment of segmental collapse in osteonecrosis of the hip. *Clin Orthop* 197: 107–12, 1983.

Micheli LJ, Browne JE, Erggelet C, Fu F, Mandelbaum B, Moseley J, Zurankowsi D: Autologous chondrocyte implantation of the knee: Multicenter experience and minimum 3-year follow-up. *Clin J Sport Med* 11: 223–8, 2001.

Milgram JW, Rogers L, Miller JW: Osteochondral fractures: Mechanisms of injury and fate of fragments. *Am J Roentgenol* 130: 651–8, 1978.

Minas T: The role of cartilage repair techniques, including chondrocyte transplantation, in focal chondral knee damage. *Instr Course Lect* 48: 629–43, 1999.

Minas T: Autologous chondrocyte implantation for focal chondral defects of the knee. *Clin Orthop* S349–61, 2001.

Muellner T, Knopp A, Ludvigsen TC, Engebretsen L: Failed autologous chondrocyte implantation. Complete atraumatic graft delamination after two years. *Am J Sports Med* 29: 516–19, 2001.

Muldrew K, Chung M, Novak K, Schachar NS, Zernicke RF, McGann LE, Rattner JB, Matyas JR: Evidence of chondrocyte repopulation in adult ovine articular cartilage following cryoinjury and long-term transplantation. *Osteoarthritis Cartilage* 9: 432–9, 2001.

Noyes FR, Bassett R, Grood ED: Arthroscopy in acute traumatic hemarthrosis of the knee. Incidence of ACL and other injuries. *J Bone Joint Surg Am* 62: 687–95, 1980.

Oakeshott RD, Farine I, Pritzker KP: A clinical and histologic analysis of failed fresh osteochondral allografts. *Clin Orthop* 233: 283–94, 1988.

Oates KM, Chen AC, Young EP, Kwan M, Amiel D, Convery F: Effect of tissue culture storage on the in vivo survival of canine osteochondral allografts. *J Orthop Res* 13: 562–9, 1995.

Ohlendorf C, Tomford WW, Mankin HJ: Chondrocyte survival in cryopreserved osteochondral articular cartilage. *J Orthop Res* 14: 413–16, 1996.

Peterson L, Minas T, Brittberg M, Nilsson A, Sjogren-Jansson E, Lindahl A: Two- to 9-year outcome after autologous chondrocyte transplantation of the knee. *Clin Orthop* 374: 212–34, 2000.

Peterson L, Brittberg M, Kiviranta I, Akerlund EL, Lindahl A: Autologous chondrocyte transplantation. Biomechanics and durability. *Am J Sports Med* 30: 2–12, 2002.

Potter HG, Linklater JM, Allen AA, Hannafin J, Haas S: Magnetic resonance imaging of articular cartilage in the knee. An evaluation with use of fast-spin-echo imaging. *J Bone Joint Surg Am* 80: 1276–84, 1998.

Rodrigo JJ, Thompson E, Travis C: Deep freezing vs. 4 degree C preservation of avascular osteocartilaginous shell allografts in rats. *Clin Orthop* 218: 268–75, 1987.

Sammarco VJ, Gorab R, Miller R, Brooks P: Human articular cartilage storage in cell culture medium: guidelines for storage of fresh osteochondral allografts. *Orthopedics* 20: 497–500, 1997.

Schachar NS, Cucheran DJ, McGann LE, Novak K, Frank C: Metabolic activity of bovine articular cartilage during refrigerated storage. *J Orthop Res* 12: 15–20, 1994.

Schachar NS, Novak K, Hurtig M, Muldrew K, McPherson R, Wohl G, Zernicke R, McGann L: Transplantation of cryopreserved osteochondral Dowel allografts for repair of focal articular defects in an ovine model. *J Orthop Res* 17: 909–19, 1999.

Steadman JR, Rodkey WG, Briggs KK, Rodrigo J: The microfracture technic in the management of complete cartilage defects in the knee joint. *Orthopade* 28: 26–32, 1999.

Stevenson S, Dannucci GA, Sharkey NA, Pool R: The fate of articular cartilage after transplantation of fresh and cryopreserved tissueantigen-matched and mismatched osteochondral allografts in dogs. *J Bone Joint Surg Am* 71: 1297–307, 1989.

Strong DM, Friedlaender GE, Tomford WW, Springfield D, Shives T, Burchardt H, Enneking W, Mankin H: Immunologic responses in human recipients of osseous and osteochondral allografts. *Clin Orthop* 14: 107–14, 1996.

Tomford WW, Fredericks G, Mankin HJ: Studies on cryopreservation of articular cartilage chondrocytes. *J Bone Joint Surg Am* 66: 253–9, 1984.

Vacanti C, Langer, R, Schloo, B, Vacanti, JP: Synthetic polymers seeded with chondrocytes provide a template for new cartilage formation. *J Plast Reconstr Surg* 88: 753–9, 1989.

Vellet AD, Marks P, Fowler PJ, Munro TG: Occult posttraumatic osteo-chondral injuries of the knee: Prevalence, classification, and long term sequelae evaluated with MR imaging. *Radiology* 178: 271–6, 1991.

Williams RJ III, Dreese J, McCarthy D, Petrigliano F, Chen C: Chondrocyte survival and biomechanical properties of fresh cold-stored condylar specimens. *Am J Sports Med* 32(1): 132–9, 2004.

Part 8. Complex Knee Injury

28

Is it best to surgically address all injured ligaments in the acute injury period?

R. Verdonk and F. Almqvist

Introduction

For any substantial and significant knee injury the attending orthopaedic surgeon should be aware of the potential for secondary or concomitant injuries which may occur or which may not be immediately apparent without careful assessment. This chapter will address the indications and advantages of treating all the injuries in the acute phase. Factors which determine the optimum management include the presence of open or closed ligament ruptures and the extent, degree and age of these lesions. The patient's age, occupation and current and potential level of sports activities, all play a role in deciding whether or not to operate. Moreover, the surgeon should realize the need for rehabilitation to regain the preinjury level of knee function. This may militate against surgical intervention.

In these complicated combined knee injuries it is of major importance to rely on a full history, examination and investigation to make the correct diagnosis, taking into account the individual's profession and level of sports involvement. Clinical examination in the hands of experienced surgeons may be able to determine the nature and extent of the injuries. However evaluation and grading of the knee joint under anaesthesia will allow more appropriate clinical grading, and may allow more accurate surgical planning and planning of rehabilitation. An arthroscopic investigation is sometimes necessary to make a final diagnosis. This may be the case in complex injuries such as anterior and posterior cruciate ligament (ACL/PCL) injuries or those in which there is articular cartilage damage. In the initial assessment of patients we use and would recommend a simple system of patient classification which categorizes the level of sports participation. The French CLAS system distinguishes between competitive athletes, leisure-time sportsmen (recreational athletes), active patients and sedentary persons, and rates the results 'C', 'L', 'A', or 'S' accordingly.

In our current practice x-ray imaging is mandatory – MRI evaluation is not currently mandatory for the investigation of these injuries but may prove to be very helpful. MRI may tend to over-rate and over-diagnose the potential soft tissue damage present. However the identification of adjacent or subchondral bone marrow oedema implies more severe trauma or articular cartilage damage which identifies the need for further investigation or inspection at the time of arthroscopy. Thus MRI is effective and helpful in allowing for a more detailed and complete diagnosis and allows better planning of any surgical or non-surgical treatment and rehabilitation.

Consideration of the early post-injury period is dependant upon the degree and extent of trauma, the injury, odema, swelling and stiffness produced. Although early presentation and management within three weeks is considered in this chapter, this time period is not an absolute cut-off period of time. The initial early and acute period following the injury where there is pain, swelling, stiffness and inflammation may take a prolonged period to dissipate. The casual reader should keep these arbitrary time periods in perspective.

Ligament injuries

Several approaches to the classification of multiple injuries of the knee are possible. One could consider the injuries according to aetiology and divide them according to varus and valgus trauma and/or a rotational component (Figure 28.1). Other approaches include consideration of the deforming force whether varus or valgus, but also categorize the position of the knee at the time of injury in terms of knee flexion and weight-bearing (Segal and Jakob 1983). A third approach is to consider the nature of multiple injuries according to sports-specific activities such as pivoting and non-pivoting sports. Thus the injury classification takes account of the desired activity

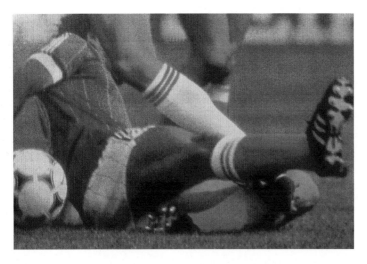

Fig. 28.1
One could consider the associated ligament injuries according to etiology, divide them according to varus and valgus trauma and add a rotational component.

required for complete rehabilitation and return to sport at the same level of competition. For simplicity this chapter will use the anatomical classification of knee injuries.

Medial collateral ligament injuries and associated lesions

In the treatment of isolated and solitary medial collateral ligament injuries (MCL) the current approach is adequate pain control, anti-inflammatory medication, rest and support. In grade two and three lesions a supporting brace and some restriction of movement in the early phase may be required. Consideration of anti-thrombotic treatment is necessary. Vigorous rehabilitation is needed but surgical intervention is not required (Figure 28.2).

Diagnosis

O'Donoghue (1950, 1955, 1973) originally described the unhappy triad of knee injuries, and the unhappy pentad when the injury was extensive and could almost be compared to a knee dislocation. The unhappy triad was a medial meniscal tear, medial collateral ligament injury and an anterior cruciate ligament tear. It has become apparent over the course of time that even though meticulous surgical techniques may be used, the acute combined surgical repair of acute intraarticular and extraarticular injuries such as these results in an increase in the incidence of arthrofibrosis, a restricted range of motion and a poor functional result. It is also clear that conservative management of MCL injuries, even in combination with extensive

Fig. 28.2
The treatment of solitary medial collateral ligament sprains and ruptures will not be considered in this chapter.

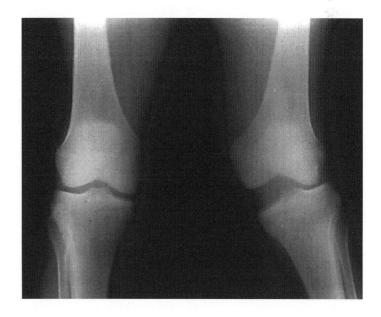

intraarticular lacerations, will result in a good result unless the ligament is completely ruptured and spontaneous end-to-end repair is not likely (Frank *et al.* 1991, Walsh *et al.* 1993). The ability to distinguish whether end-to-end apposition is present relies upon the experience of the orthopaedic surgeon, and an examination under anaesthesia. Significant MCL laxity in the position of knee extension illustrates this dramatic situation, and the requirement for surgical intervention. If laxity is only present in 30° of flexion and not in extension, only partial dehiscence of the MCL has occurred and a more conservative management would be adopted. If laxity is present in full extension the medial and posterior medial ligaments are torn and it is very often the case that the ACL is also ruptured. This extensive injury requires surgical repair of all the damaged structures.

Surgical technique

In the surgical reconstruction of the MCL a variety of surgical skin incisions can be utilized – the hockeystick approach, the reversed hockeystick or a straight medial parapatellar skin incision. All these approaches provide full visualization of the medial and postero-medial corner of the knee. After a T-shaped incision to the superficial fascia, in severe cases a traumatic arthrotomy may be evident with rupture of the collateral ligament and knee capsule. The MCL rupture is often apparent in the surgical field. However the point of damage to the deep part of the MCL may not be apparent if the superficial part of the ligament is intact. A prior arthroscopy can be helpful in determining the site of MCL rupture and obviate the need for extensive exposure. At arthroscopy the injury may be directly visualized but more commonly the meniscus will move under a valgus stress as the knee is opened. The meniscuses will either stay with the tibial plateau or the femoral condyle, dependent on which of the coronal ligaments remains intact. Commonly the ligament is either damaged at its insertion to the medial epicondyle or to the tibial insertion some distance below the medial joint line. It is important to repair the MCL in full, but also to repair the posterior oblique part of the MCL ligament. This is particularly important to provide stability to varus stress in the position of knee extension. The repair to the bone uses non-resorbable sutures anchored sub-periosteally by suture anchors, mid substance tears are repaired directly.

Anterior cruciate ligament injury and associated lesions

Can ACL rupture occur as a solitary knee ligament injury?

Extensive literature is available suggesting traumatic haemarthrosis to be a sign very commonly indicative of ACL injury (Casteleyn and Handelberg 1989, 1995, Järvinen 1997, Abbot *et al.* 1944,

Casteleyn *et al.* 1988, DeHaven 1980, Fowler 1994, Noyes *et al.* 1980). However where capsular disruption has occurred any haemarthrosis may dissipate throughout the tissues (Figure 28.3). The clinical evaluation of an ACL injury may be misleading in that instability may not be initially present due to muscle spasm, pain and swelling. Unless this is remembered and a very careful examination undertaken in the acute phase ACL injury may be missed. An examination under anaesthetic or a repeat examination after a week or two may be necessary. However clinical examination remains the standard measurement for identification and classification of these injuries and so bias remains in many of the rigid protocols and in the evaluation of results from many centres. It is worthy of note that partial ligament injuries such as grade one and two are often more painful than knees in which complete rupture of ligaments has occurred. In these cases often manifest laxity is present, but no remaining structures are intact to mediate pain through the pain and stretch nociceptors.

Surgical technique

When major AP laxity is found by clinical evaluation and also illustrated at investigation under anaesthesia, treatment with post-traumatic inflammatory measures is initiated for a brief duration of 2–3 weeks. However, if major ligament disruption to the MCL, LCL or PCL is present (see MCL rupture association), acute intervention to address these associated injuries is necessary. For patients with a desire to return to high-level activities including pivoting sports ACL reconstruction is necessary and can be planned to be undertaken after three weeks of rest, support, pain relief and regaining a degree of motion. It should however be remembered that some knees take longer than three weeks to settle down, become less swollen and regain a significant range of motion and surgery should be delayed until this has been achieved. If surgery is delayed for more than

Fig. 28.3

Massive swelling of the knee joint most often illustrates intact capsular structures suggesting intact peripheral ligament structures.

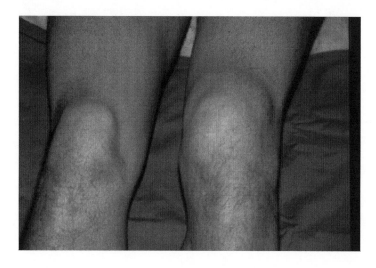

six weeks, the anatomic extraarticular structures cannot be easily recognized. With any surgical intervention vigorous rehabilitation is necessary to avoid arthrofibrosis and stiffness. The type of surgical reconstruction depends entirely on the surgeon's preference, however it is commonly recognized that ACL suturing is insufficient (Grontvedt *et al.* 1996), but that stability may be reliably achieved by autograft reconstruction of the ACL (Aglietti *et al.* 1997, Bach *et al.* 1998, Eriksson 1998, Frank and Jackson 1997, Kornblatt *et al.* 1988, Noyes and Barber-Westin 1997, Noyes *et al.* 1980, Otto *et al.* 1998, Shelbourne and Gray 1997), or by use of an allograft (Shino *et al.* 1997, Steenbrugge *et al.* 2001, Vorlat *et al.* 1999, Verdonk 1994, Stäubli *et al.* 1996, Tomford 1995, Victor *et al.* 1997).

Posterior cruciate ligament injury and associated lesions

Isolated PCL ruptures do occur, albeit uncommonly. One such injury is the avulsion of the tibial PCL insertion with a fragment of tibia from the tibia. This injury is usually produced by a traumatic hyperflexion injury. The bone fragment can be successfully reinserted, fixed with a screw and early mobilization can be undertaken (Figures 28.4 and 28.5). Otherwise PCL injury is commonly associated with other injuries including the posterior lateral complex, popliteus and the ACL.

Diagnosis

Accurate history-taking and consideration of the mechanism of injury will alert the surgeon to the possibility of a combined PCL rupture.

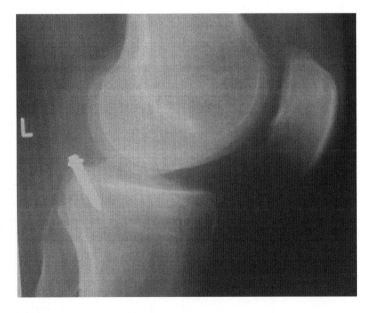

Fig. 28.4

A bony avulsion of the posterior cruciate ligament was repaired by stapling.

Fig. 28.5
The reconstructed PCL results in an almost symmetrical posterior shift on Puddu–Chambat x-ray incidence.

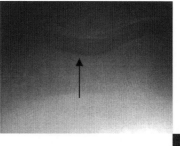

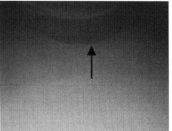

When clinical evidence of lateral corner dehiscence, injury to the popliteus or posterior lateral complex is present, this may require confirmation by examination under anaesthesia. It is thought that this combination leads to significant symptomatic posterior cruciate ligament laxity and posterior lateral rotatory laxity, therefore surgical reconstruction in the early period is undertaken in the young patient and active athlete. Refraining from early surgery is probably the most effective approach in patients who are older, less active, not involved in cutting sports or who wish to avoid potential major knee surgery.

Surgery

A straight lateral parapatellar incision provides proper visualization of the posterolateral corner and makes repair possible. The extended approach allows for open PCL reconstruction using auto- or allografts potentially in association with a posterior approach (Van Den Bossche *et al.* 1991, Eriksson *et al.* 1986, Roth *et al.* 1988). In some cases arthroscopically assisted PCL repair is advisable according to the surgeon's choice and experience. However in the acute setting where extensive capsular tearing has occurred extensive extravasation of arthroscopic fluid into the calf may restrict the duration of arthroscopy to a brief cursory inspection.

Lateral collateral ligament injury and associated lesions

Significant lateral collateral ligament rupture is uncommon. In a valgus knee or one in which there is no lateral thrust on weight-bearing repair may not be necessary (Müller 1983, Jakob and Stäubli 1992).

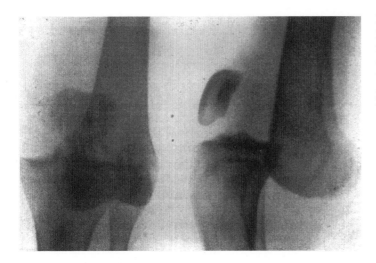

Fig. 28.6
Except in the event of open
knee dislocation and vascular
disruption, surgery could be
unnecessary once reduction
and temporary immobilization
have been achieved.

However the lateral LCL is often injured in association with a motor
vehicle accident, major knee injury and knee dislocation. In the varus
knee or one with a lateral thrust on weight-bearing surgical reconstruction and careful delayed return to weight-bearing is necessary. In
association with any LCL injury a careful assessment of the function
of the common peroneal nerve is mandatory.

Diagnosis and repair

If surgical intervention is necessary in the acute stage because of the
extent of the knee injury and extensive laxity then this should be
undertaken once limb viability has been secured (Figure 28.6).
In such injuries where the LCL has been injured damage to the
common peroneal nerve is not uncommon. This may require in
extensive injuries repair of the PCL, ACL, collateral ligaments,
nerves and vessels. In these circumstances end-to-end repair of the
LCL is unsuccessful and a reconstruction using hamstring or
bone-patellar tendon-bone graft is required. In less severe injuries
non-operative management of the LCL injury can be undertaken
with support and early range of motion. Subsequent reexamination
and assessment of the knee after two or three weeks will determine
the extent and nature of the injury and allow later reconstruction if
appropriate.

Discussion

According to the literature and personal experience, there exists no
simple obvious and straightforward surgical or non-surgical
approach for the many situations where there are multiple and
complex knee ligament injuries. Therefore each case must be
considered on an individual basis with the management based on

general principles taking account of the lifestyle, sport activities and aspirations of the individual. The patient's history and the clinical findings on examination may not be adequate for a thorough understanding of any particular knee. It is our practice to commonly utilize an examination under anaesthesia to determine the full nature of the injury. In the acute setting where the anatomy is disturbed and disguised by haemorrhage, it is mandatory to recognize the surgical difficulties and surgery in the acute situation demands considerable surgical experience and expertise. An individual program of supervised mobilization, splintage or bracing and rehabilitation should follow surgical repair.

Conclusion

The management of the acute knee with multiple ligament injuries is difficult and demands a degree of experience and expertise. The clinical evaluation is pivotal but may be helped by MRI investigation and an examination under anaesthetic. There are no universally accepted, straightforward or simple indications for the surgical treatment of multiple knee ligament injuries in the acute phase. Knee dislocation or extensive complete rupture of multiple ligaments requires stabilization in the acute phase once limb viability has been secured. This is best achieved by reconstruction of all injuries and early mobilization. Injuries in which the PCL is ruptured in association with a bony avulsion, ACL avulsion or posterio-lateral dehiscence necessitates surgical reconstruction in the acute phase. Lateral collateral ligament injuries when associated with major limb disruption, dislocation or nerve damage should be reconstructed as part of the multiple ligament repair in the acute phase. This should be undertaken by reconstruction rather than end-to-end repair other than in a valgus knee. Otherwise LCL reconstruction in the acute phase is not necessary. The medial collateral ligament rupture in association with ACL injury does not require surgery at that time unless it is associated with other ligament injuries or if the knee is completely disrupted and unstable in extension.

References

Abbot LC, Saunders JB, Bost FC and Anderson CE (1944). Injuries to the ligaments of the knee joint. *Journal of Bone and Joint Surgery*, 26A, 503–21.

Aglietti P, Buzzi R, Giron F, Simeone AJ and Zaccherotti G (1997). Arthroscopic-assisted anterior cruciate ligament reconstruction with the central third patellar tendon. A 5–8 year follow-up. *Knee Surgery, Sports Traumatology, Arthroscopy*, 5, 138–44.

Bach BR, Tradonsky S, Bojchuk J, Levy ME, Bush-Joseph CA and Kahn NH (1998). Arthroscopically assisted anterior cruciate ligament reconstruction using patellar tendon autograft. Five-to-nine year follow-up evaluation. *American Journal of Sports Medicine*, 26, 20–29.

Castelyn PP and Handelberg F (1989). Arthroscopy in the diagnosis of occult dislocation of the patella. *Acta Orthopaedica Belgica*, 55, 381–83.

Casteleyn PP and Handelberg F (1995). Place de l'arthroscopie dans le diagnostic et le traitement des luxations fraiches de la rotule. *Annales de la Société Française d'Arthroscopie*, 5, 59–61.

Casteleyn PP, Handelberg F and Opdecam P (1988). Traumatic haemarthrosis of the knee. *Journal of Bone and Joint Surgery*, 70B, 404–06.

DeHaven KE (1980). Diagnosis of acute knee injuries with hemarthrosis. *American Journal of Sports Medicine*, 8, 9–14.

Eriksson E (1998). Will we never learn? *Knee Surgery, Sports Traumatology, Arthroscopy*, 6, 67.

Eriksson E, Haeggmark T and Johnson RJ (1986). Reconstruction of the posterior cruciate ligament. *Orthopaedics*, 9, 217–20.

Fowler PJ (1994). Bone injuries associated with anterior cruciate ligament disruption. *Arthroscopy*, 10, 453–60.

Frank CB and Jackson DW (1997). The science of reconstruction of the anterior cruciate ligament. *Journal of Bone and Joint Surgery*, 79A, 1556–76.

Frank C, MacFarlane B, Edwards P *et al.* (1991). A quantitative analysis of matrix alignment in ligament scars: a comparison of movement versus immobilization in a mature rabbit model. *Journal of Orthopaedic Research*, 9, 219–27.

Grontvedt T, Engebretsen L, Benum P, Fasting O, Molster A and Strand T (1996). A prospective randomized study of three operations for acute rupture of the anterior cruciate ligament. Five-year follow-up of one hundred and thirty-one patients. *Journal of Bone and Joint Surgery*, 78A, 159–68.

Jakob RP and Stäubli HU (eds) (1992). *The Knee and the Cruciate Ligaments: Anatomy, biomechanics and clinical aspects, reconstruction, complications, rehabilitation.* Springer Verlag, New York.

Järvinen M (1997). Acute patellar dislocation – closed or operative treatment? *Acta Orthopaedica Scandinavica*, 68, 415–18.

Kornblatt I, Warren RF and Wickiewicz TL (1988). Long-term follow-up of anterior cruciate ligament reconstruction using the quadriceps tendon substitution for chronic anterior cruciate ligament insufficiency. *American Journal of Sports Medicine*, 16, 444–48.

Müller W (1983). *The Knee: form, function and ligament reconstruction.* Springer, Berlin.

Noyes FR and Barber-Westin SD (1997). A comparison of results in acute and chronic anterior cruciate ligament ruptures of arthroscopically assisted autogenous patellar tendon reconstruction. *American Journal of Sports Medicine*, 25, 460–71.

Noyes FR, Basset RW, Grood ES and Butler DL (1980). Arthroscopy in acute traumatic haemarthrosis of the knee. Incidence of anterior cruciate tears and other injuries. *Journal of Bone and Joint Surgery*, 62A, 687–95.

O'Donoghue DH (1950). Surgical treatment of fresh injuries to major ligaments of the knee. *Journal of Bone and Joint Surgery*, 32A, 721–28.

O'Donoghue DH (1955). An analysis of end results of surgical treatment of major injuries to the ligaments of the knee. *Journal of Bone and Joint Surgery*, 37A, 1–13.

O'Donoghue DH (1973). Reconstruction for medial instability of the knee. Technique and results in 60 cases. *Journal of Bone and Joint Surgery*, 55A, 941–55.

Otto D, Pinczewski LA, Clingeleffer A and Odell R (1998). Five-year results of single-incision arthroscopic anterior cruciate ligament reconstruction with patellar tendon autograft. *American Journal of Sports Medicine*, 26, 181–88.

Roth JH, Bray RC, Best TM, Cunning LA and Jacobson RP (1988). Posterior cruciate ligament reconstruction by transfer of the medial gastrocnemius tendon. *American Journal of Sports Medicine*, 16, 21–28.

Segal P and Jacob M (1983). *Le genou*. Maloine SA, Paris.

Shelbourne KD and Gray T (1997). Anterior cruciate ligament reconstruction with autogenous patellar tendon graft followed by accelerated rehabilitation. A two- to-nine-year follow-up. *American Journal of Sports Medicine*, 25, 786–95.

Shino K, Horibe S, Nakata K, Maeda A, Nakamura N and Ozkar I (1997). Allograft anterior cruciate ligament reconstruction overview and current status. *Sports Medicine and Arthroscopy Review*, 5, 112–17.

Stäubli HU, Schatzmann L, Brunner P, Rincon L and Nolte LP (1996). Quadriceps tendon and patellar ligament: cryosectional anatomy and structural properties in young adults. *Knee Surgery, Sports Traumatology, Arthroscopy*, 4, 100–110.

Steenbrugge F, Verdonk R, Vorlat P, Mortier F and Verstraete K (2001). Repair of chronic ruptures of the anterior cruciate ligament using allograft reconstruction and a ligament augmentation device. *Acta Orthopaedica Belgica*, 67, 252–57.

Tomford WW (1995). Transmission of disease through transplantation of musculoskeletal allografts. *Journal of Bone and Joint Surgery*, 77A, 1742–54.

Van Den Bossche J, Vandendriessche G, Verdonk R and Claessens H (1991). Free patellar tendon graft reconstruction of the posterior cruciate ligament. *French Journal of Orthopaedic Surgery*, 5, 279–84.

Verdonk R (1994). Les allogreffes tendineuses dans la chirurgie du ligament croisé antérieur. *Annales de la Société Française d'Arthroscopie*, 4, 47–52.

Victor J, Bellemans J, Witvrouw E, Govaers K and Fabry G (1997). Graft selection in anterior cruciate ligament reconstruction – prospective analysis of patellar tendon autografts compared with allografts. *International Orthopaedics*, 21, 93–97.

Vorlat P, Verdonk R and Arnauw G (1999). Long-term results of tendon allografts for anterior cruciate ligament replacement in revision surgery and in cases of combined complex injuries. *Knee Surgery, Sports Traumatology, Arthroscopy*, 7, 318–22.

Walsh S, Frank C, Shrive N and Hart D (1993). Knee immobilization inhibits biomechanical maturation of the rabbit medial collateral ligament. *Clinical Orthopaedics*, 297, 253–61.

29

Chronic multi-ligament knee injuries are best treated using osteotomies about the knee

T. Ait Si Selmi, Ph. Neyret, G. Schuck de Freitas,
T. Lootens, and L. Jacquot

Introduction

The exact definition of chronic complex, multi-ligament knee injuries is still not absolutely clear, because such injuries can be caused by the injury of several ligaments at the time of the accident or are the result of sequential accidents at different moments in time, or of a slow increase in knee laxity over the course of time.

Lesions to secondary structures, for example the patellar tendon, meniscus, articular cartilage or bone bruises associated with a cruciate ligament injury, can also be considered as complex ligament injuries. In the same way, after several episodes of instability an anterior cruciate ligament (ACL)-deficient knee may develop progressive laxity of the postero-medial corner or a medial meniscus injury.

In this chapter we shall consider as chronic multi-ligament knee injuries their consequence and the chronic evolution of the acute 'triad', 'pentade' and luxation about the knee (Neyret 1996).

Today we have a therapeutic arsenal consisting of ligament reconstructions and osteotomies or a combination of both for the treatment of these difficult injuries. The individual lower limb alignment and the main component of the instability will determine which technique to use.

The 'triads' (anteromedial, anterolateral, posteromedial and posterolateral) are the most frequently encountered chronic multi-ligament injuries. Their evolution is very variable according to the type of ligament injury. Anterior instabilities are most frequently associated with sports traumas whereas posterior instabilities are mainly related to road traffic accidents.

Dislocation of the knee is rare (Kennedy 1963, Johner *et al.* 1992, Meyers *et al.* 1975, Taylor *et al.* 1972, Thomson *et al.* 1984), with a frequency of occurrence ranging from 1 in 150 000 to 1 in 50 000 hospital admissions (Conwell and Allredge 1937, Neyret *et al.* 2001).

Functional anatomy and biomechanics

Each ligament is functionally linked to the other ligaments, which explains why ligament injuries are frequently of a complex nature. Two big ligament systems are distinguished from one another as the central pivot and the peripheral structures.

The central pivot is formed by the anterior and posterior cruciate ligaments. They define the axis of the knee rotation. The noticeable exception is external rotation, which is mainly controlled by the peripheral structures.

The lateral and medial peripheral structures are each formed by two entities:

- The postero-lateral corner and lateral collateral ligament (LCL)
- The postero-medial corner and medial collateral ligament (MCL).

These complex structures are the true partners of the cruciate ligaments. They control recurvatum and they participate in the antero-posterior stability depending on the degree of flexion. By themselves, they also control external rotation and prevent varus and valgus mainly at slight flexion.

Diagnosis

We have to pay a special attention in relation to the complaints of the patient and we must also interrogate them about the circumstances of the initial trauma: it sometimes helps us to understand the type of lesions encountered, their treatment and their evolution. Generally, it is impossible to identify the mechanism of trauma. We should also define what is the most important complaint at the present time. It can be either an instability disorder such as giving away or fatigability caused by pain and swelling during or after activities. It makes sense to perform an analysis in relation to the level of activity, sports motivation, and the kind of activity the patient would like to practice.

Clinical examination

The clinical examination permits us to distinguish different patterns of instability.

COMBINED LATERAL INSTABILITY

In chronic antero-posterolateral instabilities (ACL and posterolateral corner), we usually find a soft endpoint Trillat–Lachman test associated with a lateral joint-space opening and the presence of a positive Hughston external rotation recurvatum test of Hughston. These symptoms reflect a lesion of the postero-lateral corner. The dynamic tests are positive and the comparative palpation of both lateral collateral ligaments is asymmetrical.

490

In chronic postero-posterolateral instabilities (posterior cruciate ligament and postero-lateral corner), in contrast with an isolated rupture of the posterior cruciate ligament (PCL), we find a posterior translation even at 20° of flexion and a delayed firm end-point Trillat–Lachman test. We also observe a positive external rotation recurvatum test, lateral joint-space opening and an increase of external rotation. The reverse pivot-shift is not specific. When the knee is flexed the posterior translation becomes evident and we observe a positive sag test.

COMBINED MEDIAL INSTABILITY

In chronic antero-medial and postero-medial instabilities, the medial joint space opening in extension is the characteristic sign. When an extensive medial laxity is present, we must suspect a PCL insufficiency. Because the drawer sign is not always easy to distinguish in postero-medial instabilities, complementary exams are often necessary to reach the correct diagnosis.

'PENTADE' AND LUXATION

In case of medial or lateral 'pentade' the anterior and posterior drawer, dynamic tests and soft endpoint Trillat–Lachman test are positive. Dynamic tests (varus, valgus, medial and lateral translation) permit to classify pentades and luxations (Neyret 1996).

Complementary investigations

These investigations are the key to the preoperative diagnosis and they are also necessary for surgical planning.

STANDARD RADIOGRAPHIC VIEWS (AP AND LATERAL)

On the standard views we look for bony avulsions and spontaneous translation in the frontal plane. The latter is frequently observed after a reduced knee subluxation.

- Comparative monopodal stance AP views allow us to detect isolated medial femorotibial narrowing, asymmetrical lateral decoaptation, medial femorotibial narrowing with or without lateral decoaptation and hooked tibial spines.
- Comparative monopodal stance profile views at 30° of flexion allows us to measure anterior or posterior tibial translation and the tibial slope (Dejour and Bonin 1994).
- A bipodal antero-posterior view at 45° of flexion (Shuss view) permits detection of a slight femorotibial narrowing.
- Valgus and varus stress radiographs help us to evaluate medial and lateral joint decoaptation, and therefore assess frontal instability. X-Rays performed in recurvatum stress can show a posterior capsular ligament insufficiency. Other comparative dynamic views such as anterior or posterior drawer passive Lachman tests, and Puddu views allow measurement of an

abnormal sagittal translation (Dejour 1989, Dejour and Bonin 1994, Meyers and Harvey 1971).

- Long leg films are used to measure the femorotibial angle and investigate an osseous malalignment deformity.
- MRI is the investigation of choice in these injuries because of its superior imaging of ligamentous structures. It is also able to depict recent bone lesions (bone bruises). In case of knee subluxation we have to ask an MRI angiogram to look for possible vascular damage.
- Arthro CT scan is useful investigation to analyze the articular cartilage and the menisci, although MRI is equally as efficient for evaluating these structures. The latter permits a better evaluation of the subchondral bone in relation to the presence of 'bone bruise' and osteonecrosis.
- Radio-isotope bone scan can show an increase in uptake of the subchondral bone, characteristically at the medial compartment in the PCL-deficient knees, representing the first sign of osteoarthritis. MRI scanning is often sufficient to obtain this information, albeit that radio-isotope scanning provides a much more accurate and specific test for subchondral degeneration.
- Arthroscopy is only indicated as a means of investigation as a first step in the surgical management and permits overall evaluation of the knee. Diagnostic arthroscopy may be necessary and useful in certain circumstances such as in association with lateral knee decoaptation.

Physiopathology

Chronic anterior instabilities

CLASSIFICATION

We distinguish three types of chronic anterior instability:

1 Chronic evolved anterior instability (70 per cent) represents the chronic evolution of the isolated ACL rupture, which usually becomes progressively more unstable as a result of progressive stretching of the peripheral structures.
2 Chronic antero-medial instability (25 per cent) is the result of combined insufficiency of the MCL and ACL (Dejour 1989, Neyret et al. 2000).
3 Chronic antero-posterolateral instability (5 per cent) results from an insufficiency of both the LCL and ACL (Dejour 1989, Neyret et al. 2000).

CONTRIBUTING FACTORS

An ACL rupture causes a serious disorder in knee kinematics, which appears during weight-bearing conditions. Therefore, in the case of knee instability the use of monopodal-stance studies is especially interesting because they show the consequences of this instability. They also help us in the decision-making on performing an osteotomy as a treatment option for this instability in relation to the individuals' data (frontal and sagittal alignment, muscle balance, weight and height) (Dejour *et al.* 1994).

Several anatomic factors must be taken into account and they can be classified according to frontal and sagittal imbalance.

SAGITTAL IMBALANCE

The anterior tibial translation is measured on comparative profile monopodal-stance views at 30° of flexion. It allows us to define three factors that contribute to sagittal imbalance:

Anterior cruciate ligament. Analysis in weight-bearing position shows two force components: a vertical compression force on the tibial plateau and a shearing force that tends to move the tibia forward. Anterior tibial translation is a physiological phenomenon, but any asymmetrical increase (superior to 2 mm) is pathological. The main structure to restrain anterior tibial translation is the ACL.

Medial meniscus. Secondary tearing of the medial meniscus occurs during the natural evolution of the ACL-deficient knee. The posterior horn of the medial meniscus acts as a brake to control the anterior tibial translation. A differential anterior tibial translation exceeding 6 mm results in a medial meniscus tear in 70 per cent of cases. When the difference is over 10 mm, this occurs in more than 90 per cent of cases (Dejour and Bonin 1994).

Tibial slope. The slope of the tibial plateau is defined as the angle formed by the tibial shaft axis and the tangent to the medial tibial plateau, minus 90°. We consider a normal tibial slope to be 10° ± 3°. Posterior inclination beyond 13° is considered abnormal. We found a highly significant correlation between mean tibial translation and tibial slope, both in normal and affected knees. For every 10° increase in tibial slope, anterior tibial translation increased about 6 mm (Dejour and Bonin 1994).

In case of a differential anterior tibial translation between 2–5 mm, peripheral ligament injuries (medial meniscus or posteromedial corner) were found in 50 per cent of cases. When this differential value reached 6–9 mm, these lesions were presents in 70 per cent of cases and finally they were always present when the amount of anterior tibial translation was more than 10 mm (Dejour and Bonin 1994, Dejour *et al.* 1994, Dejour, Neyret and Bonnin 1994).

FRONTAL IMBALANCE

Anterior cruciate ligament. The ACL not only controls sagittal balance, but also restrains frontal instability.

Medial meniscus. Rupture of the ACL is followed by a displacement of the instantaneous centre of rotation of the tibia toward the medial compartment. As a consequence the medial meniscus becomes the most important structure in avoiding frontal imbalance.

Peripheral structures. Lesions to the medial structures may occur during the injury; these structures control valgus laxity. The MCL is the most important medial structure. The postero-lateral corner controls the tibial external rotation and protects femorotibial coaptation against varus opening forces.

Varus deformity. A constitutional varus deformity plays an important role in ACL-deficient knees. It will favour the development of osteoarthritis, particularly if the osseous deformity is greater than 6–8°.

Osteoarthritis. The presence of preoperative radiological changes is liable to influence the onset of osteoarthritis after ACL reconstruction. In the same manner, the occurrence of frontal imbalance or sagittal imbalance can also induce early osteoarthritis.

Three situations should be distinguished: medial femorotibial decoaptation (without medial compartmental narrowing) medial femorotibial narrowing (without asymmetrical lateral decoaptation) and medial femorotibial narrowing associated with lateral decoaptation. Pathological lateral decoaptation of the joint is defined as asymmetrical lateral joint-space opening in relation to the opposite knee.

The narrowing of the medial femorotibial compartment is not rare, and it translates a medial meniscal tear or cartilage lesions. Thus, evolution towards osteoarthritis can occur without lateral joint decoaptation.

FRONTAL AND SAGITTAL BALANCE RELATIONSHIP

There is a close relationship between lateral femorotibial joint decoaptation, medial femorotibial narrowing and anterior tibial translation. The anterior tibial translation affects both medial and lateral femorotibial compartments, causing mainly a progressive stretching of the postero-medial corner and wearing of the medial femorotibial compartment. Afterwards, the distance between the attachment sites of the lateral collateral ligament reduces, leading to lateral joint decoaptation during monopodal weight bearing (Dejour *et al.* 1994).

In fact, in this group, we can identify and separate several entities (Bousquet *et al.* 1991):

• *Pure lateral instability* with asymmetrical lateral opening in varus stress and lateral thrust during gait. When palpating the lateral side of the knee, with the leg placed in a 'frog leg' position, we are not able to distinguish the lateral collateral ligament. In this situation valgus osteotomy is often appropriate.

- *Pure horizontal instability* with asymmetrical external rotation, positive external rotation drawer test and a positive Hughston test. These tests mainly reflect the state of the postero-lateral complex, the popliteo-fibular ligament and popliteus. In this case, osteotomy is not appropriate.
- *Mixed instability (lateral and horizontal)*. This is the combination of the two previous instabilities. Valgus osteotomy is often necessary to provide for long-term stability.

Chronic posterior instabilities

The kinematic disorders during monopodal stance in a knee with a posterior cruciate ligament rupture are still not completely clear. Osteoarthritis shows a slow evolution and is also less apparent compared to ACL-deficient knees. Nevertheless, degenerative changes are observed in the anterior part of the medial femorotibial compartment and in the patello-femoral compartment.

CLASSIFICATION

We distinguish three types of chronic posterior instabilities:

1　The chronic isolated posterior instability that results from the chronic evolution of an isolated PCL rupture.
2　The chronic postero-postero-lateral instability reflecting the chronic state of the insufficiency of PCL and the postero-lateral corner (Dejour 1989, Neyret 1996).
3　The chronic postero-posteromedial instability which results from the chronic progressive insufficiency of the PCL and postero-medial capsule and corner of the knee (Bousquet *et al.* 1991).

CONTRIBUTING FACTORS

Sagittal imbalance. In the PCL-deficient knee we observe a progressive forward slip of the femoral condyles in relation to the tibial plateau. This forward slip is more prominent in the medial femorotibial compartment. The tibial slope is of significant influence in respect to the residual laxity (positive posterior drawer test at 70°) after PCL reconstruction. If the tibial slope decreases, residual laxity increases.

Frontal imbalance. Lateral femorotibial joint-space opening is most unlikely the result of an isolated PCL rupture. Lateral opening is only found if postero-lateral lesions are present. Evolution towards medial femorotibial osteoarthritis appears to be the rule, particularly in patients with varus malalignment. Secondary degenerative patello-femoral joint changes are less frequent and usually appear later.

Isolated chronic postero-lateral instability

In this situation the ACL and PCL are both intact. This is a rare condition (sometimes iatrogenic) representing a combination of lateral collateral ligament, popliteus tendon or muscle rupture and/or popliteo fibular ligament and lateral head gastrocnemius tears. At assessment, we find an increase in external tibial rotation, an increase in varus laxity and abnormal dynamic tests (Figures 29.1 to 29.6).

Chronic antero-posterior instabilities

Chronic antero-posterior instabilities are produced either by the chronic evolution of bicruciate ligament ruptures, or by the onset of an injury to the ACL in a PCL-deficient knee and vice-versa.

Treatment

General considerations

We have to take into account several factors. We must consider patient motivation, level of activity, patients' expectation, age and the whole of associated disorders of the knee.

ISOLATED LIGAMENT RECONSTRUCTION

The goals of treatment are to neutralize the main instability and the associated instabilities, but also to deal with articular cartilage damage. In chronic instabilities with imbalance, isolated ligament reconstruction is not able to control this imbalance. If not combined with an osteotomy, the graft or ligament reconstruction will stretch over time.

LIGAMENT RECONSTRUCTION COMBINED WITH OSTEOTOMY

The combined procedure protects the graft against the forces created by the imbalance. We obtain better results when a combined osteotomy is performed early in the osteoarthitic process. Early means before the stage of medial femorotibial articular cartilage wear exposing the subchondral bone (Dejour *et al.* 1994, Dejour, Neyret and Bonnin 1994). We call this stage pre-osteoarthritis or grade B or C according to the IKDC radiological evaluation.

ISOLATED OSTEOTOMY

Another option is to perform a stand alone osteotomy. We recommend this procedure in case of severe osteoarthritis (IKDC grade D). The osteotomy can be performed at the level of the distal femur or proximal tibia. More often proximal tibial osteotomy is performed to correct a varus limb deformity and articular malalignment about the knee (Taylor *et al.* 1972). The distal femoral osteotomy can be indicated in case of femoral valgus deformity, but presents a more difficult rehabilitation and a partial loss of mobility is often encountered as a complication. A hypercorrection in the frontal plane may occur if an osteotomy is performed in the presence of ligament reconstruction in case of osteoarthritis or asymmetrical lateral opening (Noyes *et al.* 2000, Dejour *et al.* 1994). Osteotomy is an essential procedure but should not be excessive. After correction the mechanical axis should not exceed 3° of valgus, but the amount of correction depends on the analysis of the imbalance. Excessive correction of malalignment is often associated with an inability to return to sports activities due to the modified biomechanics of weight-bearing. Asymmetrical or excessive malalignment is also aesthetically displeasing to patients. On the other hand hypercorrection may be necessary in order to obtain symptomatic relief when osteoarthritis or residual instability are present.

Osteotomy without central pivot reconstruction

High tibial osteotomy (HTO) without central pivot reconstruction is indicated in a case of symptomatic evolved osteoarthritis (IKDC grade D, or complete joint-space narrowing).

As it is very difficult to correct a deformity in both frontal and sagittal plane, we have to make a choice: either to favour correction in the frontal plane or in the sagittal plane. It is always possible to obtain a side effect, but the main goal must be determined preoperatively.

VALGUS HTO

Chronic anterior instabilities. When medial femorotibial narrowing is present, the treatment of choice is a valgus osteotomy. In a sedentary patient we can propose a total knee replacement. A unicompartimental knee replacement is contraindicated because of the anterior-posterior laxity causing excessive wear and premature loosening.

Valgus HTO is indicated when AP monopodal weight bearing films show medial femorotibial narrowing or asymmetrical lateral joint decoaptation. Others factors can also play a role in the indication of performing an osteotomy, like previous medial meniscectomy or excessive varus malalignment.

When the choice has been made in favour of an osteotomy, we then need to choose between a closing- and opening-wedge technique:

- *The closing-wedge* valgus HTO permits a good correction in patients with medial pre-osteoarthritis or osteoarthritis. We perform an oblique osteotomy in the frontal plane. During the procedure there is a tendency to decrease the backward tibial slope. By changing the bone cuts an extension component may be added to the valgus procedure if necessary, thus decreasing the tibial slope.

- *The opening-wedge* valgus HTO permits, in our experience, a more accurate correction than the closing-wedge osteotomy, moreover it can correct an excessive varus deformity. It is indicated in absent or slight medial joint-space narrowing. However, this procedure has a tendency to lower the patella and to increase the tibial slope. The latter effect can result in

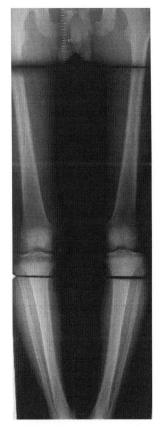

Fig. 29.1
This patient showed an increased varus alignment of the right leg after a soccer accident which happened three years before. On bipodal weight-bearing films we observe an increased varus alignment compared to the healthy side and asymmetrical lateral decoaptation.

497

an important overload of the ACL, which can lead to a 'stress rupture' of the ACL. This effect is, on the contrary, favourable in case of posterior instability.

Chronic posterior instabilities. We perform HTO at a stage before complete femorotibial osteoarthritis. However, as mentioned before, the sagittal plane deformity must be considered in cruciate ligament deficiencies. In PCL or postero-lateral complex deficiencies, the recommendation is to increase the posterior tibial slope to get better control on the posterior tibial translation. The optimal posterior tibial slope is not yet known.

TIBIAL DEFLEXION OSTEOTOMY

Tibial deflexion osteotomy is performed in case of excessive tibial slope without significant frontal imbalance. This excessive slope is constitutional and sometimes worsened by posterior femorotibial narrowing secondary to ACL deficiency.

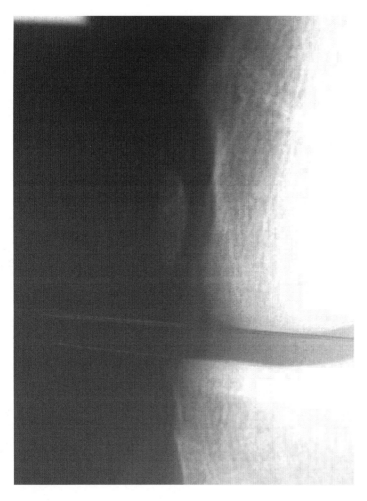

Fig. 29.2
At closer inspection of the AP film a bony avulsion of the lateral condyle is present.

Fig. 29.3
Varus stress film of the same patient showing lateral joint-space opening.

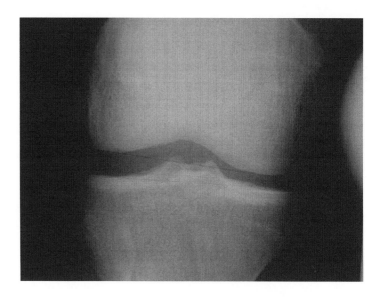

Fig. 29.4
MRI confirmed the diagnosis of isolated posterolateral instability, an abscent politeus tendon, soft tissue disruption and capsular thinning of the posterior-lateral corner.

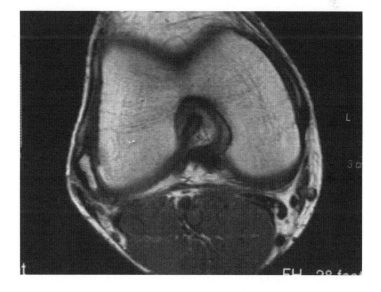

In a tibial deflexion osteotomy an anterior closing-wedge osteotomy is performed above the level of the anterior tibial tuberosity. The wedge has its base at the anterior part of the tibia and its summit at the posterior cortex into the tibial PCL fibers and above the insertion of the posterior capsule. In this way these structures avoid posterior opening.

The direction of the osteotomy is determined preoperatively on the comparative monopodal stance profile view at 30° flexion and

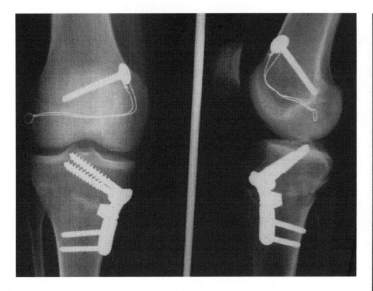

Fig. 29.5

Figs 29.5 and 29.6
Good stability and normal alignment was obtained through reinsertion of
the bony avulsed fragment with LCL and popliteus tendon attached to it,
combined with an opening-wedge valgus HTO because of the patient's
varus morphotype.

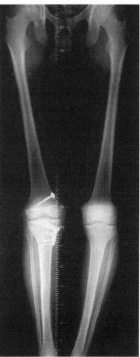

Fig. 29.6

afterwards during the procedure it is outlined with two K-wires. The
tibia is cut with an oscillating saw after gentle elevation the superficial MCL insertion and up to the patellar tendon insertion. The
posterior cortex must not be cut. The posterior cortex is weakened
by performing a number of parallel drill holes with a 3.2 mm drill.
Several osteotomes are consecutively introduced to progressively
open the tibial osteotomy. We recommend 1 mm of anterior resection to correct 1.5° to 2° of tibial slope.

If necessary, an anterior tibial tuberosity (ATT) osteotomy can
improve the approach. The osteotomy is fixed by two staples (medial
and lateral to the tibial tuberosity) and two screws in case of
osteotomy of the ATT.

In a PCL-deficient knee a closing-wedge HTO is not indicated
because it decreases the backward tibial slope creating a more
important posterior tibial translation.

VARUS HTO

A varus HTO is rarely performed in chronic instabilities because
chronic instability after rupture of the MCL is infrequent. It is
indicated in case of chronic evolution of a neglected MCL
rupture associated to central pivot insufficiency combined with a
valgus deformity. Here we can discuss performing a femoral
osteotomy to avoid an inclination of the articular line or a tibial

Fig. 29.7

Medial femorotibial narrowing on monopodal-stance view in a patient aged 40, who sustained an injury to his left knee during a martial art combat a few moths ago, resulting in chronic anterior laxity. Two years before a medial meniscectomy was performed on the same knee.

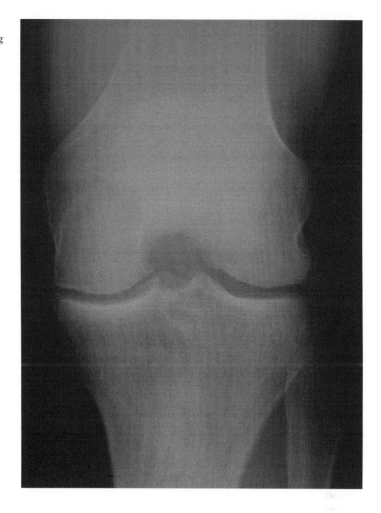

closing-wedge osteotomy and tightening of the superficial MCL. Correction of the deformity to a normal mechanical axis is the goal.

FLEXION OR ANTI-RECURVATUM OSTEOTOMY

In case of knee instability and an osseous recurvatum morphotype greater than 7°, this deformity has to be corrected by a tibial anterior opening-wedge osteotomy. The amount of the correction is obtained by comparing the angular value observed at the healthy side. The posterior capsule can be tightened in case of stretching of the posterior capsule and ligaments (Bussière *et al.* 2002). We have to be careful not to increase the tibial slope over 15° due to the risk of 'stress rupture' of the ACL. We have no experience (except in a case of femoral malunion) with anterior opening-wedge femoral osteotomy. It may be indicated in adults in those rare cases of recurvatum with a femoral origin.

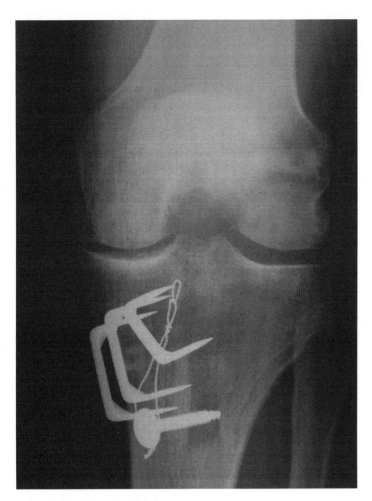

Fig. 29.8
An ACL reconstruction
(middle third patellar
tendon) combined with an
opening-wedge valgus HTO
was performed.

Osteotomy with central pivot reconstruction

We believe that any abnormality that appears on a monopodal-stance radiograph cannot be compensated for by a ligament reconstruction alone.

VALGUS OSTEOTOMY

In the chronic ACL-deficient knee valgus HTO is indicated for those symptomatic sports participants who have developed secondary medial femorotibial narrowing (Dejour *et al.* 1994, Noyes *et al.* 2000).

Lateral decoaptation reflects a condition in which any ligament reconstruction, trying to correct this deformation, will stretch. Medial femorotibial narrowing increases the risk of osteoarthritic evolution after ACL reconstruction (Dejour *et al.* 1988, 1994). In patients with medial femorotibial narrowing, an association between

Fig. 29.9

AP monopodal-stance view of
a knee after failed consecutive
reconstruction with patellar
tendon and hamstring
tendons. A distinct anterior
tibial translation was observed.
The tibial slope measured 16°.

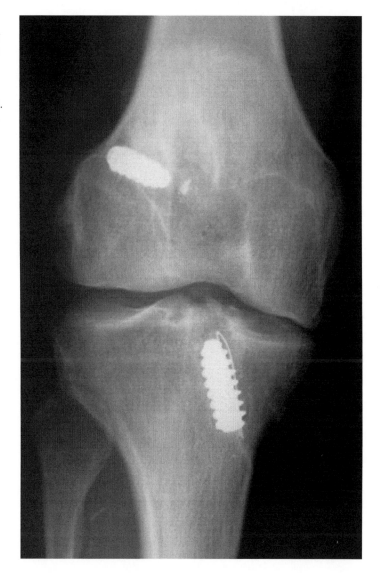

a valgus osteotomy and ACL reconstruction is preferred in the
absence of other important risk factors, such as varus malalignment,
previous medial meniscectomy and patients older than 40 years
(Figures 29.7 and 29.8). In the situation of an ACL-deficient knee
with an asymmetrical lateral joint-space opening some authors prefer to perform the osteotomy first, and to reconstruct the ACL later
(Latterman and Jakob 1996). However, this often leads to a major
valgus hypercorrection in order to control thrust when walking.
We prefer to reconstruct the ACL, the lateral structures (LCL
reconstruction using a 6 mm bone patellar tendon-bone graft, or

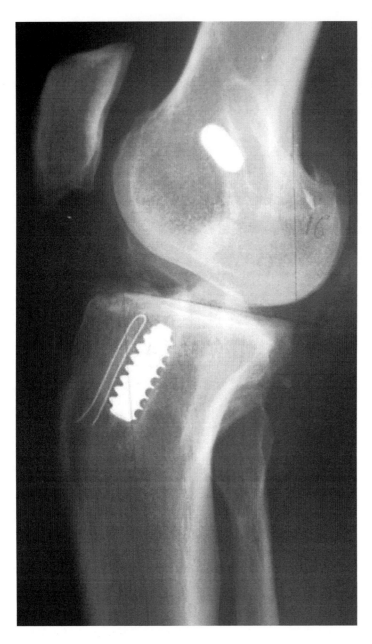

Fig. 29.10

Lateral view: a 16 mm anterior tibial translation was observed during a passive Lachmann test with the Telos device.

advancement of the popliteus and LCL complex) and to perform a slight valgus hypercorrection during the same procedure. Performing these combined gestures makes excessive hypercorrection unnecessary.

In a PCL-deficient knee with associated lateral laxity and varus malalignment we recommend reconstructing the PCL and lateral structures and performing a valgus HTO.

Fig. 29.11

An ACL reconstruction using a patellar tendon graft from the opposite knee combined with a deflexion osteotomy was performed. Intraoperative view showing fixation of the deflexion osteomy with staples.

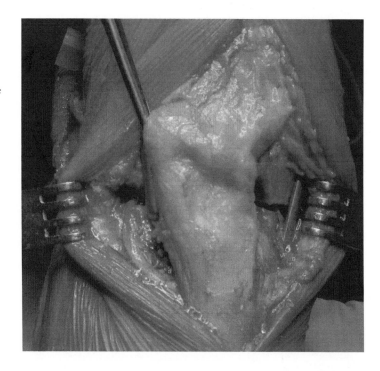

Fig. 29.12

After the osteotomy the graft is passed through the tibial tunnel and fixed with an interference screw and a wire on a post as supplementary fixation.

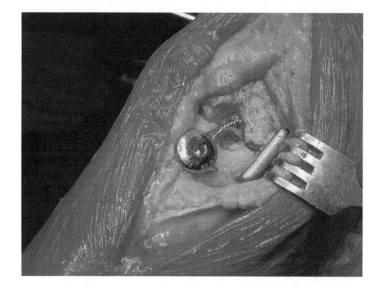

In both ACL and PCL deficiency we have to pay attention to the tibial slope because it will be modified by the osteotomy. The more the slope is increased by the osteotomy, the greater the postoperative anterior tibial translation. Conversely, if the slope is reduced, the anterior tibial translation decreases.

DEFLEXION OSTEOTOMY

Deflexion osteotomy associated with ACL reconstruction is indicated in anterior instability in the presence of an increased tibial slope, because it decreases the anterior tibial translation and prevents excessive stress on the ACL graft (Neyret *et al.* 2000) (Figures 29.9 and 29.10). Ligament reconstruction is performed in the conventional manner, but the osteotomy is performed before the introduction of the ligament graft through the tunnels (Figures 29.11 to 29.14). For the technical considerations concerning the deflexion osteotomy we refer the reader to the earlier section in this chapter on tibial deflexion osteotomy. When the middle third of the patellar tendon is harvested, elevation of the ATT must be avoided. After the osteotomy has been undertaken the graft is inserted through the bone tunnels. A tibial interference screw or a wire on a post can be used to fix the bone plug securely within its tunnel. Postero-medial reefing is necessary in case of significant recurvatum.

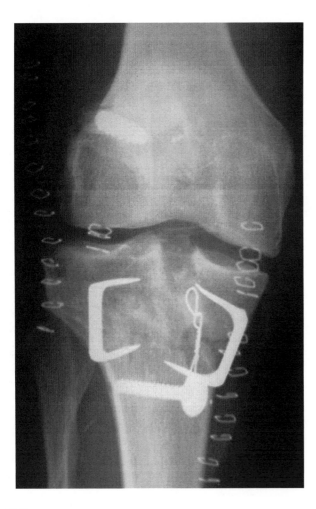

Figs 29.13 and 29.14
Postoperative AP and profile views showing the ACL reconstruction and deflexion HTO. A 6° tibial slope was obtained.

Fig. 29.14

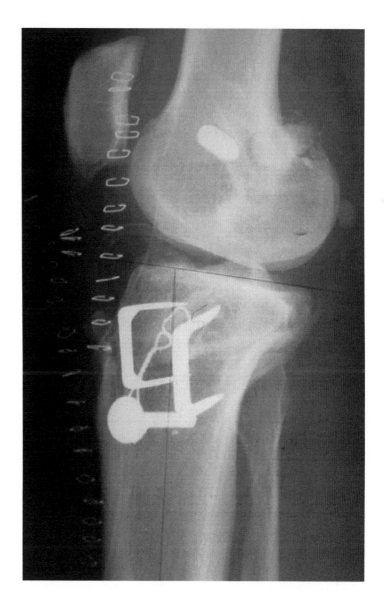

Osteotomy combined with extraarticular reconstruction

In cases of osteoarthritis and combined subjective instability, we perform the Lemaire technique combined with a closing-wedge HTO. Both the decrease in tibial slope and the lateral plasty contribute to the stabilizing effect. Our results are encouraging.

Rehabilitation

Rehabilitation is started the day after surgery. Passive motion is allowed between 0–120° using continuous passive motions. The knee is placed in a resting splint for 60 days. The splint has 10° of flexion following a deflexion osteotomy (to prevent recurvatum induced by the osteotomy) and is in full extension in the situation of varus, valgus or flexion high tibial osteotomy. Weight-bearing on the operative leg is not allowed for 60 days. In the case of a tibial tuberosity elevation, the range of motion allowed is between 0–90°. In the situation of ligamentous reconstruction, range of motion also depends on the particular type of ligamentous surgery performed (ACL or PCL reconstruction).

Conclusion

Osteotomy may have its place in the treatment of chronic instabilities. The concept of the frontal imbalance and sagittal imbalance is a recent one. The comparative analysis of radiographs in unilateral weight-bearing makes a major contribution, however, a dynamic analysis of movement is also required. When there is an imbalance, we do not recommend isolated ligamentous reconstruction. Isolated osteotomy without any ligamentous reconstruction may be the best treatment in case of osteoarthritis. The goal of an osteotomy is to correct the limb alignment in the frontal and sagittal plane and remove the unfavourable alignment. In such cases, we do not recommend a simultaneous ligamentous reconstruction.

Osteotomy can be combined with ligament reconstruction: we called it the 'combined operation'. They can be complementary, because they protect ligament reconstruction and articular cartilage. We believe that the osteotomy plays an important role in protecting not only the ligament grafts but also eventual meniscal grafts and osteochondral transplants.

References

Bousquet G, Le Beguec P, Girardin P (1991). Les laxités chroniques du genou: Physiologie, physio-pathologie, étude clinique et traitement. Medsi-Mc. Gran-Hill.

Bussière C, Aït Si Selmi T, Neyret P (2001). Genu Recurvatum. Enclyclopédie Medico-Chirurgicale. Editions Scientifiques en Médicales Elsevier SAS. Paris, App. loc. 14-327-A-10

Conwell HE, Alldredge RH (1937). Complete dislocations of the knee joint. A report of 7 cases with end-results. *Surgery Gynecology Obstetrics*, 64, 94–101.

Dejour H, Walch G, Neyret P, Adeleine P (1988). Résultats des laxités chroniques antéreures opérées: à propos de 251 cas revus avec un minimum de 3 ans. *Revue de Chirurgie Orthopédique*, 74, 637–646.

Dejour H (1989). Entorse graves du genou. Conférences d'Enseignement. In Cahier Enseignement SOFCOT, 34, 81–97. Expansion Scientifique Française, Paris.

Dejour H, Bonnin M (1994). Tibial translation after cruciate ligament rupture: two radiological tests compared. *Journal of Bone and Joint Surgery [Br]*, 76-B, 5, 745–749.

Dejour H, Neyret P, Boileau P, Donell ST (1994). Anterior cruciate reconstruction combined with valgus tibial osteotomy. *Clinical Orthopaedics*, 299, 220–228.

Dejour H, Neyret P, Bonnin M (1994). Instability and osteoarthritis. In Fu FH, Harner CD, Vince KG (eds) *Knee surgery*, pp. 859–875. Williams & Wilkins, Baltimore, Maryland.

Johner R, Baumer PM, Rogge D, Burch HB, Jakob RP, Tscherne H (1992). Dislocations of the knee. In Jakob RP, Staubli Hu (eds) *The Knee and the Cruciate Ligaments*, pp. 307–317. Springer Verlag, Berlin.

Kennedy JC (1963). Complete dislocation of the knee joint. *Journal of Bone and Joint Surgery*, 45-A, 889–904.

Lattermann C, Jakob RP (1996). High tibial osteotomy alone or combined with ligament reconstruction in anterior ligament deficient knees. *Arthroscopy*, 4, 32–38.

Meyers MH, Harvey P Jr (1971). Traumatic dislocations of the knee joint. A study of eighteen cases. *Journal of Bone and Joint Surgery*, 53-A, 16–29.

Meyers MH, Moore TM, Harvey P Jr (1975). Traumatic dislocation of the knee joint. *Journal of Bone and Joint Surgery*, 57-A, 430–433.

Neyret P (1996). Lésions ligamentaires complexes récents: Triades, Pentades et Luxations. La pathologie chirurgicale du genou du sportif. In *Cahier Enseignement SOFCOT*, 59, 37–52. Expansion Scientifique Française, Paris.

Neyret P, Zuppi G, Ait Si Selmi T (2000). Tibial deflexion osteotomy. *Operative Techniques in Sports Medicine*, 8, 1, 61–66.

Neyret P, Trojani CH, Ait Si Semi T, Versier G (2001). Acute multiple ligament injuries and dislocation in emergency. In *Surgical Techniques in Orthopaedics and Traumatology*. EFORT Bulletin. Editions Elsevier, 55–500–C-10, 6p.

Noyes FR, Barber-Westin D, Hewett T (2000). High tibial osteotomy and ligament reconstruction for varus angulated anterior cruciate ligament-deficient knees. *American Journal of Sports Medicine*, 28, 282–296.

Taylor AR, Arden GP, Rainey HA (1972). Traumatic dislocation of the knee. A report of forty-three cases with special reference to conservative treatment. *Journal of Bone and Joint Surgery [Br]*, 54-B, 96–102.

Thomsen PB, Rud B, Jensen UH (1984). Stability and motion after traumatic dislocation of the knee. *Acta Orthopedica Scandinavica*, 55, 278–283.

30

Indications and outcomes of acute, simultaneous ACL and PCL reconstruction

Hussein A. Elkousy, Jon K. Sekiya, and
Christopher D. Harner

Introduction

The management of combined anterior cruciate ligament (ACL) and posterior cruciate ligament (PCL) injury is controversial. Considerable debate exists in the following areas: injury classification, operative versus non-operative management, acute versus delayed surgical intervention, open versus arthroscopic intervention, ligament repair versus reconstruction, management of associated injuries, and use of autograft versus allograft tissue in these cases. This chapter will focus on the surgical issues involved with acute, simultaneous ACL and PCL reconstruction and how these different issues influence outcomes. We will also briefly address some of the more fundamental considerations of acute, combined ACL and PCL injuries, as they may have a significant impact on the clinical outcome.

Definition

Combined injuries of the ACL and PCL are, by definition, considered to be a type of knee dislocation. For example, some authors believe that a knee dislocation has occurred when there is bicruciate injury (Sisto and Warren 1985). In fact, most knee dislocations do have at least a ruptured ACL and PCL (Noyes and Barber-Westin 1997). Nonetheless, there have been several reports of knee dislocations wherein the PCL remains intact (Shelbourne *et al.* 1992; Cooper *et al.* 1992; Bratt and Newman 1993). In addition, classification systems of knee dislocations exist that include subgroups with an intact PCL; however, even these classification systems would define most knee dislocations as having at least bicruciate injury (Schenck 1994).

Incidence and associated injuries

Knee dislocations are a relatively rare event (Good and Johnson 1995; Shields *et al.* 1969; Meyers and Harvey 1971; Noyes and Barber-Westin 1997; Shapiro and Freedman 1995). By some estimates, knee dislocation only represents 1.2 per cent of all orthopaedic trauma (Bunt *et al.* 1990). However, many authors believe that this injury may be under-diagnosed. This may occur because many of these injuries spontaneously reduce and remain unrecognized; this is especially true in those patients who present with other more severe injuries (Kennedy 1963; Schenck 1994). Indeed, many patients who suffer from knee dislocations have sustained a high energy injury which may result in severe associated injuries (Roman *et al.* 1987; Noyes and Barber-Westin 1997; Shapiro and Freedman 1995). Often, these injuries dictate management of the bicruciate injured knee, thereby impacting the outcome.

As mentioned, knee dislocations typically result from high energy injuries (Noyes and Barber-Westin 1997; Malizos *et al.* 1997; Yeh *et al.* 1999; Kennedy 1963). The potential mechanisms of injury include motor vehicle accidents or falls from a height. However, knee dislocation may also occur following lesser energy athletic injuries (Shelbourne *et al.* 1991; Noyes and Barber-Westin 1997; Good and Johnson 1995). Knee dislocations have often been described as a rare phenomena. However, over the past thirty to forty years, athletes have become bigger, stronger, and faster, and motor vehicle accidents have increased secondary to crowded roads and larger, more speedy vehicles. These facts, considered in combination with the better recognition of these injuries by medical practitioners, may be responsible for the observed increased incidence of knee dislocation over the past two decades (Kennedy 1963; Good and Johnson 1995).

Classification and mechanism

Knee dislocations have been classified in several different ways (Good and Johnson 1995). Schenck developed a classification system based upon the constellation of injured ligaments (Schenck 1994). In 1963, Kennedy proposed a classification system based upon the direction of tibial displacement relative to the femur (Kennedy 1963). He defined anterior, posterior, medial, lateral, and rotatory knee dislocations. He also tried to reproduce these mechanisms of injury in the laboratory. Using cadavers, he was able to simulate the most common type of dislocation (anterior) through forced hyperextension (Kennedy 1963). Both of these classification systems confirm that knee dislocations are complex injuries that result from a variety of mechanisms; these injury mechanisms ultimately result in injuries to multiple structures about the knee. Isolated ACL and PCL injury is relatively rare; thus, other structures are also frequently injured and must be addressed by surgery (Fanelli *et al.* 1996; Martinek *et al.* 2000). Often, management of these associated injuries has a great impact on the eventual outcome (Fanelli *et al.* 1996).

Diagnosis

Knee dislocations may be diagnosed through a combination of history, physical examination, and imaging modalities. At the history, patients may describe a severe knee hyperextension injury or an injury in which their extremity was placed in an extremely abnormal position. More commonly, patients may be brought in by ambulance after being involved in a high energy injury (motor vehicle accident, fall) and simply present with a swollen, painful, knee. In these cases, the treating physician should have a high index of suspicion for possible knee dislocation. In some cases, the knee will still be grossly deformed, thus making the diagnosis of knee dislocation straightforward. However, in most cases, the dislocation often spontaneously reduces. If a dislocation is suspected, the physical examination should first focus on the vascular and neurological status of the affected extremity. Socks and shoes and should be removed and the foot should be examined for color, temperature, pulses, sensation, and motor function. A ligament examination is performed, and should include the Lachman test, the anterior drawer test, the posterior drawer test, and varus or valgus stability testing at zero and thirty degrees of knee flexion. It may be difficult to perform any or all of these tests secondary to patient pain, discomfort, or a large knee effusion which may make it difficult to interpret the results.

The most useful imaging in the emergency department setting is radiographs. These images may demonstrate bony avulsion injuries, associated fractures, or tibiofemoral displacement. If fluoroscopy is available, stress views may be added to further delineate the degree and extent of ligamentous injury (Figure 30.1). Magnetic resonance imaging (MRI) can be very useful; however, it may not be useful in the emergency room setting (Figure 30.2). MRI is more accurate for the diagnosis of multiple ligament injury than clinical examination (Twaddle *et al.* 1996). Computed tomography may also be a useful modality in those cases where occult fractures about the knee are suspected.

Management of associated injuries

The brief background outlined above introduces several issues which have a great impact on the outcome of patients who sustain a combined ACL and PCL injury. Management of these patients begins at the moment that the injury is sustained. Prompt recognition (a)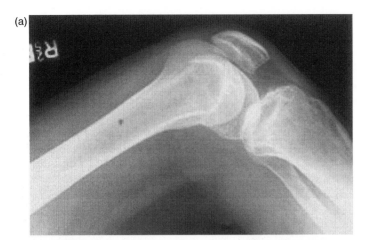

(b)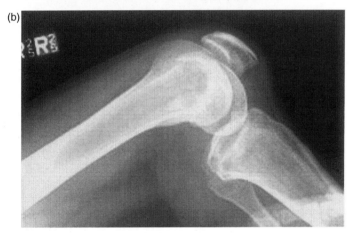

Fig. 30.1
Plain radiographs of right knee
with anterior and posterior
cruciate ligament injury.
(a) Lateral non-stress view
suggesting mild anterior
subluxation of the femur on
the tibia. (b) Lateral stress
view demonstrating moderate
subluxation consistent with
bicruciate disruption.

by on-site and emergency room personnel may have a significant
impact on the eventual outcome.

Vascular injuries

Perhaps the most important factor in optimizing the outcome of
combined ACL and PCL injuries is recognizing and appropriately
treating vascular injuries (Kennedy 1963; Green 1977; Jones *et al.*
1979; Hoover 1961; Almekinders and Logan 1992). If improperly
managed, popliteal artery injury may result in an amputation rate
as high as 89 per cent (Hoover 1961). In Kennedy's 1963 studies,
and in subsequent studies, anterior knee dislocation has been
identified as the most common type of dislocation. Kennedy
demonstrated that anterior dislocations result from a hyperextension mechanism with sequential injury to the ACL, PCL, and
eventually the popliteal artery (Kennedy 1963). The incidence of
knee dislocations with popliteal artery injuries with knee dislocation has been estimated at 25 to 35 per cent (Almekinders and

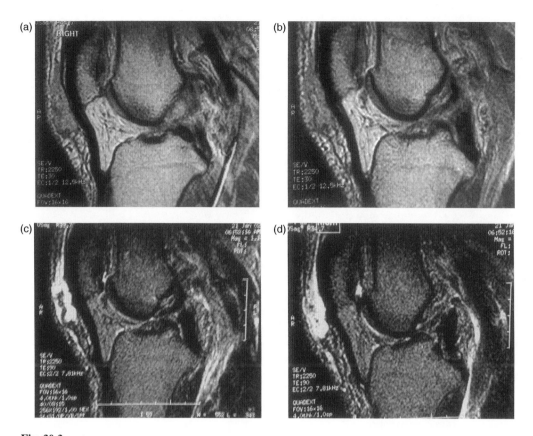

Fig. 30.2

T1 and T2 weighted magnetic resonance images (MRI) of, combined ACL and PCL injury. (a) Sagittal T1 image showing ACL disruption. (b) Sagittal T1 image showing PCL disruption. (c) Sagittal T2 image showing ACL disruption. (d) Sagittal T2 image showing PCL disruption.

Logan 1992; Green and Allen 1977; Kennedy 1963). However, vascular injury may not be as common with isolated ACL and PCL combined injuries (Martinek *et al.* 2000). A variety of algorithms still exist today for management of popliteal artery injuries associated with knee dislocations (Good and Johnson 1995; Yeh *et al.* 1999). Some authors would argue that all patients with a bicruciate ligament injury need an arteriogram regardless of physical examination (Schenck 1994). On the other end of the spectrum, some authors argue that an arteriogram is rarely necessary. A patient with a normal exam is observed; a patient with any abnormality by palpation or Doppler exam should be taken to the operating room for arterial exploration (Good and Johnson 1995). Not only does the management of the vascular injury determine the viability of the extremity, but it often also dictates the timing and approach for operative intervention of ligament injuries that will be discussed.

One common algorithm starts by first examining the foot for pulses. If the pulses are diminished as compared to the contralateral side, an arteriogram is obtained, unless the viability of the extremity is in obvious jeopardy. In that case, the patient is taken straight to the operating room in concert with vascular surgery.

The artery is then explored and an arteriogram may be obtained intraoperatively. If the pulses are symmetric with the contralateral extremity, an ultrasound is then performed. If the results of the ultrasound differ between extremities, then an arteriogram is obtained. If the ultrasound is negative, no arteriogram is obtained and the patient is observed for 24 to 48 hours with repeated vascular exams.

We prefer to routinely obtain an arteriogram on all acute patients, when feasible. This methodology clearly documents any pre-existing vascular injury prior to subjecting the patient to an involved surgical procedure. Combined ACL and PCL reconstruction procedures involve significant manipulation and positioning of the leg which may potentially complete any partial vascular injury that has not been detected due to the absence of an arteriogram.

Associated injuries

Although vascular injury may have the greatest immediate impact on combined ACL and PCL reconstructions, other associated injuries may have a more significant long-term effect on clinical outcome (Frassica *et al.* 1991; Sisto and Warren 1985; Roman *et al.* 1987; Noyes and Barber-Westin 1997; Martinek *et al.* 2000). The peroneal nerve may be injured in up to 16 per cent of all knee dislocations (Green and Allen 1977). Most authors would treat this nerve injury expectantly with delayed exploration at three months if symptoms persist (Roman *et al.* 1987; Good and Johnson 1995). However, the prognosis for recovery is poor even with delayed exploration (Roman *et al.* 1987; Good and Johnson 1995). Therefore, management of the ACL and PCL injuries may not have as great an effect on the outcome if a foot-drop persists.

We prefer to explore and release any constriction of the common peroneal nerve at the fibular neck during any surgery that addresses an injury to the posterolateral structures of the knee. Otherwise, we do not recommend peroneal nerve exploration. Any peroneal nerve deficit in the absence of a posterolateral corner injury is likely a neuropraxia; therefore, we recommend six months of clinical observation. Any residual motor deficit at that time may be treated with tendon transfers.

Bony injuries, such as tibial plateau fractures, should be addressed prior to any cruciate surgery; this may require a delay in definitive ligament reconstruction. We address the fracture acutely and delay the reconstruction based on the fracture pattern and the patient's associated injuries. Finally, injuries to the articular cartilage or meniscus may dictate whether an open or arthroscopic procedure is performed (Good and Johnson 1995). Large chondral injuries may necessitate open reconstruction.

Surgical management of combined ACL and PCL injuries

Currently, most surgeons would agree that a combined ACL and PCL injury must be addressed surgically (Kremchek *et al.* 1989). However, this has not always been the case (Good and Johnson 1995; Taylor *et al.* 1972; Myles 1967; Reckling and Peltier 1969). In 1972, Taylor *et al.* published an article asserting that combined ACL and PCL injuries could successfully be treated with nonoperative management (Taylor *et al.* 1972). However, it soon became apparent that a stiff knee, rather than instability, was often the end result. In response to publications by Myles and Taylor, Meyers published papers in 1971 and 1975 that contended that nonoperative intervention resulted in inferior outcomes when compared to operative intervention (Meyers *et al.* 1971, 1975). Most surgeons today would agree that combined ACL and PCL injury should be addressed surgically. The one exception might be older patients who be ill-affected by such an extensive knee procedure given other potential surgical risks (deep venous thrombosis, pulmonary embolus) (Malizos *et al.* 1997; Good and Johnson 1995; Kremchek *et al.* 1989).

Timing

The timing of surgery is an important factor in determining the clinical outcome. Unfortunately, the timing of surgery is often dictated by clinical circumstances that are often not directly related to the injured ligaments. For example, if the viability of the extremity is in question following a vascular repair, ligament reconstruction is usually delayed until the viability concerns are resolved. Additionally, a polytrauma patient with a severe head injury or internal bleeding may not tolerate a complex ligamentous reconstruction. In this case, the knee surgeon has no choice but to delay surgery. In both of the described circumstances, the injured extremity should be stabilized with an external fixator until the definitive reconstruction can be performed. In the absence of these other factors, most surgeons, including the authors, prefer operative intervention within the first three weeks of injury (Frassica *et al.* 1991; Good and Johnson 1995; Yeh *et al.* 1999; Malizos *et al.* 1997; Wascher *et al.* 1999; Noyes and Barber-Westin 1997). This approach facilitates the possibility that the operating surgeon might actually be able to repair injured structures as opposed to reconstructing damaged ligament (as might be necessary anyway). The early approach optimizes the surgeon's options in correcting normal knee stability following these devastating injuries. Frassica *et al.* prefers to operate within the first five days of the injury (Frassica *et al.* 1991). Some authors prefer to delay five to ten days for vascular monitoring and for range of motion therapy to aid in the prevention of postoperative stiffness (Good and Johnson 1995). The type of surgery may also dictate the timing of intervention.

For example, ligament repairs require earlier surgical intervention than reconstructions. Arthroscopic techniques may not be possible until two to three weeks after the injury as the knee capsule must regain competency prior to going forth with such an approach. If the capsule has not healed, fluid extravasation may result in lower extremity compartment syndrome (Good and Johnson 1995).

Open versus arthroscopic surgery

In the past, combined ACL and PCL reconstruction has been performed as an open surgical procedure (Figure 30.3). However, as the popularity of arthroscopic ligament reconstruction techniques has increased, knee surgeons have moved to performing combined ACL and PCL reconstructions arthroscopically (Noyes and Barber-Westin 1997). Since these changes in the 1980s, there has been some controversy as to which approach is best. Advocates of the open approach argue that arthroscopic procedures should not be performed acutely because of the high likelihood of capsular injury and the fluid extravasation associated with this method; fluid extravasation may lead to a compartment syndrome (Good and Johnson 1995). Proponents of the open approach regard the possibility of compartment syndrome as an avoidable risk that is unnecessary given the history of success in the open repair of both the ACL and PCL. Additionally, Martinek asserts that the open approach allows for a more precise repair of all knee injuries in this setting (Martinek *et al.* 2000).

In contrast, proponents of the arthroscopic approach contend that this method facilitates a complete assessment of the joint injury and more accurate reconstruction of injured structures (Marks and Harner 1993; Good and Johnson 1995). Our preference is to evaluate the joint arthroscopically first, keeping in mind that high arthroscopy pump

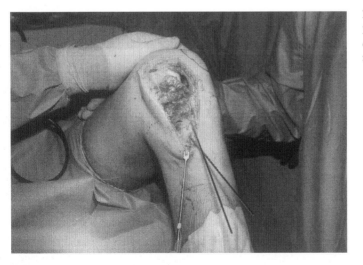

Fig. 30.3

Photograph demonstrating open combined ACL and PCL reconstruction.

pressures are undesirable. This is done with the knowledge that in the first several weeks after an injury, the capsule may be violated. However, if the capsule is intact and the joint retains the arthroscopic fluid, we prefer to perform the reconstruction arthroscopically at low fluid pressures. If the capsule is violated, we turn to an open approach with limited arthroscopic support to allow for a more accurate placement of our ligament grafts (Figure 30.4). If a repair is needed, a small incision is made to allow for open repair.

Simultaneous versus staged procedures

The primary problem with combined ACL and PCL injuries is symptomatic knee instability. Many authors feel that in order to achieve the successful restoration of knee function, both injured cruciate ligaments should be addressed simultaneously (Fanelli *et al.* 1996; Noyes and Barber-Westin 1997; Shapiro and Freedman 1995; Wascher *et al.* 1999; Twaddle *et al.* 1996; Hara *et al.* 1999). However, postoperatively the issue has not traditionally been stability, but has been stiffness (Good and Johnson 1995; Schenck 1994). This may be due, as mentioned previously, to the timing of the surgical intervention. However, some authors feel that simultaneous reconstruction or repair of both ligaments may be the cause of postoperative stiffness (Shelbourne *et al.* 1991; Yeh *et al.* 1999; Schenck 1994). Shelbourne, Schenck, and Yeh all advocate addressing the PCL first.

Fig. 30.4

Photograph of arthroscopically-assisted combined ACL and PCL reconstruction.

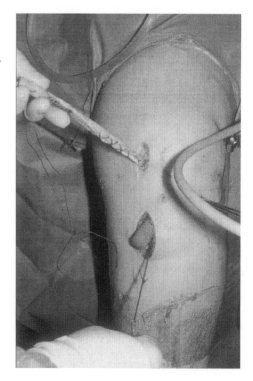

Subsequently, the patient undergoes rehabilitation to regain range of motion with a relatively stable knee. Following the restoration of full knee motion, the patient can undergo a staged, isolated ACL reconstruction. However, some authors believe that the patient will usually not require the second procedure because of sufficient stability (Shelbourne *et al.* 1991). Both Shelbourne and Yeh perform an isolated PCL reconstruction using patellar tendon autograft (Shelbourne *et al.* 1991; Yeh *et al.* 1999). In addition, Yeh advocates debriding the ACL at this initial surgery (Yeh *et al.* 1999). Unfortunately, there is little information available to guide surgeons in the application of staged versus simultaneous ACL and PCL reconstruction. One point to consider is that a staged approach might result in the application of abnormally high loads to the isolated reconstructed ligament. This, in turn, may result in graft failure. It is our contention that an appropriately timed surgery, combined with early postoperative rehabilitation, does not represent a large motion loss risk. As such, we recommend simultaneous reconstruction in the majority of cases to avoid the ultimate graft failure that might ensue with the staged approach.

Repair versus reconstruction

In general, pediatric knee injuries more often result in failure of the bony insertion of the ACL ligament as opposed to an intrasubstance rupture (Noyes *et al.* 1974; Lubowitz and Grauer 1993; Corso and Whipple 1996). The opposite is often true for adults where isolated ACL injuries more commonly occur at the midsubstance of the ligament (Corso and Whipple 1996; Noyes *et al.* 1974). However, it has been noted that combined ACL and PCL injuries present with a high percentage of avulsion injuries (Sisto and Warren 1985; Frassica *et al.* 1991; Malizos *et al.* 1997). In fact, one study noted that over half of these injuries involve bony avulsions (Marks and Harner 1993). These ACL and PCL bony avulsion injuries may be either repaired or reconstructed; these types of injuries may be more amenable to successful repair than repair of midsubstance injuries because of bone to bone healing. Consequently, many authors advocate primary repair of these injuries when possible (Frassica *et al.* 1991; Sisto and Warren 1985; Torisu 1979; Hara *et al.* 2001). In fact, Martinek advocates ligament repair even in the cases of midsubstance ACL and PCL injuries. When opting for surgical ligament repair, the surgery should be executed in the acute phase of the injury to allow for better healing (within three weeks) (Martinek *et al.* 2000). Others who advocate repair cite good outcomes and decreased morbidity; no autograft tissue is harvested and there is no risk of allograft associated disease transmission (Martinek *et al.* 2000). Conversely, many surgeons opt for primary ligament reconstruction following combined ACL and PCL injuries (Fanelli *et al.* 1996). Cruciate ligament reconstruction is a proven method of restoring knee stability and avoids the clinical concerns of stretching of the ligament that may result with primary repair (Kaplan *et al.* 1990; Feagin 1979; Shelbourne *et al.* 1991).

Many surgeons, including the authors, use a combination of repair and reconstruction (Frassica *et al.* 1991; Marks and Harner 1993; Prohaska 2001). Since we prefer to operate in the acute phase, we tend to repair bony avulsions and reconstruct midsubstance tears. If we must delay surgery beyond the initial three week post-injury interval, we prefer ligament reconstruction techniques.

Autograft versus allograft

A variety of graft choices are available for bicruciate ligament reconstructive surgery (Figure 30.5). Both ligaments may be reconstructed with allograft or autograft tissue. The grafts commonly used for the ACL reconstruction include: autogenous patellar tendon, patella–quadriceps tendon, and allografts (patellar tendon, Achilles tendon). The grafts commonly used to reconstruct the PCL include: autogenous grafts (hamstring tendons, bone-patellar tendon-bone) or allografts (patellar tendon, Achilles tendon). Good results have been obtained with all graft types, with the advantages and disadvantages mirroring those for isolated cruciate ligament reconstruction (Wascher *et al.* 1999). Autograft harvest adds donor-site morbidity to an already injured extremity; allograft use adds the risk of disease transmission as well as slower graft incorporation compared to autograft tissue. Noyes *et al.* published good results in II patients with bicruciate injuries treated with allograft (Noyes and Barber-Westin 1997). In addition, results comparing ACL reconstructions using either patellar tendon autograft versus allograft at our institution yielded similar results between the groups (Harner *et al.* 1996). For these reasons, we prefer to use allograft tissue in these circumstances. We reconstruct the ACL with allograft patellar tendon, and the PCL with allograft Achilles tendon. This avoids the problem of donor-site morbidity and it reduces operative time in an already complex surgical procedure (Marks and Harner 1993; Noyes and Barber-Westin 1997).

Fig. 30.5

Allograft patellar tendon and Achilles tendon prepared prior to implantation.

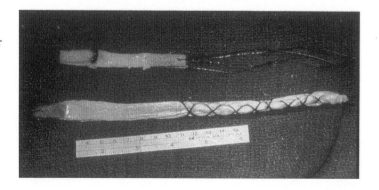

Postoperative rehabilitation

Management of combined ACL and PCL injuries is a delicate balance between the issues of instability and stiffness. Factors which play a role in this balance have been discussed. One of the arguments for acute surgical stabilization is to allow for early range of motion (Sisto and Warren 1985). Prior to stabilization, it is difficult to maintain reduction of the tibiofemoral joint, and range of motion exercises are usually delayed following a period of immobilization. However, even with surgical stabilization, arthrofibrosis is still a significant issue (Sisto and Warren 1985). Consequently, regardless of which types of surgical interventions are chosen, the postoperative rehabilitation plays a significant role in the ultimate outcome.

Some surgeons prefer to protect the reconstruction postoperatively rather than proceeding with early range of motion (Fanelli et al. 1996). Postoperatively, Fanelli et al. place the extremity in full extension for three weeks prior to initiating range of motion exercises. However, several authors advocate early postoperative motion with limited weight-bearing (Noyes and Barber-Westin 1997; Shelbourne et al. 1991; Shapiro and Freedman 1995). Range of motion exercises may be limited early in the rehabilitation protocol to prevent the application of excessive stress on the reconstructed ligaments (Noyes and Barber-Westin 1997; Wascher et al. 1999). Noyes advocates the use of a bivalved, removable cylinder cast between postoperative motion treatments. Shelbourne supports the attainment of full extension early, but he limits flexion to 90° until four weeks postoperatively. Shapiro et al. also implement an aggressive postoperative protocol. This protocol allows passive range of motion from zero to seventy degrees in a brace. The range of motion is increased by ten degrees of flexion per week. A continuous passive motion device is used postoperatively and patients are allowed to bear weight with assistive devices for four to six weeks.

In spite of all of these aggressive postoperative protocols, the incidence of arthrofibrosis is still high (Noyes and Barber-Westin 1997; Shapiro and Freedman 1995). Noyes and Shapiro both noted that several patients required repeat manipulation and arthroscopic debridement to manage postoperative stiffness.

Outcomes

Noyes and Barber-Westin (1997) published the outcomes of 11 patients treated for combined ACL and PCL injuries using mostly arthroscopically assisted techniques. Seven of those patients were treated acutely, between 7 and 28 days, and all patients were treated with simultaneous ligament reconstruction using allograft tissue. For various reasons, four patients underwent chronic bicruciate ligament reconstruction. All of the patients in the study sustained their injuries secondary to high energy trauma and most had associated injuries. None of the patients had an exclusive bicruciate ligament injury; therefore, every patient had at least three ligaments addressed surgically. Because of the concern for postoperative stiffness, all patients were placed on a postoperative rehabilitation regimen of immediate protected knee motion. Although the comparison groups were small, as they often are due to the paucity of bicruciate ligament injuries, the results demonstrated that those patients who underwent acute reconstruction (versus chronic) had better function postoperatively both subjectively and objectively at a mean follow-up of four to five years. In addition, of 22 ligament reconstructions in the acute group, only one graft failed compared with three of twelve grafts in the chronic group. The authors were pleased with the use of allograft tissue for acute, simultaneous, arthroscopically-assisted bicruciate ligament reconstruction.

Fanelli *et al.* performed a prospective study of arthroscopic reconstruction of combined ACL and PCL injuries in twenty patients. Both allograft and autograft tissue were used depending on the constellation of injuries and patient preference. In addition, timing of repair was dictated by the presence of associated injuries. Issues such as vascular status, status of the skin, and the patient's overall health were first addressed prior to reconstruction. If there was an associated MCL injury, the knee was braced for six weeks, and knee range of motion exercises were started prior to knee reconstruction. If there was an associated posterolateral corner injury, surgery was performed within three weeks. The results were encouraging at a minimum two to four year follow-up. Outcome measures, which included Tegner, Lysholm, and Hospital for Special Surgery (HSS) knee ligament scales, as well as KT-1000 arthrometer (MEDmetrics, San Diego, CA) measurements, demonstrated an improvement from the preoperative to the postoperative status. The authors also boldly concluded that there is no difference between acute and delayed reconstruction and that autograft and allograft yield equivalent results. Although the results seem encouraging, no details are given regarding the specific outcome measures of the two groups.

Shapiro *et al.* treated seven patients acutely with combined ACL and PCL injuries. The injured ligaments were reconstructed using allograft tissue in an open procedure (Shapiro and Freedman 1995). Several patients had significant associated injuries. These include a tibial plateau fracture with associated popliteal artery injury, several spine and pelvic fractures, and three peroneal nerve injuries. In spite of these association injuries, all reconstructions were performed within fourteen days. Patients were enrolled in an aggressive postoperative rehabilitation program. At a minimum two-year follow-up, most patients had a good or excellent result. These results were based upon Tegner and Lysholm scores as well as KT-1000 and physical examination evaluation. However, four patients required repeat surgical procedures for the treatment of arthrofibrosis.

Shelbourne *et al.* and Yeh *et al.* have both published reports which advocate reconstruction or repair of all structures except for the ACL. In his report, Shelbourne *et al.* notes that this type of treatment applies to low velocity knee dislocations. In addition, the 21 patients that comprise the study were all treated differently. Some patients were treated nonoperatively, while those who received operative treatment had complete or partial reconstruction or repair of all injured structures. Nine patients were treated with isolated PCL reconstruction; the ACL was not addressed in this patient group. According to this study, the isolated PCL reconstructed patients attained the greatest range of motion and were able to return to some athletics. Finally, no standardized postoperative rehabilitation protocol was implemented because the protocol changed over the seven-year period of the study. Yeh *et al.* report on combined injuries in 23 patients secondary to high energy trauma. All patients were treated with acute arthroscopic reconstruction of the PCL using patellar tendon autograft. The ACL was simply debrided. At an average follow-up of two years, patients had excellent range of motion and were satisfied with their results. Most were able to return to work and exercise, although manual labor was discouraged. Three patients still required arthroscopic lysis of adhesions for postoperative stiffness. The numbers in these studies are small, but the results do suggest that isolated PCL reconstruction can be performed in the combined ACL/PCL injured patient. Results seem to suggest reasonable short-term function with this approach. But again, caution is urged as little is understood about the long-term results of this approach, and the fate of the isolated graft reconstruction.

Wascher *et al.* addressed bicruciate injury with acute arthroscopic allograft reconstruction of both ruptured ligaments simultaneously in nine of fourteen patients. At a mean follow-up of three years, all nine patients had good or excellent results by Meyers and Lysholm scores. All patients had excellent range of motion. While only one patient reported a normal knee, several patients were able to return to sporting activities. Two of the nine patients required repeat manipulation for postoperative stiffness.

Several of the previous studies excluded patients who had avulsion injuries (Yeh *et al.* 1999; Wascher *et al.* 1999; Shelbourne *et al.* 1992). Most authors feel that avulsion injuries are best served with primary repair, but a few authors would advocate primary repair of all bicruciate injuries regardless of the site of rupture (Martinek *et al.* 2000). Martinek *et al.* report good results with acute open primary repair of bicruciate injuries. Although many patients still required postoperative manipulation, and although the objective laxity measures were not equivalent to those that underwent reconstructive procedures, this study maintains that patients have acceptable outcomes at a mean of five years post-surgery. However, of the 28 patients cited in the study, only thirteen actually underwent acute primary repair of both cruciate ligaments and no distinction was made between these patients and those who also had a reconstruction of one of the injured ligaments.

Our preferred technique

Throughout the previous discussion, the authors have stated their biases and techniques in approaching the ACL/PCL injured knee. We agree that combined ACL and PCL injuries require operative treatment to restore proper knee stability and function. We perform the procedure within the first three weeks of the injury and use all arthroscopic techniques, if possible (Figure 30.6). If fluid extravasation becomes an issue, we convert to an open procedure with arthroscopic assistance. If the cruciate ligament injuries are insertion avulsions, we perform a primary repair with a limited open technique. However, all mid-substance ligament injuries are treated with primary reconstruction using Achilles allograft for the PCL and patellar tendon allograft for the ACL. Medial collateral ligament injuries are addressed with primary repair, particularly the posterior oblique ligament if injured. Posterolateral corner injuries are all repaired acutely when possible. In cases where a repair cannot be performed or is insufficient, the posterolateral corner is reconstructed using allograft tissue. Postoperative motion begins between one and three weeks postoperatively depending on the constellation of injuries and the strength of the reconstruction and/or repair.

Fig. 30.6

Arthroscopic view from lateral portal showing ACL and PCL allografts after arthroscopic reconstruction.

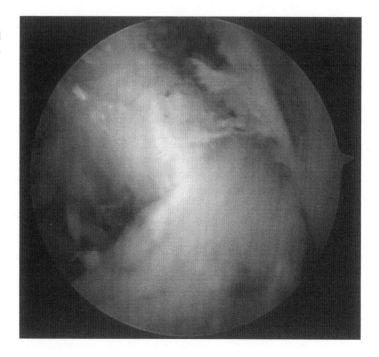

Summary

The management of combined ACL and PCL injury is very controversial. While the initial problem involves knee instability, the most common postoperative problem is knee stiffness. Early in the history of treatment of these injuries, nonoperative management was promoted. However, most current authors would agree that operative intervention is usually preferred. Because of the constellation of commonly associated musculoskeletal, vascular, nerve, pulmonary and central injuries that often occur in association with knee dislocations, the management of bicruciate ligament injuries cannot be standardized. Nonetheless, certain fundamental concepts should be considered. Vascular injury should be recognized and managed promptly. Once this is addressed, the issues of the reconstruction may be considered. In general, repair of avulsion injuries and reconstruction of midsubstance injuries best restore stability to the knee. Medial collateral ligament and posterolateral corner injuries must also be addressed surgically. Several surgical techniques exist (arthroscopic, open, or combination). Most authors advocate addressing all injured structures; most agree that surgery should be performed within a three weeks of the injury. Once the surgery has been performed, the main issue becomes attaining full range of motion without compromising graft competence and knee stability. A tailored and regimented postoperative rehabilitation protocol should be implemented with the knowledge that a subset of patients may require manipulation or arthroscopic lysis of adhesions to regain full motion.

References

Almekinders LC and Logan TC (1992). Results following treatment of traumatic dislocations of the knee joint. *Clin Orthop*, 284, 203–7.

Bratt HD and Newman AP (1993). Complete dislocation of the knee without disruption of both cruciate ligaments. *J Trauma*, 34, 383–9.

Bunt TJ, Malone JM, Moody M, Davidson J and Karpman R (1990). Frequency of vascular injury with blunt trauma-induced extremity injury. *Am J Surg*, 160, 226–8.

Cooper DE, Speer KP, Wickiewicz TL and Warren RF (1992). Complete knee dislocation without posterior cruciate ligament disruption. A report of four cases and review of the literature. *Clin Orthop*, 284, 228–33.

Corso SJ and Whipple TL (1996). Avulsion of the femoral attachment of the anterior cruciate ligament in a 3-year-old boy. *Arthroscopy*, 12, 95–8.

Fanelli GC, Giannotti BF and Edson CJ (1996). Arthroscopically assisted combined anterior and posterior cruciate ligament reconstruction. *Arthroscopy*, 12, 5–14.

Feagin JA, Jr. (1979). The syndrome of the torn anterior cruciate ligament. *Orthop Clin North Am*, 10, 81–90.

Frassica FJ, Sim FH, Staeheli JW and Pairolero PC (1991). Dislocation of the knee. *Clin Orthop*, 263, 200–5.

Good L and Johnson RJ (1995). The dislocated Knee. *J Am Acad Orthop Surg*, 3, 284–92.

Green NE and Allen BL (1977). Vascular injuries associated with dislocation of the knee. *J Bone Joint Surg Am*, 59, 236–9.

Hara K, Kubo T, Shimizu C, Suginoshita T and Hirasawa Y (2001). Arthroscopic reduction and fixation of avulsion fracture of the tibial attachment of the anterior cruciate ligament. *Arthroscopy*, 17, 1003–6.

Hara K, Kubo T, Shimizu C, Suginoshita T, Minami G and Hirasawa Y (1999). A new arthroscopic method for reconstructing the anterior and posterior cruciate ligaments using a single-incision technique: simultaneous grafting of the autogenous semitendinosus and patellar tendons. *Arthroscopy*, 15, 871–6.

Harner CD, Olson E, Irrgang JJ, Silverstein S, Fu FH and Silbey M (1996). Allograft versus autograft anterior cruciate ligament reconstruction: 3- to 5-year outcome. *Clin Orthop*, 324, 134–44.

Hoover N (1961). Injuries of the popliteal artery associated with fractures and dislocations. *Surgical Clinics of North America*, 41, 1099–1112.

Jones RE, Smith EC and Bone GE (1979). Vascular and orthopedic complications of knee dislocation. *Surg Gynecol Obstet*, 149, 554–8.

Kaplan N, Wickiewicz TL and Warren RF (1990). Primary surgical treatment of anterior cruciate ligament ruptures. A long-term follow-up study. *Am J Sports Med*, 18, 354–8.

Kennedy J (1963). Complete dislocation of the knee joint. *Journal of Bone and Joint Surgery*, 45A, 889–904.

Kremchek TE, Welling RE and Kremchek EJ (1989). Traumatic dislocation of the knee. *Orthop Rev*, 18, 1051–7.

Lubowitz JH and Grauer JD (1993). Arthroscopic treatment of anterior cruciate ligament avulsion. *Clin Orthop*, 294, 242–6.

Malizos KN, Xenakis T, Mavrodontidis AN, Xanthis A, Korobilias AB and Soucacos PN (1997). Knee dislocations and their management. A report of 16 cases. *Acta Orthop Scand Suppl*, 275, 80–3.

Marks PH and Harner CD (1993). The anterior cruciate ligament in the multiple ligament-injured knee. *Clin Sports Med*, 12, 825–38.

Martinek V, Steinbacher G, Friederich NF and Muller WE (2000). Operative treatment of combined anterior and posterior cruciate ligament injuries in complex knee trauma: can the cruciate ligaments be preserved? *Am J Knee Surg*, 13, 74–82.

Meyers MH and Harvey JP, Jr. (1971). Traumatic dislocation of the knee joint. A study of eighteen cases. *J Bone Joint Surg Am*, 53, 16–29.

Meyers MH, Moore TM and Harvey JP, Jr. (1975). Traumatic dislocation of the knee joint. *J Bone Joint Surg Am*, 57, 430–3.

Myles JW (1967). Seven cases of traumatic dislocation of the knee. *Proc R Soc Med*, 60, 279–81.

Noyes FR and Barber-Westin SD (1997). Reconstruction of the anterior and posterior cruciate ligaments after knee dislocation. Use of early protected postoperative motion to decrease arthrofibrosis. *Am J Sports Med*, 25, 769–78.

Noyes FR, DeLucas JL and Torvik PJ (1974). Biomechanics of anterior cruciate ligament failure: an analysis of strain-rate sensitivity and mechanisms of failure in primates. *J Bone Joint Surg Am*, 56, 236–53.

Prohaska DH, Harner CD (2001). Surgical treatment of acute and chronic anterior and posterior cruciate ligament medial side injuries of the knee. *Sports Medicine and Arthroscopy Review*, 9, 193–8.

Reckling FW and Peltier LF (1969). Acute knee dislocations and their complications. *J Trauma*, 9, 181–91.

Roman PD, Hopson CN and Zenni EJ, Jr. (1987). Traumatic dislocation of the knee: a report of 30 cases and literature review. *Orthop Rev*, 16, 917–24.

Schenck RC, Jr. (1994). The dislocated knee. *Instr Course Lect*, 43, 127–36.

Shapiro MS and Freedman EL (1995). Allograft reconstruction of the anterior and posterior cruciate ligaments after traumatic knee dislocation. *Am J Sports Med*, 23, 580–7.

Shelbourne KD, Porter DA, Clingman JA, McCarroll JR and Rettig AC (1991). Low-velocity knee dislocation. *Orthop Rev*, 20, 995–1004.

Shelbourne KD, Pritchard J, Rettig AC, McCarroll JR and Vanmeter CD (1992). Knee dislocations with intact PCL. *Orthop Rev*, 21, 607–8, 610–1.

Shields L, Mital M and Cave EF (1969). Complete dislocation of the knee: experience at the Massachusetts General Hospital. *J Trauma*, 9, 192–215.

Sisto DJ and Warren RF (1985). Complete knee dislocation. A follow-up study of operative treatment. *Clin Orthop*, 198, 94–101.

Taylor AR, Arden GP and Rainey HA (1972). Traumatic dislocation of the knee. A report of forty-three cases with special reference to conservative treatment. *J Bone Joint Surg Br*, 54, 96–102.

Torisu T (1979). Avulsion fracture of the tibial attachment of the posterior cruciate ligament. Indications and results of delayed repair. *Clin Orthop*, 143, 107–14.

Twaddle BC, Hunter JC, Chapman JR, Simonian PT and Escobedo EM (1996). MRI in acute knee dislocation. A prospective study of clinical, MRI, and surgical findings. *J Bone Joint Surg Br*, 78, 573–9.

Wascher DC, Becker JR, Dexter JG and Blevins FT (1999). Reconstruction of the anterior and posterior cruciate ligaments after knee dislocation. Results using fresh-frozen nonirradiated allografts. *Am J Sports Med*, 27, 189–96.

Yeh WL, Tu YK, Su J Y and Hsu RW (1999). Knee dislocation: treatment of high-velocity knee dislocation. *J Trauma*, 46, 693–701.

31

Knee motion loss: why does it happen and what does one do about it?

Thomas P. Branch and Jon E. Browne

Every surgeon is aware that complications are an unfortunate but often times unavoidable part of the surgical profession. As orthopedic surgeons, we dread the possibility of poor outcome caused by infection, vascular injury or nerve damage. Unfortunately, knee motion loss is a complication that many surgeons seem more ready to accept. Knee motion loss has been reported to occur in more than 50 per cent of total knee arthroplasty (TKA) patients (Schroder *et al.* 2001), 75 per cent of patients undergoing open reduction with fixation for distal femur fractures (Marsh *et al.* 1997), 50 per cent of patellar fracture patients (Klassen and Trousdale 1997, Smith *et al.* 1997), 40 per cent of tibial plateau fracture patients (Tscherne and Lobenhoffer 1993), 7 per cent of anterior cruciate ligament (ACL) reconstructions of Lovenhoffer the knee (Harner *et al.* 1992), and 53 per cent of patients who undergo arthroscopic repair of ACL avulsion fractures (Montgomery *et al.* 2002).

In general, knee motion loss has a profound negative affect on patient function. A knee flexion angle that is less than 100 degrees can prevent one from rising from a chair or climbing stairs in a natural, energy-efficient manner (Itokazu *et al.* 1998). For workmen's compensation patients, significant motion loss drastically increases the impairment rating; for example, significant loss of knee flexion, following TKA, increases the impairment rating from 37.5 to 50 per cent according to the fifth edition of the AMA guidelines (Cocchiarella and Andersson 2001).

Technical, structural and biological factors are relevant to the development of knee motion loss following surgery. Technical causes of knee motion loss include surgeon-based errors that ultimately lead to the knee's inability to regain full motion arc. Structural causes of knee motion loss describe those circumstances wherein the nature of the injury itself predisposes the knee to motion loss due to a loss of joint congruity or an alteration of the soft tissues about the knee. And biological causes of knee motion loss describe those circumstances wherein there is an altered local knee mileu that predisposes the knee to decreased motion (i.e. infection, arthritis and arthrofibrosis).

Technical causes of knee motion loss

Knee motion loss that is attributable to technical causes is often easy to identify. In these circumstances, radiographs or MRI can identify these problems and guide the surgeon in determining the potential cause(s) of the observed knee motion loss.

Knee soft tissue reconstruction

ACL reconstruction remains one of the most common knee reconstruction surgeries performed in the USA. Unfortunately, technical errors still occur with the placement of the neo-ligament. The identification of the potential pitfalls of ACL reconstruction allows the surgeon to anticipate these problems and to avoid them.

In 1998, Hefzy and colleagues delineated the isometric points of the femoral and tibial tunnel for ACL reconstructions (Hefzy *et al.* 1988); most surgeons use the tibial footprint and posterior superior 'over the top' position on the femur as the targets to be used in ACL reconstruction. The position of the tunnel combined with the degree of flexion used during graft tensioning and fixation determine the ultimate range of motion of the knee.

If the femoral tunnel opening is placed anterior to the isometric point within the femoral notch, and the graft is tensioned near extension, knee flexion is compromised (Figure 31.1). Conversely, if this same tunnel configuration exists but the graft is tensioned near full flexion, the knee will move fully but the ACL graft will be loose in extension. If the femoral tunnel is placed posterior to the femoral isometric point and the graft is tensioned in flexion, the knee will not achieve full extension (Figure 31.2). On the other hand, when this same tunnel configuration exists and the graft is tensioned in extension, the graft will become loose as the knee moves into flexion.

(a)

(b)

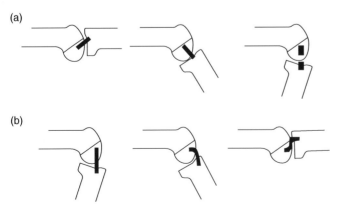

Fig. 31.1

(a) Femoral tunnel too anterior and the graft is tensioned in extension = loss of knee flexion. (b) Femoral tunnel too anterior and the graft is tensioned in flexion = loose ligament in extension.

Fig. 31.2

(a) Femoral tunnel too posterior and the graft is tensioned in flexion = loss of knee extension. (b) Femoral tunnel too posterior and the graft is tensioned in extension = loose ligament in flexion.

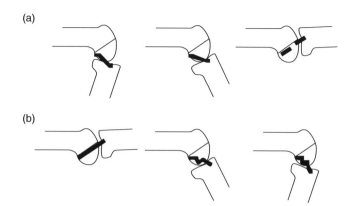

(a)

(b)

On the tibia, the position of the ACL tunnel entrance determines graft position relative to the roof of the femoral notch. ACL graft roof impingement has been identified as a major cause of failure in ACL reconstructions (Watanabe and Howell 1995). When the aperture of the tibial tunnel is placed too anteriorly the graft is forced to bend around the femoral roof when the knee reaches full extension. Thus, when the graft is tensioned in flexion with an anterior tibial tunnel, the knee will not reach full extension. Similarly, if an ACL graft is tensioned in full extension in combination with an anteriorly placed tunnel, the graft will become lax as it disengages from the roof and ultimately allow for increased femoral-tibial translation. During knee flexion, the femoral isometric attachment sites move anteriorly as the tibial attachment sites move posterior (Hefzy *et al.* 1988). There is concern that a tibial tunnel placed too posteriorly may create some impingement with the PCL, limiting flexion (Simmons *et al.* 2002). If the graft is tensioned in flexion with the tibial tunnel placed too posteriorly the knee will not reach full extension. The multiple scenarios described demonstrate that while achieving absolute graft isometry is difficult, understanding the optimal sites for graft placement is critical to achieving maximal knee range of motion following ACL reconstruction.

In addition to poor ligament placement, the formation of soft tissue lesions in the anterior compartment might also limit knee extension (i.e. cyclops lesion) following knee surgery. The cyclops lesion describes a fibrous nodule that forms in the anterior compartment of the knee usually after an ACL reconstruction. Typically, it forms immediately anterior to reconstructed ACL, and lies between the intercondylar roof and the tibial plateau as the knee moves into extension. This lesion is observed more frequently following bone-tendon-bone grafts compared to double looped semitendinosis-gracilis grafts (Watanabe and Howell 1995). In our experience the acutely repaired ACL-deficient knee has a higher risk for developing a cyclops lesion, especially if the native ACL stump is not removed during ligament reconstruction.

Knee motion loss may also follow reconstruction of the posterior cruciate ligament (PCL); PCL reconstruction remains a technically demanding procedure. This is particularly true as more complex methods of PCL reconstruction (i.e. tibial inlay procedure) are employed by knee surgeons. The isometric areas on the femoral condyle and tibial plateau have been mapped and serve as a guide for PCL reconstruction (Grood *et al.* 1988). The femoral isometric point is 11 mm posterior to the intersection of the trochlear groove and the intercondylar notch. If during single-bundle PCL reconstruction the femoral tunnel is created anterior to the femoral isometric area, graft tensioning in extension results in limited flexion; with the same construct and tensioning in flexion, the graft will become loose in extension. Positioning of the femoral tunnel posterior to the femoral isometric area combined with graft tensioning in extension, will result in graft loosening with the knee in flexion; the same construct tensioned in flexion, will limit knee extension. It has been demonstrated that the tibial origin of the PCL graft is most appropriately placed within the native tibial origin of the PCL. However, if the tibial tunnel is too anterior on the tibial plateau and the graft is tensioned in extension, the knee will lose flexion. When the graft is tensioned in flexion under these same conditions, the graft will loosen as the knee extends. It is critical to confirm full knee ROM following fixation of these grafts, especially in cases where two ligament bundles are used on the femoral side.

Improperly treated injuries to both the medial and lateral collateral ligaments (MCL, LCL) can also cause knee motion loss. These structures are not isometric ligaments and thus may be difficult to recreate surgically. The MCL is a broad ligament in the sagittal plane with anterior fibers that have increasing tension in flexion and posterior fibers that have increasing tension in extension (Arms *et al.* 1983). The LCL loosens in flexion significantly (Sugita and Amis 2001). Both the MCL and LCL rely on their posterior components to provide stability to the joint. Surgical repairs or reconstructions of the MCL or LCL that do not mimic the native positioning of these ligaments can adversely affect knee range of motion. When the attachment sites of these ligaments are placed posterior to the native isometric point and tensioned in flexion, there is limited knee extension. When the ligament repairs are placed anterior to the isometric point and tensioned in extension, the reconstructed ligament knee flexion is lost. In recent years, operative repair of the MCL has been shown to be often unnecessary following a brief period of knee rehabilitation following injury, even in those patients who may ultimately require ACL reconstruction (Woo *et al.* 2000). In contrast, repair of the LCL remains an important mainstay towards obtaining full knee function after lateral side injury (Woo *et al.* 2000). In either case, when operative repair of either the MCL or LCL is deemed necessary care must be taken to establish that the surgically identified points of graft fixation will allow full or near full knee range of motion. It is quite easy to 'capture' the knee joint by placing one's fixation points too close to the joint line; the end result of this act is usually a return trip to the operating suite for a manipulation or knee release.

Posterolateral instability (PLI) of the knee may also adversely affect knee range of motion if not properly treated. Typically, PLI is associated with a concomitant LCL, ACL, PCL tears, and lateral meniscal injury (Pavlovich and Nafarrate 2002). Reconstruction of the posterolateral corner of the knee requires knowledge of the complex anatomy in this region (Terry and LaPrade 1996). Often, these difficult cases require the use of supplemental tissue sources or the extensive repair of native knee tissue. By design, the reconstructed posterolateral knee structures should prevent excessive tibial external rotation, relative to the distal femur, and knee hyperextension. Consequently, excessive tension in a posterolateral corner reconstruction can create a functional checkrein that blocks full knee extension. Thus, it is again imperative to assess one's lateral knee soft tissue reconstructions to avoid this potential pitfall.

Meniscus repair

Meniscus repair techniques can negatively effect knee motion. For example, if the meniscal sutures are placed and tied with the knee in flexion, there exists the possibility that the posterior capsule will be tethered and prevent full knee extension. The ideal situation for repair of the posterior medial or lateral meniscus using an extraarticular suture technique would be to place and tie the sutures in extension. Unfortunately, the anatomy of the knee and the limitations of arthroscopy severely restrict the surgeon's ability to repair menisci with the knee in extension. While intraarticular only repairs of the meniscus theoretically have a reduced risk for restricting knee motion, occasionally implants can migrate causing an irritation of the posterior capsule resulting in loss of knee extension (Iannotti 2001). In the most severe cases, a frank synovitis can result and cause profound motion loss. Moreover, the loose body must be identified, and removed prior to starting treatment.

Knowledge of the anatomy and biomechanics of the menisci are critical to understanding the impact of the type of repair on the potential loss of motion after repair. The anterior horns of both menisci move anteriorly as the knee extends fully (Fu and Thompson 1992). This movement prevents the menisci from providing a mechanical block to full extension. The lateral meniscus has shown more movement during knee motion than the medial meniscus (Williams *et al.* 2002). When an extraarticular technique is used on the posterior lateral meniscus, sutures may pass through the popliteal tendon, and restrict the natural movement of the lateral meniscus. In such circumstances, tethering of the lateral meniscus could prevent the natural external rotation of the tibia during flexion; knee motion may be restricted. The same problems occur with meniscal transplantation. When the anterior horn is not positioned properly, a mechanical block to extension may occur and ultimately restrict knee motion (Chen *et al.* 1996).

Periarticular knee fractures and injuries

Knee fractures often result from high energy injuries that result in tissue damage, local bleeding, edema, and chronic inflammation. As such, these injuries are often complicated by knee motion loss if normal knee motion is not quickly facilitated. In addition, technical errors that occur during the open reduction of fractures about the knee can predispose patient to motion problems. For example, flexion or extension of distal fragment of a supracondylar femur fracture can result in movement of the joint line, and knee extension or flexion loss, respectively. The soft tissue sleeve surrounding the distal femur can be restricted by hardware used during the reconstruction. Similar problems occur with tibial plateau fractures. For instance, a tibial spine fracture that remains associated with the ACL can create a block limiting full knee extension; moreover, attempts to fix such a fragment by holding the patient's knee in extension for an extended period may also predispose the knee to permanent motion loss (Montgomery *et al.* 2002). Most of the problems associated with fracture-associated motion loss are related to the need of the orthopedist to immobilize the knee to encourage bony healing. As such, care must be taken to reduce and fix such injuries in an anatomic and stable manner. The application stable fixation should enable early knee motion following surgical repair, and should decrease the likelihood of motion problems following knee fracture.

Structural causes of knee motion loss

The structure of the joint relates to its form and function. The medial tibial plateau is concave compared to the convex lateral tibial plateau. The lateral tibial plateau's convexity increases the importance of the lateral meniscus in maintaining structural conformity between the two bones. Loss of this conformity (i.e. flattening of the normal femoral condyle due to disease) will cause knee motion loss as the normal rolling and sliding of the knee joint is impaired. Loss of anatomic conformity of the knee condyles can occur 'naturally' (osteoarthritis) or after the application of external forces (trauma). Local or subtotal structural damage to the bones of the knee joint may also impact knee motion. Isolated collapse of a femoral condyle with avascular necrosis or osteochondritis dissecans may cause local flattening of the femoral condyle and cause motion loss.

Biological causes of knee motion loss

Knee motion loss that occurs in the absence of structural abnormality or post-surgical sequelae usually has a biological basis. The biological causes of knee motion loss can be divided into intraarticular and extraarticular types. Intraarticular causes of knee motion loss include arthrofibrosis, chondrolysis, infection, synovial chondromatosis, systemic autoimmune disease, chronic joint effusion, synovitis, and arthrofibrosis. Extraarticular causes of knee motion loss include arthrofibrosis, patella infera, and lymphatic disease. By far the most challenging type of biologically based knee motion loss is arthrofibrosis.

The arthrofibrotic knee is a specific entity. Affected knees present with global swelling and restricted range of motion (Figure 31.3). The knee appears swollen, and feels warm and boggy. The periarticular soft tissues have a ruddy immobile feel; an effusion may be present, but this is not consistently found. Moreover, attempts at knee range of motion testing are met with difficulty. The clinician's initial impression might be that of an active infection; however, the clinical work-up often fails to identify an infectious agent. In its early stages, arthrofibrosis is characterized by a local inflammatory response involving the synovium and the periarticular soft tissue envelope of the knee. As time progresses, the warm boggy knee undergoes change. While the inflammatory response may subside, the knee capsule contracts and feels very firm at the end-ranges.

Patients usually experience a prolonged period of fruitless rehabilitation with little or no change in knee range of motion. Often more aggressive rehabilitation efforts will exacerbate the inflammatory process, and actually worsen the clinical condition. Similar inflammatory processes have been identified in other large joints: adhesive capsulitis (shoulder) or toxic synovitis (hip). The abnormal persistence of knee joint inflammation is the culprit in all cases of

Fig. 31.3

Clinical presentation of knee arthrofibrosis.

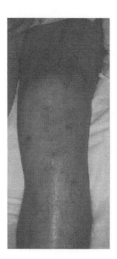
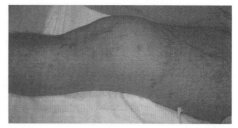

arthrofibrosis. Potential causes of arthrofibrosis include trauma, or surgery, in some cases the cause may be idiopathic and without an inciting event. Secondary arthrofibrosis (that which is caused by iatrogenic factors) is the most disturbing cause of motion loss because it can usually be prevented. Delay in the correction of technical, structural or biological causes of motion loss results in a secondary arthrofibrosis.

Analysis of arthrofibrotic tissue demonstrates the presence of a chronic inflammatory process (Bosch 2002). There is a synovial hyperplasia with fibrotic enlargement of the subintima, the infiltration of inflammatory cells (T cells), and local vascular proliferation (Bosch *et al.* 2001; Zeichen *et al.* 1999). Increased amount of Type VI collagen has also been demonstrated in arthrofibrotic knee capsule (Zeichen *et al.* 1999). Type VI collagen facilitates the cross-linkage many other types of collagen. Thus, a local increase in Type VI collagen may negatively impact the soft tissues of the knee and contribute to those findings characteristic of the arthrofibrotic knee joint.

As mentioned, the pathologic process that underlies the cause(s) of arthrofibrosis is poorly understood. Arthrofibrosis has been described as a form of reflex sympathetic dystrophy, and as a natural, but overreactive response of the patient immune response to a given injury or injury. It is known that cytokines and growth factors that are released by arterial endothelial cells in response to injury can alter the natural metabolism of knee joint synovial cells (Kasama *et al.* 2001). Inflammatory agents, including Interleukin-1 (IL-1) and transforming growth factor-beta (TGF-β), have been identified in the knee fat pad (following ACL reconstruction) and synovial cells (Murakami *et al.* 1995). Cameron and *et al.* described the typical profile of inflammatory mediators found in the synovial fluid of patients who experienced ACL rupture (Cameron *et al.* 1994). In this study, the authors found that IL-1, basic fibroblast growth factor (bFGF), TGF-β, IL-6, and IL-8 all significantly increased following ACL injury, these levels remained high even months following injury. The presence of these agents in the knee joint may be of concern as these molecules may predispose certain individuals to patella infera, or generalized capsular contracture. Cyclical stretching of human tendon and capsular fibroblasts enhances the cellular secretion of Interleukin 6 (IL-6), which then may circulate within the knee joint and act upon other tissues. Interleukin-6 causes fibroblast proliferation *in vitro* (Skutek *et al.* 2001). Thus, one can easily imagine the scenario: during 'normal' postoperative knee rehabilitation, the patient and therapist attempt to gain knee range of motion by passive flexion and extension of the knee; this results in the application of high loads across the joint capsule. These loads then result in stimulation of intraarticular fibroblasts by IL-1, IL-6, and TGF-β. These mediators then cause both knee joint inflammation and the proliferation of local capsular fibroblasts. This chain of events would explain the thickened, ruddy, capsular tissue that is observed in the arthrofibrotic knee, and the fibroblast hyperplasia that is noted histologically.

Prior to a more recent understanding of the cellularity of the knee capsule, synovial fibroblasts had been divided into two types: Type A and Type B cells. Type A cells were fibroblasts and Type B were macrophage-like cells that had immune cell properties. In addition, a Type C cell had been identified as a transition cell between the two. However, it has recently been demonstrated that all synovial fibroblasts are in fact one type of cell, the macrofibroblast. Thus, what had been known as Type A, B and C cells were merely differing forms of the same cell line. These macrofibroblasts differentiate into fibroblast or macrophage cells after exposure to cytokines and/or growth factors (Branch *et al.* 1995). This phenomena may occur in either the intraarticular or extraarticular environment. Thus, we hypothesize that arthrofibrosis is the results of an overreactive healing response that follows local knee injury. This vigorous inflammatory response ultimately results in the excessive release or activation of cytokines and growth factors by synovial fibroblasts. Thickening of the knee joint capsule, and knee motion loss are the final end-products of this process. It is also possible that certain individuals may be more sensitive to these circulating inflammatory agents, and in fact have typical levels of these cytokines following knee injury. Quite simply, we do not possess a deep understanding of this disease that would enable clinicians to more accurately predict who might be predisposed to this condition.

The cellular events that lead to the development of intraarticular arthrofibrosis also play a role in the formation of extraarticular fibrosis in affected patients. Damage to the local vascular endothelium leads to the release of inflammatory mediator cytokines into the extraarticular environment. The stimulus for this release may include the initial traumatic event or aggressive knee rehabilitation. In either case, a diffuse fibroblastic response occurs in the soft tissues about the knee. An extreme case of periarticular fibrosis is noted in cases of infrapatellar contracture syndrome (IPCS). This clinical entity is characterized by a contracture of the patellar tendon and patellar retinacular tissues, and a resultant patella baja (Paulos *et al.* 1994). The observed patellar tendon contracture limits knee flexion, and also causes difficulties in the patient maintaining full knee extension. Although IPCS is characterized by a localized fibrosis that is usually in the anterior knee, a more generalized extraarticular fibrosis can occur. In addition to the knee capsule, the surrounding retinaculum, musculature, tendons and ligaments can be affected, and may contribute to global knee motion loss. Identification of affected structures is critical to the successful treatment of the arthrofibrotic knee.

Treatment of knee motion loss

The treatment of knee motion loss is predicated on the identification the causal factors and the application of a program designed to minimize the effects of the inciting problem. Thus, the clinician must first determine if the cause of knee motion loss is structural, biological, iatrogenic or a combination thereof. The second step involves treatment: medical and/or surgical.

Treatment of knee motion loss: Iatrogenic

The cornerstone of corrective revision knee surgery is identification of the prior technical errors and the development of a pre-operative plan. Anatomic location of tunnels, grafts and hardware can be confirmed using imaging studies (radiographs, CT, MRI). Many of these cases are caused by graft malposition following ligament reconstruction surgery. The offending soft tissue (graft, scar, nodule) should be removed, and periarticular soft-tissue releases should be performed as necessary to achieve full knee range of motion (Millett *et al.* 1999). In addition to soft-tissue release notchplasty, bony debridement, and/or osteophyte resection may be needed. In fact, more severe peripatellar contractures usually involve the extensor mechanism and require extensive medial and lateral retinacular releases (skeletonizing the patellar tendon and patella) and even release of 'normal' ligaments (medial collateral, lateral collateral, anterior cruciate, posterior cruciate). The ultimate goal of these procedures is to restore the natural 'roll and glide' of the knee by the case's end (Millett *et al.* 1999). The described principles are applicable to those knee motion loss cases that are related to the placement of osteochondral allografts, unicompartmental arthroplasty, knee osteotomy, post-traumatic knee contracture or total knee arthroplasty.

Treatment of knee motion loss: arthrofibrosis

The fibroblast proliferation and soft tissue contracture that is characteristic of arthrofibrosis, results in the observed mechanical block to knee motion in affected patients. In treating these difficult cases, the orthopedic surgeon must walk a fine line between aggressive therapy (may exacerbate the biological process) and less aggressive therapy (may be ineffectual in gaining knee motion). The basic concept to consider when treating arthrofibrosis is load deformation of the tissue without vascular reinjury. In our view, the options for arthrofibrosis treatment are primarily surgical, manual and mechanical.

Surgical therapy relates to any process performed by a surgeon on a patient under anesthesia. Manual therapy is defined as a stretching program initiated and completed by a therapist with a direct hands-on application of force on the extremity. Mechanical therapy is defined as a stretching program initiated and completed by the patient with the use of a mechanical device for the application of force on the extremity.

Surgical therapy typically involves a one-time manipulation of the knee with or without arthroscopic lysis of adhesions. However, formal open releases may be necessary in those cases that fail to respond to more conservative methods of treatment. Knee motion loss that occurs within six weeks of a surgical procedure has been described as an indication for manipulation under anesthesia (Noyes *et al.* 1992). The success rates for simple manipulation have been dismal with a 14–21 per cent failure rate (Scranton 2001, Dodds *et al.* 1991). Some surgeons advocate open capsular releases and fat pad resection as an option in patients with severe knee motion loss (Lobehoffer 2002). Millett and colleagues published a series of eight patients with severe arthrofibrosis who were treated with open surgical release (Millett *et al.* 1999). Good results and a high patient satisfaction were obtained in this group of patients by using an anterior extensile approach with medial and lateral retinacular, posterior capsular, and anterior cruciate ligament releases combined with extensive fat pad and extensor mechanism debridement (Millet *et al.* 1999). Although the authors of this chapter agree that this extensive approach is sometimes necessary, the cost of such procedure at our institution approached $20,000 including fees for the surgeon, anesthesiologist, operating room, nurses, drugs, hospitalization and postoperative rehabilitation. Thus we believe that while the surgery for arthrofibrosis may be inevitable in some patients, non-operative options should be exhausted before proceeding to surgery.

Manual therapy by a physical therapist can take many forms. Proprioceptive neuromuscular facilitation (PNF) is one technique used to increase knee flexion. It is important to note that prior to the commencement of manual therapy, the local inflammatory response should be minimized in order to maximize the potential benefit of this approach. Cryotherapy, anti-inflammatory medications, and/or corticosteroid injection may used to achieve this end prior to starting such a regimen. Within the manual therapy approach there are a number of approaches that might be applied to knee motion loss patients. In the agonist contract–relax technique the patient fully contracts the extensor muscles of the knee just prior to initiating a passive flexion stretch by the therapist. This activity suppresses the Hoffman reflexes allowing more load to be tolerated by the joint during the post-contraction phase (Moore and Kukulka 1991). Furthermore, the agonist contract–relax approach results in more knee extension compared to the stretch–relax technique that is commonly used (Osternig *et al.* 1990). Passive static stretch (PSS) uses either gravity or therapist pressure to load the joint in either extension or flexion. An example of PSS is prone leg hangs with weights in an attempt to gain knee extension; this technique involves placing a five or ten pound weight on the patient's heel with his knee on the edge of a hard table and his foot hanging over the floor. There is some concern that hamstring EMG activity may prevent success in gaining full extension; however, increased hamstring EMG activity was not seen in passive stretch for 90 seconds (Magnusson *et al.* 1996). Manual therapy is effective in gaining range of motion after knee flexion loss in a high number of patients. However a sub-group of patients will not respond to what the clinician will regard as a typical postoperative 'protocol'. These patients create frustration for the treating surgeon. Consequently, we believe that there may be difficulties in using therapist-administered passive range of motion exercises in some individuals. Thus we sought out a means by which a patient my gain knee motion by controlling knee motion rehabilitation efforts and avoiding a surgical procedure.

The basic tenet of mechanical range of motion therapy is to provide individuals with knee motion loss with a means to participate in a serious, patient-controlled, home-based knee stretching program. Optimally, this program would be performed three to four times per day. Three types of mechanical therapy devices are currently available. Each device is associated with a protocol for its application. The Dynasplint®, the JAS Splint® and the ERMI® Knee/Ankle Flexionater® represent the three types of mechanical therapy devices that may be used in knee motion loss patients.

The Dynasplint® (Figure 31.4) has a spring hinge attached to an orthoses, which spans the joint to be stretched. A constant, static low load is applied across the joint, and is worn for hours at a time. The technique associated with this device has been coined Low Load Prolonged Stretch™.

The JAS Splint® (Figure 31.5) uses a worm gear attached to an orthoses that spans the joint to be stretched. The joint is moved to a static position by using the worm gear on the device creating a load across the joint. It is then kept in this position until the load decreases to the point where it can be moved into a more flexed/extended position. The technique associated with this device is called Static Progressive Stretch™.

The ERMI Knee/Ankle Flexionater® is not an orthotic device; it is a mechanical system that utilizes a seat, foot carriage and a hydraulic pump to assist the patient in the reclamation of knee flexion (Figure 31.6). This device allows the patient to have complete control of the stretching process through a hydraulic load application with a quick release mechanism. Similarly, the ERMI® Knee Extensionater® uses a high-pressure air cuff with a quick release to apply pressure across the knee in a three-point bending moment to encourage full extension. During each session the patient stretches the knee into current full flexion or extension for 1–5 minutes. The joint is then released into extension or flexion an equal amount of time for recovery and then stretched into current full flexion or

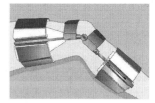

Fig. 31.4
Dynasplint Brace.

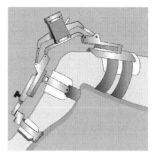

Fig. 31.5
JAS Splint.

Fig. 31.6
ERMI® Knee/Ankle
Flexionater®.

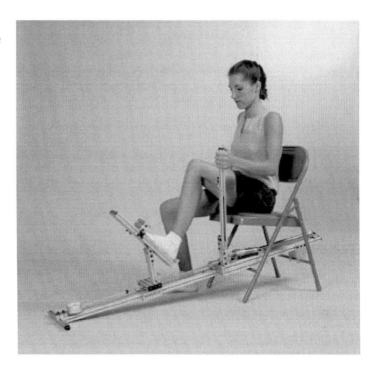

extension again for 1–5 minutes. This pattern is repeated until the
15 minutes of treatment has been completed. The load used by the
patient to achieve a maximum flexion or extension can range from
ounces up to 500 foot-pounds. The technique associated with the
ERMI® Knee/Ankle Flexionater® and the ERMI® Knee Exten-
sionater® has been termed Patient Actuated Serial Stretch™.

The results of mechanical therapy for knee motion loss have
been very good. In a series of 34 patients over a ten year period,
91.2 per cent of patients recovered functional knee flexion defined
as at least 115 degrees using the ERMI® Knee Flexionater® in five
to eight weeks (Branch *et al.* 2003). Case studies using the
Dynasplint® have demonstrated increases in knee flexion in excess
of 60 degrees in one patient and an improvement in knee extension
(average of 21 degrees) in four patients (Hepburn 1987). A case
study using the JAS® splint demonstrated a 17 degree increase in
active range of motion after a therapy interval of 29 days (Jansen
et al. 1996).

Our current peri-operative rehabilitation program begins with the
use of home mechanical therapy before surgery in those patients in
whom pre-operative knee motion is limited (fracture cases excepted).
We feel that delays in surgery related to motion loss have a significant
impact on the total downtime patients experience from injury.
Postoperatively the patient is placed back on a home mechanical therapy program if he or she does not achieve 90 degrees of flexion or full
knee extension two and four weeks postoperatively, respectively.

Both operative and nonoperative fracture patients are given home mechanical therapy as soon as fracture healing is confirmed if motion loss still exists. As a result our patients spend less time in therapy for range of motion issues and more time on muscle strengthening, flexibility and functional rehabilitation.

When a patient does not respond to the home mechanical program we implement a more intensive in-hospital program that is based on the selective use of regional anesthesia. Typically, patients are hospitalized for three days with the affected extremity anesthetized using an indwelling epidural catheter. The initial dosage completely eliminates pain at the knee followed by a lesser dosage for continuous pain management during the hospital stay. The patient uses the ERMI® Knee Extensionater® and the ERMI® Knee Flexionater® in an alternating fashion both alone and with a physical therapist's guidance allowing the patient to achieve full knee motion completely on their own without the need for surgical manipulation. Using mechanical therapy as a home therapy adjunct to formal outpatient rehabilitation has anecdotally decreased the number of knee motion loss cases observed in our clinical practice. Moreover, the success we have observed using these devices during an in-hospital approach supports our contention that most of these cases can be treated by nonoperative means.

Conclusion

Knee motion loss has many causes. The treatment of knee motion loss is predicated on identifying its cause(s) and instituting a program designed to alleviate the inciting problem. Most cases of knee motion loss are directly related to structural anatomic abnormalities and/or biological factors. Causal factor must first be identified; following this, corrective surgery or medical treatment is implemented. The third step is the administration of a rehabilitation program that focuses on the recovery of knee motion loss without aggravating the local knee inflammatory response. And while surgical procedures may be necessary to treat affected patients, our experience suggests that the use of adjunctive mechanical devices represents the best method for successfully maintaining knee motion and avoiding motion difficulties.

References

Arms S, Boyle J, Johnson R, Pope M (1983). Strain measurement in the medial collateral ligament of the human knee: an autopsy study. *J Biomechanics*, 16(7), 491–96.

Bosch U (2002). Arthrofibrose. *Orthopade*, 31, 785–90.

Bosch U, Zeichen J, Skutek M, Haeder L, van Griensven M (2001). Arthrofibrosis is the result of a T cell mediated immune response. *Knee Surg Sports Traumatol Arthosc*, 9(5), 282–89.

Branch TP, Karsch RE, Mills TJ, Palmer MT (2003). Mechanical therapy for loss of knee flexion. *Am J Orthop*, 32(4), 195–200.

Branch TP, Mosunjac M, Lackey D, Goldberg D, Subovic-Morusa M, Hillyer C (1995). The Type C synovial cell: Immunohistochemical identification. Presented at the Orthopedic Research Society 41st Meeting, Orlando, Florida.

Cameron M, Fu F, Paessler H, Schneider M, Evans C (1994). Synovial fluid cytokine concentrations as possible prognostic indicators in the ACL-deficient knee. *Knee Surg Sports Traumatol Arthros*, 2(1), 38–44.

Chen MI, Branch TP, Hutton WC (1996). Is it important to secure the horns during lateral meniscal transplantation? A cadaveric study. *Arthroscopy*, 12(2), 174–81.

Cocchiarella L and Andersson GB (2001). *Guides to the Evaluation of Permanent Impairment*. AMA Press.

Dodds JA, Keene JS, Graf BK, Lange RH (1991). Results of knee manipulations after anterior cruciate ligament reconstructions. *Am J Sports Med*, 19(3), 283–87.

Fermor B, Weinberg JB, Pisetsky DS, Misukonis MA, Banes AJ, Guilak F (2001). The effects of static and intermittent compression on nitric oxide production in articular cartilage explants. *J Orthop Res*, 19(4), 729–37.

Fu FH and Thompson WO (1992). Motion of the meniscus during knee flexion. In Mow VC, Arnoczky SP, Jackson DW (eds) *Knee Meniscus: Basic and clinical foundations*, pp. 75–90. Raven Press, New York.

Grood ES, Hefzy MS, Lindenfield TN (1988). Factors affecting the region of most isometric femoral attachments Part I: The posterior cruciate ligament. *Am J Sports Med*, 17(2), 197–207.

Harner CD, Irrgang JJ, Paul J, Dearwater S, Fu FH (1992). Loss of motion after anterior cruciate ligament reconstruction. *Am J Sports Med*, 20, 499–506.

Hefzy MS, Grood ES, Noyes FR (1989). Factors affecting the region of most isometric femoral attachments Part II: The anterior cruciate ligament. *Am J Sports Med*, 17(2), 208–16.

Hepburn GR (1987). Case Studies: Contracture and stiff joint management with Dynasplint. *JOSPT*, 8(10), 498–504.

Iannotti S, Goldberg MJ, Richmond JC (2001). Subcutaneous migration of bioabsorbable meniscal arrows. *Am J Knee Surg*, 14(2), 122–24.

Itokazu M, Uemura S, Aoki T, Takatsu T (1998). Analysis of rising from a chair after total knee arthroplasty. *Bull Hosp Jt Dis*, 57(2), 88–92.

Jansen CM, Windau JE, Bonutti PM, Brillhart MV (1996). Treatment of a knee contracture using a knee orthosis incorporating stress-relaxation techniques. *Phys Ther*, 76(2), 182–86.

Kasama T, Shiozawa F, Kobayashi K, *et al.* (2001). Vascular endothelial growth factor expression by activated synovial leukocytes in rheumatoid arthritis: critical involvement of the interaction with synovial fibroblasts. *Arthritis Rheum*, 44(11), 2512–24.

Klassen JF and Trousdale RT (1997). Treatment of delayed and nonunion of the patella. *J Orthop Trauma*, 11(3), 188–94.

Lobenhoffer P (2002). Treatment of severe arthrofibrosis of the knee by fat pad resection and posterior capsulotomy: Technique and results of 121 consecutive cases. Presented at the ACL Study Group, Big Sky, Montana.

Magnusson SP, Simonsen EB, Dyhre-Poulsen P, Aagaard P, Mohr T, Kjaer M (1996). Viscoelastic stress relaxation during static stretch in human skeletal muscle in the absence of EMG activity. *Scand J Med Sci Sports*, 6(6), 323–28.

Marsh JL, Jansen H, Yoong HK, Found EM (1997). Supracondylar fractures of the femur treated by external fixation. *J Orthop Trauma*, 11(6), 405–10.

Millett PJ, Williams RJ, Wickiewicz TL (1999). Open debridement and soft tissue release as a salvage procedure for the severely arthrofibrotic knee. *Am J Sports Med*, 27(5), 552–61.

Montgomery KD, Cavanaugh J, Cohen S, Wickiewicz TL, Warren RF, Blevens F (2002). Motion complications after arthroscopic repair of anterior cruciate ligament avulsion fractures in the adult. *Arthroscopy*, 18(2), 171–76.

Moore MA, Kukulka CG (1991). Depression of Hoffman reflexes following voluntary contraction and implications for proprioceptive neuromuscular facilitation therapy. *Phys Ther*, 71(4), 321–29.

Murakami S, Muneta T, Furuya K, Saito I, Miyasaka N, Yamamoto H (1995). Immunohistologic analysis of synovium in infrapatellar fat pad after anterior cruciate ligament surgery. *Am J Sports Med*, 23(6), 763–68.

Noyes FR, Mangine RE, Barber SD (1992). The early treatment of motion complications after reconstruction of the anterior cruciate ligament. *CORR*, 277, 217–28.

Ostenig LR, Robertson RN, Troxel RK, Hansen P (1990). Differential responses to proprioceptive neuromuscular facilitation (PNF) stretch techniques. *Med Sci Sports Exerc*, 22(1), 106–111.

Paulos LE, Wnorowski DC, Greenwald AE (1994). Infrapatellar contracture syndrome. Diagnosis, treatment, and long-term follow-up. *Am J Sports Med*, 22(4), 440–49.

Pavlovich RI and Nafarrate EB (2002). Trivalent reconstruction for posterolateral and lateral knee instability. *Arthroscopy*, 18(1), E1.

Schroder HM, Berthelsen A, Hassani G, Hansen EB, Solgaard S (2001). Cementless porous-coated total knee arthroplasty: 10-year results in a consecutive series. *J Arthroplasty*, 16(5), 559–67.

Scranton RE (2001). Management of knee pain and stiffness after total knee arthroplasty. *J Arthroplasty*, 16(4), 428–35.

Simmons R, Howell SM, Hull ML (2002). Effects of the angle of the femoral and tibial tunnel in the coronal plane and posterior cruciate ligament on ACL graft tension. Presented at the ACL Study Group, Big Sky, Montana.

Skutek M, van Griensven M, Zeichen J, Brauer N, Bosch U (2001). Cyclic mechanical stretching enhances secretion of Interleukin 6 in human tendon fibroblasts. *Knee Surg Sports Traumatol Arthrosc*, 9(5), 322–26.

Smith ST, Cramer KE, Karges DE, Watson JT, Moed BR (1997). Early complications in the operative treatment of patella fractures. *J Orthop Trauma*, 11(3), 183–87.

Sugita T and Amis AA (2001). Anatomic and biomechanical study of the lateral collateral and popliteofibular ligaments. *Am J Sports Med*, 29(4), 466–72.

Terry GC and LaPrade RF (1996). The biceps femoris muscle complex at the knee. Its anatomy and injury patterns associated with acute anterolateral-anteromedial rotatory instability. *Am J Sports Med*, 24(1), 2–8.

Tscherne H and Lobenhoffer P (1993). Tibial plateau fractures: Management and expected results. *CORR*, 292, 87–100.

Watanabe BM and Howell SM (1995). Arthroscopic findings associated with roof impingement of an anterior cruciate ligament graft. *Am J Sports Med*, 23(5), 616–25.

Williams A, Dunstan E, Robinson J, Hunt D, Gedroyc W (2002). Tibiofemoral kinematics of the weight-bearing living knee with and without the anterior cruciate ligament. Presented at the ACL Study Group, Big Sky, Montana.

Woo SL, Vogrin TM, Abramowitch SD (2000). Healing and repair of ligament injuries in the knee. *J Am Acad Orthop Surg*, 8(6), 364–72.

Zeichen J, van Griensven M, Albers I, Lobenhoffer P, Bosch U (1999). Immunohistochemical localization of collagen VI in arthrofibrosis. *Arch Orthop Trauma Surg*, 119, 315–18.

Index

accelerated rehabilitation 152–8
  acute versus chronic reconstructions 153–4
  data collection and review 152–3
  early wound healing 156
  full hyperextension 156–8
  patient 'non-compliance' 154
  preoperative 156
    knee condition 155
  regaining leg control 158
  regaining motion 153
  two-staged meniscus repair 155
ACL see anterior cruciate ligament
activities of daily living 318
aggrecanase 446
aging
  activity levels 186
  changes in ligament and tension 185–6
algodystrophy 212
allografts 521
  ACL reconstruction 62–3, 133, 200–3, 219
  banking of 413
  cryopreservation 413–14
  donors 412–14
  MCL reconstruction 243–5
  meniscal 322, 387–405
  osteochondral 455–74
  PCL reconstruction 350–1
  sterilization 412–13
American Association of Tissue Banks 413, 414
anatomy
  anterior cruciate ligament 168–9
  complex knee injuries 490
  posterior cruciate ligament 376–8
  posterolateral corner 256–60, 274–7
anterior cruciate ligament
  and frontal imbalance 493–4
  healing capacity 233
  risk equation 31
  role in knee stability 230–2
  and sagittal imbalance 493
  size 84–6
anterior cruciate ligament injury 3–14
  in adolescents see skeletally immature ACL injury
  complex 480–2
  functional impairment 3–8
  meniscal and chondral lesions 10–12
  natural history 3–14
  non-operative management 4–5
  radiographic degenerative changes 8–10
  rehabilitation 5–8

treatment see anterior cruciate ligament
    reconstruction
  see also combined ACL/PCL injuries
anterior cruciate ligament reconstruction 15–55
  allografts 133
  autografts 57–66, 133, 196, 219
    contralateral patellar tendon 197–8
    ipsilateral patellar tendon 196–7
    quadriceps tendon 200–1
    semitendinosus/gracilis 198–200
  bioabsorbable interference screws 109–28
  biochemical mediators 27–30
  bioresorbable polymers 97–108
  bone-tendon-bone autograft 57–66, 131
  combined 511–28
  early history 130–1
  failure of 211–15
  gender effects on outcome 83–95
  graft fixation see fixation
  hamstring tendon grafts 43–50, 131–2
  impaired proprioception 25–7
  meniscal pathology 17–21
  older patients 185–9
  osteoarthritis 315–17, 329–39
  osteochondral pathology 21–4
  patellar tendon graft 39–43, 196–8
  rehabilitation 139–40, 151–66
  revision see revision ACL reconstruction
  skeletally immature individuals 167–84
  timing of 238
  tunnel widening 67–81
AO washers 48
aperture fixation 45
arcuate ligament 256, 258
arthritis 213, 467
  see also osteoarthritis
arthrofibrosis 212, 535–7
  treatment 538–42
arthrometry 58
arthroscopy 518–19
autogenous tissue transplantation 460
autografts 521
  ACL reconstruction 57–66, 133, 196, 219
    contralateral patellar tendon 197–8
    ipsilateral patellar tendon 196–7
    quadriceps tendon 200–1
    semitendinosus/gracilis 198–200
  bone-tendon-bone 57–66, 130–1
  MCL reconstruction 241–3
  PCL reconstruction 350–1

autologous chondrocyte transplantation/implantation
    439–54
  clinical research 441–5
  histological evaluation 445–6
  opinions on 446–8

banking of allografts 413
basic fibroblast growth factor 246
Bi-Lok screw 120, 121
Bio-RCI screw 120
bioabsorbable materials
  basic science 111–12
  characteristics of 110–11
  clinical results 112–15
  hamstring graft fixation 115–16
  history of 109–10
bioabsorbable screws 41, 45, 48, 109–28
  biomechanical evaluation 116–18
  clinical recommendations 120
  complications of 118–20
biochemical mediators 27–30
  biochemistry of articular cartilage 27
  of osteoarthritis 27–30
biocompatibility 42
Biocryl screw 120
biomechanics
  complex knee injuries 490
  meniscal allografts 388
  posterior cruciate ligament 361–2
  posterolateral corner 277–9
bioresorbable polymers 97–108
  structural characteristics 99–106
  therapeutic uses 105
Bioscrew 73
bone bruise 172
Bone Mulch Screw 45, 72, 199
bone-tendon healing 129–49
bone-tendon-bone autograft 57–66, 130–1
  allografts 62–3
  donor site morbidity 63–4
  graft fixation 60–2
  healing within bone tunnel 76–7
  knee stability 58–60
  tunnel expansion 62
  see also tunnel widening
bone-to-bone healing 38
bucket-handle tears 20, 407, 458
bungee effect 45, 71

cartilage
  enhancement of healing 459
  resurfacing 391–2
  structure 456
cartilage injury 456–7
  diagnosis 457–8
  mechanisms of 457
  surgical treatment options 458–9

cartilage repair
  autogenous tissue transplantation 460
  autologous chondrocyte transplantation 439–54
  microfracture arthroplasty 425–37
  osteochondral allograft transplantation 455–74
celecoxib 310
chondral lesions 10–12
chondrocytes 27, 28
  autologous transplantation 439–54
Chondrogide 444
chondroitin sulfate 310
chondromalacia 410, 467
chronic anterior instability 492–5
chronic antero-medial instability 492
chronic antero-posterior instability 496
chronic antero-posterolateral instability 492
chronic evolved anterior instability 492
chronic medial instability 491
chronic posterior instability 495
Cincinnati Knee Score 78
collagen 27
combined ACL/PCL injuries
  associated injuries 512
    management 513–16
  classification and mechanism 512–13
  definition 511
  diagnosis 513
  incidence 512
  outcomes 522–5
  postoperative rehabilitation 522
  surgical management 517–21
    autograft versus allograft 521
    open versus arthroscopic surgery 518–19
    preferred technique 525
    repair versus reconstruction 520–1
    simultaneous versus staged procedures 519–20
    timing 517–18
  see also complex knee injuries
combined lateral instability 490–1
compartment syndrome 334, 518
complete transphyseal reconstruction 179–81
complex knee injuries 477–87, 488–509
  anterior cruciate ligament 480–2
  diagnosis 490–2
    clinical examination 490–2
    complementary investigations 492–3
  functional anatomy and biomechanics 490
  lateral collateral ligament 483–4
  medial collateral ligament 479–80
  pathophysiology 493–5
    chronic anterior instabilities 493–5
    chronic antero-posterior instabilities 496
    chronic posterior instabilities 495
    isolated chronic postero-lateral instability 495–6
  posterior cruciate ligament 482–3
  rehabilitation 507–8
  treatment 496–507

isolated ligament reconstruction 496
isolated osteotomy 496–7
ligament reconstruction and osteotomy 496
osteotomy with central pivot reconstruction
    502–7
osteotomy with extraarticular reconstruction
    507
osteotomy without central pivot reconstruction
    497–502
computed tomography 217
container phenomenon 113, 119
contralateral patellar tendon autografts 197–8
conventional rehabilitation 152
Creutzfeld-Jakob disease 412
cross-pins 45
cryopreserved allografts 413–14
cryopreserved cartilage grafts 462–3
cyclops lesion 212, 214, 531
cytokines 27, 29, 72

Dacron ligament prosthesis 132
deflexion osteotomy 506–7
dial test 281
dimpling 24
double gracilis and semitendinosus tendons 44
double-bundle PCL reconstruction 375–83
    comparison with single-bundle reconstruction
        379–81
dynamic posterior shift test 347
Dynasplint 540

early wound healing 156
EndoButton 43, 45, 47, 49, 199
    Continuous Loop 72
    and Mersilene tape 72, 73
epidermal growth factor 246
ERMI Knee Extensionater 540
ERMI Knee/Ankle Flexionater 540, 541
European Association of Musculo Skeletal
        Transplantation 413, 414
European Association of Tissue Banks 413, 414
extensor mechanism dysfunction 212–13
external-rotation recurvatum test 282
extracellular matrix 27, 456

fabellofibular ligament 256, 257, 275–6
failure of ACL reconstruction 211–15
Fairbank's changes 389
Fairbank's criteria 10
females
    femoral notch dimension 84
    quadriceps dominance 85
femoral condyle lesions 432–3
femoral fixation 43, 49–50
femoral notch dimension 84–6
fibrocartilage 455, 457, 459
fibrous interzone 77

fixation 72–3, 133–4
    hamstring tendon grafts 44–5, 47–50, 115–16
    patellar tendon grafts 43
    revision ACL reconstruction 221
    see also individual techniques
flexion/anti-recurvatum osteotomy 501–2
foreign body reactions 42
fractures 534
fresh cartilage grafts 463–4
    cold-storage 464–5
fresh-frozen cartilage grafts 462
frontal imbalance 493–4, 495
functional impairment 3–8
functional instability 174

gender, and ACL reconstruction 83–95
    femoral notch dimension and ligament size 84–6
    hormonal influence 86
    literature review 87
        gender difference 89–90
        no gender difference 87–9
    muscular strength and neuromuscular control
        86–7
Genzyme Tissue Repair 442
Gerdy's tubercle 259, 261
giving way 307
    see also instability
glucosamine 310
glycolic and lactic acid-based polymers see PLAGA
glycosaminoglycans 456, 463
Golgi tendon organs 25
Gore-Tex ligament prosthesis 132
grafts 193–209
    allografts see allografts
    autografts see autografts
    revision ACL reconstruction 193–209
    selection 194, 217–19
    synthetic ACL grafts 195–6
    see also fixation
granulocyte/macrophage-colony stimulating
        factor 28

hamstring strength 5
hamstring tendon graft 43–50, 131–2
    fixation 44–5, 47–50, 115–16
    knee stability 58–9
    load-elongation 44
healing capacity 233
Heberden's nodes 416
heterogeneous degradation 102
high tibial osteotomy 305–6, 329–39
    valgus 497–8
    varus 500–1
    young patients 332
high tibial osteotomy/ACL reconstruction 332–4
    complications of 334–5
history 216

HIV infection in allograft donors 412–14
hoop stress 387, 394
hormonal effects 86
Hospital for Special Surgery Knee Ligament Rating
    Form 308, 319
Hospital for Special Surgery Knee Score 308, 320

IKDC score *see* International Knee Documentation
    Committee (IKDC) rating scale
immobilization 233–4
immune reaction to donor grafts 465–6
inferolateral geniculate vessels 257
instability
    chronic anterior 492–5
    chronic antero-medial 492
    chronic antero-posterior 496
    chronic antero-posterolateral 492
    chronic evolved anterior 492
    chronic medial 491
    chronic posterior 495
    combined lateral 490–1
    functional 174
    isolated chronic postero-lateral 495–6
    ligament 392–3
    mixed 495
    posterolateral
        acute 282–91
        chronic 291–7
        and motion loss 533
    pure horizontal 495
    pure lateral 494
interleukins 28, 72, 307, 536
International Cartilage Repair Society 419
International Knee Documentation Committee
    (IKDC) score 78, 88, 308, 318, 416
Intrafix 48, 49, 199
ipsilateral patellar tendon autograft 196–7
isolated chronic postero-lateral instability 495–6
isolated osteotomy 496–7

JAS Splint 540

keratan sulfate 307
kinesthesia 25
knee abusers 215
Knee Assessment Scoring System 419
Knee Society clinical rating system 308, 444
knee stability 58–60
KT-1000 arthrometer 58, 78, 88, 347, 393

Lachman test 513
lateral collateral ligament 256, 257
    complex injuries 483–4
    repair 286–7, 290–1
    tears of 267
lateral compartment syndrome 263
ligament augmentation device 304

ligament reconstruction
    isolated 496
    see also individual ligaments
ligament-to-bone insertion 134–5
ligamentization 202
ligaments *see individual ligaments*
LinX-HT 199
Low Load Prolonged Stretch 540
Lysholm and Gillquist Knee Score 308, 320
Lysholm score 7, 88, 89, 318, 349

McMaster University Osteoarthritis Index 444
magnetic resonance imaging
    autologous chondrocyte transplantation 446
    cartilage injuries 457, 458
    complex knee injuries 478, 492
    osteoarthritis 309–10
    PCL injuries 365–6
matrix metalloproteinase 446
MCL *see* medial collateral ligament
medial collateral ligament
    complex injury 479–80
    effect of immobilization on healing 233–4
    healing capacity 233
    injury mechanisms 232–3
    role in knee stability 230–2
medial collateral ligament reconstruction 229–52
    allografts 243–5
    autografts 241–3
    clinical experience 234–8
    current recommendations 240
    future directions 246–7
    primary repair 241
    techniques 240–5
    treatment controversies 234
medial meniscus
    and frontal imbalance 494
    and sagittal imbalance 493
meniscal allografts 322, 387–405, 407–23
    biomechanical studies 388
    contraindications 394
    graft sizing and surgical technique 395–6
    mechanisms of failure 401–2
    preservation and implantation 410–19
        current practice 417–19
        donors 412–14
        meniscal reconstruction 410–11
        meniscal transplantation 411–12
        technical aspects 414–17
    rationale and indications 390–4, 407–10
        articular cartilage damage 390–1
        early meniscus transplantation 393–4
        ligament instability 392–3
        meniscus transplantation with osteotomy 392
        protection of cartilage resurfacing procedure
            391–2
    results 396–401

meniscal function 387–8
meniscal lesions 10–12
    in ACL-deficient knee 18–19
    and osteoarthritis 19–21
meniscal pathology 17–21
meniscal reconstruction 410–11
    and motion loss 533–4
    two-staged 155
meniscal structure and function 17–18
meniscectomy
    and osteoarthritis 407
    partial 408
    sequelae of 389–90
metal interference screws 41–2
metalloproteases 28
microfracture arthroplasty 425–37
    complications 434–5
    contraindications 427–8
    femoral condyle lesions 432–3
    indications 426–7
    outcome 435–6
    patellofemoral lesions 434
    postoperative management 432
    preoperative planning 428
    rehabilitation 432
    surgical technique 428–32
    tibial plateau lesions 432–3
mosaicplasty 460
motion loss 529–45
    biological causes 535–7
    structural causes 534
    technical causes 530–4
        meniscus repair 533–4
        periarticular fractures and injuries 534
        soft tissue reconstruction 530–3
    treatment 537–42
muscular strength 86–7

neuromuscular control 86–7
non-compliance 154
Noyes knee score 349

older persons 185–9
    ACL injuries 186–7
    activity levels with increasing age 186
    aging changes in ligament and tendon 185–6
    aging population 186
oligomers 102
osteoarthritis 9, 15–16
    ACL reconstruction 315–17
    ACL-deficient knee 303–27, 329–39
    biochemical mediators 27–30
    clinical approach 310–13
    diagnosis 307–10
    and frontal imbalance 494
    history 307–8
    imaging studies 309–10

meniscal allografts 322
    and meniscal pathology 19–21
    and motion loss 535
    operative technique 314–15
    and osteochondral pathology 23–4
    pathophysiology 306–7
    physical examination 308–9
    post-meniscectomy 407
    postoperative management 317–18
    preoperative evaluation 313–14
    and proprioception 25–7
    results of surgery 318–22
osteochondral allograft transplantation 459–74
    available donor tissue
        cryopreserved 462–3
        fresh 463–4
        fresh cold-storage 464–5
        fresh-frozen 462
    clinical results 467–9
    conclusions 469–70
    immunology 465–6
    technical considerations 466–7
osteochondral pathology 21–4
    and osteoarthritis 23–4
    prevalence and pattern in ACL-deficient knee
        21–3
osteochondritis dissecans 460, 467
osteonecrosis 460
osteophytes 15
osteotomy 392
    with central pivot reconstruction 502–7
    deflexion 506–7
    with extraarticular reconstruction 507
    flexion/anti-recurvatum 501–2
    high tibial 305–6, 329–39
        valgus 497–8
        varus 500–1
        young patients 332
    isolated 496–7
    tibial deflection 498–500
    valgus 502–5
    without central pivot reconstruction 497–502
Outerbridge classification 12

Pacinian corpuscles 25
partial fibrous interzone 38
partial transphyseal reconstruction 177–9
passive static stretch 539–40
patella baja 336
patellar tendon graft 39–43
    EndoButton technique 43
    fixation 43
    knee stability 58–60
    screw divergence 41
patellofemoral crepitus 88
patellofemoral lesions 434
patellofemoral ligament 256–7

Patient Actuated Serial Stretch 541
PCL *see* posterior cruciate ligament
pentade 489, 491
periosteal augmentation 137–9
physeal sparing reconstruction 176–7
physical examination 216–17
PLAGA 97–108
  degradation 100–4
  structural characteristics 99–106
  therapeutic uses 105
platelet-derived growth factor 246
poly-D,L-lactide 112
poly-L-lactic acid 98, 109, 112, 114
polyglycolic acid 97, 98, 109, 110, 112
popliteofibular ligament 256, 258
  reconstruction 286–9, 293–6
popliteus tendon 256
  reconstruction 286–9, 293–6
posterior cruciate ligament 260
  functional anatomy 360–1, 376–8
  functional biomechanics 361–2
  posterior draw resistance 378–9
posterior cruciate ligament injury 343–57
  acute isolated injuries 368–9
  chronic insufficiency 371–2
  clinical evaluation 362–5
    history 344–5, 362–3
    physical examination 345–7, 363–5
  combined ligamentous injury 370–1
  complex 482–3
  mechanism of 344, 362
  natural history 348–50, 366–7
  non-operative treatment 351–5
  radiographic studies 348, 365–6
  treatment *see* posterior cruciate ligament
    reconstruction
  see also combined ACL/PCL injuries
posterior cruciate ligament reconstruction 367–8
  allografts 350–1
  autografts 350–1
  combined 511–28
  double-bundle method 375–83
  indications 368
  technique 372–3
posterior draw resistance 378–9
posterior sag sign 346
posterior tibial subluxation 375
posterolateral corner 255–71
  anatomy 256–60, 274–7
  biomechanics 277–9
    coupled external rotation 278
    primary internal-external rotation stability 279
    primary posterior stability 277–8
    primary varus stability 278–9
  classification 280–2
  clinical overview 260–2, 280–2
  literature review 262–5

  mechanism of injury 280
  physical examination 280–2
  preferred approach to repair 265–8
  treatment of injury 282–3
posterolateral drawer test 282
posterolateral instability
  acute 282–91
    arthroscopic and surgical evaluation 283–6
    lateral collateral ligament reconstruction
      290–1
    popliteus tendon and popliteofibular ligament
      reconstruction 286–9
  chronic 291–7
    lateral collateral ligament reconstruction 296–7
    popliteus tendon and popliteofibular ligament
      reconstruction 293–6
    valgus osteotomy and posterolateral
      advancement 292–3
  and motion loss 533
  postoperative rehabilitation 297
prone tibial external rotation test (dial test) 281
proprioception 25–7
  in normal knee 25
  and osteoarthritis 25–7
proprioceptive neuromuscular facilitation 539
proteoglycans 27, 307, 456
pure horizontal instability 495
pure lateral instability 494

quadriceps active test 347
quadriceps avoidance gait 308
quadriceps dominance in females 85, 87
quadriceps tendon autograft 200–1

radiography
  ACL reconstruction 217
  ligament injuries 478
  meniscal transplantation 414
  osteoarthritis 314
  PCL injuries 348, 365–6
  tunnel widening 70
RCI screw 73
recurrent knee laxity 213–15
refocoxib 310
rehabilitation 139–40, 151–66
  accelerated 152–8
  ACL injury 5–8
    adolescents 181
  contralateral graft choice 158–9
  conventional 152
  current rehabilitation program 159–63
  current surgical procedure 151–2
  microfracture arthroplasty 432
  posterolateral instability 297
  return to sports 163–4
return to sports 163–4
reverse pivot-shift test 282

revision ACL reconstruction
  graft fixation 221
  indications for 215–16
  one-stage versus two-stage 211–26
  preoperative preparation 216–17
    history 216
    physical examination 216–17
    radiographic evaluation 217
  surgical techniques
    graft selection 218–19
    hardware and prosthetic ligament removal
      217–18
    skin incisions 217
    tunnel management 219–21
Rigid-fix 199
Ruffini endings 25

sagittal imbalance 493, 495
scintigraphy 310
screws
  bending 118
  bioabsorbable 41, 45, 48, 109–28
  fracture 118
  metal interference 41–2
  stripping 118
Segond fracture 261
semitendinosus/gracilis autografts 198–200
Sharpey's fibers 76, 134–5
Short Form-36 Physical Component Summary 444
single-bundle PCL reconstruction 379–81
skeletally immature ACL injury 167–84
  anatomy and pathogenesis 168–9
  epidemiology 167–8
  history and physical examination 170–2
  imaging studies 171–2
  indications for surgery 175
  natural history 169–70
  non-operative treatment 174–5
  operative treatment 175–81
    complete transphyseal reconstruction 179–81
    complications 181
    partial transphyseal reconstruction 177–9
    physeal sparing reconstruction 176–7
    postoperative rehabilitation 181
  tibial eminence avulsion 172–4
skin incisions 217
soft tissue to bone healing 38
Spiked Washer 48
stability of knee joint 230–2
staples 48
sterilization of allografts 412–13
stromelysin 307
suspensory fixation 45

suture/post 48
synoviocytes 28
synthetic ACL grafts 195–6

Tegner Activity Score 319, 320, 349
Tegner values 7
tendon graft-to-bone attachment 134–9
  ligament-to-bone insertion 134–5
  periosteal augmentation 137–9
  physiology 135–6
  tissue engineering 136–7
tibial deflection osteotomy 498–500
tibial eminence avulsion 172–4
  assessment of maturity 173
  functional instability 174
  intrasubstance ACL injuries 173
tibial fixation 43, 48, 50
tibial plateau lesions 432–3
tibial slope 335–6
  and sagittal imbalance 493
tissue engineering 136–7, 411
tissue inhibitor of metalloprotease (TIMP) 307
TransFix 45, 47, 199
transforming growth factor-beta (TGF-β)
  246, 536
tri-calcium phosphate 121
triad 489
Trillat-Lachman test 491
tumor necrosis factor-alpha (TNF-α) 28
tunnel management 219–21
  femoral tunnel 220
  filling tunnel defects 220
  tibial tunnel 220–1
tunnel widening 67–81
  clinical significance 78
  etiology 71–5
  healing 76–7
  timing 75–6
  variation in 74
two-staged meniscus repair 155

valgus osteotomy 292–3, 502–5
  high tibial 497–8
varus deformity 494
varus osteotomy 500–1
vascular injuries 514–16

WasherLoc 48, 49
Western Ontario Osteoarthritis Index 444
windscreen wiper effect 71, 111, 120
WOMAC knee rating scale 308

Zaricznyj classification 169